# Joyfully Gluten-Free

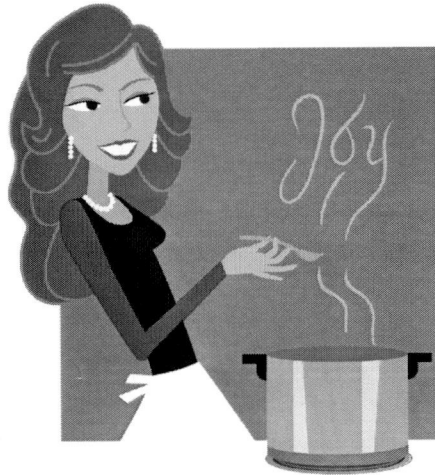

Wishing you joy!
Anita Jensen

# Joyfully Gluten-Free

## A Complete Gluten-Free Cookbook and Guide

## By Anita Jansen

Featuring an Article by Peter H.R. Green, M.D.
Professor of Clinical Medicine, Director of the Celiac Disease Center
at Columbia University College of Physicians & Surgeons

Cover Art by Terry Kubian

**Joyfully Gluten-Free  -  A Complete Gluten-Free Cookbook and Guide**
First Edition, Created and Printed in the USA

Written by:    Jansen, Anita
Published by:   Practical Publishing, L.L.C.

Library of Congress Control Number:   2010938352

ISBN 978-0-9843409-4-1

Disclaimer:  This book is <u>not</u> intended to provide medical advice or to take the place of medical advice and/or treatment from your personal physician.  The author is not a physician, and bases the medical suggestions on personal experience and her understanding of medical publications.  Readers are advised to consult their own doctors regarding their treatment and management of their medical condition.    Neither the publisher nor the author takes any responsibility for any possible consequences from any suggestion, treatment, medical application, action, supplementation, or preparation to any person reading or following the information in this book.  If readers are taking prescription medicines, they should consult their physician and not take themselves off any medications without the proper supervision of their doctor.  This book is intended to help patients discuss their care with their physician, and is <u>not</u> intended in any way to take the place of the care from their medical doctor.

Regarding gluten-free lists or products identified in recipes or anywhere in the text of this book, the author and publisher do not guarantee the gluten-free status of any product mentioned in this book. Neither the author nor the publisher is responsible for product changes or possible errors in the text of this book or gluten-free lists.  It is <u>your</u> personal responsibility to check all products to be sure they are gluten-free at the time you read this book.

In this book, people with celiac disease are referred to as "celiacs" or "celiac patients".   The designations are in no way an attempt to label people with this disease.  These references come from the medical community.  From the earliest instances of the disease being mentioned in medical journals, doctors have referred to people with this disease as celiacs, the same as they refer to people with diabetes as diabetics.

Additional copies of this book may be ordered through **www.joyfullyglutenfree.com** or by contacting **Practical Publishing L.L.C.** at the address below.  Copies are also available through **GFN Foods®**, the makers of **Gluten-Free Naturals™**, and through online book retailers.

Inquiries should be addressed to:
(P.Pub) **Practical Publishing L.L.C.**, P.O. Box 1626, Cranford, NJ 07016

*"Consider it pure joy, my brothers, whenever you face trials of many kinds, because you know the testing of your faith develops perseverance."*
*The Holy Bible, James 1:2-3* [1]

The gluten-free diet doesn't have to be a trial – it truly can be pure joy! You can live "Joyfully Gluten-Free" and this book will show you how.

Dedication:

To my wonderful husband Kai.
For your love, encouragement, and willingness
to try all of the gluten-free recipes I prepared for you.
Thank you for your constant devotion and support,
and for carefully following the gluten-free diet.

To my mother, Marian Graven;
You are a wonderful cook and you taught me
everything I know about cooking, and more.
Thank you for giving me all of your recipes
and for sharing the secrets of cooking
that have been passed down from generations.

To both my Mom and my Dad, Richard
for your encouragement to write the book
and also your encouragement to get it done!
You both always believed I could do anything.

To Linda and Frances for their friendship and assistance
with proofreading some of the medical sections and recipes;
To my brother Paul and husband Kai for help in editing sections of the book;
To Dr. Francisco Leon for reviewing the medical sections for accuracy;
And to all of the other family members and friends
who were taste-testers and proof-readers.

To my Lord and Savior, Jesus Christ.
For giving me the talent to invent these recipes,
for giving me the courage to embrace the gluten-free diet
and to not give up until I found excellent flour substitutes.
I am thankful for answering our prayers to cure my husband's illness.
I am grateful that the cure is a diet and not a lot of medications.

To the people reading this book who have celiac disease.
Remember, this is not the end of wheat,
but the beginning a whole new healthy, wonderful life for you.
It may not feel like it to you at first, but this book will show you how.
You're going to eat better than most people ever have in their entire lives.

# Preface

When I first heard about celiac disease, my impression of a gluten-free diet was that it was bland and you lived on rice cakes. But as I researched the diet, I learned that is far from the truth!

The more I learned about it and the more I experimented, I found that it was an incredibly delicious, versatile and healthy diet, where you could eat all of the foods you previously enjoyed if you were willing to substitute ingredients. It also didn't have to be as complicated as many of the books I read made it out to be. I learned that this diet could be truly sensational if you had the right knowledge and the right recipes.

Fortunately for me, my mother, Marian Graven, is a wonderful cook and she wrote an excellent cookbook for her family. When my husband was first diagnosed with celiac disease, I began converting her recipes and serving them to him. The results were phenomenal and neither of us could tell the difference between the gluten-free versions and the originals. I then developed hundreds more recipes with equally incredible results. I served them at parties and family gatherings and no one even noticed that everything was gluten-free.

I experimented with different flour blends recommended by others and found that some of the combinations of flours used in their recipes were not as good as they could be. To make matters worse, it seemed that many books were written by people who didn't remember what wheat tasted like, and no one would want to eat the foods unless they had to. So, I came up with my own blends that kept baked goods tasting fresher, improved their texture, and kept the calories close to those made with wheat. I found that other books added so many extra calories trying to duplicate something, and with my flour blends that wasn't necessary. My goal in writing this book was to only include recipes that everyone will enjoy whether or not they have celiac disease.

Since my husband is the one who must be on the gluten-free diet and I am not, I can readily compare the gluten-free and wheat versions. This is a distinct advantage that has really allowed me to create some delicious recipes. I have tested all of the recipes in this book and most of the recipes are very easy to prepare. In some cases, because we don't use wheat flour as a thickener, the recipes are much easier than the originals. You also won't waste a lot of time, money, or ingredients trying recipes that don't taste good or don't turn out right. Your entire family and guests will enjoy them, even if they don't have to be on the gluten-free diet.

I've found that by using this book a lot of stress over gluten-contamination is eliminated. In addition, if everyone in your household enjoys eating gluten-free foods there is less temptation to cheat and less work because you don't have to make separate meals. The gluten-free diet also doesn't have to be expensive. I have created a lot of meals that you can make from foods found in your local grocery store.

I have included so many recipes for different meals, so that you could go for months without eating the same thing twice! However, since you'll want to enjoy these dishes again and again after trying them, I suggest that you do make the full recipes and bring your leftovers for lunch the next day. Most places have microwaves, and you will find (like we have) that wherever you go, all the people eating their boring sandwiches will be envying your lunch!

I hope you do enjoy this book as much as I do. It has been a labor of love, and took me over 10 years to write and test. You will learn that eating gluten-free doesn't mean you can't have taste and variety.

Here's to your good health!

*Anita Jansen*

# TABLE OF CONTENTS

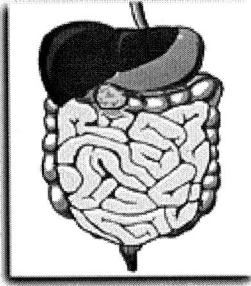

# Celiac Disease

**⟨S⟩NIDDK** | *National Digestive Diseases Information Clearinghouse*

## What Is Celiac Disease?

Celiac disease is a digestive disease that damages the small intestine and interferes with absorption of nutrients from food. People who have celiac disease cannot tolerate a protein called gluten, found in wheat, rye, and barley. Gluten is found mainly in foods, but is also found in products we use every day, such as stamp and envelope adhesive, medicines, and vitamins.

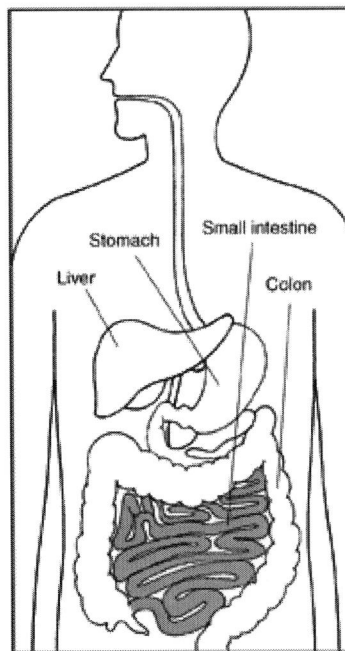

Intestine

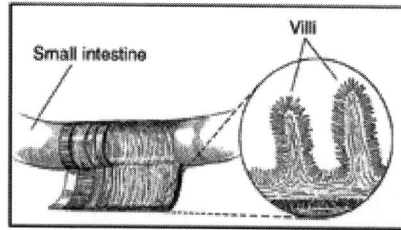

Villi on the lining of the small
intestine help absorb nutrients.

When people with celiac disease eat foods or use products containing gluten, their immune system responds by damaging the small intestine. The tiny, fingerlike protrusions lining the small intestine are damaged or destroyed. Called villi, they normally allow nutrients from food to be absorbed into the bloodstream. Without healthy villi, a person becomes malnourished, regardless of the quantity of food eaten.

Because the body's own immune system causes the damage, celiac disease is considered an autoimmune disorder. However, it is also classified as a disease of malabsorption because nutrients are not absorbed. Celiac disease is also known as celiac sprue, nontropical sprue, and gluten-sensitive enteropathy.

Celiac disease is a genetic disease, meaning it runs in families. Sometimes the disease is triggered-or becomes active for the first time-after surgery, pregnancy, childbirth, viral infection, or severe emotional stress.

## What are the symptoms of celiac disease?

Celiac disease affects people differently. Symptoms may occur in the digestive system, or in other parts of the body. For example, one person might have diarrhea and abdominal pain, while another person may be irritable or depressed. In fact, irritability is one of the most common symptoms in children.

Symptoms of celiac disease may include <u>one</u> or more of the following:

- gas
- recurring abdominal bloating and pain
- chronic diarrhea
- pale, foul-smelling, or fatty stool
- weight loss / weight gain
- fatigue
- unexplained anemia (a low count of red blood cells causing fatigue)
- bone or joint pain
- osteoporosis, osteopenia
- behavioral changes
- tingling numbness in the legs (from nerve damage)
- muscle cramps
- seizures

- missed menstrual periods (often because of excessive weight loss)
- infertility, recurrent miscarriage
- delayed growth
- failure to thrive in infants
- pale sores inside the mouth, called aphthous ulcers
- tooth discoloration or loss of enamel
- itchy skin rash called dermatitis herpetiformis

A person with celiac disease may have <u>no</u> symptoms. People without symptoms are still at risk for the complications of celiac disease, including malnutrition. The longer a person goes undiagnosed and untreated, the greater the chance of developing malnutrition and other complications. Anemia, delayed growth, and weight loss are signs of malnutrition: The body is just not getting enough nutrients. Malnutrition is a serious problem for children because they need adequate nutrition to develop properly. (See Complications.)

## Why are celiac symptoms so varied?

Researchers are studying the reasons celiac disease affects people differently. Some people develop symptoms as children, others as adults. Some people with celiac disease may not have symptoms, while others may not know their symptoms are from celiac disease. The undamaged part of their small intestine may not be able to absorb enough nutrients to prevent symptoms.

The length of time a person is breastfed, the age a person started eating gluten-containing foods, and the amount of gluten containing foods one eats are three factors thought to play a role in when and how celiac appears. Some studies have shown, for example, that the longer a person was breastfed, the later the symptoms of celiac disease appear and the more uncommon the symptoms.

## How is celiac disease diagnosed?

Recognizing celiac disease can be difficult because some of its symptoms are similar to those of other diseases. In fact, sometimes celiac disease is confused with irritable bowel syndrome, iron-deficiency anemia caused by menstrual blood loss, Crohn's disease, diverticulitis, intestinal infections, and chronic fatigue syndrome. As a result, celiac disease is commonly under diagnosed or misdiagnosed.

Recently, researchers discovered that people with celiac disease have higher than normal levels of certain autoantibodies in their blood. Antibodies are protective proteins produced by the immune system in response to substances that the body perceives to be threatening. Autoantibodies are proteins that react against the body's own molecules or tissues. To diagnose celiac disease, physicians will usually test blood to measure levels of

- Immunoglobulin A (IgA)
- anti-tissue transglutaminase (tTGA)
- IgA anti-endomysium antibodies (AEA)

Before being tested, one should continue to eat a regular diet that includes foods with gluten, such as breads and pastas. If a person stops eating foods with gluten before being tested, the results may be negative for celiac disease even if celiac disease is actually present.

If the tests and symptoms suggest celiac disease, the doctor will perform a small bowel biopsy. During the biopsy, the doctor removes a tiny piece of tissue from the small intestine to check for damage to the villi. To obtain the tissue sample, the doctor eases a long, thin tube called an endoscope through the mouth and stomach into the small intestine. Using instruments passed through the endoscope, the doctor then takes the sample.

## Screening

Screening for celiac disease involves testing for the presence of antibodies in the blood in people without symptoms. Americans are not routinely screened for celiac disease. Testing for celiac-related antibodies in children less than 5 years old may not be reliable. However, since celiac disease is hereditary, family members, particularly first-degree relatives-meaning parents, siblings, or children of people who have been diagnosed-may wish to be tested for the disease. About 5 to 15 percent of an affected person's first-degree relatives will also have the disease. About 3 to 8 percent of people with type 1 diabetes will have biopsy-confirmed celiac disease and 5 to 10 percent of people with Down syndrome will be diagnosed with celiac disease.

The Web contains information about celiac disease, some of which is not accurate. The best people for advice about diagnosing and treating celiac disease are one's doctor and dietitian.

## What is the treatment?

The only treatment for celiac disease is to follow a gluten-free diet. When a person is first diagnosed with celiac disease, the doctor usually will ask the person to work with a dietitian on a gluten-free diet plan. A dietitian is a health care professional who specializes in food and nutrition. Someone with celiac disease can learn from a dietitian how to read ingredient lists and identify foods that contain gluten in order to make informed decisions at the grocery store and when eating out.

For most people, following this diet will stop symptoms, heal existing intestinal damage, and prevent further damage. Improvements begin within days of starting the diet. The small intestine is usually completely healed in 3 to 6 months in children and younger adults and within 2 years for older adults. Healed means a person now has villi that can absorb nutrients from food into the bloodstream.

In order to stay well, people with celiac disease must avoid gluten for the rest of their lives. Eating any gluten, no matter how small an amount, can damage the small intestine. The damage will occur in anyone with the disease, including people without noticeable symptoms. Depending on a person's age at diagnosis, some problems will not improve, such as delayed growth and tooth discoloration.

Some people with celiac disease show no improvement on the gluten-free diet. The condition is called unresponsive celiac disease. The most common reason for poor response is that small amounts of gluten are still present in the diet. Advice from a dietitian who is skilled in educating patients about the gluten-free diet is essential to achieve best results.

Rarely, the intestinal injury will continue despite a strictly gluten-free diet. People in this situation have severely damaged intestines that cannot heal. Because their intestines are not absorbing enough nutrients, they may need to directly receive nutrients into their bloodstream through a vein (intravenously). People with this condition may need to be evaluated for complications of the disease. Researchers are now evaluating drug treatments for unresponsive celiac disease.

## The Gluten-Free Diet

A gluten-free diet means not eating foods that contain wheat (including spelt, triticale, and kamut), rye, and barley. The foods and products made from these grains are also not allowed. In other words, a person with celiac disease should not eat most grain, pasta, cereal, and many processed foods. Despite these restrictions, people with celiac disease can eat a well balanced diet with a variety of foods, including gluten-free bread and pasta. For example, people with celiac disease can use potato, rice, soy, amaranth, quinoa, buckwheat, or bean flour instead of wheat flour. They can buy gluten-free bread, pasta, and other products from stores that carry organic foods, or order products from special food companies. Gluten-free products are increasingly available from regular stores.

Checking labels for "gluten-free" is important since many corn and rice products are produced in factories that also manufacture wheat products. Hidden sources of gluten include additives such as modified food starch, preservatives, and stabilizers. Wheat and wheat products are often used as thickeners, stabilizers, and texture enhancers in foods.

"Plain" meat, fish, rice, fruits, and vegetables do not contain gluten, so people with celiac disease can eat as much of these foods as they like. Recommending that people with celiac disease avoid oats is controversial because some people have been able to eat oats without having symptoms. Scientists are currently studying whether people with celiac disease can tolerate oats. Until the studies are complete, people with celiac disease should follow their physician's or dietitian's advice about eating oats. Examples of foods that are safe to eat and those that are not are provided in the table below.

The gluten-free diet is challenging. It requires a completely new approach to eating that affects a person's entire life. Newly diagnosed people and their families may find support groups to be particularly helpful as they learn to adjust to a new way of life. People with celiac disease have to be extremely careful about what they buy for lunch at school or work, what they purchase at the grocery store, what they eat at restaurants or parties, or what they grab for a snack. Eating out can be a challenge. If a person with celiac disease is in doubt about a menu item, ask the waiter or chef about ingredients and preparation, or if a gluten-free menu is available.

Gluten is also used in some medications. One should check with the pharmacist to learn whether medications used contain gluten. Since gluten is also sometimes used as an additive in unexpected products, it is important to read all labels. If the ingredients are not listed on the product label, the manufacturer of the product should provide the list upon request. With practice, screening for gluten becomes second nature.

## The Gluten-Free Diet:  Some Examples

Following are examples of foods that are allowed and those that should be avoided when eating a gluten-free diet. This list is *not* complete, so people with celiac disease should discuss gluten-free food choices with a dietitian or physician who specializes in celiac disease. People with celiac disease should always read food ingredient lists carefully to make sure that the food does not contain gluten.

| Food Categories | Foods Recommended | Foods To Omit | Tips |
|---|---|---|---|
| **Breads, cereals, rice, and pasta:  6-11 servings each day** | | | |
| Serving size = 1 slice bread, 1 cup ready-to-eat cereal, ½ cup cooked cereal, rice, or pasta; ½ bun, bagel, or English muffin | • Breads made from corn, rice, soy, arrowroot corn or potato starch, pea, potato or whole-bean flour, tapioca, sago, rice bran, cornmeal, buckwheat, millet, flax, teff, sorghum, amaranth, and quinoa<br>• Hot cereals made from soy, hominy, hominy grits, brown and white rice, buckwheat groats, millet, cornmeal, and quinoa flakes<br>• Puffed corn, rice or millet, and other rice and corn made with allowed ingredients<br>• Rice, rice noodles, and pastas made from allowed ingredients<br>• Some rice crackers and cakes, popped corn cakes made from allowed ingredients | • Breads or baked products containing wheat, rye, triticale, barley, oats, wheat germ, bran, graham, gluten or durum flour, wheat starch, oat bran, bulgur, farina, wheat-based semolina, spelt, kamut<br>• Cereals made from wheat, rye, triticale, barley, and oats; or made with malt extract, malt flavorings<br>• Pastas made from ingredients above<br>• Most crackers | • Use corn, rice, soy, arrowroot, tapioca, and potato flours or a mixture of them instead of wheat flours in recipes.<br>• Experiment with gluten-free products. Look for gluten-free products at the supermarket, health food store, or direct from the manufacturer. |

| Food Categories | Foods Recommended | Foods To Omit | Tips |
|---|---|---|---|
| **Vegetables: 3-5 servings each day** | | | |
| Serving size = 1 cup raw leafy, ½ cup cooked or chopped, ¾ cup juice | • All plain, fresh, frozen, or canned vegetables made with allowed ingredients | • Any creamed or breaded vegetables  (unless allowed ingredients are used), and canned baked beans<br>• Some French fries | • Buy plain, frozen, or canned vegetables seasoned with herbs, spices, or sauces made with allowed ingredients. |
| Food Categories | Foods Recommended | Foods To Omit | Tips |
| **Fruits: 2-4 servings each day** | | | |
| Serving size = 1 medium size, ½ cup canned, ¾ cup juice, ¼ cup dried | • All fruits and fruit juices | • Some commercial fruit pie fillings and dried fruit | |
| Food Categories | Foods Recommended | Foods To Omit | Tips |
| **Milk, yogurt, and cheese: 2-3 servings each day** | | | |
| Serving size = 1 cup milk or yogurt, 1½ oz natural cheese, 2 oz processed cheese | • All milk and milk products except those made with gluten additives<br>• Aged cheese | • Malted milk<br>• Some milk drinks, flavored or frozen yogurt | • Contact the food manufacturer for product information if the ingredient is not listed on the label. |
| Food Categories | Foods Recommended | Foods To Omit | Tips |
| **Meats, poultry, fish, dry beans and peas, eggs, and nuts:** | | | |
| Serving size = 2 to 3 oz cooked: count 1 egg, ½ cup cooked beans, 2 Tbsp peanut butter, or ¼ cup nuts as 1 oz of meat | • All meat, poultry, fish, and shellfish; eggs<br>• Dry peas and beans, nuts, peanut butter, soybeans<br>• Cold cuts, frankfurters, or sausage without fillers | • Any prepared with wheat, rye, oats, barley, gluten stabilizers, or fillers including some frankfurters, cold cuts, sandwich spreads, sausages, and canned meats<br>• Self-basting turkey<br>• Some egg substitutes | When dining out, select meat, poultry, or fish made without breading, gravies, or sauces. |
| Food Categories | Foods Recommended | Foods To Omit | Tips |
| **Fats, snacks, sweets, condiments, and beverages** | | | |
| | • Butter, margarine, salad dressings, sauces, soups, and desserts made with allowed ingredients<br>• Sugar, honey, jelly, jam, hard candy, plain chocolate, coconut, molasses, marshmallows, meringues<br>• Pure instant or ground coffee, tea, carbonated drinks, wine (made in U.S.), rum, alcohol distilled from cereals such as gin, vodka, whiskey<br>• Most seasonings and flavorings | • Commercial salad dressings, prepared soups, condiments, sauces, seasonings prepared with ingredients listed above<br>• Hot cocoa mixes, nondairy cream substitutes, flavored instant coffee, herbal tea<br>• Beer, ale, malted beverages<br>• Licorice | • Store all gluten-free products in your refrigerator or freezer because they do not contain preservatives.<br>• Avoid sauces, gravies, canned fish, products with hydrolyzed vegetable protein or hydrolyzed plant protein (HVP/HPP) made from wheat protein, and anything with questionable ingredients. |

2001, the American Dietetic Association. "Patient Education Materials: Supplement to the Manual of Clinical Dietetics." 3rd ed. Used with permission.

## What are the complications of celiac disease?

Damage to the small intestine and the resulting nutrient absorption problems put a person with celiac disease at risk for malnutrition and anemia as well as several diseases and health problems.

- **Lymphoma and adenocarcinoma** are cancers that can develop in the intestine.
- **Osteoporosis** is a condition in which the bones become weak, brittle, and prone to breaking. Poor calcium absorption contributes to osteoporosis.
- **Miscarriage and congenital malformation** of the baby, such as neural tube defects, are risks for pregnant women with untreated celiac disease because of nutrient absorption problems.
- **Short stature** refers to being significantly under-the-average height. Short stature results when childhood celiac disease prevents nutrient absorption during the years when nutrition is critical to a child's normal growth and development. Children who are diagnosed and treated before their growth stops may have a catch-up period.

## How common is celiac disease?

Data on the prevalence of celiac disease is spotty. In Italy, about 1 in 250 people and in Ireland about 1 in 300 people have celiac disease. Recent studies have shown that it may be more common in Africa, South America, and Asia than previously believed.

Until recently, celiac disease was thought to be uncommon in the United States. However, studies have shown that celiac disease is very common. Recent findings estimate about 2 million people in the United States have celiac disease, or about 1 in 133 people. Among people who have a first-degree relative diagnosed with celiac disease, as many as 1 in 22 people may have the disease.

Celiac disease could be under diagnosed in the United States for a number of reasons including:

- Celiac symptoms can be attributed to other problems.
- Many doctors are not knowledgeable about the disease.
- Only a small number of U.S. laboratories are experienced and skilled in testing for celiac disease.

More research is needed to learn the true prevalence of celiac disease among Americans.

## Points to Remember

- People with celiac disease cannot tolerate gluten, a protein in wheat, rye, barley, and possibly oats.
- Celiac disease damages the small intestine and interferes with nutrient absorption.

- Without treatment, people with celiac disease can develop complications like cancer, osteoporosis, anemia, and seizures.
- A person with celiac disease may or may not have symptoms.
- Diagnosis involves blood tests and a biopsy of the small intestine.
- Since celiac disease is hereditary, family members of a person with celiac disease may wish to be tested.
- Celiac disease is treated by eliminating all gluten from the diet. The gluten-free diet is a lifetime requirement.
- A dietitian can teach a person with celiac disease food selection, label reading, and other strategies to help manage the disease.

## Diseases Linked to Celiac Disease

People with celiac disease tend to have other autoimmune diseases. The connection between celiac disease and these diseases may be genetic. These diseases include:

- thyroid disease
- systemic lupus erythematosus
- type 1 diabetes
- liver disease
- collagen vascular disease
- rheumatoid arthritis
- Sjögren's syndrome

## Dermatitis Herpetiformis

Dermatitis herpetiformis (DH) is a severe itchy, blistering manifestation of celiac disease. The rash usually occurs on the elbows, knees, and buttocks. Not all people with celiac disease develop dermatitis herpetiformis. Unlike other forms of celiac disease, the range of intestinal abnormalities in DH is highly variable, from minimal to severe. Only about 20 percent of people with DH have intestinal symptoms of celiac disease.

To diagnose DH, the doctor will test the person's blood for autoantibodies related to celiac disease and will biopsy the person's skin. If the antibody tests are positive and the skin biopsy has the typical findings of DH, patients do not need to have an intestinal biopsy. Both the skin disease and the intestinal disease respond to gluten-free diet and recur if gluten is added back into diet. In addition, the rash symptoms can be controlled with medications such as dapsone (4',4'diamino-diphenylsuphone). However, dapsone does not treat the intestinal condition and people with DH should also maintain a gluten-free diet.

## Hope Through Research

The National Institute of Diabetes and Digestive and Kidney Diseases (NIDDK) conducts and supports research on celiac disease. NIDDK-supported researchers are studying the genetic and environmental causes of celiac disease. In addition, researchers are studying the substances found in gluten that are believed to be responsible for the destruction of the immune system function, as happens in celiac disease. They are engineering enzymes designed to destroy these immunotoxic peptides. Researchers are also developing educational materials for standardized medical training to raise awareness among healthcare providers. The hope is that increased understanding and awareness will lead to earlier diagnosis and treatment of celiac disease.

The U.S. Government does not endorse or favor any specific commercial product or company. Trade, proprietary, or company names appearing in this document are used only because they are considered necessary in the context of the information provided. If a product is not mentioned, the omission does not mean or imply that the product is unsatisfactory.

## For More Information

**American Dietetic Association**
120 South Riverside Plaza, Suite 2000
Chicago, IL 60606–6995
Phone: 1–800–366–1655 or 1–800–877–1600
Email: hotline@eatright.org
Internet: www.eatright.org

**Celiac Disease Foundation**
13251 Ventura Boulevard, #1
Studio City, CA 91604
Phone: 818–990–2354
Fax: 818–990–2379
Email: cdf@celiac.org
Internet: www.celiac.org

**Celiac Sprue Association/USA Inc.**
P.O. Box 31700
Omaha, NE 68131–0700
Phone: 1–877–272–4272 or 402–558–0600
Fax: 402–558–1347
Email: celiacs@csaceliacs.org
Internet: www.csaceliacs.org

**Gluten Intolerance Group of North America**
15110 10th Avenue, SW., Suite A
Seattle, WA 98166
Phone: 206–246–6652
Fax: 206–246–6531
Email: info@gluten.net
Internet: www.gluten.net

**Gluten-Free Living** (a bimonthly newsletter)
P.O. Box 105
Hastings-on-Hudson, NY 10706
Phone: 914–969–2018
Email: gfliving@aol.com

**National Foundation for Celiac Awareness**
124 South Maple Street
Ambler, PA 19002
Phone: 215–325–1306
Email: info@celiacawareness.org
Internet: www.celiacawareness.org

**North American Society for Pediatric Gastroenterology, Hepatology and Nutrition (NASPGHAN)**
P.O. Box 6
Flourtown, PA 19031
Phone: 215–233–0808
Email: naspghan@naspghan.org
Internet: www.naspghan.org www.cdhnf.org

---

## National Digestive Diseases Information Clearinghouse

2 Information Way
Bethesda, MD 20892–3570
Email: nddic@info.niddk.nih.gov

The National Digestive Diseases Information Clearinghouse (NDDIC) is a service of the National Institute of Diabetes and Digestive and Kidney Diseases (NIDDK). The NIDDK is part of the National Institutes of Health under the U.S. Department of Health and Human Services. Established in 1980, the Clearinghouse provides information about digestive diseases to people with digestive disorders and to their families, health care professionals, and the public. The NDDIC answers inquiries, develops and distributes publications, and works closely with professional and patient organizations and Government agencies to coordinate resources about digestive diseases.

Publications produced by the Clearinghouse are carefully reviewed by both NIDDK scientists and outside experts. This fact sheet was reviewed by Ciaran Kelly, M.D., Beth Israel Deaconess Medical Center; Mitchell Cohen, M.D., Cincinnati, Children's Hospital Medical Center; Walter Reed Army Medical Center; National Foundation for Celiac Awareness; Celiac Disease Foundation; Celiac Sprue Association/USA Inc.; and Centers for Disease Control and Prevention staff.

---

NIH Publication No. 06–4269
October 2005

The NDDIC is a service of the <u>National Institute of Diabetes and Digestive and Kidney Diseases</u>, <u>National Institutes of Health</u>

National Digestive Diseases Information Clearinghouse
2 Information Way
Bethesda, MD 20892–3570
Phone: 1–800–891–5389
Fax: 703–738–4929
Email: <u>nddic@info.niddk.nih.gov</u>

Web page: http://digestive.niddk.nih.gov/ddiseases/pubs/celiac/index.htm

---

Feel free to go to the above web page and print out copies of this NIH document. On their web page they state that it is not copyrighted and may be distributed freely. In fact, they encourage users to "duplicate and distribute as many copies as desired." This is an excellent article to give to family members and friends so they better understand celiac disease. Also, this article has been updated many times over the years to reflect the most current knowledge on celiac disease. You may want to check back again for an up-to-date version. If the link is no longer active, go to: http://www.niddk.nih.gov and click on health information and then digestive diseases.

Or go to the Celiac Disease Awareness Campaign for healthcare professionals and patients at: http://www.celiac.nih.gov/ for more information on celiac disease from the National Institutes of Health. The articles on this website are also not copyrighted, so that you can distribute them freely.

## How Prevalent is Celiac Disease?

A recent study suggests that 1 in 133 Americans have celiac disease (CD). "In at-risk groups, the prevalence of celiac disease was 1:22 in first-degree relatives, 1:39 in second-degree relatives, and 1:56 in symptomatic patients. The overall prevalence of CD in not-at-risk groups was 1:133."[2]

Historically, celiac disease was thought to have been only a European disorder. Celiac disease was previously known to have a high prevalence in those of Irish and Italian descent. However, doctors have found it is not limited to those countries. For example, a recent study in Spain found 1 in 118 Spanish newborns have celiac disease[3].

Doctors are finding high instances of celiac disease worldwide, and not just in Europe. Studies recently have shown that it may be more common in Africa, South America, and Asia than previously believed. "...celiac disease is a common disorder not only in Europe but also in populations of European ancestry (North and South Americas, Australia), in North Africa, in the Middle East and in South Asia, where until a few years ago it was historically considered extremely rare."[4] In Argentina one study found it was 1:167[5]. In the Middle East, celiac disease is more prevalent than previously thought. For example, in Iran it found to be 1:166[6]. In Israel, celiac disease is "relatively common".[7] In another recent study done in Turkey from healthy blood donors, celiac disease was found to be as high as 1.3%, which is relatively high compared to the Western World.[8]

A chart compiled by the CDHNF (www.celiachealth.org) written using study details from Drs. Fasano and Catassi[9] shows the high prevalence and under-diagnosis of celiac disease around the world:

| Country | Prevalence on Screening Data | Prevalence Screening by Symptoms |
|---|---|---|
| Brazil | 1:400 | ? |
| Denmark | 1:500 | 1:10,000 |
| Finland | 1:130 | 1:1,100 |
| Germany | 1:500 | 1:2,300 |
| Italy | 1:184 | 1:1,000 |
| Netherlands | 1:198 | 1:4,500 |
| Norway | 1:250 | 1:675 |
| Sahara | 1:70 | ? |
| Slovenia | 1:550 | ? |
| Sweden | 1:190 | 1:330 |
| United Kingdom | 1:112 | 1:300 |
| United States | 1:133 | 1:10,000 |
| Worldwide Average | 1:266 | 1:3,345 |

Many people do not have classic symptoms (like digestive complaints), and are therefore not being diagnosed. In the previous NIH article in this book they discussed the possible symptoms, and some patients may have only one symptom from that list. Some symptoms can easily be thought to be caused by something else. Some patients may have no symptoms until a complication occurs such as bone fractures from osteoporosis. For this reason, I believe that more screening for celiac disease is needed worldwide.

*This article is written by Dr. Peter H.R. Green of Columbia University College of Physicians & Surgeons. It explains the possibility that JFK had celiac disease and the complications he could have avoided, if he were diagnosed.*

# Did A President Have Celiac Disease?

### Was JFK the Victim of an Undiagnosed Disease Common to the Irish?
by Dr. Peter H.R. Green, Professor of Clinical Medicine, Director of the Celiac Disease Center
at Columbia University College of Physicians & Surgeons
(Reprinted by permission of the author)

New revelations that have appeared in the New York Times and the Atlantic Monthly, about John F. Kennedy's health have raised questions about his physical condition during his presidency. Robert Dallek, in the December Atlantic Monthly, described in "The Medical Ordeals of JFK" long standing medical problems that started in childhood. In Kennedy's adolescence, gastrointestinal symptoms, weight and growth problems as well as fatigue were described. Later in life, he suffered from abdominal pain, diarrhea, weight loss, osteoporosis, migraine and Addison's disease. Chronic back problems, due to osteoporosis resulted in several operations and required medications for chronic pain. He was extensively evaluated in major medical centers including the Mayo Clinic and hospitals in Boston, New Haven and New York. Among the multiple diagnoses were ulcers, colitis, spastic colitis, irritable bowel syndrome, and food allergies. His medications included corticosteroids, antispasmodics, Metamucil and Lomotil. However it is not clear that his physicians obtained a definitive diagnosis.

Review of this medical history raises the possibility that JFK had celiac disease. Celiac disease is caused by ingestion of gluten, which is the main protein component of wheat and related cereals, rye and barley. The small intestine develops villous atrophy that results in difficulties in the absorption of nutrients. Diarrhea and abdominal pain are common symptoms. Elimination of gluten from the diet results in resolution of the inflammatory condition in the intestine and the associated symptoms and prevention of the complications of the disease. A life-long gluten-free diet is then required. People with celiac disease, providing they adhere to the diet have normal longevity.

Celiac disease can present at any age. In infancy and childhood it may cause chronic diarrhea, abdominal pain, and growth, behavioral and development problems. In older individuals the presentation of celiac disease is frequently due to the development of complications of the disease. These include anemia, osteoporosis, skin rashes or neurologic problems. The neurologic problems include neuropathy, epilepsy, ataxia (balance disorders) and migraine. While the disease is more common in females, men are affected as well. Osteoporosis is common in patients with celiac disease; men often are more severely affected than women. Gastrointestinal symptoms in celiac disease persist for many years prior to diagnosis and are often attributed to an irritable bowel syndrome or spastic colitis. Patients typically see many physicians prior to the diagnosis of celiac disease.

Autoimmune disorders occur more frequently in patients with celiac disease than the general population by a factor of ten. Frequently the autoimmune disorder assumes greater clinical significance than the celiac disease and as a result is diagnosed first. The associated autoimmune disorders include thyroid dysfunction, psoriasis, dermatitis herpetiformis (an intensely itchy skin rash), Sjögren's syndrome, and Addison's disease. Relatives of patients with celiac disease have a greater risk, not only of celiac disease, but also of other autoimmune diseases.

*This article is written by Dr. Peter H.R. Green of Columbia University College of Physicians & Surgeons. It explains the possibility that JFK had celiac disease and the complications he could have avoided, if he were diagnosed.*

## THE IRISH CONNECTION

Celiac disease was formally considered a rare disease of childhood. It is now recognized as being very common in those of European descent, one of the most common genetically determined conditions physicians will encounter. Recent studies have demonstrated the country with the greatest prevalence to be Ireland. In Belfast one in one hundred and twenty two have the illness.

The prominent familial association of the disease indicated by the occurrence in one of ten first degree relatives and in 80 percent of identical twins points to a genetic component of the disease. However the actual genes responsible for the disease have not been discovered though there are many groups working on the problem. It is known that there is a strong association with specific HLA genes that are required for the disease to occur, but are themselves not sufficient for the disease to be manifested.

Kennedy's Irish heritage, long duration of gastrointestinal complaints (since childhood), diagnosis of irritable bowel syndrome and migraine, presence of severe osteoporosis, and the development of Addison's disease all lead to a presumptive diagnosis of celiac disease. Kennedy was given steroids for his problems. Steroid use is associated with the development of osteoporosis and Addison's disease. However steroids were initially used in clinical practice in the 1930s and 1940s for many indications, not considered appropriate now. In the case of Kennedy, if he did in fact have celiac disease, the steroids would have suppressed the inflammation in the intestine and reduced his symptoms, making diagnosis of celiac disease less likely to be established. The occurrence of Addison's disease in his sister, however, argues for a familial cause of his Addison's disease, rather than an iatrogenic one.

Could celiac disease have been diagnosed in Kennedy during his lifetime? Possibly. The disease was first recognized in 1887 as well as its treatment with an elimination diet. It was recognized to occur at all ages. However, it was not until the 1950s that the shortage of bread during the Second World War and its subsequent reintroduction in Holland prompted recognition of the role of wheat as a cause of this malabsorption syndrome. While it was in the 1970s that physicians became aware of the more subtle presentations of the disease. The diagnosis of celiac disease initially requires consideration that it may be present in an individual patient; even now many physicians do not consider the diagnosis.

It would however be possible to diagnose celiac disease in JFK now, if biopsies taken during his life, or autopsy material of the small intestine had been archived and was now made available. Frozen blood samples could also provide diagnostic material for there are serologic tests now available that are sensitive and specific for the condition.

**A diagnosis of celiac disease, if it had been made could have been treated by diet alone. This would have prevented all the manifestations of the disease and its complications.** Because of the strong genetic component of celiac disease, Kennedy's family may well be interested in obtaining the diagnosis as well.

*Peter H.R. Green, MD*

## Complications and How to Treat or Avoid Them

You just learned that celiac disease is a disease of malabsorption (which means you're not absorbing food and nutrients properly). A simple way to think about what is happening in your body is that when you eat gluten, your body's immune system attacks the gluten, and in so doing damages its own small intestine.

Studies show that even small amounts of gluten (about 0.1 gram per day)[10] may cause a reaction. In Italy, a study showed 1 milligram of gluten a day kept a patient from healing[11]. Medical researchers have shown that approximately ⅛th of a teaspoon of gluten or the equivalent of ¹⁄₁₀₀₀ of a slice of bread has had a negative impact on the villi.[12] Another study noted that "the threshold for gluten contamination can safely be set at 100 parts per million" that can be tolerated by celiacs.[13] This is not a lot of gluten at all, which is why food manufacturers need to be careful of cross contamination in products for people with celiac disease.

> (Note: the FDA is working on a new guideline defining "gluten-free" in the U.S. as below 20 parts per million gluten contamination. Good gluten-free companies already follow this guideline. Studies show 20 ppm is a safe limit for celiac patients. I applaud this guideline. Lab tests are available for this standard. It provides more products for celiac patients. As nice as a zero gluten guideline would appear to be, it would be impossible to maintain, would mean less available products, and would mean even higher prices.)

Celiac disease may be difficult to diagnose, because the symptoms may vary. Many people have symptoms that are not gastrointestinal symptoms; celiac disease "involves organs other than the gut"[14]. Half of the adults with celiac disease do <u>not</u> have gastrointestinal symptoms.[15] Another example of the variety of the disease is that some people can be very thin, while others can be obese[16].

The symptoms of celiac disease may vary for the following reasons:

1. **The extent of the damage to your intestines** – Untreated celiac patients absorb some nutrients but not <u>all</u> of the nutrients. Your body may be damaging some parts of your intestines more or less than others.

2. **The location of the damage** – Different nutrients are absorbed in different areas of the small intestine. For example, iron is absorbed in the duodenum, which is the first part of the small intestine into which the stomach empties. Most untreated celiac patients have some damage in the duodenum, which is why most are anemic and experience tiredness before going on the diet. But some celiac patients may be more anemic than others, depending on how intensely your body attacks gluten and also the years of damage.

3. **The number of years of malabsorption** – More years means more possible damage. Not having a mineral like calcium for a few days may not adversely affect your bones. Not having enough calcium for 10 years may do serious damage. Some

patients may not feel any symptoms until the damage is severe from the lack of the nutrient. For example, if calcium is a nutrient you are not absorbing, you may not know it until you develop osteoporosis or bone problems (explained later in this section).

Many problems experienced by celiac patients result from not absorbing vitamins and minerals. **You could eat a lot of the foods containing those nutrients or even be taking vitamin/mineral supplements, but until you are on the gluten-free diet and your small intestine heals, your body may <u>not</u> absorb the nutrients properly.**

Below is a list of problems you may be experiencing from malabsorption. Assuming that celiac disease is the primary cause, many of these problems may disappear as you continue on the diet. This chart explains some symptoms caused by deficiencies using definitions from Stedman's™ Medical Dictionary [17]. This chart is based primarily on the work of Dr. Pruessner and Dr. Nelson, from their articles about celiac disease.

### Some Signs and Symptoms of Celiac Patients Caused by Malabsorption[18-21]

| Symptom | Possible Reason |
|---|---|
| Anemia | Deficiency of iron (most common), folic acid, vitamin $B_6$ and vitamin $B_{12}$ |
| Bleeding caused by blood coagulating more slowly (hemorrhagic diathesis) | Deficiency of vitamin K |
| Bone Pain, osteoporosis, abnormal bone growth in children | Calcium, vitamin D, and protein not being absorbed properly |
| Bulky and greasy stools (steatorrhea) | Fats are not absorbed properly |
| Cholesterol levels are abnormally low or "too good" | Fats are not absorbed properly. Less lipoprotein production in the liver. |
| Diarrhea | Carbohydrates, protein and fats are not absorbed properly. Transit time in the gastrointestinal tract is accelerated. |
| Fatigue, tiredness, lethargy, weariness or malaise | Anemia (see above) and/or immune system activation |
| Gait unsteadiness or spastic gait | Deficiency of Copper (causing copper deficiency myeloneuropathy)[138] |
| Gas (flatulence), bloating (abdominal distention), foul-smelling stools | Bacteria in the large intestine ferment the carbohydrates and proteins that are not absorbed properly in the small intestine. This creates gas and bloating. |
| Hair follicles inflamed (follicular hyperkeratosis) | Deficiency of vitamin A |
| Hair loss (alopecia) or patchy hair loss (alopecia areata) | Nutrients not absorbed properly. In alopecia areata, the immune system attacks hair follicles. |
| Hyper-pigmented inflammation of the skin | Deficiency of niacin |
| Hypoglycemia | Glucose absorption delayed |
| Infertility, loss of menstrual period (amenorrhea), and impotence | Malnutrition caused by proteins and calories not absorbed properly. Also possibly deficiency of vitamin D and calcium. Regarding infertility, also possibly iron, folic acid and/or zinc not being absorbed properly. Others suggest all of |

| Symptom | Possible Reason |
|---------|-----------------|
| | the above, as well as vitamin K, vitamin B-6, and Vitamin E.[6] |
| Irritability/forgetfulness | Low folate[6] |
| Mouth problems – scaling and cracks around the lips (cheilosis), inflammation of the tongue (glossitis), and inflammation of the mucous membranes of the mouth (stomatitis), and mouth ulcers (aphthous ulcers) | Deficiency of iron, riboflavin, niacin, folic acid and vitamin $B_{12}$ and other nutrients. |
| Muscle twitches and cramps (tetany). (When tetany is very severe, it could lead to seizures) | Calcium, magnesium, and vitamin D not absorbed properly |
| Nail malformation, outer surface concave (koilonychia or spoon nails) | Iron deficiency. |
| Nerve damage – numbness, pain, burning, tingling, pins and needles in the arms and legs (peripheral neuropathy) | Deficiency of vitamin $B_{12}$ |
| Night blindness and eye dryness of the cornea and conjunctiva (xerophthalmia) | Deficiency of vitamin A |
| Red lesions on the skin (purpura) | Deficiency of vitamin K |
| Scaly rash or inflammation of the skin (scaly dermatitis) | Deficiency of zinc and essential fatty acids |
| Short stature, failure to thrive | Nutrients not absorbed properly |
| Swelling/fluid retention – a collection of fluid under the skin and in the abdomen (edema) and or ascites (fluid in the peritoneal cavity) | Protein not absorbed properly |
| Tooth Problems – Dental enamel defects, discoloration | Enamel defects caused by demineralization of teeth as a child, due to not absorbing minerals properly. Malabsorption of calcium may also cause discoloration of the teeth or a greater susceptibility to tooth decay. |
| Weight loss | Nutrients not absorbed properly |

NOTE: Celiac disease is <u>one</u> cause of malabsorption, and the focus of this book. If your doctor has not diagnosed you as having celiac disease, you may have a different medical condition that may cause malabsorption. Malabsorption may be a very serious condition, and needs to be investigated by your physician.

These are just a few of the problems you may avoid if you have celiac disease and follow the diet carefully.

To help with the healing process, I recommend taking a multivitamin/mineral supplement daily that is gluten-free. Most physicians recommend taking a multivitamin, but check with your doctor <u>before</u> taking <u>any additional</u> supplements. Some people choose to take additional vitamin C because it is not stored by the body. <u>Other vitamins in excess may be very dangerous</u>. For example, too much vitamin A may cause liver damage. Some celiac patients may already have liver damage, so it is important to check with your doctor before taking too much vitamin A. Your doctor is your best source for what you should take. As you continue on the diet and you heal, your vitamin/mineral needs may change. Another caution: check when purchasing vitamin E since it may possibly be made from wheat germ oil.

As you begin on the diet and heal, you will start to absorb not only vitamins but also medications normally. That may mean in some cases that medications may be absorbed differently. Some prescription medications such as thyroid medication may need to be adjusted as you heal. The same may be true for hormones, seizure medication, antipsychotic medication, or any medication you take where the amount is adjusted based on your body's absorption. Diabetes patients should also work with their doctor. Their medication or insulin may need to be adjusted, since some patients may manifest acute hyperglycemia with the initiation of the diet.[22] Others may manifest hypoglycemia with initiation of the diet. In all of these cases inform your physician and get yourself monitored as you heal on the diet during the first 6 months to a year. Most people start to see some improvements in their health within two weeks, but complete healing may take 6 months or longer. For some elderly patients or slow healers it may take a year or two.

The Merck Manual Home Edition has an excellent chart explaining each nutrient and what happens when there is either a deficiency or toxicity. Understanding what you are lacking may help you talk to your doctor to get you the right supplement or help you choose foods that may replenish nutrients you need. Both the Merck Manual Home Edition and the Merck Manual of Diagnosis and Therapy for Physicians [more technical than the home version] are available on the web page http://www.merck.com/pubs/, with many chapters on-line. The chart I am referring to is in the hard-copy of the Home Edition book, but you may look up each nutrient individually on-line if you choose.

Here is some brief information on some of the nutrients that I think are most important:

- Folic acid is important. For some people a lack of it may cause calcifications to form in the brain. In some cases these calcifications may cause seizures.
- Potassium is needed if you have significant diarrhea, but check with your doctor before taking more than what is in a multivitamin. According to the Merck Manual, "The level of potassium in the blood must be maintained within a narrow range. A potassium level that is too high or too low can have serious consequences, such as an abnormal heart rhythm or even cardiac arrest."[20]
- Extra iron may be needed initially if you have anemia. Your doctor can tell you what you need. (Note: some iron pills may cause constipation as a side-effect.) Too much iron may be harmful, so work with your doctor to get the right dosage.
- B vitamins may help clear up cracks at the side of the mouth (angular cheilitis) and may help with mouth sores (aphthous ulcers). Malabsorption of $B_{12}$ may also lead to nerve damage. The amount in your multivitamin is usually sufficient. Only take additional amounts if your doctor tells you to do so.

Another complication caused by malabsorption of calcium and bone building nutrients is osteoporosis. In order for your body to function, it needs calcium. If it is not getting what it needs, it may pull calcium from your bones so your levels will remain normal in your blood. That is why a blood test for calcium levels may not indicate possible osteoporosis. For many celiac patients, during their years of undiagnosed celiac disease their body took the calcium it needed from their bones in order for their body to function and their bones may be much weaker than they realize.

(Note: In some cases there may be low levels of calcium in the blood, a condition called hypocalcemia. In one case, a patient with hypocalcemia was diagnosed with celiac disease and doctors found that, "The initiation of a gluten-free diet resulted in correction of all biochemical abnormalities and a substantial increase in bone mineral density.")[23]

I suggest that <u>all</u> people with celiac disease be checked for osteoporosis. A very high percentage of people with celiac disease do have osteoporosis (or the beginnings of osteoporosis which is called osteopenia), and most don't know it. One article suggests 100% of celiac patients have some form of bone loss[18]. Others suggest 90% of patients. Osteopenia is not limited to adults: "Children with celiac disease are at risk for reduced bone mineral density. A strict gluten-free diet improves bone mineralization, even in 1 year. Early diagnosis and treatment of celiac disease during childhood will protect the patient from osteoporosis."[24]

The longer it takes for you to be diagnosed with celiac disease, the greater your chances of having bone loss. It is much better to be diagnosed early before it happens. Since many people with celiac disease are not being diagnosed early, a recent study suggests that all osteoporosis patients should be screened for celiac disease. "The prevalence of celiac disease among osteoporotic individuals (3.4%) is much higher than that among non-osteoporotic individuals (0.2%). The prevalence of celiac disease in osteoporosis is high enough to justify a recommendation for serologic screening of all patients with osteoporosis for celiac disease."[25]

Osteoporosis is often called a "silent" disease because most people are unaware anything is happening to their bones. The first sign of osteoporosis could be bone pain or worse problems, such as bone fractures. Bone fractures in your spine (also called vertebral fractures) are incredibly painful and could possibly lead to chronic pain the rest of your life. If you get a compression fracture in your back, it will heal crushed and you may lose height. When it affects the lower back, it may possibly cause not only back pain but rib pain. This may happen if the loss of height brings your ribs closer to your pelvis. Your abdomen area may stick out because your internal organs need a place to go, because of the loss of height. A fracture in the upper back may cause back curvature (called kyphosis or a dowager hump). This may also be very painful, and you may no longer be able to stand up straight.

You may potentially avoid these problems if you get yourself tested early, and stay on the diet. The sooner you get diagnosed and follow the diet, the sooner you may build bone. If you wait too long, some bone may never be restored. One study found that untreated celiac patients had a higher prevalence of bone fractures, and found that, "...early diagnosis and effective treatment for celiac disease were the most relevant measures to protect patients from the risk of fractures."[26]

Ask your doctor to prescribe a Bone Mineral Density (BMD) test or a DEXA scan for you. Those are two names for the same test. It is a painless, very low-level radiation x-ray that reveals bone density. Some doctors use a test that checks the spine and arm, while others use a test that checks the heel. Both tests can show if there is bone loss.

If you are an adult and your bone density level is low, your doctor may recommend taking either Miacalcin® nasal spray (calcitonin-salmon, a polypeptide hormone) or Fosamax® pills (alendronate sodium, a bisphosphonate) to help further build bone. As of this writing these two products are gluten-free. Some doctors feel that you should begin these medications <u>after</u> you are on the diet a while so that you are not only absorbing the drug normally, but also calcium normally and nutrients. <u>This is very important</u>. Some recommend waiting as long as a year. This is also mentioned on the website www.celiacdiseasecenter.columbia.edu. If your bones are not too severe and your doctor says you may wait, there is the possibility that your body may be able to rebuild bone on its own during that year and the medication may not be needed!

Other doctors are recommending the Miacalcin® to celiac patients, because it is absorbed through the blood vessels in the nose and not absorbed through the digestive system. If you have very severe osteoporosis that must be treated before your small intestine to heals, this may be an option for you. I know a celiac patient who used this medication for a year, and it seemed to "jump-start" their bone building. The physician felt it was no longer needed after that. The bone density continued to increase by following the diet carefully and is within the normal range now.

If you use any bone building medication, be sure to get periodic check-ups as there may be side-effects. Fosamax® and other bisphosphonates in particular, may possibly cause burning pain in the esophagus in some patients. If this burning condition (called GERD) continues a long time, it may possibly cause other problems like Barrett's esophagus, a pre-cancerous condition. For patients on Miacalcin®, you may get irritation in your nose if you don't switch the nostril you spray it in each day.

Another possible complication with bisphosphonates is "jaw death" or osteonecrosis if you have a tooth pulled. It is a very rare and "very painful condition that can lead to serious complications, including ulcerations within the bone lining of the mouth, infection, and breakdown of the jawbone with disfigurement."[27] The jaw bone cannot regenerate itself and heal. Since these medications remain in the bone for years, it is believed that stopping the drug is not a solution. Once the jaw bone dies there is little that can be done to reverse it. To prevent this complication, see your dentist regularly for preventative care. If needed, a root canal may avoid a tooth extraction. Most cases were reported in patients using intravenous bisphosphonates but there were cases in women who had teeth pulled while taking Fosamax®.[27, 28]

A problem that may also be associated with long-term use of Fosamax® is atypical fractures of the femur (leg bone). Some small studies "suggested a link between prolonged bisphosphonate therapy and atypical fractures… Theoretically bisphosphonates suppress bone turnover and thus might be associated with accumulated micro-damage in bone."[29, 30] It is a rare side-effect, and in the cases described the leg fractures occurred from low trauma incidents.

If you are using bone building medication, be sure to speak to your doctor about taking additional calcium, vitamin D, and magnesium in addition to a multivitamin. (Note: Magnesium can be very important to bone building. Magnesium deficiency impairs parathyroid hormone secretion, and contributes to osteoporosis caused by malabsorption.)[31] Be sure to drink plenty of water with calcium supplements since you may develop kidney stones from taking calcium pills without enough fluids. Some people who are building bone rapidly may experience involuntary twitching of the thumb or other places on the body which may be a signal that more magnesium is needed. Check with your physician, to confirm the right amount for you. Some doctors recommend taking smaller dosages of these additional supplements twice a day rather than taking them all at once so that more of the calcium is absorbed by the body.

You may also want to consider limiting your intake of carbonated beverages each day. Carbonation in beverages may not be good for your bones because of the phosphorus content. Also, the caffeine may inhibit calcium absorption. There is still some debate about this. One study suggested that after consumption of caffeinated beverages, there was a reduction in calcium and magnesium renal re-absorption[32]. In other studies "high phosphorus intake has been associated with altered calcium homeostasis and hypocalcemia in animals and humans."[33-36] However, other doctors have suggested these findings may be the result of carbonated beverages replacing calcium-containing beverages in the diet. So I think moderation may be the key. My suggestion is to enjoy carbonated beverages (many are gluten-free) but also choose some more healthful beverages that provide calcium for your bones, instead of possibly depleting it.

Another bone problem caused by the lack of calcium and vitamin D is osteomalacia (softening of the bones with pain, tenderness, muscle weakness, and often weight loss/anorexia). A recent study suggests that "osteomalacia symptoms may be the only presenting feature of celiac disease" and doctors should test for celiac disease in patients with bone pain, muscle weakness and musculoskeletal pain.[37] If celiac disease is the cause, the sooner you get diagnosed and follow the diet, the better it is to help this condition.

Disturbed gastric motility, or the inability of food to move spontaneously in the gastrointestinal system, is another problem that celiac patients may have in the esophagus, stomach, small intestine, gallbladder and colon. According to an article by Dr. Tursi, "In fact, esophageal transit, gastric and gallbladder emptying, and orocecal [mouth to gut] transit time are delayed while colonic transit is faster. These findings are related to the complex interactions among reduced absorption of food constituent (in particular, fat), neurologic alternation, and hormonal derangement. Motility [movement] disorders of the gut are also a predisposing factor in the development of small intestinal bacterial overgrowth and may contribute both to development of symptoms in some untreated celiacs and to the persistence of symptoms after gluten-free diet in some of them. All of these alterations fortunately disappear after gluten-free diet, and patients return well being status."[38] (Note: further discussion about bacterial overgrowth is addressed in the Chapter "What if the Diet Doesn't Seem to Be Working for Me?")

Dr. Tursi mentions hormone disturbance. Estrogen is important to bone health, and malabsorption may affect estrogen levels. Men normally have a very small amount of estrogen and a study in which men had no estrogen showed decreased bone mass.[39] Bone mass improved when the right amount of estrogen was administered. Although that study was not about men with celiac disease, some men with celiac disease may have no estrogen until following the gluten-free diet. The hormone levels return to normal by remaining gluten-free. This may possibly be due to low cholesterol levels, because estrogen is a steroid hormone made from cholesterol within the body. Many celiacs have cholesterol levels that are too low before going on the diet. By following the diet the cholesterol levels may return to normal. Then the normal amount of estrogen may return and then bone mass may increase. The lack of estrogen may affect both men and women. That is another reason that the diet is so important to good health.

The complications of miscarriage and infertility for celiac patients may be caused by malnutrition. Both problems usually subside if you remain on the diet and are still of child-bearing age[18]. In some cases, celiac disease may be silent your entire life and come out <u>during</u> pregnancy. Celiac disease may be dormant in a person and come out after changes in the body from pregnancy, surgery, puberty, menopause, or infection. If you have a family history of celiac disease and become pregnant, it is wise to get a blood test for celiac disease because malabsorption issues may affect your baby. If celiac disease is discovered, following the gluten-free diet may improve pregnancy outcome.[40] Untreated celiac disease in the mother is associated with low birth weight of the child, so it is very important to remain on the diet. "A gluten-free diet is considered crucial for a normal birth in coeliac [celiac] women."[41] [Coeliac is the British spelling for celiac]. In another study, they found that pregnant women with undiagnosed celiac disease were associated with "intrauterine growth retardation, very low birth weight, preterm birth, and caesarean section. In contrast, a diagnosis of celiac disease before the birth were not associated with these adverse fetal outcomes." This study concluded that the risks are reduced when celiac disease has been diagnosed and the diet is followed by the pregnant mother.[42] Men also may have fertility issues from untreated celiac disease, which may be resolved with the diet. It is well known that "male gonadal function is reduced in celiac disease".[41]

Short stature in children is also caused by malnutrition and depending on how early the child is diagnosed; often children with treated celiac disease grow and catch-up in stature to children their own age.[18] A recent study suggested in addition to malnutrition, a cause may be the "high prevalence of positive antipituitary antibodies" that correlated with height impairment in newly diagnosed celiac patients.[124,125] Children are commonly diagnosed because they have "failure to thrive" or are "late bloomers" with delayed puberty.

There are several neurological complications that may be caused by celiac disease when diagnosis is delayed. Seizures are one of them. Some celiac patients with seizures are fortunate because when they get on the diet and stay on the diet, their seizures don't ever return. In some rare cases, some celiac patients have unknowingly had seizures during their sleep. Some patients with Type 1 diabetes may have nocturnal hypoglycemia with seizures[6]. Others without diabetes may have these seizures. The next morning they may feel muscle pain or bone pain but have no knowledge that a seizure happened, unless someone witnessed it and told them. Patients with nighttime seizures may also have the possibility of their problem resolved by staying on the diet. The sooner a celiac patient follows the diet, the better the chances of being cured by diet alone[18]. If you suspect you are having seizures, you should see your doctor immediately. Seizures may be a serious problem and may sometimes break fragile bones in celiac patients with osteoporosis. The cases in which seizures are reversible are usually those caught early. In other cases when caught late, the gluten-free diet has shown to significantly reduce seizures.[43]

Unfortunately, for others their seizures may not be resolved, especially if the problem was caught later. If you are already on seizure medication you will need to work with your doctor as you begin the diet, and continue on it. As your intestines heal from the diet, very often you may begin to absorb the medication differently, and therefore less may be needed. This needs to be monitored. If your doctor does not see calcifications in the brain, you may be able to be slowly weaned from the medication as you heal on the diet. Each case is different, so you should work closely with your doctor. In one article, a celiac patient with difficult-to-control seizures went on the gluten-free diet and seizures became controllable and they were able to reduce their medication[44]. Do not stop your seizure medication without approval from a doctor. Most medications must be cut back slowly and can't be discontinued abruptly. Your doctor will most likely recommend an EEG during the process and monitor you carefully as your medication is reduced.

> Note: some seizure medications like Dilantin® have a side-effect that affects the bones, since it appears to block vitamin D absorption and may make osteoporosis worse. If you are on this seizure medication you should discuss it with your doctor, especially if your bones are weak.

Another symptom of untreated celiac disease may be neuropathy (disorder affecting the nervous system). "Approximately 10% of CD patients have an associated neurologic disease, most often peripheral neuropathy or ataxia but also seizures, dementia or psychiatric illness."[15]

A different study concluded that peripheral neuropathy occurs in about 8% of celiac patients[45]. Symptoms of peripheral neuropathy are problems such as burning, tingling and numbness of legs and hands. Some people who have been diagnosed too late have problems the rest of their lives. Others are fortunate that when diagnosed early their symptoms remit, or they avoid this complication altogether with the diet. (Some patients may need supplementation with Vitamin $B_{12}$ until digestion returns to normal.) In another study, a patient had neurological problems including myopathy [abnormal condition of muscular tissue], polyneuropathy [disease involving a number of peripheral nerves], and ataxia [inability to coordinate muscle activity] as well as a Vitamin E deficiency. "A gluten-free diet and vitamin E supplementation reversed both the clinical neurological manifestations and the abnormalities in the muscle biopsy."[46]

Another study noted that "coeliac [i.e. celiac] disease can sometimes present in the guise of a neurological disorder, which may greatly improve when a gluten-free diet is started promptly. Therefore, the possible presence of coeliac disease needs to be carefully considered in patients with cerebellar ataxia [loss of muscle coordination caused by the brain], epilepsy [seizure disorder], attention/memory impairment or peripheral neuropathy."[47]

Migraine headaches, another neurological complication, may clear up with the diet if the patient has celiac disease. In one article, the patient's migraine headaches disappeared once they followed the gluten-free diet[48]. According to a recent study, "the variability of neurologic disorders that occur in celiac disease is broader than previously reported and includes 'softer' and more common neurologic disorders, such as chronic headache, developmental delay, hypotonia [condition with loss of muscle tension or tension in the body], and learning disorders or ADHD [attention deficit hyperactivity disorder]."[45]

According to the NIH Consensus Conference in 2004, "in addition, a variety of neuropsychiatric conditions such as depression, anxiety, peripheral neuropathy, ataxia, epilepsy with or without cerebral calcifications, and migraine headaches have been reported in individuals with celiac disease."[49] Another article noted that "Celiac disease (CD) long has been associated with neurologic and psychiatric disorders including cerebellar ataxia, peripheral neuropathy, epilepsy, dementia, and depression."[50] Untreated celiac disease affects the brain.

Thyroid disease is also another complication that may affect mood and behavior. "Patients affected by celiac disease tend to have a high prevalence of panic disorder and manic depressive [bipolar] disorder, and association with sub-clinical thyroid disease appears to represent a significant risk factor for these psychiatric disorders."[51] Studies show in some cases the problem may be reversed with the gluten-free diet. "The greater frequency of thyroid disease among celiac disease patients justifies a thyroid functional assessment. In distinct cases, gluten withdrawal may single-handedly reverse the abnormality."[52] Another study suggests that anyone with autoimmune thyroid disease should be tested for celiac disease[53].

Some people with "anxiety, depression, irritability and poor school performance"[21] may actually have untreated celiac disease. For them, there may be a possibility that the diet could resolve their problems and they may be able to be weaned off their medications. "Psychiatric symptoms and psychological behavioral pathologies are common in patients with untreated coeliac [celiac] disease. There are several case reports of coexistence of coeliac sprue and depression, schizophrenia and anxiety... Coeliac disease should be taken into consideration in patients with psychiatric disorders, particularly if they are not responsive to psychopharmacological therapy, because withdrawal of gluten from the diet usually results in disappearance of symptoms."[54] This article further suggested that physicians check for celiac disease because in many cases patients have "silent" celiac disease and behavior problems may be the only clinical symptom.

Dermatitis herpetiformis (DH) is another possible complication of celiac disease. It is an itchy rash that is commonly on elbows, knees and buttocks, but could be other places as well. It is a rash that may blister. It is an immune-mediated reaction to gluten. Even though most DH patients do not have any gastrointestinal symptoms, they must follow the diet carefully because they are susceptible to all of the same complications. The only cure for this rash is to remain gluten-free. In some severe cases, your doctor may prescribe Dapsone®, a medicine for leprosy that may help with symptoms, but the rash will not clear up without the diet. Also, Dapsone® does have side-effects, and is not without risk. The drug carries warnings that there have been some deaths from severe anemia, and problems with jaundice and liver function. Some DH patients may already have anemia and damaged liver function as a complication of celiac disease, and therefore cannot use Dapsone®. Complete blood counts must be done while you are using this medication. According to the Physician's Desk Reference "The patient should be warned to respond to the presence of clinical signs such as sore throat, fever, pallor [paleness of the skin], purpura [patches of purplish discoloration], or jaundice [yellowish pigmentation of the skin]."[55]

For patients with dermatitis herpetiformis, eating gluten may cause a rash flare. (The rash may come within an hour after eating gluten or come days later.) However, taking too much iodine daily may also cause a rash flare. A flare from iodine is <u>not</u> a gluten reaction and does not affect the small intestine[56]. Iodine is important to have in your diet and should not be eliminated from it, unless directed by your doctor. I suggest that if you take a multivitamin with 100% of your daily iodine requirement that you use plain salt instead of iodized salt. On days when you eat a lot of foods containing iodine (like shrimp, sea salt, or seaweed) choose a multivitamin with a lower percentage of iodine. Then the next day go back to your multivitamin with 100% iodine. Ask your physician what is best for your situation. Some celiac patients may have thyroid problems, and iodine plays an important role in thyroid function. If you have thyroid problems, be sure to check with your doctor about the right iodine levels for you.

Keep in mind that some anti-inflammatory medications like ibuprofen may worsen a DH rash[20]. If you have a DH rash flare from gluten or from iodine, be aware that anti-inflammatory drugs may make it worse.

Other skin disorders are associated with celiac disease such as psoriasis. One study found that 4.34% of psoriasis patients had celiac disease.[57] Another study found that psoriasis patients with antibodies to gliadin can be improved by a gluten-free diet.[58, 59]

Undiagnosed celiac disease may be a cause of liver problems or autoimmune hepatitis. Doctors should screen for celiac disease when the cause of chronic liver disease is unknown. Studies have shown that liver damage has been reversed and/or progression prevented from the gluten-free diet in some cases where celiac disease is the cause. In one study it was noted that "celiac disease may be the underlying cause of unexplained elevations of liver enzyme levels ... moreover in the majority of patients, liver enzyme levels will normalize on a gluten-free diet."[60] In another study, "The possible presence of celiac disease should be investigated in patients with severe liver disease. Dietary treatment may prevent progression to hepatic failure, even in cases in which liver transplantation is considered."[61] A 19 year old woman was referred for emergency liver transplantation, and fortunately her doctors' diagnosed celiac disease. Instead of surgery, the patient recovered within 1 week on the diet, and within 5 months her liver tests normalized.[62]

Undiagnosed celiac disease is associated with the development of cancer. "Enteropathy associated T-cell lymphoma is widely recognized as a complication of celiac disease, and gluten restriction has been shown to significantly decrease the risk of this malignancy to the level of the general population."[63] A study in Finland found that a group of dermatitis herpetiformis patients who got T-cell or B-cell lymphoma were the ones who had "adhered to a gluten-free diet <u>significantly less strictly</u> than the dermatitis herpetiformis patients in the control group without lymphoma."[64]

Another type of cancer associated with celiac disease is non-Hodgkin's lymphoma. "Patients with celiac sprue carry a considerable risk of gastrointestinal malignancies, in particular non-Hodgkin's lymphoma. These malignancies represent the most serious of complications of celiac disease."[65] In another study, it was noted that "small-intestinal malignancies are rare. Major risk factors for the development of these malignancies include celiac disease, which predisposes to both carcinoma and lymphoma."[66]

The thought of cancer as a possible complication is very frightening, but the good news is that cancer may be avoided if you stay on the diet. To understand why cancer is a complication, think about the damage happening inside you when you eat gluten. Every time your body damages your small intestine, it then tries to heal itself. All of this damage and then healing causes a lot of new cells to be created. Because so many cells are constantly being created in the same tissue with constant turnover of damage and healing, there is a greater chance that the tissue cells will begin to uncontrollably replicate and create a cancerous growth or tumor. If your intestine stays undamaged, you may dramatically lower your risk.

Untreated celiac disease may be a potential trigger for other autoimmune diseases in the future. Some believe this happens because "increased intestinal permeability may permit entry of other toxins which might induce autoimmune diseases."[6] In autoimmune diseases the body's immune system attacks its own tissues. Celiac disease is an autoimmune disorder because your body attacks its own small intestine. Other autoimmune diseases are rheumatoid arthritis (the body attacks joints and tissues) and type 1 diabetes (the body attacks beta cells of the pancreas). Both of these diseases are associated with celiac disease.

Also associated with celiac disease are; Down Syndrome, Turner Syndrome (a disorder with a chromosome count of 45 and only one X chromosome causing development problems such as dwarfism, webbed neck, elbows that point outward, pigeon chest, abnormal sexual development), Williams Syndrome (a disorder causing facial deformities), selected IgA deficiencies, and first degree relatives with celiac disease.[6] Many physicians recommend that if you have any one of these problems or are related to someone with celiac disease that you be tested for celiac disease. See "Diseases Linked to Celiac Disease" for other diseases/problems associated with celiac disease.

A study in Australia reported that, "Identification and dietary treatment of coeliac [i.e. celiac] disease in children with diabetes improved growth and influenced diabetic control. Evaluation of the outcome of treatment of coeliac disease in diabetes should include assessments of gluten intake."[67]

The sooner you get diagnosed and on the diet, the sooner you may eliminate your risk of other autoimmune diseases. A recent study showed that patients who had their celiac disease diagnosed as children less than 2 years of age carried only a 5% risk of coexisting autoimmune disorders. The risk when diagnosed between ages 2 and 10 was 17%. If diagnosed in an individual over age 10 years was celiac was associated with a 25% risk of other autoimmune diseases. The data showed that "... the prevalence of autoimmune disorders in celiac disease is related to the duration of exposure to gluten".[68]

You'll also have a much longer life by being diagnosed and following the gluten-free diet. A recent study showed that "during 45 years of follow-up, undiagnosed (i.e. untreated) celiac disease was associated with nearly 4-fold increase risk of death."[67]

Throughout this book, I have referred to celiac disease as an autoimmune disorder. This is different from an allergy. Celiac disease is not an allergy. Although it's convenient when you're with people to say you're allergic to wheat because people understand allergies, celiac disease is quite different. With an allergy, the immune system creates a histamine response to something. In an allergic reaction, each encounter with the food allergen may cause a more severe response. Some food allergies may cause hives, swelling, and even difficulty breathing.

In my opinion, the diet for celiac disease can be easier to deal with than an allergy to wheat. For some people with wheat allergies, it is possible for them to become allergic to other grains if they do not constantly vary what they eat. If you were one of those people who kept developing more allergies, you would most likely have to rotate the grains you ate about every 3 to 4 days depending on your physician's instructions, because having the same thing too often could possibly cause you to become allergic to it. That would mean if on Monday you ate rice, you could not eat rice again until Thursday or Friday. That's a lot to keep track of. Also, for some people with allergies (such as a peanut allergy), an allergic response may be life threatening due to difficulty breathing or even anaphylactic shock. Although ingesting gluten is not good for your body, when mistakes happen the situation is not immediately life-threatening as it sometimes is for some people with allergies.

One of our relatives did not rotate her foods after she was diagnosed with a wheat allergy. She frequently ate wheat at restaurants or family gatherings. Now she is allergic to <u>seven</u> foods instead of one, including soy and corn. Her doctor said that if she doesn't rotate rice, then she would become allergic to that as well. (Rice is usually the least allergenic grain.) Since you have celiac disease and not an allergy, you can eat the same grains every day (although prepared in different and delicious ways as described later in this book!) Much like those without celiac disease eat wheat every day, you can have your safe flours every day.

There are some people with both celiac disease and food allergies. If you do have allergies to grains, talk to your doctor to find out if you need to rotate your gluten-free grains or not. If you are someone who needs to rotate them, you can still use my recipes. Not all recipes (especially main dishes) use my gluten-free blends so there is flexibility. I prefer the fine white rice flour as a thickener, but you can also rotate the grains used and it will work. For example, cornstarch, arrowroot, tapioca starch, or potato starch may be used.

After you start the gluten-free diet, it will take some time to heal. Most people do start seeing positive results in 2 weeks. You will find that many annoying problems you had (that you most likely didn't associate with celiac disease) will go away. It may start with the clearing of mouth ulcers and smaller problems. From there usually you start having much more energy and a sense of well-being. With time, larger problems will clear up too. For many who are lactose intolerant, after 3 to 6 months of being on the diet they are surprised to find they are able to drink milk again without problems. (For many celiac patients it takes 3 to 6 months for the intestines to completely heal. For some elderly patients it may take as long as a year. In some cases very slow healers can take up to two years.) Lactose digesting bacteria cannot live in a damaged small intestine. For many people once the small intestine heals, this good bacterium has the right environment and is able to return and digest lactose again.

*Note: If you were lactose intolerant before going on the gluten-free diet, and your lactose intolerance went away after you followed the gluten-free diet; but then later the lactose intolerance returned – that is a sign to check for hidden gluten in your diet. Some people don't experience painful immediate gastrointestinal symptoms that tell them they ingested gluten, so this may be an indicator for you. Damage from gluten may affect lactose digestion.*

Proper nutrition is important for your health. You may eliminate many problems by staying on the diet. Many people have a lot of symptoms when they are diagnosed, but instead of needing many pills with side-effects and many treatments to cure their problems, all they need is the gluten-free diet. As in the previous article, it is possible that all of John F. Kennedy's symptoms could have been avoided if he knew about the gluten-free diet. The good news is that you have the knowledge, so you can do something about it. You don't have to suffer needlessly like he did.

---

*If you like to read medical documents, or want to see photos of what Dermatitis Herpetiformis looks like, there is an excellent article to on the web, entitled "Detecting Celiac Disease in Your Patients" by Harold T. Pruessner, M.D. http://www.aafp.org/afp/980301ap/pruessn.html, published by AAFP. (You can also find it by doing a search of his last name and the article name). It has several photos of DH and the other complications. This article is copyrighted, but you may print out the information for your personal use. It also explains medical test results, and what your doctor should be looking for to early-diagnose patients. If you prefer an explanation with less technical information, click on the patient information handout link. Another excellent site with photos is at www.celiachealth.org. Just be prepared before you look at the photos on the physician's page, because there are some rather graphic photos of body parts there.*

## Diseases/Problems Related to and/or Associated with Celiac Disease

Some physicians feel that patients with these problems should be tested for celiac disease. In other cases, physicians have found that the gluten-free diet has helped ease symptoms. For further information and to understand the relationship, see www.celiachealth.org and www.celiac.com. Some information in the listings below comes from information on these sites, unless otherwise footnoted. Other information comes from journal articles, as noted.

Note: Some diseases are listed more than once, because of listing both the technical and more common names. Also, I have tried to make this list as up-to-date as possible, but every week as I check journal articles I notice that doctors are finding more and more diseases and/or problems associated with celiac disease.

Adenocarcinoma[69]

Abdominal Distention (especially in children; also called bloated belly)

Abdominal Pain

Addison's Disease (an autoimmune-induced disease of the adrenal glands. Symptoms may include weight loss, increasing fatigue, and lack of appetite, anemia, darkening of skin, increased sensitivity to the sun, low blood sugar, low blood pressure, nausea, vomiting, diarrhea or constipation. and dehydration[70].)

Adrenal Failure

Alopecia (hair loss/baldness)

Anemia; folate, iron or pernicious — 3% of people with iron deficiency anemia have celiac disease.. 5-8% of adults with unexplained anemia have celiac disease.[6] In Pernicious Anemia B$_{12}$ is not absorbed properly and symptoms may include fatigue, sore tongue, yellow skin, tingling of hands and feet, depression, memory loss, difficulty with balance, shortness of breath, and occasionally heart palpitations[70]. Since men are rarely anemic, they should be tested for celiac disease if anemic. Men or women who have anemia that does not respond to supplementation should be tested for celiac disease.

Anxiety and Depression

Aphthous Stomatitis, recurrent[71]

Aphthous Ulcerations, recurrent

Arthralgia or Arthropathy (pain or disease affecting a joint)

Arthritis — cases of arthritis in a child resolved once diagnosed and on the gluten-free diet.[131,132]

Arthritis — Rheumatoid

Asperger's Syndrome — some websites suggest a gluten-free and casein-free diet help people with this condition and improves behavior. Casein is found in milk. They do not necessarily have celiac disease, but the diet may be helpful. The theory behind it is that both gluten and casein seem to have an opiate-like effect from gluten exorphines and gliadorphin peptides formed in the digestion of gluten[72]. This reaction can affect socialization and behavior.

Asthma — a recent study showed 25% of children with celiac disease had asthma, compared with about 3% of children without celiac disease[73]

Ataxia (nerve disease)

Attention Deficit Disorder and Attention Deficit Hyperactivity Disorder (ADD and ADHD) — some claim a gluten-free diet helps with these conditions & improves behavior.

Autism — some websites claim a combination gluten-free and casein-free diet improves this condition and behavior. Casein is a protein found in milk. Some suggest "all children with autism should be screened, even if no gastrointestinal symptoms are present."[74] Some claim even those without celiac disease are helped by this diet.

Autoimmune disorders

Autoimmune liver disease or Autoimmune Chronic Active Hepatitis, Primary Biliary Cirrhosis and Primary Sclerosing Cholangitis[75]

Autoimmune hemolytic anemia[21]

Autoimmune thrombocytopenia[21]

Autoimmune thyroiditis

Bird Breeder or Bird Fancier's Lung — journal articles showed a connection in 1977/1978 but I could find no new information on the subject.

Bone Density — some studies show that 90% of patients with celiac disease have bone loss. Other articles suggest 100% of celiacs should be tested for bone loss[18].

Bowel adenocarcinoma (a type of cancer)

Brain Perfusion — (brain blood flow) abnormalities are more common in patients with celiac disease and may be improved by a gluten-free diet.[76]

Brain White-Matter Lesions

Captivating Lymph Node Syndrome[69]

Carcinoma of the Esophagus, small bowel or oropharynx

Cardiomyopathy — The Mayo Clinic reports of a patient with cardiomyopathy and celiac. Their cardiac function improved on the gluten-free diet [139,140]

Cerebellar Atrophy

Cerebellar Ataxia[77] (loss of muscle coordination caused by disorders of the brain)

Cerebral Calcifications (sometimes in the occipital region causing visual disturbances and seizures)[78]

Cerebral Vasculopathy — (disease of the blood vessels in the brain) and may cause recurrent transient strokes in children. Since celiac disease is a treatable cause for cerebral vasculopathy, they suggest testing be included for cryptogenic (obscure) stroke in childhood, even in absence of typical gut symptoms.[79]

Chilblains or Pernio — "cutaneous lesions that may accompany systemic illnesses including states of malnutrition and autoimmune diseases" [128]

Chronic Fatigue Syndrome — myalgic encephalomyelitis or ME, PVS, PVFS

Cleft Lip and Palate — It is suggested that undiagnosed celiac in the maternal and paternal parents could be a cause. It is known the lack of folate is a cause.[123]

Colitis — microscopic and collagenous

Collagen Vascular Disease

Collagenous sprue

Collagenous colitis — "collagenous colitis may be the presenting clinical and pathologic feature of celiac disease. Diagnosis of collagenous colitis should lead the clinician to consider exclusion of underlying occult celiac disease."[80]

Congestive Heart Disease

Constipation — In an article by Dr. Joseph Murray posted on the internet, called "the Widening Spectrum of Celiac Disease" he said about 20% of his celiac patients have constipation instead of diarrhea. Also some celiac patients are not thin, have never been thin, and may even be obese.

Crohn's Disease

Cystic Fibrosis

Dementia

Dental-Enamel Hypoplasia (under-developed tooth enamel due to a deficiency)

Depression (a recent study in adolescence showed that untreated celiac disease "may play a role in vulnerability to depressive and behavioral disorders")[81]

Dermatitis Herpetiformis of DH (An itchy rash that usually goes away with the gluten-free diet.) According to the Merck Manual Home Edition, 10% of people with celiac disease have DH.[20] Approximately 90% of patients with DH do not have any gastrointestinal symptoms[6]

Dermatomyositis[130]

Diabetes (type 1) insulin dependent diabetes mellitus (also called IDDM) — Celiac disease is 20 times more likely for patients with Type 1 diabetes; 5% of children with diabetes also have celiac disease. In a study done in the Czech Republic, a 3.8% frequency of celiac disease was found in the siblings of diabetic children.[82] Symptoms of Diabetes Mellitus may be excessive thirst, hunger, weakness, frequent urination, blurred vision, trembling, confusion, weight loss, and coma (if left untreated).[70]

Diarrhea

Dilated cardiomyopathy [141,142]

Down Syndrome — 10% of all children with Down Syndrome have celiac disease[6].

Dyspepsia

Enteropathy-associated T-cell lymphoma (intestinal lymphoma) – remaining strictly gluten-free is protective and significantly lowers risk[83]

Epilepsy — with or without cerebral calcifications. "Prevalence of celiac disease was increased among patients with epilepsy of unknown etiology."[84]

Erythema nodosum[129]

Eosinophilic Esophagitis – 4% of children with celiac had eosinophilic esophagitis[143]

Failure to thrive in children

Farmer's Lung

Fatigue[136,137]

Fibromyalgia

Fibrosing Alveolitis[21]

Follicular Keratosis

Gall Bladder Disease

Gastroparesis (delayed emptying of bowels)

Grave's Disease — An overactive thyroid. Symptoms may include weight loss, rapid pulse, protruding eyes, feeling too warm, restlessness, insomnia, diarrhea, irritability, palpitations.[70]

Hashimoto's Thyroiditis — An underactive thyroid. Symptoms may include weight gain, slow pulse, red puffy eyes, feeling too cold, mental slowness, drowsiness, confusion, constipation, enlarged thyroid gland in the neck, and thick/course hair.[70]

Head Aches/Migraines

Hepatitis, autoimmune and chronic active — Up to 9% of patients with active ALT, AST may have silent celiac disease. Liver biopsies showed non-reactive hepatitis and which may normalize with a gluten-free diet.[6]

Hypertransaminasemia (a gluten-free diet normalizes liver enzymes and histologic changes in most patients)[75]

Hyposplenism (absent or reduced spleen function. Patients with hyposplenism have a higher risk of bacterial infections, especially pneumonia. For these patients, some doctors may recommend getting a pneumovax inoculation)

Hypothyroidism, hyperthyroidism[21]

Idiopathic dilated cardiomyopathy — 5.7% have celiac disease[6].

Idiopathic pulmonary hemosiderosis[21]

Idiopathic Thrombocytopenic Purpura (ITP)[144]

IgA Deficiency

IgA Mesangial nephropathy

IgA Nephropathy — 3.6% have celiac disease[6]

Impotency

Infertility

Inflammatory Bowel Disease — (particularly ulcerative proctitis)[21]

Interstitial lung disease, including chronic fibrosing alveolitis[21]

Intussusception (usually intermittent)[69] (enfolding of one segment of the intestine within another)

Iridocyclitis, choroiditis[21] (possible association)

Irritable Bowel Disease (IBD)

Irritable Bowel Syndrome (IBS) — a recent study shows that 4.6% of IBS patients have celiac disease

Juvenile Chronic Arthritis — up to 3% of these children have celiac disease

Kidney Disease

Lactose Intolerance — Some doctors suggest that patients with lactose intolerance be screened for celiac disease. One study found 24% of those that were positive for a H2-lactose breath test had celiac disease.[85]

Liver Disease

Low Bone Mass

Lung Cavities

Lymphoma — Non-Hodgkins, T-cell, B-cell

Macroamylasemia[133,134]

Microscopic colitis[21]

Migraine Headaches — 4.4% of those with migraines have celiac disease[6]

Monoarthritis[131]

Multiple Sclerosis — some websites claim some people have improved on a gluten-free/casein-free diet. Studies show there is a link between neurological disorders and celiac. In one study some celiac patients had an MS like disorder[86].

Myasthenia Gravis (a disease involving muscle function, with symptoms of muscle weakness, fatigue, difficulty swallowing, droopy eyelids, unsteady walk, double vision, enlarged thymus gland, high pitched voice. Sixty-six percent of patients are female.[70])

Nerve Disease

Neurological Disorders such as peripheral neuropathy, postural instability, gluten ataxia.

Osteoarthritis

Osteoporosis, osteomalacia, osteopenia

Pancreatic Disorders and Exocrine Pancreatic Insufficiency

Pancreatitis[87, 88]

Panic disorder/major depressive disorder (may be a possible role of thyroid autoimmunity and celiac)[51]

Pernio or Chilblains — celiac may also be a cause of « blue toe » syndrome[127]

Peripheral Neuropathy

Polymyositis

Polyneuropathy

Post viral fatigue syndrome (PVFS)

Primary Biliary Cirrhosis[21]

Psoriasis — association observed. "The presence of CD-associated antibodies in psoriasis patients correlates with greater disease activity"[89] Other doctors found a higher prevalence of celiac disease in patients with psoriasis (4.34%)[57]

Pulmonary Hemosiderosis[140]

Raynaud's Phenomenon — Often seen in combination with other autoimmune diseases (i.e. lupus, rheumatoid arthritis, or Sjögren's syndrome) Symptoms may include sensitivity to the cold such as painful spasms with exposure to cold or hand/feet changing colors from white to purple or blue to red.[70]

Recurrent Pericarditis[21]

Reflux Oesophagitis — "Coeliac patients have a high prevalence of reflux oesophagitis. That a gluten-free diet significantly decreased the relapse rate of GERD symptoms suggests that coeliac disease may represent a risk factor for the development of reflux oesophagitis."[90]

Refractory Sprue

Restless Leg Syndrome (caused by low serum iron/ferrin)[91]

Rheumatoid Arthritis

Sarcoidosis[92]

Schizophrenia

Scleroderma — a diseases that causes fibrosis (scar tissue) to form in the skin or organs. Symptoms may be leathery skin, swollen red fingers, heartburn, indigestion, constipation, diarrhea, muscle pain/weakness, and shortness of breath. Eighty percent of patients are female.[70]

Sclerosing cholangitis[21]

Selective IgA deficiency

Short stature and delayed puberty — About 10% of children with short stature have celiac disease[6]

Sjögren's Syndrome — a disease involving reduction of excretions by mucus glands. It can cause dryness of eyes, mouth, skin, vagina, lungs, brain, sinuses, blood vessels and cells, digestive track, bladder, kidneys and joints. Some symptoms are caused by dryness such as dry eye, sores in the mouth/tongue/throat, gum inflammation, tooth decay or loss, dry skin, rashes, vaginal dryness, yeast infections, shortness of breath, and chronic sinusitis. Other symptoms may include confusion, tingling/numbness in hands/feet, seizures, stroke, kidney disease, fatigue, joint/muscle pain, blood clots (vasculitis), diarrhea/constipation/ abdominal pain. Ninety percent of patients are female[70].

Small-intestinal adenocarcinomas

Spontaneous Abortion and Fetal Growth Retardation

Squamous cell carcinoma[69]

Steatorrhea (fat in stools)

Stroke, Ischemic and Pediatric[79, 93]

Systemic Lupus Erythematosus — Lupus may affect many organs of the body such as joints, muscles, skin, heart, brain, lung, blood vessels, intestines, hearing & balance. Symptoms vary but may include fatigue, fever, anemia, rashes from the sun, muscle aches, painful/stiff joints, confusion, seizures, inflammation of heart or lungs, mouth sores, vasculitis, blood clots & changes in urine; 90% of patients are female.[70]

Systemic Sclerosis[94]

Thrombocytopenic Purpura (ITP)[144]

Thrombocytosis (an increase in platelets in the blood)

Thrombosis (deep vein and cerebral vascular)[95, 96]

Thyroid Disease (autoimmune)

Thyroiditis

Thyrotoxicosis

Turner Syndrome — 4-8% have celiac disease[6]

Type 1 Diabetes Mellitus

Ulcerative jejunoileitis[69]

Urticaria — a case was reported of a child with chronic urticaria that had celiac disease. It is suggested in chronic or refractory urticaria to check for celiac disease.[126,135]

Vasculitis

Vitiligo (de-pigmented white patches of skin)

Vitamin K Deficiency

Williams Syndrome — 8.2% of patients have celiac disease

## Lessons Learned on My Journey to Discover Good Gluten-Free Food

Now you know what celiac disease is, and that you're not alone in this diagnosis. One in 133 Americans are believed to have it[2]. Even a president may have had it! Another article says that "Celiac Disease is among the most common inherited diseases with a worldwide prevalence of almost 1% of the population."[97]

But how do you go about following this life-saving diet? Well, fortunately you don't have to follow the same path that I took. I was completely overwhelmed when I first learned of my husband's diagnosis. I loved good food, but I was committed to keeping our house completely gluten-free. I read as many gluten-free cookbooks as I could find and tried scores of gluten-free products. What I found was that most of these foods were terrible! The breads fell apart and most baked goods were stale, heavy, gritty or gummy. Some products left you with rice-grit stuck in your teeth. The flavor, texture, and mouth-feel of many of the baked goods were downright awful. The food was horrible, and I was not going to put up with it!

I knew that people with celiac disease could eat better. They did not need to add bad food to their list of worries. Someone just needed to take the time to figure out where to find the right ingredients and how to adapt the recipes to make them work, and so I set out to do just that.

In the beginning, I experimented a lot and many of my creations were thrown away. It turns out that it is really difficult to get all of the right properties in baked goods without being able to take advantage of the elastic properties that gluten provides. Without gluten, breads, cakes, and other baked goods don't always rise properly, and can often crash. Some gluten-free flours have unusual flavors that can affect your final product. Others are just dense or too wet, which create heavy baked goods that go moldy very quickly. Through trial and error I set out to learn every property of every type of gluten-free flour available, and use that knowledge to make my creations.

Slowly but surely, I began having success by developing specific flour blends that were tailored for specific baked goods. I found that the best flour blend for a cookie was not necessarily the best flour blend for a cake. And those two blends didn't work that well in pies or breads. I often read about others who have claimed to have developed an All-Purpose gluten-free flour, but when I tried their recipes and their flour blends, I found that their flour blends only worked well in a few of their recipes and their other recipes were not good. There was always something wrong, either the taste, texture, final product height, or something else wasn't quite right. I hoped that there might be a correct formula for a gluten-free All-Purpose flour, but it was clear to me that no one had found it.

So I experimented for months, which turned into years, to develop the various flour blends and recipes. And one day in 2010, to my husband's surprise, I discovered a way to create a flour blend that worked wonderfully in breads, pie crusts, cakes, all types of cookies, and even cinnamon buns – it could do everything! I tested this blend in other things just to see if it could possibly work in other recipes and it did. In many cases it worked even better than my original flour blends tailored for a specific recipe. And in a lot of cases it was easier to make than the gluten versions because I didn't have to worry about overworking the batter/dough and bringing out the gluten. (For example, I could blend muffins in a mixer and over-mix it without it getting tough. I could re-roll pie crust over and over without it getting tough.) I started serving these creations to people and they thought they were just regular food. Some celiac taste-testers initially found the food "scary" because it was just too good and too "real." I got a lot of people rechecking with me and asking, "Are you sure this is gluten-free?"

When I first started writing this book a decade ago, I told people that a good-tasting gluten-free All-Purpose flour was a myth; I looked and it just didn't exist. But 10 years later I've come to eat my own words because I invented one that actually worked! And on top of that, I was able to create this flour blend without soy which can be an allergy problem for many people. It was a "eureka" moment and an answer to prayer.

At the time of the discovery, we were just about to go to press with the original book. But this discovery was too good not to publish. And the ability to create "real" foods like pie crust opened up even more recipes and foods for people to enjoy. So I retested all of the recipes I originally had in this book, and added some of our other family favorites that I previously wasn't able to convert. I then decided that for the sake of those who need as many options as possible (perhaps to deal with specific allergies in addition to celiac disease) to include the new recipes using my new All-Purpose flour blend as well as some of my original recipes using the other blends. That way you have the choice to make foods that are best for your needs.

I've also included other recipes that don't need any special gluten-free ingredients. You may want to start with those until you're able to purchase the special gluten-free flours. And I have included many variations to recipes to give choices. Sometimes you don't have all the ingredients on hand, but I've suggested how you can make it without all of the ingredients. Other times you are short on time and need an easier or faster way to prepare it, and I've included easier versions. Maybe there is an ingredient you don't like or are allergic to, so the variations can help you to know if it will work without it. Since many people with celiac disease have never cooked before in their lives, I've given very detailed directions and tried to make things easy to prepare. I've also provided cooking secrets that I've learned from my mother and I've learned along the way so you can benefit from that expertise.

My hope is that in by sharing my knowledge and creativity with recipes, you will learn how to be more creative in your cooking, making cooking more enjoyable and fun. There is no need to feel deprived and depressed on this diet; there is a whole world of good gluten-free food out there for the making – armed with a little knowledge you can truly be Joyfully Gluten-Free!

## The Power of the Right Flour – Helpful Hints about Gluten-Free Flours

Getting the flour right can make all of the difference between a delicious recipe and something that you will regret making. Here are some of the issues I had to deal with early on in while inventing new flour blends:

- <u>The grind is important.</u> I found that there was no consistency in the fineness of the grind between brands of flour. Course flours yielded heavier products and some too fine flours created breads that fell after coming out of the oven. Many brands of rice flour produced grainy/gritty results. Some brands of tapioca starch yielded heavy, gummy baked goods. The differences in flour grinds made a huge difference in how things turned out.

- <u>Watch out for contamination.</u> Flours can look safe on ingredients lists, but there may be contamination. Just because it says corn flour, it doesn't mean it wasn't milled, grown or packaged in a place that also processes wheat products. Anyone who has ever transferred flour from one container to another knows that flour can easily become airborne and go everywhere. In factories, this is even more of a problem than at home – imagine truckloads of flour being dumped into bins next to each other, or machines sifting flour next to gluten-free items, and you get a good idea of the problem. Often times, factories run many items in one large room at the same time and they also sometimes share processing equipment. Various parts of equipment that contact flour, like augers or mixers, may be difficult to clean and can be sources of contamination. To reduce the possibility of contamination from a previous run containing an allergen, some companies may throw out the first batches of the next item they run, but this adds to costs. So does the extra cleaning needed. So, make sure that you buy your flour from a source that is aware of these dangers and has taken the proper precautions to avoid contamination – contact them to verify the information.

- <u>Buy safe, high quality flours that will work with your recipe.</u> It is not worth any savings if you either get sick or if your recipe is a flop. You need to make sure that you will enjoy the food that you make and it improves your health. In my search, I've always looked for flours that are safe, fresh, not too expensive, and have a consistent grind. Keep in mind that many of the gluten-free flours are whole grains which means they can go rancid more quickly. Buy from stores that sell a lot so their stock is rotated and things are fresh. I remember buying rice bran from a health food store. I went through all of the work to make a gluten-free bread, only to find out it was inedible because the bran was rancid. I also remember buying gluten-free flours with a heavy grind and went through all of the work only to have a bread that was as dense as a hockey puck. And I remember the time I made my husband sick because I purchased inexpensive rice flour that turned out to be contaminated because I didn't check first to be sure it was safe. The money I saved on that less expensive flour was no savings at all. (Now with the new labeling law, many companies tell you if their product was produced in a facility with wheat, but 10 years ago that labeling did not exist.)

- <u>The recipes you use are important for success with gluten-free flours.</u>  I feel that if people are going to invest the time and money to make gluten-free food, it should turn out right.  In many of the gluten-free cookbooks that I've read, it seems like some of the recipes were never tested – or if they were, the writer didn't know how to cook, or maybe they just didn't know what good flavor or texture was…  I have tested everything in this book for you.  This book is not like other books that are copies of other people's recipes that are reprinted and never tried.  I have made the recipes over and over again to guarantee your success.  Many of these recipes my mother or I invented and these recipes don't exist elsewhere.

To ensure that people would have success with my recipes, I did a careful search to find flours with just the right qualities that were needed.  I talked with farmers, processors, and distributers all over the country to find the very best available.   After finding the flours, I tested them again and again to make sure that the recipes were foolproof.  I was very pleased to find that using these flours, I've been able to recreate virtually any kind of food imaginable – and based on the reaction from my party guests, the gluten-free versions are just as good, if not better, than the traditional versions.

Since I am aware that some of these flour blends are not available to the general public in local grocery stores, I have teamed up with GFN Foods™ so that people using my recipes can achieve the same consistency and flavor that I have enjoyed.  Flour blends and mixes are available at www.gfnfoods.com or www.glutenfreenaturals.com on the internet and at stores listed on their website.  There are additional sources for other ingredients listed in the back of this book.  I primarily did this to give you the consistency you need to make these recipes.  If I just gave you the flour blends like in other books and didn't tell you the specific flours to use, your results would be different.  And since many of the ingredients are not available to the general public, but only to manufacturers (in very large quantities), it just made sense to have them blended together for you to make it easy and consistent, rather than selling the individual ingredients.

If you don't want to shop on the internet to purchase gluten-free flours, or can't find stores carrying these products, you can still make these recipes and use other sources for gluten-free grain ingredients.  With so many recipes in this book you have a lot to choose from.   I have broken down a lot of recipes so you don't have to use the flour blends I have created.  Just remember that your results might differ from mine if you swap flour blends or ingredients.  For some recipes (like baked goods), having just the right flour properties is critical.

## Gluten-Free Flours/Products can be Expensive – What Can I Do?

Over the years in working with gluten-free foods, I found that gluten-free flour usually costs more than wheat flour; this is very understandable. For one, gluten-free flour is not produced on the same scale as wheat flour. This will be true until a lot more people are diagnosed and companies see the need to mass produce gluten-free products. Having separate gluten-free rooms in their manufacturing plant, designated gluten-free equipment, and extra liability insurance all add to the cost. Good companies purchase grain from dedicated farmers, with dedicated mills and dedicated packaging facilities. Employees have to continually recheck the status of ingredients. In addition, gluten-free food companies that test their products for gluten have to charge more because the specialized gluten tests are very expensive and the consequences for contamination are high. Even though they confirm the gluten-free status with their suppliers, many test the ingredients as soon as they come into their plant to be absolutely sure. Many also do expensive lab tests of the final product to prove beyond a doubt that it is safe before selling the product, and to have proof that each product lot is gluten-free. Beyond that, if they choose to have the GF certification symbol on their package, it adds even more to the cost of the final product. (All symbols such as GF, Kosher, Whole Grain, etc. on products cost companies lots of money to use and you have to pay for it.)

However, being gluten-free doesn't have to be outrageous in price, especially if you're a smart shopper or can shop as part of a group. Many gluten-free support groups purchase items in bulk to keep costs low. Case quantities are much cheaper than single items. If you are willing to purchase case quantities, contact the company and ask. Many companies are willing to give you a discount if you place a minimum bulk order. You might be pleasantly surprised to find that for many gluten-free companies a case consists of 6 items instead the previously common dozen. Some require as few as 4 cases to receive a discount. You will save shipping costs on bulk orders too. After a little legwork, you may find that you don't have to purchase as much as you think in order to save big.

Many gluten-free companies offer monthly specials on celiac listserv, such as free shipping. Check (http://listserv.icors.org/SCRIPTS/WA-ICORS.EXE?A0=CELIAC) to get the code needed, or ask the company if they are running a special before you place your order. At the beginning of the month this website allows free advertising to gluten-free companies.

You can also buy quite a lot of regular food items in your local grocery store (see lists at the end of the book) that so happen to be gluten-free. For example, you may not need to spend extra money on a special gluten-free sauce or salad dressing when there are many regular brands that are already gluten-free. As always, choose brands that you know are safe. If you want to purchase store-brands, it can be done, but you will need to contact them. Many stores have gluten-free lists on their websites and others have 800 numbers that you can call to check. Just keep in mind with store brands that suppliers may change, so if the packaging or ingredients list looks different, check it again. Some stores have wonderful return policies and in those stores I take chances and buy the product and check it when I get home. Some other stores do not and some fresh food items can't be returned, so in those cases it is more prudent to check before you buy. If it's not gluten-free, you're wasting money instead of saving it.

Some health insurance plans permit you to deduct the additional cost of gluten-free items from your flexible spending account, so that is something else that may be worth checking into to try to save money. The bookkeeping can be very time consuming; but may be worth it if you have more than one family member with celiac disease.

Another way to save money is to go for quality instead of quantity. Get the gluten-free treats you really enjoy and enjoy them in smaller quantities. This will help to keep costs down and also trim your waistline. The expensive gluten-free foods often are the "treats" or "junk food" items. For good health, it is best to limit those anyway.

Another option to reduce costs is to purchase your own grain mill and grind some of the grains yourself, but I don't recommend it unless you have the budget to purchase a professional type of mill that is capable of a fine grind. I tried that option with an inexpensive home grain mill, but I found that it yielded a much heavier, grittier and inconsistent product. (It was also time consuming and the machine was very noisy!) Until I found a source for brown rice flour, I used to grind my own. I admit I did not enjoy the breads made with my grittier home-ground flour. A fine grind of flour makes a huge difference in how your baked goods turn out. (My husband used to call breads made with my home-ground flours "lead-bread" because they were so heavy.) Some brands of cornmeal can be ground into a finer flour, but I found that the commercial corn flour is finer, and this makes a difference. I haven't gotten rid of the grinder (yet) because it does make good cream of rice cereal from rice, and it can grind buckwheat groats, but I admit that I rarely use it anymore. Most home grain mills can't grind as well as a professional one.

Some celiacs who like bean flours tell me that they use a grinder especially designed for Indian/Asian cuisine to make dal flour. They were able to order these grain mills on-line or get them in Indian specialty markets. I personally have not tried this option because we don't like the taste of bean flours. It may be something worth looking into if you enjoy those types of products.

You can find some of the gluten-free flours in health food stores, Asian markets, gluten-free specialty stores, and some grocery stores. However, there are several safety precautions you need to observe when buying from these sources.

1.  Do not purchase from open bins because of possible contamination. (When workers refill bins, flour may go everywhere and shoppers may not careful with the scoops.)

2.  Use the same caution with repackaged items from stores. When we were first learning about the diet, we experienced product contamination from an Asia/India food market that repackaged 50-pound bags of rice flour into 4-pound bags.

3.  Use caution with some products from other ethnic stores too. Their flours may be cheaper, but you need to be sure they're safe. In one Chinese food store, I couldn't read the company name on a label of flour (let alone the ingredients list) since it was all in Chinese! Since I can't read Chinese, I had to pass on getting a good deal on that flour. I might have considered buying it in spite of my language problem if I could have called them, but there was no phone number or address to contact anyone. So, I recommend

that you choose brands that have a way to contact them so that you can verify that there is no contamination.  Packages with 800 numbers and/or web pages listed make life much easier.

4.  Don't just take word of mouth advice.  Some people at health food stores have no idea what gluten-free really is.  In one store, I was told to try kamut but it contains gluten! Review the safe and forbidden lists in this book so that you will know right away if a grain is safe for you or not.

I hope this advice has been helpful to you and will allow you to avoid some of the mistakes that I have made.  It has been a long but fruitful journey in our home to find a way to recreate all the foods that we loved – and now you can learn from my successes (and failures) so that you can enjoy good food that "just so happens to be" gluten-free.
In the next section I list the flours that I use, and I also included their calories.

## Special Flours/Ingredients for Gluten-Free Recipes

Here is my list of special ingredients you can use to replace wheat. My goal in writing this book was to make gluten-free foods easy to make, delicious tasting, and the same or lower calories as wheat. All of the ones I created are lower calories than wheat which is 455 calories per cup. To extend shelf life of all gluten-free flours, I suggest you store them in the refrigerator or well wrapped in the freezer. Or vacuum package them to double their shelf-life. Baked goods can also be frozen. (To save time, make full batches and freeze leftovers.)

### Gluten-Free Flour Blends Used in This Book
(These are available ready-mixed through www.gfnfoods.com)
With these 4 flour blends, you can make almost every baked good imaginable!

Gluten-Free Naturals™ All Purpose Flour – If you only want to use one flour blend, this is the one to use. This flour blend replaces wheat cup for cup and is the first flour blend that works well for dough and pastries that can be rolled out with a rolling pin. You can make excellent pie crusts with this flour and it is actually easier to use than wheat flour. It also works well for biscuits and cookie cutter cookies. It can be used in quick breads, yeast breads, cakes and cookies. You can coat meats and brown them. You can make sauces the same way you would as with wheat flour.

It took me almost 10 years to develop this flour blend. When I started this book I didn't think an all purpose flour could exist in the gluten-free world because all of the other ones I tried did not work or did not taste good.

Baked goods made with this flour are light and springy. They are not gritty. (Most other gluten-free products are grainy, heavy, dense, low in protein, and low in fiber which causes you to get hungry again quickly.) It not only provides better nutrition than white rice flour breads, but also better taste and texture. It contains whole grains. (Gluten-Free Naturals™ Bread flour is about 400 calories per cup.)

Gluten-Free Naturals™ Cookie Blend – This is a blend of flours that replaces wheat cup for cup in cookies. Cookies made with this flour freeze well. If you wrap cookies well and put them in a freezer bag, my experience is that they keep for months.

I find that cookies made using this flour blend taste the same as wheat flour cookies. They also do not fall apart easily like those made with rice flour. This blend is lower in calories than other blends you may have tried. You can easily convert most of your favorite cookie recipes using it cup for cup. It works well in traditional cookie recipes, but doesn't work well in cookies using sugar substitutes or those with low sugar content. It does contain soy flour. It contains whole grains. (Gluten-Free Naturals™ Cookie Blend is about 440 calories per cup.)

Gluten-Free Naturals™ Sandwich Bread Flour and Multi-Grain Bread Flour – These are blends of flours that replace wheat cup for cup in yeast breads, and contain whole grains.

Breads made with these flours are light and springy. (Most other gluten-free breads are grainy, heavy, dense, low in protein, and low in fiber which causes you to get hungry again quickly.) These flours not only provide better nutrition than white rice flour breads, but also have much better taste and texture. Breads will keep for 3 or 4 days, the same as homemade wheat breads without preservatives. If you want to keep breads longer, slice and freeze any leftovers you don't plan to eat right away. Leftover breads also make excellent breadcrumbs.

You can also make rolled out breads, pie crusts, biscuits, etc. with Gluten-Free Naturals™ Sandwich Bread. Gluten-Free Naturals™ Multi-Grain Flour does contain soy; the Sandwich Bread does not. (Gluten-Free Naturals™ Bread flour is about 400 calories per cup.)

## Other Gluten-Free Flours
Listed in Alphabetical Order

Note: Many of these flours are made from whole grains which are much more nutritious for you. As I said earlier in this book, most people with celiac disease who follow the diet properly eat healthier than most Americans who can eat wheat. However, the reason that these healthful grains are not used often by manufacturers is that their shelf-life is more limited. Many of these flours go bad much more quickly than processed white wheat flour. White wheat flour was developed to be shelf-stable a long time.

With the exception of white rice flour, cornstarch, arrowroot starch, and tapioca starch, (easy to remember since they are all very white in color) – if you are not going to use gluten-free flours quickly, I do not recommend that you store them in your pantry. Store them in the refrigerator or freezer to prevent them from possibly going rancid. To extend the shelf life of the flour blends, also store them in the refrigerator or freezer. Or vacuum package them to double their shelf-life.

Storing whole grain flours for long periods of time in warm or hot temperatures in a paper bag that exposes them to air is especially bad. Many of these grains have the outer hull containing fiber and oil, which are more nutritious but can make them go rancid. Eating rancid food is not good for your health, and it tastes bad too. Storing flours at hot temperatures (especially past their expiration date) also increases the chances of getting bugs in them. All grains (even the "white" ones listed above) are susceptible to bugs such as grain moths and grain beetles if stored improperly in a hot place. Most of these flours will keep one year if stored in a cool dry place. I recommend that you refrigerate, freeze, or vacuum seal them to extend shelf-life. (Vacuum sealing can double shelf-life.)

Almond Meal – This is ground almonds and used in flourless cakes, tortes, almond paste and some cookies. You can make your own by grinding almonds in a food processor. It can go rancid quickly and lose flavor once exposed to the air. I store it in the refrigerator or vacuum package it. If grinding it yourself, grind it right before you use it. (Almond Meal is about 640 calories per cup.)

Amaranth Flour – If it is fresh, it has a mild flavor. After it is exposed to air it can have what I call a "grassy" flavor. I keep it in an airtight container, since exposure to air affects the flavor. It can go rancid. Most health food stores don't sell it quickly, which is why I think I experienced some bad tasting amaranth a few times and threw baked goods away. Be careful to check that it is not contaminated with gluten since it may be grown or milled with other gluten containing grains. Some health foods stores carry brands that say they are "wheat-free" but that does not mean gluten-free. There are other brands that are free of contamination. Manufacturers say it is a very nutritious grain. (Amaranth flour is about 440 calories per cup.)

Arrowroot Starch – If you are allergic to cornstarch, arrowroot may be a good choice for you. It is a good thickener for sauces and gravies. It can be used in baked goods. I don't use it because it is expensive, harder to find, and other starches work just as well. (Arrowroot is about 440 calories per cup.)

Bean Flours – There are many bean flours to choose from and they are a good source of fiber and protein. Some finely ground bean flours like garbanzo bean (chickpea) can give a nice texture to breads. However, it has a strong taste that you either love or hate. I only like garbanzo bean flour in Panelle (see index). I don't like the flavor of most bean flours, so I rarely use them. Some have a course grind which produces heavy/dense baked goods. Some other bean flours are fava, lentil and mung bean. Mung bean flour is the same ingredient that is used to make Chinese bean threads which are a noodle that has a clear appearance. For some people with sensitive digestive systems, bean flours can be gaseous because bean flours are not soaked and rinsed the way that dried beans are cooked. Some people grind their own bean flours using grinding mills for Indian cooking. (Most bean flours are about 440 calories per cup.)

Buckwheat Flour – Despite the name, buckwheat is gluten-free and is a member of the rhubarb family. Buckwheat flour has a unique flavor with a similar texture as wheat. When my husband first started the diet and gluten-free pasta was hard to find, I used to make buckwheat pasta with a pasta machine and the dry the pasta in a dehydrator. Once boiled, buckwheat pasta I made had a milder flavor. Since I've found excellent brands of gluten-free pasta (see product list), I rarely make this anymore since it was too much work. Note: Soba noodles are buckwheat noodles, but most often they either contain wheat or they are made in facilities that make wheat pasta. I have not found a safe brand in the U.S. as of this writing, which is why we avoid it. (I only found one safe brand, King Soba®, in the U.K.) Also use caution as some products like buckwheat pancake mixes contain wheat.

For a milder flavor, you can use buckwheat groats and grind them yourself into flour. Use what you grind right away. Groats are available in health food stores and some grocery stores. The whole grain can be cooked up as a pilaf or side dish. Kasha (roasted buckwheat) is an acquired taste because it has a much stronger flavor. There are recipes on the package if you want to make kasha. We tried it, but the flavor of kasha was a little strong for us. (Buckwheat flour is about 480 calories per cup.)

Corn Flour – This is a corn flour ground to the same consistency as wheat flour. It is not coarse like cornmeal. You can make your own by grinding cornmeal finer in a mill, but it may not be as fine as the commercially ground corn flour. Use caution with purchasing some brands of corn flour because corn is frequently milled with wheat and may be contaminated. Corn flour can be white or yellow, and I prefer the yellow variety. Corn flour in this book is not the same ingredient as listed in many British recipes. In England, Canada and Australia, the term "cornflour" refers to cornstarch. These are two different things.

Also, do <u>not</u> substitute Masa Harina (yellow corn flour treated with lime to make tortillas) for yellow corn flour in my recipes. The grind is not as fine, and the lime treatment can affect the texture of your baked goods. (Corn Flour is about 470 calories a cup.)

On another note, when "corn gluten" is listed on a product, they are referring to a gummy or sticky part of the corn; it is not the gluten that triggers celiac disease. Corn is gluten-free.

<u>Cornmeal</u> -There are many different grinds of cornmeal available on the market. Course cornmeal is good for polenta. Finer cornmeal is good for baked goods or for a cornmeal coating on meats.

Don't purchase cornmeal that is milled in the same factory where they mill wheat. For example, I checked with Indian Head Cornmeal from Washington Quality Foods (Wilkins-Rogers www.wrmills.com) in 2006. Here is their response: "The Indian Head Cornmeal itself is gluten-free. It is, however, packed on equipment that also packs wheat flour products. The lines are cleaned out between products, but if you or your family member is extremely sensitive to wheat gluten, then please be aware that this packaging situation exists." These disclaimers make it hard to know what to do, but I suggest you err on the side of caution. I personally would choose another brand that is safer. If you're going through the work to follow the diet, it is best to make sure it is safe. I recheck products in the future, because the gluten-free status may change. I have found that many manufacturers changed their products because of so many requests for gluten-free foods. (Cornmeal is about 470 calories per cup.)

<u>Cornstarch</u> – You can get this in any grocery store and I have listed some safe brands in the list in the back of this book. You may also be able to find cornstarch for less money in bulk packaging on the Internet, but be sure there is no contamination. Cornstarch is a component of standard cake flour, so using some cornstarch in your cakes will make them lighter. It's also a wonderful ingredient for Chinese foods, and for pudding type desserts. It works well as a thickener in gravies or sauces but it does not freeze well. Sauces made with cornstarch will separate when frozen. Textures of baked goods containing high amounts of cornstarch may become grainier after freezing, so I do not recommend freezing a cake that uses 100% cornstarch as the flour. (Cornstarch is about 480 calories per cup.)

<u>Flax</u> – Flax seeds or flax meal can be added to breads and other baked goods. It is a good source of healthful Omega 3 Fatty Acids and fiber. It has a nutty flavor that some people like and others don't. It can go rancid quickly so store it in the refrigerator or freezer or vacuum package it. Like other grains, the whole grain doesn't go rancid as quickly as the flour. I grind flax seeds into flax meal and use it immediately after I grind it using my food processor. I add 1 or 2 Tablespoons to breads to add fiber and nutrition.

Flax can also be used as an egg substitute in baked goods, for those allergic to eggs. (For 1 egg use 1 Tablespoon flax plus 3 Tablespoons water, blend, let sit 2 minutes and add to baked goods. The volume will be lower and the final product will be chewier/denser.) (Flaxseed meal is 480 calories per cup, and flax seed is about 853 calories per cup.)

<u>Millet Flour</u> – When you think of millet, you may think of birdseed, but this is a different variety for human consumption. It has a nice flavor if it is fresh and good nutrition, but

since it is a whole grain it can go rancid quickly. I have purchased it at health food stores and it was already rancid, so check dates. Make sure you choose a brand not contaminated with wheat. I have produced some nice baked goods with it, but like some of the other flours there is a lot of inconsistency between brands because some grinds are not fine and produce heavier products. (Millet flour is 440 calories per cup.)

Montina® Flour – This is a flour from a wild grass that is gluten-free. It is not rice, just as wild rice is a grass and not rice. Montina® is a good source of fiber. They recommend using about 15% of it in baked goods. It is expensive because they have put a lot of research into producing this new grain. My personal experience with this was that I found their yeast bread was a little time-consuming to make. I gave some to a friend who is allergic to many grains and she enjoyed it. The recipe was similar to other gluten-free rice breads I have tried. (Montina® is about 570 calories per cup.)

Potato Flour – This is flour made from ground dehydrated potatoes. You may substitute potato flakes if you cannot find the flour, but the final product may be a little heavier/denser. Just make sure that the flakes are gluten-free. You can also substitute Potato Buds® which are gluten-free as of this writing, and pulverize them. Potato flakes frequently contain Mono and Diglycerides, which is a fat. There is some concern in the celiac community about these fats containing a wheat binder, but with the new labeling law in the U.S. they would have to declare if it contained wheat and I have not found this to be an issue. (Potato flour is about 640 calories per cup.)

Potato Starch – This starch is made from the starchy part of potatoes. I usually find it in my grocery store where they have specialty foods and items for Passover. This flour is good for thickening. It is also very smooth without grit and bland in flavor. The downside is that for some brands it can be about 900 calories per cup! Some other brands say they are 640 a cup. Compared to wheat at 455 per cup, that is a large calorie difference. So I use potato starch sparingly. I find that too much potato starch seems to make baked goods more crumbly. Check the labels for calorie content if you plan to use it, and look at the calories and grams per cup. Some brands are denser than others because of the way they are manufactured. The lighter starch produces lighter baked goods. I've also noticed that many brands of gluten-free baking mixes that contain potato starch don't show you the "prepared" calories, because the mix alone calories are already high and you may not purchase the product if you knew how high calorie it really is.

Quinoa – It is a grain that can be added to breads or used as a side dish, and is touted as very nutritious. It is also an ingredient in some gluten-free pastas. I find it has a little bitter flavor to it. (The outer shell of the grain tastes a little bitter. It should be rinsed well before using to remove that shell. There are brands that are pre-rinsed and dehulled and have a milder flavor.) Some people like it cooked up as a breakfast cereal or as a pilaf. Some like it as part of a salad with oil and vinegar dressing and grilled vegetables. It is a healthful grain that many people like. However, we don't like the flavor so I don't use it. This grain can also go rancid. Perhaps the reason we didn't like it the few times we tried it may be that it wasn't very fresh. (Quinoa flour is about 640 calories per cup.)

<u>Rice Flour, Fine White</u> – There are quite a few brands of rice flour being sold, and most are safe because factories that manufacture rice usually don't do wheat (but check to be sure). Unfortunately, there is no consistency in the grinds from one manufacturer to another, and the grind can affect baked goods. I prefer a fine grind, but some can be too fine and cause baked goods to fall. You can find some fine grinds at Asian Markets, but if you buy it from these stores, choose packages that are from a manufacturer (not repackaged) and also check for contamination. Be careful if buying from bulk bins at health food stores for the same reason.

Rice flour is excellent in sauces and sauces will freeze very well and not separate like wheat flour or cornstarch. Color and texture in sauces is close to wheat, but it is much easier to cook with because you can sprinkle and blend the flour right into the liquid. Traditional cream sauces made with wheat require that you to melt butter and blend in the flour with the butter. For rice flour sauces you can eliminate the butter (and the butter calories) and that step. Rice flour is good as part of a blend of gluten-free flours for baking. I find if you try to substitute flour using 100% rice flour that it yields a gritty/heavier product, so I don't recommend it. White rice flour has a longer shelf-life because it doesn't have the outer bran part. It should be stored in a cool dry place. In sauces I use the same ratio of rice flour as I would wheat flour, although some books say you can use less. (Rice flour is about 560 calories per cup.)

<u>Rice Flour, Fine Brown</u> – Fine brown rice flour has almost all of the properties of white rice flour with more fiber. In breads, brown rice flour makes a product that is less crumbly than those made with white rice flour.

Brown rice flour may go rancid more quickly than other flours because it contains the outer bran part of the rice kernel. If you are planning to keep this flour for a long period of time (especially 6 months or longer), refrigerate or freeze it to extend shelf-life. You can use it cold in your recipes. If you use it quickly, store in a cool, dry place. Purchase brown rice and brown rice flour only from places that sell their products quickly. I have tried brown rice flour from some small health food stores where products didn't move, and it was rancid. There is not a lot of consistency in the grinds between brands, and I prefer this flour with a finer grind. (Rice flour is about 560 calories per cup.)

<u>Rice Flour, Sweet (or Gummy Rice)</u> – This flour is very good for thickening sauces. I rarely use it because white rice flour also works for sauces, and I find it easier to keep one type of white rice flour on hand instead of two. If I do use it, the product sold under the Mochiko® Blue Star Brand that is found in most Asian food stores is gluten-free as of this writing. It is like the fine rice flour mentioned above, except that it is made from "sticky rice" or glutinous rice instead of regular white rice. (Glutinous means gummy in this case and does not contain gluten.) If you have an Asian market in your area, you may be able to find this flour locally. (Rice flour is about 560 calories per cup.)

<u>Sorghum Flour</u> – You may think of sorghum syrup when you hear the name, but the flour is made from a different variety. Although you can find it a lot cheaper in Indian food markets, I do not recommend that you purchase it from there. Some are bitter tasting, too heavy a grind, and in my local store I found it had wheat contamination. If it doesn't move quickly, it may also be rancid. To extend the flour's shelf-life (it has the same shelf life as

whole wheat flour); keep it in the refrigerator or freezer. You can use it cold from the freezer in your recipes. If you plan to use it quickly, store it in a cool, dry place. Some websites suggest that this flour may be good for people with diabetes since it metabolizes more slowly than other flours. Other names for sorghum are juwar and milo. (Sorghum is about 480 calories per cup.)

Soy Flour – In my recipes I use low fat or defatted soy flour. Whole fat soy has a very strong flavor, in my opinion, and goes rancid more quickly.

Soy flour can help improve texture, but many people don't like the strong "beany" taste. Many brands are safe but there are a few companies that grow soy as a cross rotation crop for wheat. Soy flour works well in baked goods that have fruit or nuts. Soy has a nutty flavor that may enhance the flavor of nuts. It also has excellent protein, so you won't feel hungry as quickly after eating it. If you are allergic to soy, you may substitute other bean flours that are suitable for you. I suggest that you keep soy flour in your refrigerator or freezer to keep it fresher longer, especially if you want to store it longer than 6 months. Like other whole grain type flours, it may go rancid more quickly, especially if not kept in a cool, dry place. Soy flour has fewer calories than wheat. (Soy is about 330 calories per cup.)

Tapioca Starch or Tapioca Flour – In my recipes, I use tapioca starch. Both tapioca starch and tapioca flour are interchangeable, and can be used. According to the Thailand Tapioca Council, they are made from the same product (root of cassava plant) but manufactured differently. The starch uses more modern methods. You can purchase tapioca starch in Asian stores, and I have found that most brands are free of contamination, but check. Most brands of tapioca starch are flavorless and odorless, but I have tried some less inexpensive brands that have an unpleasant taste and smell that I don't like.

Tapioca starch or tapioca flour can help provide some chewiness to breads and pizza crusts. Even if you don't like tapioca pudding, you will probably like it in recipes. It is also called cassava flour or manioc flour. When you fill a canister or container with this flour or when you measure it, I recommend you do it gently as it can get airborne and make a mess. Don't pour it in the bowl or it will "poof" up and spill out on the other side of your bowl. (Tapioca Starch is about 360 calories per cup.)

Teff – This in an Ethiopian grain that is used to make a sourdough flat bread called injera. There are recipes on the internet for this sour pancake/crepe-like bread, but some recipes contain wheat flour. The traditional bread uses 100% teff and is fermented for several days. Injera definitely is an acquired taste. I personally prefer my crepe recipes because they are easier to make, mild in flavor and you don't have to ferment them.

Teff flour has good nutrition and can be added to gluten-free breads. It is also sold as a tiny grain, which can also be added to breads or cooked as a cereal. It can be expensive and hard to find. Store it in the refrigerator or freezer since it is a whole grain flour. Be careful of contamination since it may be grown with wheat. (Teff flour is about 450 calories per cup.)

## Other Gluten-Free Flour Blends

I don't use the traditional gluten-free flour blend found in other books that contains rice flour, potato starch and tapioca starch. At the time it was developed, this blend was a wonderful breakthrough for celiac patients, because there weren't baked goods available. I am grateful to the author, who originally developed this blend, because it showed that there could be gluten-free substitutes for people with celiac disease. However, my experience with it is that this blend doesn't work well in all things. It can be heavy or grainy in some baked goods, and since I can eat wheat I really notice the difference. It also is higher in calories than wheat, so it is harder to gauge your calorie intake when you eat foods made with this blend. Yes, you can try this blend in my recipes, but keep in mind that the final product won't have the same flavor and won't be as light in texture. As far as the newer bean flour blend, I don't use that one either. The garbanzo/fava bean flour does have a flavor that can be strong for some people. Neither my husband nor I liked breads made with this blend. Yes, you can try substituting it in some of my recipes, but the results also won't be the same. If you want results that even non-celiacs will enjoy, then I recommend you do not substitute.

## Other Special Ingredients

<u>Egg white powder</u> – This is not a necessity, but I like the convenience. It is usually cheaper and easier than buying eggs and separating them. I use them in breads, coatings, and to make angel food cake. I also like adding a little egg white powder to chicken before stir-frying it for Chinese dishes. You can substitute egg whites in my recipes. Egg white powder is available in some grocery stores and on the Internet. Be sure to read ingredients. Most brands contain 100% egg whites.

<u>Xanthan gum</u> – This is the "glue" that holds gluten-free breads and baked goods together. It's an excellent gummy thickener with no flavor. You can find it in health food stores, specialty stores, or on-line. If you find that your products seem too gummy, you may have to adjust the amount of gum you are using or try a different brand. One of the reasons we came up with the flour blends is so that your baked goods will turn out right every time and you won't need to purchase this expensive ingredient.

Xanthan gum has other uses. You can add a pinch to thicken salad dressings, but if you do use it very sparingly and add only a pinch at a time. You will be surprised how little it takes to thicken liquids.

Xanthan gum is a natural ingredient. If you spill it on your counter, I suggest you wipe off as much as you can with a <u>dry</u> cloth or paper towel. Use a wet cloth or sponge only to get the last residue. Otherwise, you will have a slimy mess that is difficult to clean. Stir xanthan gum into your dry ingredients for easier blending. My experience is that the texture of baked goods turns out better if you add it to the dry ingredients rather than the wet ingredients. I suggest using 1 teaspoon to 1 cup of gluten-free flour.

Whenever you measure xanthan gum, do it gently because it can get airborne and make a mess. Using the flour blends avoids the problem of airborne xanthan gum, since the gum is already mixed in.

<u>Guar Gum</u> – I tend to use xanthan gum in most of my recipes, since it is readily available in health food stores and xanthan is a superior thickener. Guar is less costly, harder to find, and for some people it has some laxative effect. Some people think some brands of guar gum changes the flavor of baked goods. You can substitute guar in my recipes but the texture may be a little different. In some recipes it will be a little harder to mix your batter because it will be thicker. In other recipes it will give a slightly more moist texture. I suggest using 1 teaspoon guar gum to 1 cup of gluten-free flour. If your products are not holding together well or have an unusual aftertaste, then it may be the guar gum and you should try a different brand.

The choice is yours whether to use xanthan or guar. Guar gum is also a natural ingredient. As with xanthan gum, if you spill any on your counter, wipe it up dry (same as noted above with xanthan gum) or you can have a difficult gummy mess to clean up.

Another way to save money is to put together a mixture of ½ xanthan and ½ guar gum. I suggest trying this in a small amount first to be sure it is to your liking in baked goods. To blend, put it in a sealed container and shake. It is very important to let it rest a while before opening the container.

Both xanthan and guar gums can get airborne and can make a mess. You also do not want to breathe in these gums, since in large amounts they can be a lung irritant. (I learned this from experience when handling a large amount. Thankfully the irritation is temporary and non-carcinogenic, but it was very unpleasant and I recommend avoiding this!) Using the flour blends avoids this problem, since the gum is already mixed in. (Once mixed in with the flours in baking mixes it doesn't get airborne like it does when you take it directly out of the package.)

# Tips for Converting Recipes

Now that you know the ingredients, how do you convert your favorite recipes?

Follow these simple guidelines for your main dishes.

- For main dishes, a good substitute for thickening is fine white rice flour or sweet rice flour. Rice flour freezes well. White rice flour has a long shelf life. It browns well when used on the outside of meat for stews. It gives that creamy white color in gravies like wheat flour. It is not as goopy or gel-like as cornstarch is in gravies. You can slowly sprinkle in rice flour, mix it in with a whisk, and thicken a sauce gradually. This makes it easier to use than wheat flour. You can also eliminate the fat used in making cream sauces. Instead of melting butter and adding the flour to the fat, just add the rice flour to the liquid. It is easiest to blend in the rice flour using a small amount of liquid and then adding more liquid. It is easiest to blend in using a whisk.

- Gluten-Free Naturals™ All Purpose Flour works the same way as flour when browning meats or making sauces. Use the traditional method of melting butter and then mixing in the flour and making your sauce.

- Using a lot of white rice flour can cause constipation for some people. If you need to add fiber to your diet, use brown rice flour instead of white rice flour. Just be sure to store brown rice flour properly so it doesn't go rancid. Or instead of rice flour use Gluten-Free Naturals™ All Purpose Flour. It contains whole grains and no rice flour. Some people find it easiest to fill their flour canister with this All Purpose Flour and use it for everything.

- For chicken that is tender and is easy to cut with a fork, coat it in tapioca starch or tapioca flour, instead of rice flour before cooking. Unfortunately, you will not be able to freeze the dish well and your gravy will be a little goopy, but the meat will be delicious and juicy. Note: Tapioca starch does not brown well like rice flour. If brown gravy is needed, coat in rice flour.

- Cornstarch can also be used to coat meat and make it seem like it is more tender. When used to coat meat to be fried, it can make a light and crispy coating. However, leftovers will lose all the crispiness. Cornstarch does not freeze well. Frozen cornstarch gravies do not have good texture and the gravies will separate.

- Brown rice flour, fine white rice or sweet rice flour work well as a substitute for plain bread crumbs in meatballs and meatloaf. I substitute it Tablespoon for Tablespoon. If your recipe specifies flavored bread crumbs, add some additional herbs and spices based on the bread crumb recipe in this book.

- When making bread crumbs or croutons from gluten-free breads, do not attempt to dry the bread first and then cut or pulverize the bread. Always cut or pulverize the bread first and then dry it. Not only will your end product not be as good, but it will be too difficult to do.

- Breads made with Gluten-Free Naturals™ bread flour can be used to make bread crumbs that are wonderful in main dishes or as a coating. Take day-old bread and pulse it until fine in a food processor. Spread in a layer on baking sheets and bake at 200°F for about 1 hour or longer until dry. Once dry, store it in an airtight container or jar. This bread can also be used to make bread cubes for croutons or for turkey stuffing. Cut day-old bread in cubes and dry using the baking method. If desired, when you initially bake the bread, add some herbs and garlic powder to the batter so you have herb flavored croutons. (Note: do not attempt to dry the bread first and then pulverize it afterwards. It not only is more difficult to do, but the end product will not be as good.)

- Bread crumbs from Gluten-Free Naturals™ Bread can also be made by air drying them. Make a very thin layer of crumbs on a baking sheet or plate. This works well in homes with low humidity. I find within one day the crumbs are dry and there is no need to bake them. I make crumbs from the ends of every loaf I make. Since it is a smaller quantity, they dry quickly on a plate. I store the dried crumbs in a jar. Before I know it I have a jar full of wonderful gluten-free bread crumbs.

- When a recipe calls for fresh bread crumbs, pulverized day old bread made with Gluten-Free Naturals™ bread flour in the food processor and use it in your recipe.

- Gluten-Free Naturals™ Cornbread can be used to make a delicious turkey stuffing. Spread batter on a large greased jelly roll pan. Bake 20 to 25 minutes. Remove from oven. Cut into cubes and follow stuffing recipe. (See recipe in this book).

- If you are allergic to a flour in any of my recipes, I suggest you substitute flours. For example for soy flour, substitute another bean flour. For cornstarch, substitute arrowroot starch or tapioca starch. For best results I recommend the GFN Foods™/Gluten-Free Naturals™ products because they were used to develop the recipes in this book. Gluten-Free Naturals™ All Purpose Flour doesn't contain soy.

- To find gluten-free flours locally, I telephone stores and ask if they carry what I need, which saves me time. Many grocery stores will special order items for you.

- Experimenting can be fun. I usually make ½ the recipe the first time I make something to see if I like it. If I like it, from then on I make the full recipe, and freeze the rest. Leftovers are great for lunches and for travel.

Here are tips for converting baked goods:

- Gluten-Free Naturals™ All Purpose Flour can be substituted cup for cup for almost every baking recipe, and no special pans are needed. Some other gluten-free flour blends require special pans, or baked goods become too browned or burned.

- Instead of using all butter in cakes, breads, and quick breads, substitute some oil. Oil is the same calories as butter, has less saturated fat, and the oil will help improve the texture to make baked goods seem less gritty. (Oil is also casein-free.)

- For some cake recipes you are converting using Gluten-Free Naturals™ All Purpose Flour, you may have to add some additional liquid so that the batter is not too thick and rises properly. Try the recipes in this book first, so you get a feel for what your batter consistency should be. Then try converting your own recipes. You can compare the flour to liquid ratios in the recipes in this book, and then apply it to your recipe. Sometimes I had to increase the liquid and found that it resulted in higher rising, moister cakes. Too much liquid can make your cake fall after it is baked, so I don't recommend adding more than double the liquid.

- A heavy duty mixer (such as a KitchenAid®) can help beat thick mixes, and improve the texture of baked goods. If you plan to bake a lot, I think it's worth the expense.

- Have your pan greased <u>before</u> you mix your batter. Once mixed, put it in the pan, smooth the dough, and get it in the oven. Gluten-free batters that sit will get thicker and be difficult to work with because of the gums. If you wait to grease the pan after blending the ingredients you will often find that it is difficult to spread the batter in the pan.

- If your pancake batter seems too thin, wait a few minutes before adding more gluten-free flour. Often times the gum will thicken the batter and the extra flour may not be needed.

- It is easier to convert your wheat recipes to gluten-free if they are not high in flour. Initially try to select ones that use only 1 or 2 cups. After you have more experience baking gluten-free baked goods, then you can try converting recipes with higher levels of flour.

- Baking recipes using gluten-free buttermilk or plain yogurt often have better texture/higher volume.

- If possible, use smaller baking pans especially if your recipe is high in rice flour. I often use three small loaf pans instead of one large one. You will save baking time and produce a product that holds together better.

- If converting cookie recipes using Gluten-Free Naturals™ All Purpose Flour, slightly pack the measuring cup when measuring. If you have too little flour drop cookies will turn out more crispy than chewy.

- When converting your own cookie recipes using Gluten-Free Naturals™ Cookie Blend, I suggest you don't pack your measuring cups full, thus eliminating about 1 Tablespoon per cup. Gluten-free flours are too difficult to sift so this trick gives you the amount as if you had sifted. I find that the cookies turn out with a more moist texture with a little less flour.

- For easy handling of cookie dough, refrigerate the dough before rolling it out or making dough balls. Cookies turn out moister and higher if the dough is refrigerated. They turn out drier and flatter if the dough is not refrigerated. This gives you flexibility to create the kind of cookies you like. If you want a crunchy molasses cookie, don't refrigerate the dough first (see index for recipe). Drop cookies are the easiest and most successful cookies to convert to gluten-free using Gluten-Free Naturals™ Cookie Blend. Cookie cutter cookies and bar cookies with crusts are easier to convert with Gluten-Free Naturals™ All Purpose Flour.

- For cookie-cutter cookies using Gluten-Free Naturals™ All Purpose Flour, you may want to roll out the cookies first between 2 sheets of waxed paper. Then put it on a cutting board so it lays flat and put it in the refrigerator to get firm. It will make it easier to roll out and your dough will chill faster so you can bake the cookies faster. Since there is no gluten in the dough, feel free to re-roll it and repeat the process. They won't get tough like wheat cookies do when you re-roll them.

- Cookies made with Gluten-Free Naturals™ All Purpose Flour will be a little sweeter than those made with Gluten-Free Naturals™ Cookie Blend. You can add a little more flour to avoid this.

- For best results when baking cookies, use a gray nonstick pan especially when using Gluten-Free Naturals™ Cookie Blend or rice flour blends. Sometimes cookies can burn when using dark black colored pans, especially at higher temperatures especially if they contain rice flour. Gluten-Free Naturals™ All Purpose Flour is not affected by the pan color, so dark or light non-stick pans may be used.

- For cookie recipes that call for powdered sugar in the cookie (such as Russian tea cakes), use granulated sugar for better results. Cookie Blend works best in cookies that contain white granulated sugar or brown sugar. (See index for recipe.)

- For pie crusts, you also don't have to worry about overworking your pie crust dough as you would a traditional crust. Gluten-Free Naturals™ All Purpose Flour makes an easy pie crust and doesn't need a pie shield because it doesn't over-brown like some other gluten-free flours. However, crusts made with rice flour or Gluten-Free Naturals™ Cookie Blend will brown faster than wheat flour, so use a pie crust shield to stop the crust edges from burning.

- For an easy way to roll out pie crusts, I recommend rolling out your pie crusts between 2 pieces of waxed paper. There is no need to chill the dough first if using Gluten-Free Naturals™ All Purpose flour.

- For an easy way to get your pie crust into the pan after rolling it out, use an extra pie plate as a mold following this method: Roll out your crust and remove the waxed paper on the top. Put it back on and flip the crust over. Remove the waxed paper on this side and replace it. Take an extra pie plate and turn it upside down on your counter, and slide it under the bottom waxed paper under the crust. You now have the upside down pie plate (using this one as a mold), a layer of waxed paper, your rolled pie crust and the top layer of waxed paper. Center the pie crust on the pie plate and shape it to form the plate. Remove the top waxed paper. Place the pie plate you will bake the pie in upside down on top. Now flip the whole thing over and remove the top pie plate. Remove the other piece of waxed paper. Viola – a perfectly shaped pie crust and no difficulty getting it in the pan! Now flute the edges, add your filling.

- For roll-out dough to make biscuits, sometimes you have to reduce the water in the recipe to make dough that you can roll out. I suggest after you roll it and get it in the pan, brush the biscuits with cool water and cover with plastic wrap. The dough will absorb the extra water and create a lighter product. Once most of the water is absorbed, bake the biscuits.

- You can knead dough made with Gluten-Free Naturals™ All Purpose Flour. If you made your roll-out dough too wet, you can knead it and incorporate more flour so you can roll it out.

- Using blends of flours makes the most delicious products with the best texture. Trying to use only one gluten-free flour (instead of a blend) as a wheat substitute usually yields products that are very heavy, dense, or grainy.

- We have had great success converting wheat bread recipes with Gluten-Free Naturals™ Bread Flours, but we suggest you work with the recipes in this book first before you try to convert your own. Gluten-free bread dough has a different texture. Once you learn what the consistency is like, you will have a better sense of the water/flour ratio needed.

- You can substitute 1 Tablespoon of baking powder for the yeast in some pizza recipes and bake it right away instead of letting it rise. Baking powder breads made with Gluten-Free Naturals™ Bread Flour will have a more biscuit-like flavor. Those made with yeast will taste like traditional bread.

- Quick breads using baking powder and Gluten-Free Naturals™ All Purpose Flour will have a lighter texture and are easier to make than those made with yeast.

- Many gluten-free yeast breads made with mostly rice flour turn out flat on the top or dome slightly. Breads made with Gluten-Free Naturals™ Bread Flours or Gluten-Free Naturals™ All Purpose Flour and yeast will be light in texture and dome like regular bread.

- Do not attempt to convert wheat bread recipes to gluten-free breads using other gluten-free flour blends suggested in other books. Our experience is that it won't work. The chemistry for gluten-free breads can be very complicated. You can't do a second punch down because there is no gluten and the xanthan gum is only able to hold the air bubbles in one punch down and loses elasticity if punched down again. Our experience is that converting a wheat bread recipe cup for cup using gluten-free flour blends in other books (rice flour or bean flour blends) will not work. Use a tried and true gluten-free recipe and substitute flours if you need to. For rice or bean blends, try the recipes recommended on the Red Star Yeast Bread web page (www.redstaryeast.com).

- Since gluten-free breads tend to have some starch to replace wheat flour, your bread will tend to go stale more quickly. For wheat products, the staling process begins when the starch begins to convert in the wheat, which happens immediately after it's baked. However it is a slower process for wheat than it is for gluten-free breads made using starch. To preserve freshness, you may want to freeze whatever you're not going to eat in 3 or 4 days. Just like homemade wheat bread goes stale quickly without preservatives (usually lasting no more than 3 days); the same will be true of most gluten-free breads.

- Leftover gluten-free pizza can be refrigerated for several days (just like wheat pizza) and either heated in a clean toaster oven or microwave. It can also be frozen. Reheating and toasting can restore some of the freshness to day-old gluten-free breads and pizzas.

- Rice Breads made without some added starches, tend to be heavy, gritty, and grainy in texture and do not slice well. They don't usually hold well together for sandwiches. Breads made with pure rice flour tend to get moldy quickly because they are wet and dense. When making breads using rice flour, use a blend of flours for best results. Brown rice flour breads hold together better than white rice flour breads. Brown rice flour also adds more fiber and nutrition. It also works best blended together with other flours.

- Recipes with flour blends freeze well, but recipes with 100% cornstarch as the flour do <u>not</u> freeze as well and freezing may change their texture. My experience is that they become ruined and are grainy and fall apart.

- It's nice to have muffins, cakes and breads in the freezer for a quick breakfast or snack. For best flavor and texture, reheat breads and muffins in a toaster oven or a microwave oven.

- When I experiment making cakes, I make one layer. When cool, cut the layer in half like a half-moon. Top one layer with frosting, and then top with the other. (There are a few brands of pre-made frosting that are gluten-free, but not all are, so read ingredients.) Then frost the rest of the cake. I find that half layer cakes are more than enough for a small dinner party.

- For best results, use different pans for different applications:

- For Gluten-Free Naturals™ All Purpose Flour, almost any type of pan can be used. It is not affected by pan color or shininess like other gluten-free flours.

- For breads made with a combination of gluten-free flours, glass Pyrex® or metal non-stick loaf pans are the best to use. Although glass pan manufacturers may tell you to reduce the oven temperature when using glass, I do not do this. I find that the outside of the bread browns better and the center cooks better.

- Breads and Pizzas with high rice flour content that are found in other books (75% rice flour or more, based on flour) tend to burn using a very dark pan, so in that case a silver pan works better.

- Corn muffins and muffins using Gluten-Free Naturals™ All Purpose Flour turn out best in a non-stick type muffin pan. A shiny aluminum pan can also be used with Gluten-Free Naturals™ Cornbread mix or Gluten-Free Naturals™ All Purpose Flour.

- For best results, use gray colored non-stick pans for cookies using Gluten-Free Naturals™ Cookie Blend. Very dark non-stick pans may cause your cookies to burn, or your baking time may have to be adjusted. Silver pans may also be used, but baking times may need to be increased by a few minutes.

- For pizza crusts using a combination of gluten-free flours, dark non-stick type pans brown better than silver pans. They work best for Gluten-Free Naturals™ Pizzeria Style Crust Mix. Bakers Secret® pans work well. A silver pan may be used but you may have to lengthen the baking time.

- A glass Pyrex® pan or a metal non-stick type pan works best for Gluten-Free Naturals™ Homemade Brownie Mix and also some of the cake recipes in this book. Using a glass pan with the brownies makes them chewier and I like the texture better, although a non-stick type pan also works well. (If you like gooey brownies, reduce the baking time by 5 minutes.) A shiny silver pan doesn't work as well for brownies, and you may have to increase baking time.

- For cakes, I use two Baker's Secret® or KitchenAid® non-stick 9" round pans. For cupcakes I also use a non-stick muffin pan.

- Regarding silicon pans, I have had success making cakes with dark blue or black pans, but not with red pans. The red pans didn't absorb enough heat to bake gluten-free items properly. I have also had success with Silpat® for cookies but you have to bake them longer.

- Do not use Corningware® white casserole dishes or white loaf pans for baking gluten-free baked goods. It will not conduct enough heat for gluten-free baking and your baking will be raw at the bottom. Use glass Pyrex® or metal non-stick pans instead. The new Corningware® Simply Lite™ is glass and works well too.

- A non-stick metal mini-muffin pan works well for mini-quiches and mini-muffins. If using Gluten-Free Naturals™ All Purpose Flour, a shiny aluminum one may also be used.

- I prefer glass Pyrex® pie pans for pies.  Non-stick metal may also be used.

- In this book if it makes a difference, I tell you the pan I use.  In the next section I suggest pans and tools that I find work best when making gluten-free foods. When converting your own recipes, you may have to experiment to figure out what is best for your recipes.

## Tools of the Trade

Here is a list of the special tools I use to make gluten-free cooking easier, in my order of preference.

<u>Whisk</u> – I find they work well for blending the flours together. (Or, you can use a sealed Tupperware® type bowl and shake the flours together. Let them settle a moment before opening the lid.) A whisk also works well to blend the gluten-free flour into liquids to make sauces and gravies without lumps.

<u>Loaf pans</u> – I find that glass Pyrex® pans and non-stick metal pans brown better and work best for breads. I use a glass loaf pan to make meatloaf. I often use three mini non-stick loaf pans by Ecco®, instead of one large one to make breads that slice better and bake in about half the time. They can be used for mini appetizer sandwiches or quick breads. For yeast breads in this book a large non-stick 10 inch by 5 ½ inch non-stick loaf pan works really well.

<u>Pie plates</u> – Glass Pyrex® works best for pies but non-stick metal may also be used. A deep dish glass pie plate (the type with ridges along the edge) works best for "crustless" pies.

<u>Pizza pans</u> – Non-stick pans work best for pizzas made with combinations of flours. They conduct the heat better and allow the bottom to brown. Baker's Secret® non-stick pans are a good choice. Silver pans may be used, but the bottom of your pizza crust won't brown without using longer baking times and lower temperatures. Silver pans are better only for pizza crusts made with a high content of rice flour (75% of flour used), since rice flour tends to brown more quickly than other flours. Don't choose the Airbake® pizza pans with the holes in it. Gluten-free dough may drip through the holes and make a mess. Even thicker doughs may get stuck in the holes and be hard to remove.

<u>Mini Muffin and Regular Muffin Pans</u> – Your muffins will bake faster using mini-muffin pans. They are especially good for company so people can try different muffins. You can also use them to prepare mini cakes to substitute for ladyfingers in dessert recipes. Mini-quiches are nice appetizers. Regular muffin pans are very good too. They're also great for cupcakes. Mammoth muffin pans or "top of the muffin" pans are good for making bread rolls. For all muffins, I use the non-stick variety of pans.

<u>Cookie sheets</u> – For cookies using Gluten-Free Naturals™ Cookie Blend, I use a light gray non-stick cookie sheet. For a cookie to be very brown/dark on the bottom, choose the dark non-stick variety. Watch carefully as they can burn more easily when using dark pans. For Gluten-Free Naturals™ All Purpose Flour, you can use a light or dark metal non-stick pan. To use an Airbake® pan, you may have to raise the temperature or extend the baking times, as your cookies may be underdone and thus fall apart/crumble more easily. A silver pan with a Silpat® (non-stick silicon pad) also works but you have to increase the baking time.

<u>Cake Pans</u> – I use the non-stick variety such as Baker's Secret®. Non-stick pans work well with the Gluten-Free Naturals™ All Purpose Flour. Regarding a spring-form pan, I use a shiny silver pan if the recipe contains a crust using Gluten-Free Naturals™ Cookie Blend.

Otherwise a non-stick one may be used for most cakes. I have tried silicon cake pans for all of the flour blends and have had success with dark blue or black ones, but not red colored ones because the red didn't absorb as much heat. For Angel Food cake I use an aluminum tube pan; don't use a non-stick pan because it must cling to the side of the pan or it won't rise properly.

<u>Hand Blender</u> – These are very inexpensive and I find them to be a time-saver. I use it to puree soups, make refried beans, to blend drinks, and to make sauces. They don't take up much space and they are easier to clean than a regular blender. The blender I use is made by the Braun® Company. If you splurge for the upgraded model, it has a nut chopper and whipping attachment. (I have had it a long time so there may be better models available.)

<u>Mixer</u> – I recommend a heavy-duty model like a KitchenAid® with a 325 watt motor. I have the Artisan®, but other models are also very good. If you are going to do a lot of baking, a mixer makes it a lot easier. The mixer does help to make lighter gluten-free baked goods. Recipes containing xanthan gum can be difficult to mix by hand. If you are going to purchase any kitchen appliances, I would say that the heavy duty mixer is probably the best thing to invest in.

<u>Food Processor</u> – This is a luxury item that can chop, make nut meal for flourless cakes, and whip up liquids. Choose one with a powerful motor and a plastic center tube high enough so liquids don't pour out. The cutting blade of a food processor can usually whip cheesecakes and "crustless" pies better than a traditional blender. Most bowls and blades can go in the dishwasher for easier clean up.

<u>Pie Crust Shield</u> – This is an aluminum ring that covers the edge of your pie crust so it doesn't over-bake. This is not needed with Gluten-Free Naturals™ All Purpose Flour. It is only needed with other gluten-free flours so that it doesn't over-brown or burn. For example, you need to cover the crust edges if your pie crust contains rice flour or Gluten-Free Naturals™ Cookie Blend. This is not a necessity, as you can make your own using aluminum foil.

<u>Insulated Lunchbox</u> – great for carrying those wonderful meals you've made.

<u>Crock-pot®</u> – Many crock-pot recipes are gluten-free. You can thicken gravies using rice flour, or by adding a couple of tablespoons quick cooking tapioca at the start of cooking. (See index for recipes). Some people have successfully made gluten-free breads in Crock-pots. My best success was with the older models without removable crocks. This is because older models have coils inside the sides that heat more uniformly. (Some older models also have removable baking inserts.) See the basic bread recipe for suggestions to use one. Be forewarned that some models don't work well to bake bread. The temperature of the different models can vary, and some models have uneven heat. This can make the bread rise unevenly and bake improperly.

<u>Bread Machine</u> – A bread machine is not a necessary item, but can be extremely convenient to use. This is by far the easiest and most fool-proof way to make bread. I have a Zojirushi® that I am able to program to eliminate the second punch down and second rise. That is very important for gluten-free breads to rise properly. I have included recipes with

and without a machine. I suggest if you are new to the diet to try the recipes that don't use a bread machine, or try the mixes I developed for www.gfnfoods.com first. If you find you are eating a lot of breads and enjoying them, then invest in a bread machine. It is worth it to get the programmable model. Some bread machines make you do a dough cycle with rise cycle, and then you have to press bake. Some bread machines have short bake cycles so you will have to press bake more than once, and you have to do so before your under-baked bread cools down and falls. The 2-pound loaf size of the Zojirushi® makes nice sandwich slices. I often pack my lunch and my sandwiches look totally normal. This can be important for children's school lunches.

Bread machines take out the guesswork by timing the rise and then baking the bread for you, which is very convenient. Especially in the winter when temperatures are colder, bread machines will make your breads rise higher because they have a heat cycle to help them rise. If you keep your home cold in the winter, or have a home that is drafty, a bread machine will enable you to successfully make breads during the winter months.

A word of caution when trying new recipes in bread machines: I recommend that you be at home and occasionally check the machine during the first time you're trying a new recipe. Gluten-free bread dough is different than wheat dough. I had one bread experiment go over the top and start to burn on the baking unit. I had added too much liquid by mistake, and the thin bread dough rose more than it was supposed to; it went up and over the pan and onto the heating element. My kitchen started to fill with smoke! Fortunately I was there to smell the smoke and unplug it. It was a mess!

Yeast breads in a bread machine take some practice. (This is true for regular or gluten-free breads.) For new recipes check the bread as it starts to bake, paying particular attention to the level of the dough as it rises, as I mentioned above. Keep in mind that it will rise a little more when it just begins to bake. If the level is too high, it may be because that there is too much liquid, too much batter, or too much yeast. Breads without gluten seem to be more prone to rising and pouring over the top, since there is no gluten to hold them together. Once you know your machine and have used the recipes, I do leave the house after it is mixed and I let the bread machine do its thing! I like to set up the machine on Saturday or Sunday morning, and then come home to warm baked bread at lunch.

FoodSaver® Vacuum Packaging System – This is not a necessary item, but a wonderful way to keep all of your gluten-free ingredients fresh. The one I use has a jar sealer. I use the large ½ gallon Ball® wide-mouth canning jars and store all of my gluten-free flours in those. They seal and reseal very well. (Your grocery store can order these jars for you or you can buy them on-line.) By removing the air, you can keep most flours fresh for 2 years. This method keeps grains bug-free because bugs need air to survive, and bugs cannot get into airtight sealed jars. Many gluten-free flours such as soy, sorghum, brown rice flour, rice bran, bean flours, millet, amaranth, teff, quinoa, flax, and nut flours contain oils that can go rancid. Seeds and nuts can also go rancid. By vacuum packaging, you remove the air that causes these grains to go rancid more quickly. I even use the FoodSaver® to vacuum package corn tortillas since I purchase them in packages of 100 and this keeps them fresh a long time. Without vacuum packaging I have found them to go moldy quickly.

If you want an inexpensive way to vacuum package that uses less storage space, choose the WineSaver® and get the wide mouth canning jar sealer top. Use this with the Ball® canning jars. The WineSaver® is less expensive than the FoodSaver®. You can also use the WineSaver® to vacuum package oil and wine. Canning jars are dishwasher safe and easier to clean than the FoodSaver® plastic bags or canisters. But do not try sealing FoodSaver® canisters with the WineSaver®, because my experience is that it can cause the canisters to crack and render them unusable. That is because the WineSaver® doesn't have automatic shut off like the FoodSaver®.

Even without the vacuum packaging system, I find the large wide mouth canning jars seal better than regular canisters. The tall size fits well in side by side refrigerators, and they are inexpensive to buy. Even without the vacuum packaging, I like using them to store brown sugar in my pantry because the rubber seal lid keeps the sugar moist. I even these jars to store cleaned/dried lettuce in my refrigerator.

Alternatively, these flours can be stored in the refrigerator or freezer to extend their shelf life without vacuum packaging. I have successfully stored them in freezer bags. But if you have limited refrigerator and freezer space, the vacuum packaging can be a way to keep your grains shelf-stable.

## Know Your Other Ingredients

You've learned about the new flours you will be using, but you also have to think about the rest of your diet. In the U.S., especially in packaged foods, there can be hidden gluten where you least expect it! Once you know the brands and what to look for, it becomes very easy. But if you're a newly diagnosed person with celiac disease, it's time to look through your refrigerator and cupboard to find out if you need to replace foods with other brands that are safe.

If you are unsure about any product, call the manufacturer. Most have 800 numbers on the packages or on their web pages. Many store brands also have telephone numbers and will check for you. Your telephone calls may make a difference! I understand that companies like McCormick® had so many telephone calls about their product's gluten-free status that the formulations of their vanilla and their curry powder were changed to make them safe for people with celiac disease. Telephone calls have changed the policies of many companies to have better listings on food labels too. When I call I try to be very patient, I ask questions, and I am always grateful and courteous whatever their response. I believe that a lot of phone calls from a lot of courteous people can make these companies want to make more foods that meet our needs.

If you enjoy the computer, many companies provide gluten-free lists on-line. I believe it's because they have received so many phone calls that they are now making these lists available.

Most companies prefer giving the information by phone or on-line, so it is the most current information. Some companies will send lists in the mail. (Keep in mind that lists can get outdated and product ingredients can change. If the package looks different, I check it again.) Other companies send coupons for their products with the lists, and some have included coupons for free products or $5.00 off several of their products. I have found that checking can be financially beneficial as well as beneficial to your health.

Products can change at any time, and the status of those on my list may have changed since this book went to print. You need to check for yourself. In the back of this book there is a listing of products and also some web pages that maintain gluten-free lists. I have included these lists because I didn't like books that told you to get a gluten-free item (for example the recipe lists gluten-free sour cream), but didn't tell you what brand to use. What good was it to me? I didn't know where to begin with the diet when we first started with it. I was overwhelmed thinking about the number of product ingredient lists I'd have to read at the grocery store. I needed a place to start. So to help you, I have provided a list of the gluten-free ingredients that I used to create the recipes for this book.

Keep in mind that in the U.S. in 2006 a new allergen labeling law went into effect. The 8 allergens (all proteins) are wheat, milk, soy, fish, shellfish, peanuts, tree nuts, and eggs. Under the ingredients lists on packages, many products will now print in bold "contains wheat", which makes it more helpful in choosing products. Unfortunately, rye, oats, barley, and barley malt are not included in this allergen list so you have to be watchful for those in the ingredients list. But as this diet is getting more popular, I am noticing more companies are labeling their products "gluten-free."

Let's look at the other food groups that you need to think about when you are shopping.

## DAIRY PRODUCTS

When we think of dairy foods we think of calcium. Since many people with celiac disease have osteopenia or osteoporosis and need extra calcium, dairy products can be a good source, if you can tolerate them. As we discussed before, calcium is very important for all celiac patients because approximately 90 to 100% have some form of osteoporosis[18]. If you can't eat dairy, look for other sources to add calcium to your diet. Products like canned salmon or fresh green leafy vegetables can be good sources. Also, many products are enhanced with calcium. Just be sure to check the status of those products because I found that some orange juices with calcium added were not gluten-free. Milk substitute beverages such as soy milk are enhanced with calcium and many brands are gluten-free.

Many people with celiac disease are lactose intolerant. For most, once they are on the gluten-free diet from 3 to 6 months their lactose intolerance will disappear. Once the villi heal, the dairy digesting bacteria have the right environment and they may come back.

For those who are lactose intolerant, you may be able to tolerate yogurt better than milk because the yogurt culture breaks down some of the lactose (but not all.) You can substitute yogurt for milk in most of my recipes for baked goods like breads or cakes. You can use part yogurt and part water if your yogurt is very thick. Other people may tolerate evaporated milk better than whole milk, so I have used that in many of my soup recipes. Others may tolerate goat cheese without problems because of its low lactose content. (My favorite is a soft goat cheese [fromage de chèvre] that I like crumbled on salads.) Other products you may consider are very hard cheeses made from cow's milk like cheddar because they have much lower lactose content than soft cheeses like mozzarella. There is also Lactaid® milk which is gluten-free as of this writing. (Or you can use Lactaid ultra® or Lactaid Fast Act® or DairyCare® or Digestive Advantage® pills so you can tolerate lactose. These products are gluten-free as of this writing. This is mentioned in the medical section of this book.)

If you find that cow's milk is not for you, or you are on a gluten-free casein-free diet (many people with autism or Asperger's Syndrome, as well as some people with ADD and ADHD choose to be both gluten and casein free), then substitute the milk in my recipes. You can substitute soymilk, rice milk, almond milk, or potato milk in most of the recipes. Just be sure to read labels carefully to be sure they are gluten-free. See the list at the back of this book. Some brands of rice milk and soy milk contain barley enzymes or extract. Barley and barley malt contain gluten. (Rice Dream® has such a low amount that their product tests below 20 ppm so it is considered safe. Some other products on the market are not.)

Most grated mozzarella cheese is gluten-free. Check your ingredients. Many brands use rice flour or cellulose or potato starch to keep it from sticking, which are safe ingredients.

Most ricotta cheese is gluten-free. When it lists vinegar, in the U.S. that usually means corn vinegar. Corn is the cheapest vinegar. Distilled vinegar is also safe. (Malt vinegar contains gluten, but it is not usually used in ricotta because of its stronger flavor.) Check that the cheese doesn't contain modified food starch. If so, you will have to find out the source of the starch from the manufacturer. I find it easier to buy only those without this ingredient, unless they specify the source.

Plain yogurt is usually gluten-free. I buy ones that don't contain unspecified modified food starch, to make it easier rather than rechecking the source. For flavored yogurts you will most likely have to check with the manufacturer to find out if they contain gluten, because flavorings may contain gluten. (See list at the back of this book for some safe brands. As of 2010, many brands are now labeled gluten-free!) If you can't find safe brands in your area, one solution is to add some jam or fruit to the plain yogurt. I also like to have plain yogurt on hand for baking. You can substitute plain yogurt for buttermilk in baking recipes.

Beware of some imitation cheese foods. Some contain unspecified modified food starch or fillers which may be unsafe. If you can tolerate dairy foods, I think it's easier to choose real cheese. Some cheeses contain annatto coloring, which unto itself is gluten-free. (It comes from the pulp around a seed.) Annatto also may be made with alcohol (i.e. ethyl alcohol which is distilled alcohol. Distilled alcohols are safe no matter what the grain source, if they are distilled properly). So far, all of the companies that I called did not use annatto with alcohol or with a binder, which some celiacs were concerned about. If you have a reaction to products with annatto there is a good chance you're allergic to it. If so, try products without annatto. There are good cheeses without it, since it's a coloring and doesn't affect the flavor.

Some "veined cheeses" such as blue cheese, Gorgonzola cheese, Roquefort, and Stilton cheese may grow the mold used in the cheese on wheat bread. (There are some safe brands available, so if you love blue cheese you just need to choose those brands. I have listed some brands that were safe as of this writing, in the back of this book.) A good substitute for blue cheese is goat cheese or Feta cheese for most recipes. If you choose Feta cheese, you may have to use less salt in the recipe. (Or, rinse the feta cheese in cold water to remove some of the salt.) For people with lactose intolerance, they may find goat cheese to be much easier to digest than those made from cow's milk.

Read labels when purchasing whipping cream or heavy cream. Most canned creams in aerosol cans that I checked are gluten-free, and I have listed some safe brands in this book. Plain whipping or heavy cream is safe. Some companies are now adding chemicals so they may add milk and give you less cream, since cream is more expensive than milk and it can enhance whipping. I check the source if there are additives. When I called Land O'Lakes® years ago about their premium whipping cream, at that time they couldn't confirm the gluten-free status so they said don't use it. I checked back in 2010 and their website says, "to the best of our knowledge" their creams are gluten-free. After reading that I decided to choose Hood® brand which says it is safe. I try to support companies that go the extra mile and are willing to say they are safe, rather than choose the ones who go for the legal disclaimers, and probably don't test their products to be sure.

Sour Cream without additives, such as Friendship® and Breakstone® brands are gluten-free.

MEATS

All fresh meats with nothing added are gluten-free. That is good news. However, I personally don't like the new trend by companies to add solutions to meat. They not only add salt, chemicals, and possibly gluten, but they add water so you are getting less for your money. I am noticing this trend with lower priced meats. Read the vacuum packages (cry-o-vac) types carefully. They often write out the numbers so you'll miss or overlook it. For example "contains a twelve percent added solution..." in fine print and elsewhere on the package there will be an ingredients list. I am finding that solutions are added mostly to chicken, pork, and turkey. If it says "added solutions" those are the ones I check. If it just says "contains solution" that is the blood from the meat and nothing to worry about. (Note: The meats to really be concerned about are the meats with marinades added. Usually anything with teriyaki flavor contains wheat.)

I prefer meats without solutions/nothing added because I think they are not only better quality but also fresher. Recently when my local store had pork on sale, the whole tenderloin was labeled that it contained added solutions. However, the sliced and repackaged did not have an ingredients list! When I asked the butcher, he said it was the same meat and the boneless pork chops contained added solutions. He explained that the solution was gluten-free. However, I didn't want the added tenderizers in my meat. I then asked if they had one without solutions, and they substituted Hormel® pork tenderloin (with nothing added) at the sale price. I'm glad I asked!

Some brands of turkey contain hydrolyzed vegetable protein, which could possibly contain wheat. With the new labeling law, if it contains wheat it should be stated. I check with the manufacturer anyway to find out the source to make sure it is safe. I prefer turkey that is minimally processed with nothing added. I've listed some gluten-free brands in the back of the book. I find it easier to use the fresh items (not marinated) to be sure that it's safe. Some brands of turkey include seasoning packets. I have found that those usually contain wheat so you should not use them.

Some frozen chicken parts have flavorings or solutions added, so be sure to check. There are several major brands that are not adding solutions, which is good news. Some just have some added water from processing which is fine. I've listed some safe brands and products in the back of the book.

Some meats like ground turkey have flavorings added. So far the brands I have checked did not have flavorings that contained wheat. If it did it should be listed because of the new labeling law. I check those anyway to be sure. (I have listed some safe brands in the back of this book.)

In addition to some fresh pork products getting added solutions, you should check ingredients when purchasing hams. I have listed some safe brands in the back of this book. When these brands of gluten-free boneless hams go on sale, I ask the butcher to cut them into ham steaks and I keep them in my freezer and use them when I need a quick dinner. They are good grilled or pan fried. (The butcher will also spiral cut and tie it for me if I wish. He knows me and always thoroughly cleans the slicing machine with a clean cloth before he cuts my meat.) I also cube some ham to use in omelets, salads, soups, or fried potatoes. I keep it frozen in small freezer bags so it is ready to be added into recipes. Many people don't realize that a lot of grocery stores have this free service available from the butcher. I have found my butcher to be very helpful in selecting the right items and keeping them free from contamination. I admit that I am not good at selecting tender steaks, but the butcher is able to help me with that too.

Many products like hot dogs, kielbasa or smoked sausage, and bacon can be gluten-free, but you have to purchase the right brands. I have listed a few brands that I use in this book, but there are many others. You should always call and check with the manufacturers. Beware of some with fillers that contain wheat. Some hot dogs have added farina which is wheat. You may have to check flavorings. Some bacon and sausages with maple flavoring may contain wheat. Some fresh corned beef may contain unsafe ingredients in either the meat or the seasoning packets.

Sausages can have added wheat. I called about several store brands of Italian sausage and was told they were not gluten-free. There was gluten in the flavorings and a possible contamination issue. The ingredients list looked fine but the product was not safe for celiacs. Some brown and serve type sausage and sausage patties can also contain gluten. See the list in this book for some safe brands. As of this writing, Jones Dairy Farm® brand is labeled gluten-free. Check other sausages like Bratwurst for additives. As of this writing, Boar's Head® brand is labeled gluten-free.

Some frozen meat products contain gluten. Check the ingredients lists. Many frozen meat items contain breading. For example, plain frozen fish is fine but fish sticks contain gluten.

Regarding Deli or cold cuts, I purchase only those in packages that I know are safe from the manufacturer. I suggest that you stay away from the deli counter, as there may be contamination. Some make sandwiches and slice breads in those areas. Many roast beefs are coated with wheat to make them brown. Most olive loaf contains wheat. The person working there may wipe down the slicing machine with a contaminated rag. I personally think it's too risky to buy at the deli counter, so I choose prepackaged items. They also have a longer shelf life than deli counter items, and many are labeled gluten-free. However, if you do love deli items, it can be done safely if they understand your needs, they are willing to check ingredients, and they clean the equipment/area for you. Choose a time when they are not too busy so that there are no distractions or mistakes. Some stores do have a separate slicer and separate area just for gluten-free cold cuts, which is the right way to do it.

## VEGETABLES

All fresh vegetables are gluten-free. Beware of canned or frozen vegetables with sauces. It is better to purchase plain ones and to make your own sauces. You'll find it is easy with this book.

Beware of "natural flavors" in some frozen potato products. This ingredient was in a package of frozen toaster hash browns and it fooled me. The natural flavoring in that product was wheat. The new labeling law now discloses any wheat in natural flavorings, so it is easier to make the right choices than it was in years past.

Check the modified food starch source in canned cream corn. Some brands list the source and some do not. A lot of brands now list corn or tapioca which are both safe. For pickled vegetables check that it doesn't contain malt vinegar. Malt vinegar contains gluten, and it would be listed on the label. Other vinegars are safe.

All dried beans are gluten-free. Many canned beans are also safe, but check ingredients. For example, plain kidney beans are safe but sometimes the ones that say they are for chili have unsafe ingredients.

## CONDIMENTS

You probably will find that most of the condiments you already use are gluten-free. For example, I always purchased Hellmans® (Best Foods®) Mayonnaise, Heinz® Ketchup, French's® mustard, and Vlasic® pickles and all of those products are gluten-free. The LaChoy® brand Soy Sauce is the one my husband liked best and that is also gluten-free. Check the lists at the end of this book and I think you will be pleasantly surprised to find that a lot of the products that your family already purchases are safe. Just keep in mind that with products like mayonnaise that "double-dipping" (putting a knife back in the mayonnaise that has gluten crumbs) will contaminate it. So if you have family members that eat gluten in your home, you may want to purchase the squeeze bottles to prevent this problem. Check products like salad dressings, marinades, and sauces as those may contain gluten.

---

In conclusion, there are a lot of foods that you can have, and the gluten-free diet is very versatile. For more detailed food lists, see the next section of Safe and Forbidden Lists in this book.

Also, don't think store brand products are always off-limits. For example, I call 1-800-ShopRite and they provide the gluten-free status of many of their store brand food and vitamin products. Discount grocery stores like Aldi are carrying more gluten-free products too. Wal-Mart's store brand has a policy to clearly label if the item is gluten-free. Safeway, Kroger's, and Winn-Dixie provide lists on their web pages. Check web pages or 800 numbers on products from the stores in your area.

Keep in mind that when choosing store brands it is important to notice ingredient changes, because sometimes suppliers may change. The method I use is to check the gluten-free status and stock up on the item when they have a sale. Before stocking up on it again, I re-check the ingredients and the label. If they look different, I call and re-check it again. One way to double-check is to cut off the label from the last one you verified and purchased. Compare it at the store to the new one before you buy it again.

Most store brands are made by the major manufacturers, and you'll be surprised to find out that many of them are gluten-free. By doing some checking, you will have more products to choose from and save money too.

## Safe List (Includes additives/ingredients seen on food labels)

Note: This list was created using information from www.celiac.com, www.clanthompson.com, and www.glutenliving.com, as well as my own research. I recommend subscribing to their publications to get the most up-to-date information, and checking their websites. This safe list is for pure ingredients. Manufacturers may change products at any time so read labels.

**Note: For flours/grains you purchase for baking or cooking, it is always a good idea to check with the manufacturer regarding possible contamination. They may grow, or mill, or package their grains in the same equipment that contained wheat, making them unsafe. Grain mills are particularly difficult to clean. Those with a ✓ are the ones to check. Thankfully many brands of alternative grains are now labeling whether or not they are gluten-free.**

Acacia Gum

Acesulfame K or Potassium (Sweet One® or Sunett® artificial sweetener)

Acetanisole

Adipic Acid

Adzuki Bean

Agar or Agar Agar (made from red algae)

Agave

Albumen or egg white

Alcohol (specific types & brands. Added flavorings may contain gluten. According to Gluten-Free Living Magazine and the American Dietetic Assoc., alcohol distilled properly is safe for celiacs.)

Alfalfa

Alfalfa sprouts

Algae

Alginate, Potassium (extract of seaweed)

Alginate, Sodium (extract of algae)

Almonds (check the added ingredients on roasted/salted or flavored almonds)

Amaranth Flour ✓

Annatto & Annatto Color (a safe ingredient derived from the pulp around seeds. Some people report allergic reactions to annatto. It can be made with ethyl alcohol, a distilled alcohol, which is safe.)

Apple Cider Vinegar (Pure Apple Cider Vinegar is safe. Some brands of vinegar with added flavors may not be safe. As of 2008, Heinz cider flavored vinegar is now gluten-free.)

Arabic Gum

Arachis Oil (peanut oil)

Arborio Rice (purchase plain rice without seasonings. Caution: in restaurants risotto may contain unsafe broth or bouillon).

Arrowroot

Arrowroot Starch

Artichokes

Artificial Butter Flavoring

Artificial Flavoring

Ascorbic Acid (vitamin C)

Aspartame (NutraSweet® artificial sweetener)

Baking Powder (check labels, most are safe but some may contain wheat)

Baking Soda

Balsamic Vinegar (Real balsamic vinegar is safe. I found a cheaper imitation type with caramel color in a discount brand, so check that. Some brands in Italy with added flavorings are not safe, so use caution in Italy. It appears these unsafe brands are not being imported in the U.S.)

Bean flour ✓

Beans such as Adzuki, Kidney, Pinto, Lentil, Mung, Romano, Navy, Lima, Black Eyed Peas, Dried Peas, and Chickpeas

Benzoic acid

Bergamot oil (ingredient in Earl Grey tea)

Besan (Indian for chickpea)

Beta Carotene

Beta Carotene

BHA

BHT

Bicarbonate of Soda or Baking Soda

Biotin

Brandy (Specific brands only. Made from fruits but added flavorings may make them unsafe.)

Brazil nuts

Brown Sugar

Buckwheat flour ✓ (despite the name, pure buckwheat is gluten-free and in the rhubarb family.)

Buckwheat groats

Butter (check flavorings in unsalted butter - wheat would be declared)

Buttermilk (check for additives)

Calcium Carbonate

Calcium Caseinate

Calcium Chloride

Calcium Disodium

Calcium Lactate

Calcium Pantothenate

✓ = check for possible wheat contamination, when purchasing this flour or grain.

Calcium Phosphate
Calcium Proprionate
Calcium Silicate
Calcium Stearate
Calcium Stearoyl
  Lactylate
Calcium Sulfate
Calrose Rice
Cane Sugar
Canola Oil (also called
  Rapeseed Oil)
Capers (check pickling
  ingredients)
Capsaicin (hot component
  of chili peppers)
Carbonated Water
Carboxymethylcellulose
Carnauba Wax (from a wax
  palm tree)
Carob Bean
Carob Bean Gum
Carob Flour ✔ (check
  ingredients; some report
  that it could contain malt.)
Carrageenan (made from
  red seaweed/algae.
  According to
  www.foodallergy.org it is
  not related to fish or
  shellfish.)
Casein (a derivative from
  milk. Safe for a gluten-free
  diet but those on a casein-
  free diet must avoid it.)
Cassava (tapioca)
Cellulose
Cellulose Gum
Cetyl Alcohol
Champagne (real
  champagne or Asti
  Spumante are safe. Some
  sparkling wines with
  additives may not be.)
Cheeses (Almost all natural
  "real" cheese are safe,
  except some blue type
  veined cheeses like
  Gorgonzola, Roquefort,
  Blue & Stilton which may
  utilize bread mold in their
  manufacturing process.
  Check the source of

modified food starch,
  additives, and flavorings in
  some processed cheese
  foods. Some imitation
  cheeses may be unsafe.)
Chestnuts
Chickpea Flour ✔
Chickpeas
Chicory
Chocolate Liquor (the
  ingredient found in candies
  such as chocolate chips and
  chocolate bars; not the
  liquor drink)
Cider (Cider is squeezed
  apples. Check ingredients;
  some processed cider may
  contain flavoring additives)
Cider, hard – (Specific
  brands only.)
Citric Acid – (Most U.S.
  tomato products use citric
  acid made from corn or beet
  which is safe. On the
  internet I have read claims
  of imports from China
  being unsafe but according
  to Gluten-Free Living
  Magazine citric acid is a safe
  ingredient.)
Cocoa (Cocoa powder used
  in baking. Use caution with
  the beverage; it may contain
  gluten.)
Coconut and Coconut
  Flour
Coffee (beware of some
  instant coffee with barley
  grains, and some flavored
  coffees because of possible
  gluten additives.)
Cognac (made from grapes.)
Cold cuts (only certain
  brands, and it is safer to use
  prepackaged. I suggest you
  stay away from deli items
  unless you know how clean
  and careful the deli is.
  Slicing machines can cause
  contamination if not
  cleaned. Roast beef often
  has wheat to make it brown
  on the outside. Olive loaf
  usually has wheat.

Sandwiches are often made
  in store deli areas.)
Corn
Corn Flour ✔
Corn Gluten
Corn Masa Flour
Corn Oil
Corn Sugar
Corn Sweetener
Corn Syrup (check for
  added flavorings; when
  listed on food labels as just
  corn syrup it is safe.)
Corn Syrup Solids
Corn Vinegar
Cornmeal ✔ (In 2003 I was
  told by Goya® that their
  polenta cornmeal may have
  possible contamination.)
Cornstarch (US brands are
  safe. Check imported; I saw
  a package of Maizena in the
  Hispanic food section that
  contained wheat)
Cotton Seed Oil
Cowpea
Cream of Tartar
Curds
Dal or Dahl (Indian name
  for lentils and beans. Use
  caution when prepared as a
  stew because of additives.
  A celiac friend who travels
  in India warns that some
  asafoetida added to Dal may
  contain wheat flour.)
Dasheen (Caribbean name
  for Taro)
Dates (Plain dates are safe,
  but beware of those dusted
  with oats to prevent
  sticking.)
Demineralized Whey
Dextran
Dextrose
Diglycerides
Dioctyl Sodium
  Sulfosuccinate (laxative
  ingredient)
Dipotassium Phosphate
  (sometimes added to non-
  dairy creamers)

✔ = check for possible wheat contamination, when purchasing this flour or grain.

Disodium Guanylate

Disodium Inosinate

Disodium Phosphate

Distilled Vinegar (according to Gluten-Free Living & the American Dietetic Association Distilled Vinegar is safe if distilled properly. Beware of added flavorings.)

Dutch Processed Cocoa

EDTA (Ingredient in some soft drinks)

Egg white powder (check labels; it should only contain dried egg white)

Egg Yolks

Eggs, fresh (there are reports that some scrambled egg type products may contain gluten, so check ingredients on those products & in restaurants.)

Ester Gum

Ethyl Alcohol

Ethyl Maltol

Ethyl Vanillin

Expeller Pressed Canola Oil

Fava Bean Flour ✓

Fava Beans (These beans are safe for people who only have celiac disease. Some people of Mediterranean, African and Southeast Asian decent may also have C6PD deficiency or "Favism", a hereditary condition with symptoms usually in males. For these people, fava beans cause hemolytic anemia (anemia from destruction to blood cells) with jaundice. The website www.g6pd.org gives more information.)

FD&C Colors Blue #1 Dye & Lake, Blue #2 Dye & Lake, Green #3 Dye & Lake, Red #3 Dye, Red #40 Dye & Lake, Yellow #5 Dye, Yellow #6 Dye & Lake

Ferrous Fumerate

Ferrous gluconate (an organic iron salt used in ripe olives to maintain color)

Ferrous Lactate

Ferrous Sulfate

Filberts (or hazelnuts)

Fish – all fresh. (Beware of additives or breading in frozen fish. Check canned fish ingredients. Beware of products like imitation crabmeat and lobster, which may contain a wheat starch binder.)

Flaked Rice

Flax, flour, meal, seeds and oil

Folate

Folic Acid or Folacin

Frankfurters (certain brands only)

Fructose

Fruits, all fresh

Fruits, Dried (beware of wheat/oats on some dried dates and apricots)

Fumaric Acid

Gelatin

Ghee (rendered butter used in the cooking of India. Check for additives.)

Gin (Specific brands only.)

Gluconolactone or d-delta-gluconolactone

Glucose and Glucose Syrup – it can be made from wheat. If processed properly, it is safe. Because of possible contamination, it is a good idea to check. Some brands like Odense® told me in 2004 not to use their Almond Paste.

Glutamic Acid

Glutinous Rice or Gummy Rice

Glycerides

Glycerin

Glycerol Monooleate

Glycol

Glycol Monosterate

Glycolic acid

Grappa (a distilled wine, with no grain alcohol)

Grits, Corn ✓ (Check for contamination. We had a problem with some brands of instant grits. When I checked Quaker® Brand years ago they said there could be contamination.)

Guar Gum

Gum Acadia

Gum Arabic

Gum Tragacanth

Hazelnuts

Herbs

High Fructose Corn Syrup

Hominy (corn)

Honey

Hops

Horseradish (this root by itself is safe, but sometimes is combined with other ingredients that may contain gluten, so check.)

Hot Dogs (certain brands only)

Hydrogen Peroxide

Hydrolyzed Caseinate

Hydrolyzed meat protein

Hydrolyzed soy protein

Hydroxypropyl cellulose

Hydroxypropyl methylcellulose

Inulin – (usually made from Jerusalem artichoke or chicory root.)

Invert Sugar

Iodine (safe, but may cause Dermatitis Herpetiformis rash to flare up in large doses. Products like seaweed contain iodine.)

Iron

Isolated soy protein

Isomalt (a sugar substitute that doesn't contain malt; it is a fiber. For some it may cause some GI distress.)

✓ = check for possible wheat contamination, when purchasing this flour or grain.

Jerusalem Artichoke

Job's Tears

Jowar or Juwar Flour ✓
(A type of sorghum flour)

Karaya Gum

Kasha ✓ (roasted buckwheat groats)

Kidney Beans

Kudzu and Kudzu Root Starch

Lactase

Lactic Acid

Lactose

Lactulose

Lard

Lecithin

Lemon Grass

Lentil Flour ✓

Lentils

Licorice Root & Licorice Extract (caution: most licorice candy contains wheat)

Liqueurs (specific types and brands only)

Locust Bean Gum

Magnesium Carbonate

Magnesium Hydroxide

Maize or waxy maize (this is corn in the U.S. Note: in the U.K. they sometimes use the word Maize to refer to any grain, and it may be wheat.)

Malic Acid

Maltitol (sugar substitute; may have a laxative effect)

Maltodextrin (In the U.S., this ingredient when listed on <u>food</u> labels is safe. It must be corn or potato, unless specifically noted that it is from wheat. In vitamins they <u>are</u> permitted to use maltodextrin made with wheat, and it does not have to be labeled as from wheat. In Canada in food or vitamins, maltodextrin can be from wheat, and it does not have to be specified on label. Note: a different ingredient called Dextrimaltose may or may not be safe.)

Maltol (a synthetic flavoring that does not have malt and is safe)

Manioc (tapioca)

Mannitol (derived from seaweed)

Margarine (certain brands only, check ingredients)

Masa Flour ✓ (corn flour treated with lime.)

Masa Harina ✓ (corn flour treated with lime.) Note: in Spanish the word Harina means flour. If only the word Harina is on a Spanish product it may be wheat flour and is not safe.

Mead (distilled from honey. Check if flavoring were added).

Meats, fresh and unprocessed (Be careful because some pork, chicken, and turkey have marinades, additives, solutions or fillers. Stay away from precooked items that have wheat to brown them.)

Meats, processed (certain brands only. Be careful because some ham, bacon, cold-cuts, sausage and hot dogs may have added gluten fillers or flavorings.)

Methylcellulose

Microcrystalline Cellulose

Milk (Real milk is gluten-free. Check ingredients on enhanced milk products — some report enhanced skim milk products with oat additives. Check ingredients on low-fat half and half.)

Milk Protein Isolate

Millet

Millet Flour ✓

Milo Flour ✓ (a variety of Sorghum.)

Mineral Oil

Molasses (check ingredients – it should be made from sugar.)

Mono- and Diglycerides (these are fats that could possibly have a wheat binder, but in 2006 it must be declared because of the new labeling law. In the name brand chocolate and instant mashed potatoes I checked they were safe.)

Monopotassium Phosphate

Monosodium Glutamate or MSG (if made in USA it is safe; there are some reports that imported may possibly contain gluten but with the new allergen labeling law, wheat would have to be declared.)

Monostearates

Mung Bean

Mung Bean Threads or Cellophane Noodles (Used in Asian cooking, and found in Asian stores)

Mushrooms

Mustard Flour, Powder or Ground Mustard (Without added ingredients this is gluten-free. Some brands may use wheat flour in ground mustard to make it free-flowing, but with the new labeling law this would be listed. I checked mustard flour in the past, and was told it is mustard seed ground fine as flour. If there is no ingredient list on a spice package, it is just the spice. At one time Coleman's® dry mustard contained wheat flour, but I believe this has changed. However, their prepared mustard still contains wheat the last time I checked.

Mustard Seeds

Natural Smoke Flavor

Navy beans

Niacin & Niacinamide

✓ = check for possible wheat contamination, when purchasing this flour or grain.

Nitrates

Non-Fat Dry Milk

Nuts (except wheat, rye & barley. Use caution with some flavored nuts as they may have gluten added.)

Oils (all varieties including olive, canola or rapeseed, corn and soy.)

Oleyl Alcohol/Oil

Olives (Ferrous gluconate is a safe ingredient. Some marinated olives or those with additives may be unsafe.)

Ouzo (alcohol from grapes and anise)

Palmitate – Vitamin A

Papain

Paraffin (wax)

Pea Flour ✓

Pea Starch

Peanut Butter (check ingredients, most are safe.)

Peanuts

Peas

Pecans

Pectin

Pepper

Pepsin

Pickles (certain brands only. Distilled vinegar is a safe ingredient. Most pickling spices are safe.)

Pigeon Peas

Polenta Cornmeal ✓ (Caution: in restaurants unsafe bouillon or broth may be added to polenta).

Polydextrose

Polyethylene Glycol

Polyglycerol

Polysorbates 60, 80

Popcorn

Port wine (most port wines are safe, but check.)

Potassium Benzoate

Potassium Caseinate

Potassium Citrate

Potassium Iodine

Potassium Lactate

Potassium Sorbate

Potato Flakes (most mono and diglycerides used are safe, and with the new labeling law if wheat were used as a binder it would have to be declared.)

Potato Flour ✓

Potato Starch

Propyl Gallate

Propylene Glycol Monosterate

Psyllium (plain psyllium is safe but check additives in laxatives)

Quinoa (read packages carefully, as some Quinoa noodles contain wheat.)

Quinoa Flour ✓

Ragi (finger millet)

Rape and Rapeseed oil

Red wine vinegar

Rennet and Rennet Casein

Reticulin

Riboflavin (vitamin)

Rice Flour, white or brown ✓ (In 2003 I was told by Goya® that their rice flour may have possible contamination).

Rice Noodles

Rice Starch

Rice Vinegar

Rice, all types (including white, enriched white, brown, jasmine, basmati, arborio [used to make risotto], & wild rice. Beware of pilafs & packaged rice mixes with flavorings. In restaurants, order plain rice. Risotto in a restaurant may contain gluten from the broth used to make it.)

Romano Bean (chickpea)

Rosin

Royal Jelly

Rum (Specific brands, made from cane sugar).

Saccharin

Saffron

Sago Flour ✓

Sago Palm

Sago Starch

Saifun (bean threads)

Sake (Specific brands only).

Salt

Seaweed

Seeds (Sesame, Poppy and Sunflower are safe, all except wheat, rye & barley.)

Shea (a fat from a shea tree)

Sherry (most are fine because they are distilled from grapes. Check.)

Silicon Dioxide

Sodium (salt)

Sodium Acid Pyrophosphate

Sodium Alginate

Sodium Ascorbate (or Ascorbic Acid)

Sodium Benzoate

Sodium Bicarbonate

Sodium Caseinate (gluten-free, not casein free)

Sodium Citrate

Sodium Erythrobate

Sodium Hexametaphosphate

Sodium Lauryl Sulfate

Sodium Nitrate

Sodium Phosphate

Sodium Saccharine

Sodium Silacoaluminate

Sodium Stannate

Soft drinks (check ingredients; only certain brands/flavors are safe).

Sorbic Acid

Sorbitol-Mannitol

Sorghum

Sorghum Flour ✓

Soy Flour ✓

Soy Lecithin

Soy Protein

Soy Protein Isolate

Soybean

✓ = check for possible wheat contamination, when purchasing this flour or grain.

Sparkling Wines (Most are safe. Check additives).

Spices – pure spices (check ingredients in spice blends and ground spices. If no ingredients are listed on the spice bottle that means it's pure spice.)

Splenda® (sucralose)

Stearamide

Stearates

Stearic Acid

Succotash (corn and beans)

Sucralose (Splenda®)

Sucrose (sugar)

Sugar, brown (Some report added caramel color that could possibly contain wheat. The companies I contacted said they use cane sugar, which has no gluten. Some say if invert syrup [may have caramel color] or additives are listed, you should check. To date, I have not seen brown sugar with these additives.)

Sugar, confectioners (check ingredients; in the U.S. most have cornstarch, which is a safe ingredient.)

Sugar, invert

Sugar, white granulated

Sulfites

Sulfosuccinate

Sulfosuccinate

Sulfur Dioxide

Sweet Chestnut Flour

Sweet Potatoes

Tallow (beef fat)

Tapioca

Tapioca Flour or Tapioca Starch

Tarro or Tarrow Root

Tartaric Acid

TBHQ or Tetra or Tributylhydroquinone

Tea (Tea bags are not glued together with gluten, so they are safe. Plain tea is safe.

Beware of some flavored teas and herb teas that contain gluten.)

Tea, iced (homemade from plain tea bags is safe. Beware of some mixes, and some canned or bottled may contain gluten. Some flavored teas/herb teas may contain gluten.)

Tea-Tree Oil

Teff

Teff Flour ✓

Tequila – (specific brands only; most are made with agave and agave is safe.)

Thiamine Hydrochoride

Tofu or Soy Curd or Soya Curd (check ingredients)

Tragacanth

Tragacanth Gum

Tri-Calcium Phosphate

Turmeric (Kurkuma)

Tyrosine

Vanilla, pure (distilled alcohol is safe).

Vanillin (distilled alcohol is safe).

Vegetables – All fresh (beware of sauces in frozen vegetables, additives, and sauces in some canned vegetables)

Vermouth (distilled from grapes).

Vinegar (red, white, balsamic, and cider; vinegar distilled properly is safe. Malt vinegar contains gluten. In U.S. product ingredients, when it lists just vinegar it is usually corn vinegar. Beware of some flavored vinegars. For example, in 2004 Heinz® cider flavored was unsafe, but in 2008 it was changed to be gluten-free. Tarragon vinegar may contain gluten due to added flavorings. Real balsamic vinegar is

safe. Some report cheaper versions with caramel color/additives that should be checked. On the Italian celiac site, some balsamic vinegars not imported to the U.S. are unsafe due to additives.)

Vitamin A (retinol), A Palmitate, $B_1$, $B_{12}$, $B_2$, $B_6$, D

Vodka (Specific types; many are from potato or corn. Distilled alcohol is safe if distilled properly. Check with manufacturer.)

Walnuts

Waxy Maize

Whey

Whey Protein

Whey, Demineralized

White wine Vinegar

Wild Rice

Wild Rice (use caution in purchase rice mixes which may contain wheat)

Wine (almost all wines are safe, including port wines and most sherry wines.)

Wine Coolers (Specific types and brands only; beware of barley malt)

Wine Vinegar (& Balsamic)

Xanthan Gum

Xylitol

Yam Flour ✓ (Use caution if purchasing FuFu mix; an African yam flour mix. It often is not pure yam flour.)

Yams

Yeast

Yellow Corn Flour ✓

Yogurt (plain, unflavored; some flavored yogurts are now labeled gluten-free/check labels)

✓ = check for possible wheat contamination, when purchasing this flour or grain.

## Possibly Safe Ingredients

It is recommended that you check the following ingredients if the source is not specified. They are possibly safe, but it's a good idea to check to be sure. The new food labeling law should help to make things easier, since wheat is one of the major allergens (all of these allergens are proteins). January of 2006 it went into effect. **Most of these items on the list are there because wheat could possibly be used, and now with this new law wheat would be disclosed. There are a few items on the list that may contain barley or malt, and unfortunately those ingredients are not affected by the law and those items should be checked.**

This list was created using information from www.celiac.com, www.clanthompson.com, and www.glutenliving.com, as well as my own research. I recommend subscribing to their publications to get the most up-to-date information, and/or checking their websites. I also suggest you mark up this list as things change.

Some brands already have a policy that they will note any of the 8 food allergens on their labels, and some companies also include rye, oats and barley. (For example, Kraft® Foods says that they will not hide gluten in any additives, and puts the source in parenthesis). If not from one of these companies with this policy, these are some food additives many people suggest you check.

My hope is that the need to check almost all of these ingredients will no longer be necessary because of better labeling. The diet is so much easier now than years ago. When we started nothing was disclosed and we had to check everything. Alcohol/spirits still do not have ingredients labels, so check those. Medications often do not have labeling, so those should be checked as well.

Amylase Enzymes — a bread improver (food additive) that can be made from barley and is usually used in wheat breads. If it is food additive E1100 it is from fungus or from pigs; in dishwasher soaps it is made from bacteria and is gluten-free.

Artificial Color — most are safe but it's good to check. It could possibly utilize a gluten-containing grain. The new U.S. labeling law should disclose any wheat.

Blue Cheeses — some may be unsafe because the mold used to make it is grown on wheat bread. Some do not use bread mold at all. The new U.S. labeling law should disclose any wheat. In Canada their Celiac Society found most blue cheese was not made on bread mold & the few that were, tested below 20 ppm.

Bouillon — check manufacturer; many brands contain gluten, especially those used in restaurants.

Brown Rice Syrup (may contain gluten, check)

Caramel Color — in soft drinks it is usually from sugar. In some products it can be wheat or barley malt. If made in the US it is usually <u>not</u> from wheat or barley. Imported may or may not be safe.)

Coloring — artificial coloring such as Red #2 is safe. However, possibly a natural brown color as in a gravy or sauce could be unsafe. If unsure, check the source.

Dextrimaltose — may utilize wheat in manufacturing but the labeling law should expose it; check labels

Dextrins — I check if not specified. In the USA it is usually corn, but it can be made also made from wheat, potato, rice, etc. The law should disclose wheat.

Edible coatings (may contain gluten)

Flavored Spirits — some flavored brandies or spirits

may have gluten from the added flavorings.

Flavoring(s) — wheat can be a part of the flavoring. I was surprised to find gluten in mint flavoring. I also found unsafe flavoring in frozen French fries. Barley malt can be in flavorings and does not have to be declared since barley is not a major allergen.

French Fries — if fried in contaminated oil it would be unsafe. In addition, some french fries are coated with flour and flavorings.

Glutamate — The new labeling law should disclose if any wheat were used.

Glutamic Acid — The new labeling law should disclose if any wheat were used.

Glutamine — an amino acid, check manufacturer. The new labeling law should disclose if wheat were used.

Hydrolyzed Plant Protein or HPP — wheat is a plant and may possibly be used.

The new labeling law should disclose if wheat were used.

**Hydrolyzed Vegetable Protein or HVP** – It may be wheat. The new labeling law should disclose if any wheat were used.

**Lip Balm** – some brands may be unsafe. Check.

**Maltodextrin** – In vitamins, it may be made from wheat. In foods in the U.S. it is made from corn or potato and is safe. There are different rules for vitamins and food.

**Maltose** - May use wheat in the manufacturing process but the labeling law should expose it.

**Medications** – check all of your medications because many contain gluten.

**Milk variety that is a new no fat no & cholesterol** – may utilize a new process of super-skimming that contains oats as a fiber rich fat replacement. Some non fat products contain starches or flavorings which may contain wheat.

**Modified Food Starch** – check source if not specified. Often in the U.S. corn is used, but it may possibly be wheat. In the name brand canned pie fillings I checked it was corn or tapioca. The new labeling law should disclose if wheat were used.

**Modified Starch** – check if source is not specified. For example, modified tapioca starch is safe. Often it is corn or tapioca. The new labeling law should disclose if any wheat were used.

**Natural Flavoring** – wheat is natural and so is barley malt! It is a good idea to check the flavor source. I was fooled a few times with this ingredient. Most

natural flavor added to meat is gluten-free, but it's a good idea to check.

**Natural Juices/Meat** – can contain hydrolyzed vegetable protein or HVP.

**Non-Dairy Creamer, Sour Cream & Whipped Topping**- check ingredients, especially at restaurants.

**Oat Gum** – if processed properly and the protein completely removed, it would be safe. Since there is still controversy about oats for celiacs, I do not recommend eating oats until research is complete.

**Pasteurized Cheese Spreads** – may contain gluten, check labels.

**Prescription Medications** – some medication have gluten-containing ingredients added as binders or fillers. Check all medicines.

**Scotch Whiskey** – Double distilled spirits are safe if distilled properly as long as no wert or mash is put back into the alcohol. Check regarding contamination or added flavorings.

**Seasonings** – according to glutenfreeliving.com, seasonings could be anything. The new labeling law in 2006 should disclose if it contains wheat. I was fooled by this ingredient because malt does not have to be declared.

**Spice Blends** – If spices are pure, they are gluten-free. Some spice blends contain wheat to make them free flowing. The new labeling law should disclose if it contains wheat.

**Stabilizers** – may be derived from gluten.

**Starch** – check if source is not specified. It may be

wheat. In the U.S. most often they use corn starch. The new labeling law should disclose if wheat were used.

**Stilton cheese** – may be made with wheat bread mold. The new labeling should disclose this. (See blue cheese)

**Stock Cubes** (check manufacturer, many brands contain wheat).

**Textured Vegetable Protein** – Usually soy, but possibly could be wheat. The new labeling law should disclose any wheat.

**Vegetable Gum** – it could be wheat or it could be carob, xanthan, guar, gum arabic, locust bean, cellulose, etc. The new labeling law should expose if it is wheat.

**Vegetable Protein**– Usually made from soy but possibly wheat. The new labeling law should disclose any wheat.

**Vitamins** – check manufacturer, many brands contain wheat as binders or fillers.

<u>In Europe</u>: Celiac societies (such as www.celiacos.org) suggest that the following starch additives found on food labels in Europe may or may not contain gluten. The e-number descriptions are from http://www.eufic.org. The 1400 series numbers are starches

| E-1404 | oxidised starch |
|---|---|
| E-1410 | monostarch phosphate |
| E-1412 | distarch phosphate |
| E-1413 | phosphated distarch phosphate |
| E-1414 | acetylated distarch phosphate |
| E-1420 | acetylated starch |
| E-1422 | acetylated distarch adipate |
| E-1440 | hydroxy propyl starch |
| E-1442 | hydroxy propyl distarch phosphate |
| E-1450 | starch sodium octenyl succinate |

# Forbidden List – Foods/Ingredients <u>Not</u> Safe for a Gluten-Free Diet

This list was created using information from www.celiac.com, www.clanthompson.com, and www.glutenliving.com, as well as my own research. I recommend subscribing to their publications to get the most up-to-date information, and checking their websites.

Note: There are a few items that may be on both safe and forbidden lists, <u>since certain brands may be safe and others are not</u>. If it says check, you should check before using. All other items listed are <u>unsafe</u> and not suitable for the diet, unless of course a product is made by a gluten-free company to replace it such as gluten-free beer).

As a general rule, anything that has the name "wheat" (except for buckwheat) is unsafe. Malt is also unsafe unless specified. There is a malt made from corn, but most companies use the malt made from barley because it makes a much better tasting product. Corn malt is usually specified.

Abyssinian Hard Wheat
Alcohol/Liquor/Spirits with unsafe flavorings
Asafoetida or Hing (An Indian spice; if pure it would be safe but many brands contain wheat flour.)
Atta Flour (whole wheat flour used in India cuisine)
Avena (Spanish for oats)
Avena Sativa Extract (from oats)
Barley
Barley Grass (may have contamination with seeds, and seeds contain gluten. Pure barley grass without contamination would be gluten-free).
Barley Malt
Beer (beer is unsafe, with the exception of some gluten-free beers made especially for celiacs).
Bleached Flour
Bouillon containing wheat
Bran
Bread Flour
Brewer's Yeast (a byproduct of beer and beer is unsafe).
Bromated Flour
Brown Flour
Bulgur
Bulgur Nuts

Bulgur Wheat
Cebada (Spanish for barley)
Centeno (Spanish for rye)
Cereal Binding
Chapati (Indian wheat flatbread)
Communion Wafers (only special ones made especially for celiacs are safe).
Couscous
Cracked Wheat
Cream of Wheat
Dinkle
Durum wheat or flour
Edible Starch
Einkorn (related to wheat)
Emmer (a variety of wheat)
Enriched Flour
Farina
Farro (Spelt)
Filler
Flour ("Flour" on food labels that is unspecified is always wheat flour).
Food Starch (if unspecified, check – it may be made from wheat)
Fu (dried wheat gluten)
Germ (wheat germ)
Graham Flour
Granary Flour
Gravy Cubes and Mixes
Groats (barley, wheat)
Gum Base (check, often is wheat or oats)

Hard Wheat
High Gluten Flour
Hing or Asafoetida (Indian spice that often contains wheat)
Hordeum Vulgare Extract (from Barley)
Hydrolyzed Wheat Protein
Imitation Crabmeat and Lobster (Most contain a wheat binder. Crabmeat and Lobster dishes at restaurants [e.g. crabcakes, lobster or crabmeat salad, lobster bisque] often contain imitation).
Kamut (Pasta wheat)
Kaploid (Australian wheat)
Koji
Licorice candy / red & black (Products like Twizzlers® contain wheat)
Macha Wheat
Maida (all purpose wheat flour used in Indian cuisine)
Malt
Malt Beverage (drinks such as Zima®/Sparks®)
Malt Extract
Malt Flavoring
Malt Syrup
Malt Vinegar
Malted Milk
Malted Milk Balls

Matzo or Matzoh Meal

Matzo Semolina

Miso

Naan (Indian wheat flatbread)

Non-Dairy Creamer, Sour Cream & Whipped Topping (check ingredients; many consumer products such as Coffee-Mate® and Cool Whip® are safe as of this writing, but some products used by restaurants are unsafe.)

Noodles (made from wheat)

Oat Bran (contains oats)

Oatrim® fat replacer (made from hydrolyzed oat flour)

Oats (Research is ongoing about oats and their safety. Oats are normally grown with wheat. Most physicians consider U.S. oats to be unsafe due to contamination. European oats may or may not be safe. I recommend that you avoid oats until the research is complete. But if you want to try oats, work with your doctor and purchase only safe brands. There are conflicting studies about oats, and it is very controversial. As of 2006, some doctors suggest that some celiac patients may tolerate ½ cup of cooked oats per day and not more than that amount. These patients must get blood tests as they add oats back to their diet to be sure they are not adversely affected. They usually have to wait at least 6 months on the diet to be sure it is working for them, and then be monitored to add oats. Some celiac patients may tolerate non-contaminated oats and others may not.

New companies such as www.glutenfreeoats.com sell wheat-free uncontaminated oats. They are expensive. On the package they give suggestions on how to add oats slowly into your diet.)

Oriental Wheat

Orzo (pasta made from wheat. Don't be fooled; orzo pasta can look like rice but it is made from wheat.)

Pasta (made from wheat or semolina)

Pearl Barley

Persian Wheat

Phosphated Flour

Plain Flour

Polish Wheat

Poulard Wheat

Puri (Indian wheat flatbread)

QK-77 Kamut

Rava (semolina in Indian cuisine)

Rice Malt (contains barley or Koji)

Rice Syrup (may contain Rice Malt. Check with manufacturer. There are some safe brands available.)

Roti (Indian wheat flatbread)

Roux (a mixture of fat and wheat flour; used in sauces)

Rye

Rye Flour

Seitan (wheat gluten)

Self-Rising Flour

Semolina (durum wheat)

Semolina Triticum

Seviyan (Vermicelli noodle used in Indian cuisine)

Shot Wheat

Shoyu (soy sauce) Watch out for this ingredient especially in food in Hawaii and Japan.

Sirimi (imitation seafood created with a starch binder that may be wheat. Check source; most sirimi contains wheat).

Small Spelt

Soba Noodles (although buckwheat is a safe ingredient, most soba noodles contain wheat or are contaminated with wheat. I only found one safe brand on the internet, from www.kingsoba.com)

Soy Sauce (check manufacturer, most brands contain wheat, especially imported ones. Most Chinese restaurants use soy sauce containing wheat).

Spaghetti (made from wheat or semolina)

Spelt (don't be fooled! Spelt is unsafe for celiacs. It may be called wheat-free on products, but it is not gluten-free. It has the gluten protein in it).

Spirits (Some have added unsafe flavorings. Some have contamination from mash in distillation process.)

Sprouted Barley

Sprouted Wheat

Strong Flour

Suet in Packets (may be coated with wheat starch)

Suji (Semolina in Indian cuisine)

Tabbouleh

Teriyaki Sauce (most always contains soy sauce with wheat in it).

Textured Vegetable Protein or TVP (Check manufacturers, many brands contain gluten).

Timopheevi Wheat

Trigo (Spanish for wheat)

Triticale (a cross between wheat and rye)

Triticosecale

Triticum

Triticum Vulgare (wheat germ oil)

Udon (wheat noodles)

Unbleached Flour

Vavilovi Wheat

Vegetable Protein (may contain wheat; the new labeling law should disclose if any wheat were used).

Vegetable Starch may contain wheat; the new labeling law should disclose if any wheat were used).

Wheat

Wheat Bran

Wheat Germ

Wheat Germ oil

Wheat Grass (may contain seeds. Pure wheat grass with no contamination from seeds may be gluten-free.)

Wheat Nuts

Wheat Starch (in the USA/Canada it is <u>not</u> considered safe. Wheat starch from China is <u>not</u> safe. In Europe only a specially processed Codex Alimentarius wheat starch made for especially for celiacs is considered safe in those countries. It was not recommended in the U.S. since it was previously permitted to have wheat contamination up to 200 parts per million. In 2008 Codex Alimentarius changed their standard to 100 ppm for foods rendered gluten-free (i.e. this wheat starch) and 20 ppm for foods naturally gluten-free. The U.S. recommended guideline is 20 ppm for both. See more about this under "travel" and our experience in Norway.)

Wheat, Abyssinian Hard triticum durum

Wheat, Bulgur

Wheat, Durum

Wheat, Monococcum

Wheat, Triticum

White Flour

Whole Wheat Flour

Whole-Meal Flour

Yogurt, flavored (many brands add modified food starch and gluten in the flavorings. For example on the Dannon® yogurt website in 2010 they said they don't consider their flavored yogurt to be "gluten-safe". The good news is there are other safe brands that are labeled gluten-free, so as of 2010 not all flavored yogurt is forbidden, only some brands.)

# Warning – Hidden Gluten Where You'd Least Expect It!

These tips are important to remaining gluten-free. In the U.S., these are hidden gluten sources that you need to know about. Remember – gluten is only a problem if you ingest it.

### At home or office

- Don't lick stamps, envelopes or other gummed labels because very often the glue contains wheat. Use a damp sponge to seal them, or get the self-sticking kind. The stamp hinges that stamp collectors use also may contain gluten.

### Kitchen Appliances/Utensils/etc.

- There can be contamination from the toaster and toaster oven. Get separate toasters and do not share with someone who uses wheat. Also do not share bread machines. Have one dedicated to gluten-free baking.

- Don't reuse plastic bags that contained items that have gluten. Gluten containing crumbs and film are very difficult to completely wash away.

- Clean pans and grills thoroughly. If someone just made a gluten-containing grilled cheese sandwich, you cannot make your gluten-free one without cleaning the grill first. Gluten will transfer to your sandwich and contaminate it.

- For outdoor grills, if wheat-containing rolls or buns were grilled on it, or if gluten-containing barbeque sauce was used on it, the grill is contaminated. Either put foil down and cook your food on that, or clean the grill thoroughly.

- Wooden kitchen utensils, cutting boards, and rolling pins may harbor gluten. So can some iron pots, colanders, and some Teflon® pans. In some cases the gluten can be difficult to remove, so clean carefully or you may want to purchase new ones. Pans with seams can also have gluten that is difficult to remove. Clean pots and pans are safe pans.

- Baking stones are very porous and can harbor gluten that cannot be cleaned away. I recommend if you plan to use one, that it be dedicated to gluten-free foods.

- Keep your can opener blade clean, especially if others are opening cans containing gluten.

- Use clean potholders and have ones designated for removing your gluten-free baked goods from the oven. You don't want to use a potholder that handled wheat bread (especially snowflake rolls) to handle your gluten-free bread. It is inevitable that potholders touch the food and may have wheat flour on them. Wash all potholders when you start the diet.

- Clean your mixer, blender, and all kitchen appliances carefully as gluten can hide around the blades or in crevices.

- If you can invest in getting a good dishwasher, I highly recommend it. With some cheaper dishwashers you will notice that all of the crumbs end up on the glasses. If your home has both gluten and non-gluten items, you want a dishwasher that gets dishes really clean. Also, don't overload your dishwasher when you use it. Good water flow ensures cleaner dishes.

- I like to use wash cloths and disposable sponges for dish washing. For heavily soiled gluten containing pots and pans, I suggest you clean them using a sponge dedicated for gluten. Clean the sponge well and put it in the dishwasher to clean it again. Or, if very dirty throw the sponge away. You don't want to start rubbing gluten onto everything you're trying to clean. When you wash gluten-containing washcloths in your washing machine, make sure you don't overload the washer so that they will get really clean. Good water flow cleans better. Tightly packed washing machines don't clean as well.

- If you can invest in a double-sink it is also a good idea. Have one side for gluten and the other side gluten-free. That way if you are making pasta, you don't have to worry about contamination from the sink. It makes it easier for cooking and washing foods. You can soak gluten containing items on one side and not on the other. Once dishes are thoroughly cleaned, they are safe.

- We suggest having a separate colander/strainer for gluten-free pasta. It's not a good idea to share one used for gluten pasta, as all of the holes are difficult to get clean.

- Keep counters clean when preparing foods. Crumbs can contaminate foods.

- Clean knives that slice gluten breads. Some people put them back into the knife holder without washing them, so wash them before using them. Keep utensil drawers crumb-free.

- Some brands of paper towels may contain gluten in the glue to seal the rolls and hold them to the cardboard center. Don't use those glue containing sheets on food.

Medicines

- Medicines and vitamins may contain gluten. Check with the manufacturer. Look for vitamins that say gluten-free and also check the list of ingredients. If your prescription contains gluten and there is no substitute for that medication, you may be able to get it compounded (reformulated) through www.stokesrx.com. They are a pharmacy that caters to celiac patients. They recommend having your doctor write "DAW" (Dispense as Written) on all of your prescriptions. Generic brands may change as often as once a year. Most major U.S. brands have 800 numbers you can call and check. You can get the phone number from the pharmacist, from on-line phone directories, the internet, or from a PDR book in the library. (A PDR is the Physician's Desk Reference, which lists all prescriptions and their side effects.) Another resource list to check medications is www.glutenfreedrugs.com. This website, created by a pharmacist, is a service to help people with celiac disease. It has an extensive listing of gluten-free medications, with links to contact manufacturers yourself.

- Laxatives may contain gluten. Check ingredients.

- Beware of some health food nutritional items that say they are gluten-free but contain things like barley grass, which may have contamination from seeds. Some also claim that wheat starch is gluten-free, but only a special codex wheat starch from Europe is considered safe in some countries. In the U.S. the wheat starch available is not considered safe; (see "unsafe list" for reasons why).

## Personal Care

- Some toothpaste and mouthwash made outside the U.S., including some store brands, may not be safe. Use the major brands in U.S.A. and check ingredients. Also, check with your dentist regarding the polishing cream they use. In 2005, our dentist found out that only the Pina Colada flavor was safe, but all other flavors contained gluten. Our dentist uses Sultan Dental Products – Topex® Prophylaxis Polish/Cleaning Paste, www.sultandental.com, telephone: 201-894-5500. Since it is possible to swallow some of the paste or mouthwashes by mistake, use safe dental care products. As of this writing, Crest® (www.pg.com) and Colgate® (www.colgate.com) toothpastes are safe (gluten-free status listed under FAQ). Listerine® (www.pfizer.com 1-800-223-0182) and Scope (www.pg.com) are also gluten-free as of this writing. Also, if you are getting a fluoride treatment at the dentist, or using fluoride rinses, check to be sure that is gluten-free.

- Check that denture adhesives and denture cleaning products are gluten-free.

- Lipsticks and lip balm products may contain gluten. There may be wheat germ oil or wheat containing Vitamin E in the products.

- Lotions, creams, and other cosmetics can contain gluten (for those with dermatitis herpetiformis, a skin condition caused by celiac disease), which may irritate the condition. Also, if you use a hand lotion containing gluten, you would not want to put your hands in your mouth. Keep gluten-free hand lotion in the kitchen, because your hands may touch food. For the same reasons, we choose soaps that do not contain gluten (some soaps contain oatmeal or wheat germ). It is also suggested to use hair spray that does not contain gluten, as it is possible to breathe in the spray and ingest gluten.

- Laundry spray starches I checked do not contain gluten, but there is a possibility that the more natural type products could. If you have dermatitis herpetiformis, gluten on the skin may irritate the rash. If you have this condition, ask the Drycleaner to confirm the starch they use on shirts is wheat free. (Skin contact may irritate but will not cause damage in your gut.)

- The glue on some toilet paper rolls contains wheat. Don't use the end piece to blot lipstick.

## Shopping for Food

- Health food store employees may not understand the diet and give you incorrect advice. (For example, they may say that spelt and kamut are safe for people with celiac disease – when they are absolutely not! Wheat-free does not mean gluten-free.)

- There can be cross-contamination between food store bins selling flours and grains. It is usually from scoops or flour getting airborne when bins are filled. Beware of repackaged items for the same reason. Others unaware of the gluten-free diet will not be careful.

- Some people have worried about stickers on fresh fruit, but the glue used is gluten-free.

- Some conveyor belts in grocery stores can have gluten on them from flour leaking from bags. For this reason, I put fresh fruits and vegetables in bags instead of putting them directly on the belt. It's always a good idea to wash these foods before eating them.

- Some cash register receipts contain gluten in the printing, so make sure small children with celiac disease do not put them in their mouths.

- Until you get used to shopping, I suggest you bring some safe lists with you. There are some excellent up-to-date lists on the internet or use the one in the back of this book.

For Children – at School or Play

- Some play dough or modeling clay for children may contain gluten. Some finger paints may contain gluten. (In 2009, Elmer's® Finger-paints contained gluten.) Since young children may put things in their mouths, choose safe brands and discuss art supplies with their preschool and elementary school teachers. Colorations® brand gluten-free play clay can be ordered from www.discountschoolsupply.com (or see index for clay recipe).

- If you have a young child who might put things in their mouth, check other school supplies. In 2009 Elmer's® Craft Bond Tacky Glue was gluten-free, but some other glues were not. Crayola® Crayons are gluten-free.

- Gluten can be more of a challenge for preschool children with celiac disease, as they are frequently on the floor and put their hands in their mouths. Floors should be free of crumbs.

- Keep pet food away from crawling children since most brands contain gluten.

- Most stickers have self-adhesive which is safe. Stickers you lick are usually not safe.

- You will need to work with your child and their teacher to make sure they do not get unsafe foods. You want to be sure they are only given safe snacks. Sometimes children want to share or trade food items. My goal with this book is to make food items so close to their gluten counterparts that children will feel completely normal about their food and not feel the need to try others or have to explain why theirs looks so different. Even so, you will still have to work with teachers so they learn what is needed.

- There are books, camps, and clubs especially devoted to children's issues and it is a good idea to get involved to help your child make the right choices in dealing with gluten. They also won't feel alone in their situation.

- Babies and young children may put fabrics in their mouths. If the child has celiac, you may want to wash their bibs, clothing, etc. separately from highly soiled gluten-containing washables.

<u>At Church</u>

- Communion wafers contain gluten. Don't take communion unless you special order acceptable ones (for example: Ener-G® foods makes communion wafers), or make arrangements to be able to use your own bread. Do not dip your bread in wine/grape juice where others have dipped gluten-containing bread.

<u>Foods and Beverages</u>

- Be careful with cereals. Most contain malt flavoring (malt is from barley and unsafe), or other unsafe ingredients. Some are also made on the same manufacturing lines as wheat and there may be contamination. Check with the manufacturer.

- Beware of some rice and soy beverages, because their manufacturing process uses barley enzymes or extract. Barley contains gluten. Most EdenSoy® beverages contain barley extract. (Rice Dream® beverages contain barley enzymes but the level is so low [below 20 ppm] so they say their product is gluten-free.)

- Beware of wheat bread crumbs that get into butter, jams, spreads, mayonnaise, and peanut butter or on the counter, etc. Have your own separate butter dish, and use squeeze bottles for mayonnaise, ketchup, etc. Spreading condiments onto wheat bread with a knife and going back for more causes contamination. For family gatherings we bring packets of ketchup, mustard, mayonnaise and pats of butter. If others in your family eat gluten, get in the habit of putting your food on a clean dish instead of on the counter.

- Some sauce mixes and sauces contain gluten (for example, soy sauce, fish sauce, ketchup, mustard, mayonnaise, salad dressings, etc.) Check with the manufacturer to find out if they are safe (see list in the back of this book).

- Ice creams may have gluten. Check with the manufacturer.

- Many packet & canned soups contain gluten. Check with the manufacturer.

- Some brands of rice paper (used to make Asian Spring Rolls) contain gluten.

- Dried meals, gravy mixes, and frozen meals often have gluten. Sometimes I have found that although the ingredients looked fine that gluten was hidden in natural flavorings or in modified starches. (The new labeling law in 2006 helped expose hidden wheat in these types of ingredients.)

- Snack foods may have wheat contamination. Check with the manufacturer. Often corn chips are not made on dedicated equipment. Nacho type flavorings contain wheat and are used on the same equipment line as the plain version. Some flavored/seasoned or dry roasted nuts may have gluten. Some flavored potato chips may contain gluten. Do not just go by the ingredients list without checking with the manufacturer. Our experience is that snack foods can be one of the most contaminated foods.

- Ground spices may contain wheat flour that is used to prevent clumping. Read labels when purchasing dry mustard and spice blends. (Note: in the last few years many companies have removed the wheat because of so many telephone calls to them.)

- Some flavored coffees and teas (some contain barley), packaged rice mixes (flavorings or bouillon could contain gluten), some frozen potatoes (flavorings could contain gluten), some creamed vegetables (in the starch to thicken sauce), some tuna in vegetable broth (usually the broth in cheaper store brands), some puddings (may have wheat starch), and some commercially prepared salads, vegetables and salad dressings contain gluten. Since gluten is natural, it could be in natural flavoring. Also beware of meat in marinade or meat that is injected with added solutions (found in some brands of turkey, chicken, or pork). Again, the new labeling law is exposing a lot of hidden wheat in these types of products.

- Candies made outside the U.S. can use wheat flour to prevent them from sticking together, but they do not have to list it on the label. (For example, MackIntosh's® toffee from Canada would seem to be safe from reading the label, but when we called years ago they told us it is not gluten-free because of the wheat they use to prevent sticking.)

- Some studies in Europe showed that gluten-free oats may be safe for celiacs. Almost all regular oats in the U.S. are grown and milled with wheat, except for special gluten-free oats. If you want to add them to your diet, doctors suggest you start slowly (after several months of healing on the diet) and get blood work done to be sure you are not reacting to them. I suggest you get your doctor's approval before adding gluten-free oats to your diet. Oats are still controversial. Some additional studies have yielded different results. For example, one follow-up study of 9 patients said oats were <u>not</u> safe.[98] Some celiacs can't tolerate oats.

- Don't just think of what you eat but also what you drink. Some beverages may have gluten. I was surprised to find that lemon Snapple® iced tea used to contain gluten years ago. (As of 2004 I understand this has changed and now all flavors are safe for celiacs.) Some brands of orange juice contain unsafe flavorings or additives. For example, Tropicana® Pure Premium that just contains 100% orange juice is safe, but some of the varieties with additives may not be safe for celiacs. In another instance, I purchased root beer from a company called Cold Spring Brewery®, because the ingredients list looked safe. I then went to their website and discovered that they only advertised beer, which made me wonder about possible contamination. My suspicion was confirmed when I called the company and they said that their root beer was not gluten-free.

<u>On the Job at Home or Work</u>

- Some brands of wallpaper paste sold in plastic buckets contain wheat. I suggest you choose a product without wheat just to be safe, especially if you're wallpapering a kitchen as it may drip on places where you prepare food. (Note: I called several major brands of pre-pasted wallpaper and was told they use glue containing potato starch and an antifungal. You do not need to be concerned about having your hands in the glue on the back of pre-pasted wallpaper, but I recommend cleaning hands thoroughly because of the antifungal.)

- Walking by a bakery and smelling bread baking is not a problem. However, if you are close enough to inhale flour that may cause a problem. Some people want to continue to bake using wheat flour for their non-celiac family members. If so, you need to use caution because if you've working with wheat flour it may potentially get airborne. Breathing wheat flour dust may be a problem because if you taste it you're ingesting it. Some professional bakers have had to wear breathing masks for this reason. Also, if you have your hands in flour, thoroughly clean hands and nails afterward to avoid ingesting it from your hands. This may seem extreme but some people who thought they had refractory sprue (not healing with the diet) found this was the cause.

In the Hospital

- If you are going to be in the hospital, it is <u>very important</u> for you to take charge of your diet. By that, call the hospital beforehand and speak to the dietician. Bring the dietician's phone number in case you're getting the wrong foods once you are there. Use the GIG Document and forms from this website (www.gluten.net) to help you get the right care: http://gluten.net/downloads/print/Hospital%20Stays%20Made%20Safe.pdf

- Bring some foods like gluten-free crackers and gluten-free bouillon that are safe.

- Speak to your doctor and whoever else is caring for you. Get your family involved and if possible to visit you during meals. Ask family members to bring you some safe items that you know you can have. Hospitals can be one of the <u>worst</u> places as far as helping to maintain your diet. You would think it would be the best place, but often the staff members who deliver the meals are not familiar with the diet. There can be mix-ups. There can be volunteers that don't know. You may have a different staff member preparing and delivering each meal.

- Question <u>all</u> of your medication. Appoint a family member or a friend as an advocate for you. The last thing you want to do when you're ill is fight about your diet, so have someone do it for you. This is really important to maintain your health. With so many people coming in and out of your room doing things for your care, they may not realize your gluten-free status. You don't need gluten damage in addition to whatever else you're in the hospital to heal from. A healthy gut with healthy digestion and proper absorption of nutrients can only help your healing process. Damage from celiac disease may also hinder medication and absorption needed for healing. It may cause more damage to your body and further weaken it. It may set your immune system into haywire mode, when you need it working right.

- There have been some concerns about latex gloves and rubber party balloons since they have a white powder inside. The ones I checked were safe and contained talc or cornstarch. I have not found a name brand with a problem, but it's a good idea to check if you plan to use either of these.

In a Restaurant – See next section for "Eating Out Cautions"

# Eating Out Cautions

Eating out can be a little difficult at first, but it can definitely be done. To avoid disappointments, I suggest you contact the restaurant before you go, just to make sure they can accommodate your diet. If you can, take the time to speak to the chef to educate him/her about your needs. It is easier to do it on the phone before you arrive rather than getting there and finding out they are unable to provide anything for you.

Calling beforehand usually reduces the amount of discussion needed once you are in the restaurant. Telephone the restaurant early or in-between standard meal times, so they have time to talk to you. If possible, get the name of the person that you spoke to. It may help you get better service once you are there. We have found this method dramatically improves the quality of the food my husband receives. In some cases the restaurants have purchased special food normally not on the menu to accommodate his diet. A little planning and contact beforehand can make you feel like an expected guest rather than an inconvenience.

Especially when you travel, it pays to do some homework to find an accommodating restaurant. Websites like www.glutenfreerestaurants.org list restaurants with gluten-free menus. Also search for the local celiac societies, because they often list their favorite gluten-free restaurants and often provide suggestions for a good meal. Books are available that list gluten-free restaurants, such as the Triumph Dining Guide.

Ten years ago when we started the diet, eating out was so much more difficult than today. Not only did they not understand the diet, but often they would make mistakes and think it was fine to remove the offending wheat item after it contaminated everything. For example, one restaurant tried to remove the croutons from the salad and re-serve it to my husband. Another time my husband was served the perfect gluten-free meal, but then the waitress quickly came back and put a roll on top of it and contaminated it! (It was a "snowflake" roll coated in wheat flour, and it sprinkled flour all over his food!) In those days we used to always bring back-up food because we often weren't sure about what we were being served. People were unfamiliar with the diet and would routinely do what they always did, not realizing the consequences for someone with celiac disease.

Fortunately, with more media attention about the gluten-free diet, restaurants are becoming much more knowledgeable and we've noticed that these types of mistakes don't happen as frequently. Celiac societies have been working with restaurants to education and improve dining for celiacs.

My husband likes to present a dining card to the waiter or waitress to help to make explaining the diet easier. You may want to make up your own restaurant card depending upon your preferences. The cards have worked well for us when we've traveled in the U.S. For overseas travel, you can find cards in many languages on the Internet, and on celiac society web pages. (See a sample one under "Travel Suggestions" in this book.) As more and more people are learning about the diet, it will keep getting easier and easier.

Other times my husband doesn't want to deal with it. He wants to join friends at a restaurant but doesn't want to explain and doesn't want to worry about his food. At those times he brings his own food. He orders a beverage. He prefers that at office parties, and most people don't even notice.

Eating out is always risky, but it can be done. I am detailing the safest, most conservative approaches to eating out. I have provided some sample cards on the next page that my husband has used, based on his meal preferences. He feels more confident that the food is safe if it is simple. He would rather not worry about what is in a sauce or spice blend.

This is a business sized card that is easy to keep in your wallet.
This one is good for a simple meal from a busy chef since it is quick to read:

> I suffer from a very <u>severe</u> allergy to wheat, rye, oats and barley.
> Could you please prepare me the following meal:
> - Plain Grilled meat. Do <u>not</u> cook on a surface/grill where you have grilled bread items. Please put aluminum foil down first to prevent contamination. No meats with marinade, tenderizer, added solutions, breading, flour, sauces, soy sauce, gravy, or juices containing bouillon.
> - Baked potato or plain rice. No spices please. Real butter pats, salt and pepper on the side.
> - Tossed salad. Fresh vegetables only. No croutons or crumbs. Oil & Red Wine Vinegar on the side.
> - Steamed vegetables. No spices or sauces.
>
> Please ask the chef to speak to me. Thank you very much!

Here is a larger card with more detail.
We use this one for longer stays at B&Bs, so that meals can be more varied.

> ### I HAVE A <u>VERY SEVERE</u> ALLERGY TO GLUTEN, A.K.A. CELIAC DISEASE
>
> I CANNOT eat anything made from Wheat, Rye, Oats, Barley or Malt. This includes: Breads, Bread crumbs, Croutons, Pastas or Orzo, Bouillons, Sauces or Gravies, Dressings, Beer, Processed Cheeses, Soy Sauce, Deep fried foods cooked in the same oil as breaded or floured foods, Marinated foods, Cakes, Cookies, Pies and other Baked Goods. Also, Natural Flavors, Modified Food Starch, Artificial Flavors, Spice Blends, MSG, Tenderizers, Malt, and HVP are a problem for me.
>
> PLAIN or "naked" foods are best for me. I CAN eat: Meat, Poultry, Seafood, Eggs, Vegetables, Fruit, Milk, Rice, Corn, Cornstarch, Potatoes, most Cheeses, Wine, Real Butter (new pats to ensure no contamination), Wine Vinegar, and Oil. Foods must be cooked in a separate clean pot or pan, or in an area of the grill that has been cleaned, with separate cleaned utensils used. I will get very sick from only traces of gluten. Gluten can transfer from an unwashed pan, or from reused frying oil onto my food, or from crumbs getting on my plate.
>
> Plain broiled meat, baked potato or plain rice, plain steamed vegetables, salad with oil and wine vinegar (no croutons), and fruit are good foods for me as a meal. My meat and vegetables may be seasoned with salt and garlic powder. You may cook my meat on a new piece of aluminum foil.
>
> Please ask the chef to come and speak to me so we can create a meal to meet my needs. Thank you.

Restaurant cards can be very helpful in noisy, crowded restaurants. They can help you to get the chef to come out to get the conversation going to meet your needs. The last time we presented this restaurant card, the chef came out and explained that he was just certified in preparing gluten-free foods. He told us he could do something much more elaborate than this. He talked about many options and my husband received a wonderful meal. I did too because I decided to order something different that was gluten-free so we could share it. My husband asked the chef if he would be willing to serve us the meals himself so we would be sure that we received the correct ones. The chef agreed and he served it immediately after he prepared it. It was a great dining experience!

## POINTS TO KEEP IN MIND WHEN ORDERING AT A RESTAURANT:

I suggest you keep these points in mind so you know what to ask your server to get it right. (Better yet, ask the chef to come out and speak directly with you, so the one making the food gets the information first-hand.) Eating out can be done safely with the following tips:

- Fried restaurant foods may have gluten because of gluten contaminated grease. French fries that are fried in the same oil as onion rings or breaded foods are contaminated with gluten. Also be sure they are not putting meat in a fryer to thaw it before putting it under the broiler.

- Ask about the grill when ordering grilled restaurant food. If any bread item was grilled, and then they grilled your food on it, it will be contaminated. They should put clean aluminum foil down before grilling your food.

- Some restaurants cook or reheat Prime Rib, beef, and other meats in canned aus jus sauce which may contain gluten. This can especially be a problem if you order a steak and it is too rare. To reheat it without it becoming dry they may use this method. Some restaurants use pre-seasoned meats that may contain gluten. Use caution ordering roast turkey since some self basting turkeys may contain gluten.

- Some restaurant meats contain marinades and other ingredients that contain gluten. Often they use soy sauce which contains wheat. Items cooked in beer are also not safe for celiacs. (Cajun cooked shrimp is usually prepared by boiling it in beer.) Some barbeque sauces contain beer. Sauces and bouillons usually contain gluten too. Some spice blends may contain gluten.

- Salads are usually a safe choice but be sure it was prepared in a clean area away from croutons and breads. If they used a cutting board used for bread to prepare your salad there could be contamination. Imitation bacon bits may contain gluten.

- Restaurant salad bars may have contamination from croutons, gluten-containing dressings, and from people mixing items with contaminated spoons. For the same reason, be careful at buffets. If they have made special items for you, try to go first before others put contaminated spoons into your safe items.

- It is too risky to order crabmeat salad or lobster salad. Restaurants frequently supplement these salads with the imitation kind (sirimi), and it contains gluten. Sushi restaurants may also use it, or may use soy sauce for flavoring which contains wheat. Crab cakes may also contain gluten.

- Some restaurant food items are unsafe because they reuse foods. For example, they didn't sell all of the hamburgers they made so they take the meat out of the buns and make chili. This was a problem for us at a hamburger place that had the chili listed as gluten-free on the web site, but at the local place it was contaminated.

- A hamburger made on a clean grill without the bun can be a good choice as long as the hamburger meat is 100% beef without fillers. Some restaurants use unsafe fillers. (This is especially a problem in Europe.)

- Most soups and sauces in restaurants are unsafe. Many use soup bases or bouillon containing gluten. Many soups and sauces are thickened with wheat flour. A "roux" contains wheat flour. Some restaurants may use leftover ingredients in soups which may contain gluten.

- Some Italian restaurants use the water that pasta was boiled in to thin sauces, which contaminates the sauce. If they are going to make gluten-free pasta for you, check that the sauce is safe, that your pasta is boiled it in a separate pot with clean water, and that your pasta is drained in a clean colander and kept separate from the other wheat products in the kitchen. If they offer gluten-free bread, make sure it is cut on a clean board away from wheat bread items and crumbs.

- Some safe items to order are a salad without croutons, steamed rice or baked potato with butter on the side, and perhaps some fruit. As a back-up (in case they don't have much gluten-free food for you or make a mistake) bring one of those foil packets of gluten-free tuna or salmon, or bring meat and cheeses to top your salad or baked potato. Use oil and vinegar or the juice of lemons for the salad dressing or bring your own. Beware of the sour cream for the potato (many restaurants use non-dairy sour cream which may be unsafe), and only use packets of sour cream with safe ingredients listed or use pats of butter with safe listed ingredients. If you want to order meat, question them about their grill and ask to have the chef see you. Some meats come to them pre-seasoned or with added tenderizer so you need to ask about that. Poached salmon could be a good choice, but make sure they aren't poaching it in water with gluten-containing bouillon. Plain rice is a good choice but rice pilafs or those with added bouillon and spices may contain gluten. Some restaurants make polenta using bouillon or may fry it in contaminated oil.

- For breakfast I suggest ordering boiled eggs, fruit and beverage for a simple meal. (Ask about the eggs if you want scrambled fried eggs. Some restaurants are using an egg mix that contains wheat, or adding some pancake batter to scrambled eggs.) Some restaurants make their own hash brown potatoes, but many use frozen potatoes which contain wheat, or have a wheat coating or seasoning on them. Most bacon without added flavorings is safe, but you need to check if it is safe. Some flavored bacons contain gluten. Bacon bits added to omelets may contain gluten. Some sausage contains gluten or is cooked on the same griddle with gluten-containing items. Use caution using non-dairy creamers in coffee or tea since some of those may contain gluten. In Spain, most orange juice is unsafe (unless they make it for you fresh from oranges). Sometimes I pack some gluten-free Muesli (see index for recipe) just in case the restaurant can't accommodate my husband for breakfast. He asks for a bowl and orders milk.

- Another suggestion is to try a Chinese restaurant. Request that they steam your entire meal, add no soy sauce and serve it with plain rice. Just make sure the chicken is real, (i.e. not chicken roll) and that the steamer is clean (no soy sauce). Plain rice is safe but fried rice may contain gluten. Most soy sauce packets from restaurants contain gluten. Bring your own with you. (It is a good idea to bring a restaurant card in Chinese to help you when you order. You can find free translation cards on-line at www.celiactravel.com or buy them from www.triumphdining.com). You could also try a Thai restaurant if you know their food. There are quite a few safe Thai dishes. (For example, Pad Thai uses rice noodles and fish sauce instead of soy sauce which is usually gluten-free but you have to check.)

- Most Indian cuisines utilize beans and rice, but check carefully with the restaurant because some spices like hing or asafoetida (also spelled asafetida) may contain wheat. Some restaurants thicken curries with wheat flour. (At home they are often thickened by being cooked down and reducing.) Some prepare non-wheat flatbreads/crepes/pancakes (ragi/millet rotis or dosas crepes made of lentils and rice, or appam fermented rice crepe/pancakes) on the same griddle as those made from wheat (naan/wheat flatbread). (At home dosas and appams are usually made in special pans, but sometimes restaurants cook them all on the same grill/griddle.) A tandoori oven can be a cause of possible wheat contamination; because of the preparation of naan. (It may be safer to choose a restaurant that doesn't use a tandoori oven for naan. According to Triumph Dining, some restaurants toss the naan on the sides of the tandoori oven creating flour dust that contaminates other foods cooking in the oven.) Some restaurants fry wheat items (like samosas/wheat stuffed pastries) and non-wheat (like pakoras/vegetables dipped in chickpea batter) in the same oil. [Note: Some add wheat flour to pakoras, so make sure they are 100% gram/chickpea flour.] Wheat items to stay away from are chapati, roti, naan, and puri. Wheat flour is atta (whole wheat) and maida (all purpose flour). Other unsafe items are suji or rava (semolina), rava dosa (crepe made of wheat), and seviyan (vermicelli). Use caution ordering kofta (these meatballs usually contain rice but may contain bulgur wheat) and gravies (may be thickened with wheat). Saag paneer (spinach cheese dish) is usually gluten-free but sometimes may contain wheat to thicken it, so check. Make sure masalas do not contain hing/asafoetida. Bringing a restaurant card can help you get a safe meal. (See www.triumphdining.com for a card in English and in Hindi, or get a free card from www.celiactravel.com/restaurant-cards.html). Or better yet, bring a friend who speaks the language!

- If you want bread with your meal, I suggest you bring your own bread wrapped in foil. Often the restaurant can warm it in the oven for you. Ask them to keep it wrapped. Or bring some gluten-free crackers and some form of protein, such as peanut butter or cheese. Corn cakes by RealFoods® (imported from Australia) are very tasty, thin and crispy. We keep a package of them and a jar of peanut butter in our car for "hunger emergencies".

- A new item called Toastabags® (www.toastabags.com) is a bag that can help keep toast contamination free when using a non-dedicated toaster. We have used it on trips because it is small for travel. Usually toasters are available at hotel continental breakfasts. Be careful removing the toast because the <u>outside</u> of the bag may be contaminated with gluten. Don't put the bag on the plate that you put your toast on. When cooled, we store the used bag in a zip lock bag to be sure that the gluten does not contaminate anything else while in storage.

- At ice cream parlors, most servers do not wash the scoops after filling the cones. They also usually fill cones over the ice cream containers and crumbs can get into the ice cream. Or, they dip scoops into water containing gluten before going to another flavor which just contaminates everything. We solved this problem by frequenting a place that sells not only dipped ice cream but also prepackaged pints. We get the pint and share it. We like that we can verify the ingredients with them. The soft serve type machines can be safer than the dipped ice cream for this reason. Check ingredients before you order.

- Some flavored coffees and teas have gluten. Order plain or do your homework before going to a coffee shop, so you know which flavors are safe and which are not. If they grind their own coffee in the shop, there also may be possible contamination if they sell some coffees that are unsafe. Grinders are often very difficult to clean. Some non-dairy creamers may contain gluten. Some non-dairy whipped cream toppings may also contain gluten. Restaurants may use unsafe whipped toppings on coffee drinks or desserts.

- Most waiters/waitresses/chefs do not understand the gluten-free diet. You send food back because they put onion rings on your steak or croutons on your salad and they try to remove the item instead of preparing you a new meal. They often don't understand what items are unsafe. Beware of sauces, bouillon, flavorings, and spice blends they use in restaurants.

- Don't be careless in ordering at a restaurant by just trusting the staff, or yielding to peer-pressure from friends or family that "it will be fine". Until you learn the restaurant and the staff, I find it best to bring your own main dish or entire meal, and just order a beverage. Most restaurants can microwave your food in your container. Restaurants can be especially accommodating when you tell them your doctor has you on a special diet or you have extreme allergies. (People don't understand celiac disease, but they do know about allergies.) If you don't want to ask, or are unsure if they have a microwave, microwave it before you leave and put it in an insulated lunch box. (Try using a microwavable heat pack to keep your food warm). You can also heat a gluten-free frozen entree, if you don't want to cook ahead of time.

- Some restaurant chains now have gluten-free menus on-line. Do your homework. Call ahead to be sure they follow that menu. When you're there, ask to speak to the chef to be sure you get what you ordered. Reconfirm your meal when it is served. I have received the wrong meal several times at restaurant chains. You don't want to go through the effort and receive the wrong food!

The safest approach is to bring your own meals. My husband usually does this because he knows he will like what he's eating and he doesn't have to worry if they will have something for him. He feels the experience is more relaxed this way. Every restaurant we have gone to where we brought his meal has been very accommodating. As long as they've got at least one paying customer (i.e. me), the restaurants don't seem to mind that he brings his own food. Of all the restaurants we've gone to there was only <u>one</u> 4-star restaurant in a hotel in Washington D.C. that refused us, and they said that was because they were expecting a food critic and they didn't want that person to see different food on someone's plate.

For weddings and banquets, even if the caterer says they will provide a gluten-free meal I suggest you bring a back-up meal in a small cooler or lunch box. I'll never forget the time that my husband was reassured he would have a gluten-free meal at a family wedding, only to find out upon arrival that there was nothing there for him. The caterer apologized but there was nothing there that he could eat. The bride and groom apologized and they were upset he didn't receive the food they ordered. Unfortunately, there were no restaurants or stores conveniently located to pick up something else, so my husband had to go hungry. At another wedding they did have the gluten-free meal, but a server gave it to a non-celiac by mistake. That person started eating it so it couldn't be retrieved. They were able to make something else but it was a long wait and it wasn't as nice as the original meal. At a catered conference dinner in a museum, my husband made arrangements for a gluten-free meal, but there was a mix-up and the meal was given to another celiac. The person who received the meal was from Europe and didn't know that in the U.S. you often have to request a gluten-free meal in advance. Her server heard the request for gluten-free and assumed that she was the one who ordered the meal. Another time we purchased tickets for a luau because we were promised a gluten-free meal. The salad was brought out and it was safe. But the main course got lost in the kitchen. A server told my husband to go in the buffet line and he could have anything there, but we noticed that many of the signs on the food said "shoyu" which is soy sauce. I questioned another server who confirmed the buffet food was unsafe. So my husband only had the salad that night. They never found his gluten-free dinner in the kitchen.

From these experiences we have learned to bring food in a cooler with ice packs. It never hurts to have a back-up plan. If we don't want to carry the meal, we leave it in the car or check it at the restaurant's coat-check stand. If we don't need it, we bring it home. Having a back-up meal eliminates the stress when mistakes happen, so you can enjoy the party. It is particularly good to have a back up meal at a wedding – the last thing a new bride and groom needs to worry about on their wedding day is why did their caterer forget to prepare your special meal. We found it best to express our sincere appreciation to the bride and groom for requesting a special meal, regardless of whether we needed to resort to our back up meal. Often times my husband has found that his back-up meal was better than the catered meal anyway, and so he is happy that he has a good meal.

Sometimes I think restaurants are relieved that he brings his own meal so that they're not responsible for any mistakes. Recently at a banquet, my husband brought his food because he didn't want to take the time to describe the gluten-free diet to the server and chef. The waitress said, "Why didn't you call us, we would have made you a special meal." He responded, "Do you have a gluten-free kitchen and can you guarantee against any type of gluten contamination in my meal?" "No" was the reply. "I'm really sensitive to gluten, so it's best that I brought my own." "I understand. Can I get you a clean plate?" was the reply. Seeing the food from that kitchen, he was really glad that he brought his own. Every single item served from salad, to entree, to vegetables and dessert had gluten in it.

Whether you bring your own food or you order your meal at a restaurant, I suggest that you do tip well. This will help you and other celiac patients get good meals and good service there in the future. Money talks!

## POINTS TO KEEP IN MIND FOR FAMILY GATHERINGS OR PARTIES

- To avoid contamination when food is served "family style", it's a good idea to serve yourself first. You can't expect others unfamiliar with the diet to know about contamination. You'll see people get butter and put it on their bread and get more butter and dip back and forth. You'll see people cut your gluten-free cake with a knife that cut a gluten-filled dessert. They don't realize and don't understand. Most people don't even realize what is in what they are eating. (I have had so many people suggest eating potato bread to avoid wheat because they thought it was made from potatoes, but the first ingredient is wheat!) If your host has really gone through the trouble to prepare dishes that are gluten-free, then take your food first while they're still gluten-free. Don't expect seconds to be safe, so take enough the first time. If it's a buffet containing gluten-free and some gluten items, don't take home the leftovers unless someone watched the food very carefully because your gluten-free foods probably got contaminated.

- Be more involved with your diet. See what's going on in the kitchen. It's not safe to eat slices of turkey from a bird that has been stuffed with bread stuffing. The stuffing will contaminate the bird and the gravy. Bring food and have a back-up plan so you don't end up hungry. People who don't know the diet and don't often prepare gluten-free foods can and will make mistakes. We've learned to expect it. The mistakes usually happen during the last minute preparations. (Oops, I just put butter that has bread crumbs on it in the mashed potatoes!) You can graciously turn down their food if you have something else to eat. (If the food you brought needs refrigeration, use an ice pack in an insulated lunch box so you can bring your food home if you don't need it as a backup.)

- Beware of pressure by others to cheat on the diet. This diet is for life – in fact it is saving your life! My husband's doctor suggested that you think of the amount of rat poison that you would like to eat, and that is the amount of gluten you should risk eating. Gluten is toxic to a celiac patient. Complications can be serious and for some people healing can be weeks or months after ingesting a little gluten. Don't allow peer pressure to destroy your health. If you stay gluten-free, you can avoid all complications.

- Some people prefer to eat before they arrive at events, because then they are full and not tempted to eat anything or cheat. The choice is up to you. My husband prefers to be a part of the party, and be eating while everyone else is. I often find out ahead of time what the menu is, and try to duplicate it for him. He gets a clean plate, microwaves his food which looks like everyone else's so no one is even aware that he has something different. (You'd be amazed how unaware people can be!) He just slips away into the kitchen and takes care of it. He prefers to choose a seat near the end of the table so he's not passing a lot of gluten-containing foods over his plate.

- Plan ahead to be spontaneous! Sounds funny, but a person with diabetes wouldn't think of leaving the house without their insulin. Have meals ready in the freezer that you can grab at a moment's notice. Or have snacks like gluten-free crackers, cheese, peanut butter, beverage or fruit ready to go. Or have some shelf-stable gluten-free Hormel® microwave meals on hand. (They're better heated but they can be eaten cold.) When you're going out put some food in an insulated lunchbox. If it needs refrigeration use one of those freezer packs to keep it cold. When you're out for the day, you're ready for anything because you've got a back-up plan, if needed.

# Travel Suggestions

Travel is possible, and not difficult if you do your homework before you travel. In the last section you just learned some healthy ways to eat in restaurants. Here are some examples and ideas from our trips in the U.S. and overseas. You <u>can</u> travel and remain healthy!

<u>U.S. Trips:</u>

- Check the internet for local celiac groups who will give you a lot of ideas/suggestions before you go. They often recommend gluten-free friendly restaurants and stores. We found that having this information takes the stress out of traveling. Do an internet search of the state or city and "celiac support" or "celiac group" and you can usually find what you need. For example, in Florida we found several groups and chose one near where we would be traveling. From their list, we found a very good gluten-free bakery nearby. Most U.S. groups list restaurants and stores that carry gluten-free foods.

- Many restaurants now have gluten-free menus on-line! Call your hotel and find out what is nearby. Or, many hotels have free internet access and you can check after you arrive. By looking at menus, often it is easier to tell if they can accommodate your needs.

- Some hotel chefs will meet with you and accommodate your diet – especially if you are staying at a resort. We contacted our hotel in Hawaii two weeks in advance of our trip. They special ordered gluten-free items (breads, rolls, bagels, pancake mix, etc.) and prepared wonderful meals for us. They didn't charge us any extra for this service. Many cruises will do the same thing for you, but they have to know in advance so that they can order the ingredients needed for you.

- If you want to supplement restaurant meals with your own foods, then request a hotel room with a refrigerator. Some hotels also have microwave ovens available that can be delivered to your room. (Some hotels will waive any extra fees for a refrigerator if it is for a medical condition, so you may want to bring a note from your doctor.) When you travel, bring a few empty microwave containers and plastic utensils to use for cooking. I also bring a small sample size of dish washing soap. Some hotels have kitchens in the rooms, but you need to be sure you wash pans carefully. Most hotels can tell you where health food stores or grocery stores are so you don't have to pack a lot of food for your trip.

- Check gluten-free lists on the internet before you go, to supplement restaurant meals. Items you can find in grocery stores are sometimes easier to find, since some areas have limited health food stores. Here are some examples we have used:

  - Hormel® has many products that are shelf-stable and gluten-free.
    - ◆ Hormel® chili with beans is gluten-free as of this writing. You can make a stuffed baked potato with it, or top a gluten-free hot dog on a corn tortilla with some cheese. (There are microwave versions, some with pop-top lids, or buy a can opener at a dollar store.)
    - ◆ Hormel® Dinty Moore® stew and Hormel® "ComplEats" chicken and rice and several other microwave shelf-stable meals are gluten-free. (See list on their web page.)
    - ◆ Hormel® sliced pepperoni is labeled gluten-free on the package. It's great on a salad and you refrigerate it only after it's opened.

- Hormel® and Jennie-O® have some refrigerated microwaveable fully cooked entrees. (See list on web page.)

- The Laughing Cow® and Mini-Baby Bel® are shelf-stable gluten-free cheeses. They are in single serving sizes, and no need to refrigerate unless they are opened.

- Those new foil shelf-stable easy-open packets of Bumble Bee® or Starkist® Tuna or Salmon are good to supplement salads that you order in restaurants. I brought some of these to Europe since they are easy to pack in my suitcase. We were glad to have them when we arrived since the first day we were too tired to shop for food or find a restaurant. (Note: for travel to Germany they suggest you put a doctor's note stating you have celiac disease in your suitcase with any shelf-stable food in your luggage.)

- Valley Fresh® (www.valleyfresh.com) has new foil shelf-stable packets of pre-cooked chicken breast that are good on a salad or in a tortilla. You can find them in the grocery store near the tuna packets.

- Tyson® Foods has some fully cooked refrigerated meats like roasted chicken or chicken strips that are safe as of this writing. The strips are good on a corn tortilla or on a salad. You have to call to verify which products, as ingredients may change.

- Purdue® chicken also has some fully cooked refrigerated chicken strips that are labeled gluten-free.

- Some flavors of Uncle Bens® ready rice are gluten-free, and can be prepared in the microwave.

- Kraft® foods won't hide gluten ingredients in their products, so there are many safe items you can have. We purchased their packaged Oscar Mayer®/Louis Rich® turkey cold cuts. Their feta cheese is good for a Greek salad. Kraft® cheese may also be a good choice. We like it on top of the ready-to-eat bagged tossed salads.

- Those small flip top cans of Underwood Deviled Ham® are gluten-free as of this writing and travel well. We bring those and some gluten-free crackers for a nice appetizer or snack. Spam® is also gluten-free as of this writing.

- Some Weight Watcher's® Smart Ones® frozen entrees from Heinz are gluten-free. You can confirm by calling 1-800-255-5750. In 2009 the Broccoli & Cheddar Potatoes, Lemon Herb Chicken Piccata, Fiesta Chicken, Santa Fe Rice & Beans, Creamy Tuscan Chicken, Grilled Chicken in Garlic Herb Sauce, Home-Style Chicken, and Chicken Santa Fe are gluten-free. Amy's® also has some frozen entrees labeled gluten-free.

- Wal-Mart® and Aldi® store brand items are clearly labeled if they are gluten-free. If you can find nothing else while traveling, try those stores. You will find something to eat.

- Some Progresso® Soups are labeled gluten-free. Since they have flip-top cans they are easy to open while on a trip.

- For dessert, there are many brands of safe gluten-free ice cream (see list). The new pint sizes are convenient and fit in small hotel refrigerator freezers.

- For some of our U.S. trips to National parks where there were few restaurants, we brought a small 6 inch electric fry pan with us to cook some meals in our hotel room. I cooked meat in the fry pan, and meanwhile cooked vegetables, rice or potatoes in the microwave. Some people bring a small George Forman® Grill and a small rice cooker on road trips. (I bring less and microwave rice – see index for recipe.)

- On some U.S. road trips where I don't think I'll easily find foods, we bring lots of frozen meals in a cooler so we don't have to cook while we're away. Weeks before the trip when I prepare food I put extra meals away in microwave containers and freeze them. You can get ice at your hotel for your cooler (or use those frozen cold packs). We found that many hotels were willing to store our food in their large freezer for us. I put my microwave containers of food in large freezer bags that seal, to not only keep them together but keep them free from water if I have to use ice in the cooler and it melts. It's a little bit of work to prepare before a trip, but this method of bringing frozen meals works well, and we found that some restaurants would heat them for us as long as we ordered a beverage. You will find you have a lot more time for touring when you don't have to think about your meals. This worked well for us when visiting family too.

- In Colorado we were staying in a small town. We asked the hotel to provide a refrigerator and a microwave, which they did. We found that when there are no restaurants nearby that can accommodate your diet, you usually can find a health food store or grocery store. We called our hotel in advance so we knew they had a Whole Foods® Store and Wild Oats Market® nearby. After we arrived, we bought gluten-free frozen entrees, gluten-free cereals for breakfast, milk, bags of salad, cheese, meat, gluten-free salad dressing and gluten-free bread. We had coffee and cereal in our room. We ate some picnic lunches. When the restaurant selected for a meeting could not accommodate a gluten-free entree, we would microwave a frozen gluten-free entree at our hotel room and put it in an insulated lunchbox. We ordered a salad and beverage and they gave us an extra plate for the entree.

- In Seattle we found lots of health food stores, and we also had wonderful smoked salmon at the Seattle fish market (check ingredients). When we got close to Canada, some restaurant menus listed that they served breads for gluten-free sandwiches. Some don't use designated toasters for the gluten-free bread, so ask before they prepare your sandwich. They will defrost the gluten-free bread in the microwave if you request it.

- Disneyland® and Disneyworld® are now catering to people on the gluten-free diet. E-mail or call in advance and give them a two-week notice. You will have to make reservations and alert them at the time of your reservation that you need gluten-free food.

Foreign Trips – Foreign travel is sometimes easier than in the U.S., especially if you travel in a country that has a high incidence of celiac disease. Here are some suggestions from our experiences:

- England: We stayed in a B&B in London that prepared wonderful meals for us. We contacted them by e-mail in advance with our needs. We found the U.K. celiac support website (www.coeliac.co.uk) and located stores that carried gluten-free foods. Sainsbury's® stores had the shelves labeled, so we knew which items were safe. This made it much easier to shop for groceries than at home. You will probably have an easier time traveling in the U.K. and Canada because they seem to know the diet better than in the U.S. We also ordered gluten-free foods from U.K. companies by web pages and had them shipped directly to our hotel so they were there when we arrived. (We did find a lot of local shops that carried gluten-free foods, but this was helpful to have something there upon arrival.) We found that a small B&B can be an excellent place to stay because they gave us a lot of service and accommodation for the diet.

When we were traveling around, I carried a backpack with some food items. When there wasn't much on a restaurant menu that was gluten-free, we ordered a "jacket potato" (i.e. a baked potato) and a plain salad. We supplemented that with food from the backpack. Most restaurants were very accommodating. We even went to a Chinese restaurant that knew the diet and prepared a nice stir-fry without soy sauce. We stayed away from beef on that trip because of mad cow disease, but found that there were a lot of other menu options to choose from.

- Spain: In Barcelona and Valencia we e-mailed our hotels before our trip. When my English e-mails were not being answered, I used http://babelfish.yahoo.com to get a free translation of my message. I wrote in my last paragraph that I did not speak Spanish and would appreciate if they could reply in English or simple Spanish. They responded in English and said that another person who stayed during the previous week had celiac and they would take care of us. Free breakfast was included with our hotel room. They purchased gluten-free baked goods for us for breakfast at no extra charge! They also gave us fresh squeezed orange juice since some orange juice mixes in Spain may be unsafe. We brought printouts from their Celiac Societies that were written in Spanish (www.celiacscatalunya.org for Barcelona, acecova.org for Valencia, and celiacos.org for Spain). This made it very easy to explain the diet to the restaurant manager who spoke very little English. (I have provided a copy of one of the charts in this book.) They provided excellent gluten-free breads, fruits, cheeses, ham, natural yogurts, and beverages. They checked on the status of everything we were unsure about. The term in Spain is "sin gluten" meaning "without gluten". The celiac society told us that the store El Corte Ingles® carried a lot of gluten-free products. On the top level of the store, we found that they now have a "Celiacos" menu in their cafeteria and we enjoyed gluten-free meals there. In the lower level we found the "Super Mercado" where we purchased breads and items to supplement other meals. Trigo is wheat in Spanish, so check labels carefully if purchasing other foods that are not in the gluten-free section. (We were surprised to find Trigo in Cola Cao® hot chocolate mix. Avena is oats and is found in some herbal teas.) Also check products for E-1400 starch additives which may or may not be safe. (See the possibly gluten-free list in this book for the exact numbers.) If you want to supplement meals with any canned items, we found that canned foods had pop top lids so you don't need can openers. We liked the tuna packed in olive oil on a salad. You can pay by credit card at El Corte Ingles but they will ask for identification such as your passport or U.S. photo driver's license. You can exchange U.S. dollars (not traveler's checks) at a special "banco" in their stores, and we found that the exchange rate was better than at the local banks. If you are going to bring extra cash, you may want to use a money belt. I found Barcelona to be very safe, except near the old medieval tourist section. I almost got my pocket picked by some children (gypsies?) who were trying to get me to sign a petition to "help children". Meanwhile they were trying to help themselves to my wallet. Use caution at train stations too.

- Norway: Bakeries and grocery stores carried wonderful gluten-free items and they knew the diet very well there. They do not accept credit cards for food purchases and take debit cards or cash only; so be aware of this before you shop. Most people do speak English and most people we met knew about celiac disease and the diet. Many gluten-free products are similar as in the U.S. but some products contain a special Codex wheat starch. If you want to try some of the wheat starch breads, we recommend that you do <u>not</u> overdo it. They are good and your initial reaction will be to eat a lot. Keep in mind that this wheat starch is permitted to have gluten contamination of up to 100 parts per million. *(Prior to 2008 it was 200 ppm. In 2008 they changed their standard to 100 ppm for products rendered gluten-free [i.e. wheat starch]; and 20 ppm for products naturally gluten-free.)* So, why do they allow this starch and why the difference in the standard from the U.S.? (1) Norwegians seem to eat less than typical Americans. Their portions are smaller, their bread slices are smaller, and they eat open faced sandwiches with one slice of bread instead of 2. (2) In Norway, they have low contamination in everything else because factories are small and dedicated. Their overall diet seems more limited than what we have in the U.S. (3) They don't eat so many processed foods that have a high risk of contamination. They eat more plain fresh foods. (4) They rarely eat out in restaurants. Most Norwegians eat at home. So, if you don't overdo the wheat starch breads and eat Norwegian sized portions, you can tolerate them while you're in Norway. If you have a larger appetite and want to eat several open faced sandwiches, then it would be better to purchase some flatbreads without wheat starch and have additional sandwiches on that. Eat more fresh vegetables and fruits like they do. We didn't eat more than 2 wheat starch items in a meal; for example, no more than 2 small slices of bread, or 1 roll, or 1 small slice of bread and 1 small slice of cake. They do have flourless nut cakes made with hazelnuts that do not have wheat starch. (Just don't bother discussing the contamination issue with Norwegians, because if you try, they will just think you are a crazy American! …although that humorous misunderstanding might have been avoided if we actually could speak Norwegian….) When checking food ingredient lists, Hvete is wheat. (Easy to remember because if you mispronounce it phonetically in English – it sounds like wheat.) Bygg is barley, Rug is Rye, and Havre is oats. If you want to eat in restaurants it can be done, and most restaurants and fast food places can accommodate you. You can get a gluten-free hamburger at McDonald's or Burger King, or pizza at Dolly Dimples restaurants. Their gluten-free society can give you more suggestions via their website.

- <u>Italy</u>: We had terrific meals because their celiac society has a restaurant program. They train the restaurants to prepare foods in a separate area, in separate pots, etc. They have wonderful gluten-free pastas and breads. On their web page they list restaurants all over Italy (www.celiachia.it). We tried several restaurants and were very pleased with the meals that we had. When we were unsure of the bread and pasta (because it was so good); they brought out the packages to show us. Participating restaurants have a sticker near their doorway that shows they are part of the program, and they have to re-certify to continue in it. An important tip: Have your hotel concierge make dinner reservations for you in Italian and explain that you need gluten-free food. That way when you arrive they are expecting you and have the food needed for you. We don't speak Italian so this was very helpful. Other suggestions to guarantee a safe meal are on their website. Some restaurants did have a separate menu but most would suggest items from the menu that they made gluten-free. The celiac society also has lists of ice cream shops (gelato) and hotels participating in the program. When we went into Switzerland we stayed in a hotel near the Italian Lake District area that we found through the Switzerland celiac society (www.celiachia.ch the Italian-speaking site). They prepared wonderful gluten-free German and Italian meals for us. The term for gluten-free in Italian is "senza glutine". (Senza is pronounced the same way as in English, but the "e" at the end of glutine is pronounced ay, like in hay, or "gluten ay"). Other Italian words to watch out for on labels are Frumento (wheat), Grano (grain), segale (rye), orzo (barley), avena (oats), farro or spelta (spelt), kamut, and triticale. Most hotels don't have microwaves available in the guest rooms, but many have them in their offices or restaurants and they will heat something for you. I was able to bring some foods to the front desk and they heated them for me. The word for microwave oven is microonda, pronounced "me crow on day". We found that this pronunciation worked in Italy and in Spain.

- <u>Anywhere outside the U.S.</u>: I recommend that you always search the internet to find the celiac society website for the country you plan to visit. Through these websites we have found not only restaurant cards (in both English and their language), but also places to buy gluten-free foods, suggested restaurants that have foods for celiacs, and suggested products available that are gluten-free. Some even suggested hotels that accommodate the diet. We have e-mailed society members and they have provided very helpful advice. There is a list at the end of this section with the web addresses for many of the celiac societies that I found on the internet. If you don't speak the language, use Google translator. (See the chart of foreign celiac societies later in this section).

Here is an excellent restaurant card prepared by the Norwegian Coeliac Society (NCF) from their website at: www.ncf.no. It is reprinted here with their permission. We have found that the best foreign restaurant cards are those prepared by celiacs in that country. They know the unsafe foods to watch out for in their own country. (We sometimes found that the list of unsafe foods can be different than those the U.S.)

| ENGLISH | NORSK |
|---|---|
| **To the person who prepares my food**<br>(should be handed to the kitchen): | **Til den som skal tilbrede mitt måltid**<br>(bør leveres til kokken): |
| I suffer from coeliac disease and cannot therefore eat prepared food that contains gluten. Gluten is found in wheat, barley, rye and oats and therefore in normal bread, biscuits, pasta etc. Even small quantities of gluten (crumbs, flour dust etc.) can make me ill. Rice, vegetables, fruit, pure fish and pure meat are naturally gluten-free and can therefore be used in the preparation of gluten-free meals. | Jeg har sykdommen cøliaki og kan derfor ikke spise matretter som inneholder gluten. Gluten finnes i hvete, bygg, rug og havre og dermed i vanlig brød, kjeks, pasta osv. Selv små mengder gluten (smuler, meldryss osv.) kan gjøre meg syk. Ris, grønnsaker, frukt, ren fisk og rent kjøtt er naturlig glutenfritt og kan med fordel brukes i et glutenfritt måltid. |
| **Preparation of gluten-free food:** use kitchen utensils that have been cleaned and are free from gluten residues. | **Tilbreding av glutenfri mat:** bruk kjøkkenredskap som er rengjort og uten rester av gluten. |
| **Serving gluten-free bread:** Remember that gluten-free bread must not be mixed with normal bread and that it must be cut on a breadboard that has been cleaned.<br>**Sauces:** gluten-free flour, potato flour or maize flour can be used instead of normal flour. Remember that all ingredients in the sauce must be gluten-free. | **Servering av glutenfritt brød:** husk at glutenfritt brød ikke må blandes med vanlig brød og at det må skjæres på rengjort skjærefjel.<br>**Saus:** istedet for vanlig mel kan glutenfritt mel, potetmel eller maizenamel brukes. Husk at også alle andre ingredienser i sausen må være glutenfrie. |
| **Serving mixed products such as minced products, hamburgers, minced beef, ketchup, dressings etc:** check the ingredients. | **Servering av blandingsprodukter som farseprodukter, hamburgere, karbonader, ketchup, dressinger osv.:** sjekk varedeklarasjon. |
| **Spices:** some types of spices can contain gluten (flour). Please check the ingredients. | **Krydder:** enkelte kryddersorter kan inneholde gluten (mel). Vennligst sjekk varedeklarasjonen. |
| **French fries:** must be fried in fat that has not been used to fry other foods that contain gluten such as breaded foods. | **Pommes frites:** må stekes i fett som ikke er brukt til å steke andre retter som inneholder gluten f.eks. panerte retter. |
| Please do not use the product if the list of ingredients is inadequate or missing. | Dersom varedeklarasjon mangler eller er mangelfull, vennligst ikke benytt produktet. |
| I look forward to a gluten-free meal! | Jeg ser frem til et glutenfritt måltid! |
| This information is provided by The Norwegian Coeliac Society (NCF) www. ncf. no | Denne informasjonen er laget av Norsk Cøliakiforening (NCF) www.ncf.no |

Here is a document from www.celiacscatalunya.org that we found very helpful when we traveled to Barcelona and Valencia, Spain. (Keep in mind that foods in Spain are different than in other Spanish speaking countries.) I added the English translation to their chart using translation web pages. The "list from Association" is on their web page.

## La Dieta Sin Gluten – The Diet Without Gluten

| | Sí puede comer | Yes, you can Eat | No puede comer | No, you cannot eat |
|---|---|---|---|---|
| | Ensaladas, verduras y patatas hervidas, legumbres y arroz hervido | Salads, vegetables [such as tomatoes] and potatoes boiled, vegetables [such as peas/beans] and rice boiled | Verduras y arroz precocinado, legumbres cocinadas (ver Lista de la Asociación) | Vegetables and precooked rice, cooked vegetables (see list from Association) |
| | Carne y pollo a la plancha o fritos (sin harina) | Meat and chicken cooked on a griddle or fried (without flour) | Carne con salsas o elaboración no controlada | Meat with sauces or uncontrolled processing |
| | Pescado a la plancha, hervido o frito (sin harina) | Fish cooked on a griddle, boiled or fried (without flour) | Pescado con salsas o elaboración no controlada (ver Lista de la Asociación) | Fish with sauces or uncontrolled development (see list from Association) |
| | Huevo frito o tortilla (sin aditivos) | Fried egg or omelet [a Spanish tortilla] (no additives) | Algunos restaurants ñaden harina a las tortillas | Some restaurants add flour to egg omelets [a Spanish tortilla] |
| | Todo tipo de fruta y zumos naturales | All kinds of fruit and natural juices | | |
| | Leche, mantequilla, quesos, yogurts naturales y de sabores (sin trozos) | Milk, butter, cheeses, natural yogurts and flavored (without pieces [of fruit]) [such as plain or vanilla yogurt] | Yogurts con trozos u otros alimentos añadidos | Yogurts with pieces [of fruit] or other food additives |
| | Todo tipo de aceite | Any kind of oil | | |
| | Sopas y salsas hechas en casa, sin harina de trigo ni aditivos | Soups and sauces made at home without wheat flour or additives | Sopas y salsas (ver Lista de la Asociación) | Soups and sauces (see list from Association) |
| | Café y bebidas, except las derivadas de la cebada | Coffee and drinks outside those derived from barley | Whisky, cerveza, Baileys | Whisky, beer, Baileys |
| | Harina y derivados: los especiales para celíacos y maizena | Flour and derivatives: especially for celiacs and cornstarch | Harina y derivados: Pan, Galletas, Pasteles | Flour and derivatives: Bread, Biscuits, Cakes |
| | Pasta y rebozados: los especiales para celíacos | Pasta and coatings: those especially made for celiacs | Pasta normal (macarrones, espaguettis) y rebozados | Normal Pasta (macaroni, spaghetti) and coatings |
| | Jamón tipo "serrano" | Ham type "Serrano" | Embutidos y patés (ver Lista de la Asociación) | Sausages and patés (see list from Association) |
| | Conservas de verduras y legumbres hervidas, y conservas en aceite | Preserved/canned vegetables and boiled vegetables, and preserved in oil | Conservas (ver Lista de la Asociación) | Canned (see list from Association) |

## CHART OF WORLDWIDE CELIAC SOCIETIES

Many of these sites are in the language of that country.  To be able to read them, go to www.google.com.  Put the web page address in the search section.  After it locates your web page, click "translate" and it will translate it into English.  Once you find the section of the site that explains the diet, you can open that site in the original foreign language version.  Print that page and bring it with you to restaurants so that they will understand your needs in their own language.  (I often print the English translated version on the back.)  If you can't find what you need on the web page, e-mail the society.  Most will respond within a week.  For the United States, I have not listed all of the local celiac societies.  I have found that doing a web search with the name of the state and "celiac" or "celiac support" locates what you need.

| Country | Website(s) |
| --- | --- |
| Argentina | www.celiaco.org.ar |
| Australia<br>New South Wales<br>Queensland<br>Southern Australia<br>Tasmania<br>Victoria<br>Western Australia | www.coeliac.org.au<br>www.nswcoeliac.org.au<br>www.qld.coeliac.org.au<br>www.sa.coeliac.org.au<br>www.tas.coeliac.org.au<br>www.vic.coeliac.org.au<br>www.wa.coeliac.org.au |
| Belgium | www.coeliakie.be and http://vcv.coeliakie.be |
| Canada | www.celiac.ca and www.fqmc.org |
| Croatia | www.celiac.inet.hr |
| Czech Republic | www.volny.cz/coeliac and http://coeliac.cz/en |
| Denmark | www.coeliaki.dk |
| Finland | www.keliakia.org |
| France | www.afdiag.org |
| Germany | www.dzg-online.de |
| Ireland | www.coeliac.ie |
| Israel | www.celiac.org.il |
| Italy | www.celiachia.it |
| Netherlands | www.coeliakievereniging.nl |
| Norway | www.ncf.no |
| Portugal | www.celiacos.org.pt/ |
| Spain<br>Aragon<br>Barcelona (Catalunya)<br>Cantabria<br>Madrid<br>Palmas Province/Canarias<br>Seville<br>Valencia | www.celiacos.org<br>www.celiacosaragon.org<br>www.celiacscatalunya.org<br>www.odriozola.org/celiaquia<br>www.celiacosmadrid.org<br>www.asocepa.com/<br>www.celiacossevilla.org<br>www.acecova.org |
| Sweden | www.celiaki.se |
| Switzerland<br>French Speaking Area<br>Italian Speaking Area | www.zoeliakie.ch<br>www.coeliakie.ch<br>www.celiachia.ch |
| Uruguay | www.acelu.org |
| United Kingdom | www.coeliac.org.uk |
| United States<br>Celiac Disease Foundation<br>Celiac Sprue Association<br>Gluten Intolerance Group | www.celiac.org<br>www.csaceliacs.org<br>www.gluten.net |

WORDS OF ENCOURAGEMENT

- ♦ It may seem overwhelming at first when reading these suggestions, but rest assured that the gluten-free diet gets easier and you'll get healthier with each passing day. It's worth it! You can avoid so many complications by sticking with the diet. Most people say they have never felt better in their lives once they are on the diet and follow it properly.

- ♦ Scientists <u>are</u> working on a cure, so you may not have to be on this diet forever if their research is successful. Until then, take care of your health. If you have too much damage from cheating on the diet, these medical solutions may not work for you.

  There are many approaches to the research, and here are some of them: (1) The University of Maryland worked on "tight junction regulators" which they believe will stop intestinal permeability and help to manage or control celiac disease. Alba Therapeutics (www.albatherapeutics.com) is in clinical trials of this compound called AT1001 (larazotide acetate). You can read more at www.albatherapeutics.com or at www.clinicaltrials.gov. (2) A group at Stanford (www.celiacsprug.org) worked on an enzyme called PEP (prolyl endopetidase) that would break down the gluten so you could digest it. Alvine Pharmaceutical acquired it and it is in clinical trials and the compound is called ALV003-0812. More information is on their web page: http://alvinepharma.com. (3) In Finland, ChemoCentryx is testing their compound CCX282-B to prevent migration of activated lymphocytes to the gut. (4) In Australia, NexPep is starting trials of a vaccine that may prevent celiac disease. You can read more about these compounds on www.clinicaltrials.gov. Another interesting point I read about in a journal article was that celiac patients have rod-shaped bacteria that normal patients do not have[99, 100]. Scientists are learning more, and perhaps eliminating these bacteria could be another possible road to a cure.

  Taking a different approach, other researchers are trying to find out if ancient forms of wheat do not cause celiac disease. Results have been very exciting, and in the future there may be a special wheat for celiacs.[101-103]. The NIH Celiac Awareness Spring/Summer 2008 newsletter reported that researchers at Washington State University discovered a mutant form of barley that lacks the gliadin-type of protein. These researchers have partnered with Arcadia Biosciences. The NIH has given them a grant to help their research in the hopes that this work will provide a safe grain for celiacs.[104]

  There are many developments that point to a cure, so stay strictly on the diet until your doctor advises you that a new treatment is available.

- ♦ You may want to consider supporting celiac research and education. More awareness will help companies see the need and create more products. Three Universities/Hospitals that are trying to create more awareness are: Columbia University (web page: http://www.celiacdiseasecenter.columbia.edu), the University of Maryland (web page: http://www.celiaccenter.org), and Beth Israel Deaconess (web page: http://www.bidmc.harvard.edu). You can also find other celiac societies to support listed at the end of the NIH article in this book.

♦   Helping others helps you!  Take the time to educate restaurants and stores, so that more products will be carried and it will become easier to get the foods you need.  In doing so, you are not only helping yourself, but helping others.  Also, help others get diagnosed so that they will become healthier.  Celiac Disease is a much bigger problem than people realize.   Since my husband has been diagnosed, I have helped several friends and acquaintances get diagnosed.   For example, a friend of mine was tired, recently developed thyroid problems, had irritable bowel syndrome, and sometimes had anxiety.  It seemed as if there was one health problem after another.  I convinced my friend to get the blood test and it was positive for celiac disease.  Although not thrilled about a new diet at first; now they are thankful for it.  I was there to help with the diet, and now their good health has returned.

If you are feeling alone or frustrated about having celiac disease, find a support group, get onto the internet (there are some great chat groups), and reach out.  Sharing your experiences may not only help you, but help someone else.

♦   Don't give up.  This book is filled with delicious gluten-free recipes that are so good that you won't miss out on any of the foods you love!  I have served these recipes to people who have raved about my wonderful cooking and had no idea it was gluten-free.  You will have all the food you love, and you will stay healthy at the same time!

## What if the Diet Doesn't Seem to Be Working for Me?

You've been diagnosed with celiac disease. Your doctor has confirmed the diagnosis by both blood test and biopsy. You know all about what you can eat. You've been on the diet a couple of weeks. If you are like most people you should be feeling better already. However, maybe you're one of the people whose symptoms have not gone away. Why isn't the diet working? Here are some suggestions, based on our experience. Note: your experience may be different from ours, but these suggestions may help to open up a conversation with your doctor.

### <u>You may be eating hidden gluten, and not know it.</u>

This is the most common reason. My husband was not doing well at one point and it turned out to be hidden gluten in corn chips. The bag's ingredients looked right, but when I called the manufacturer I was told that there was no way they could be gluten-free. The grain was delivered in a bin next to wheat flour that could easily mix with the corn, and wheat flour was often airborne in that room. The machine made tortilla chips and nacho flavored tortilla chips, and the nacho chip flavoring contained wheat. That phone call solved a mystery and my husband started to improve once we eliminated that brand. It took being a detective, writing down what he was eating, and calling to figure out why he was not doing well. Now I always check with manufacturers. There are brands that do not have contamination (see list at the end of the book), so don't despair. It's worth taking the time to be sure. Many companies list safe products on their web pages so usually I check there first.

Another way to determine hidden gluten in your diet is to start with a very simplified diet and once you feel good, add foods one at a time. If you add a food that brings back your symptoms, you know it is a problem. One difficulty is that some people's reactions may not be immediate (for example, a dermatitis herpetiformis rash may not flare immediately but may take several days). You may have to think back to several days before the reaction to figure out which food caused the problem. As you are learning the diet, it may help you to keep a food diary.

> *Note: dermatitis herpetiformis may flare either because of gluten, or because of too much iodine in the diet. Iodine is important, so if you are getting 100% in your multivitamin, use salt without iodine and cut back on high iodine foods like shrimp to see if the flare subsides. Flares from iodine do not affect the villi, but flares from gluten do, so you need to find out what is causing the problem. If you like a lot of high iodine foods in your diet like kelp, sea salt, and shrimp, perhaps try a gluten-free vitamin with a lower percentage of iodine. Check with your doctor to determine what is best for you.*

Check the "unsafe and possibly safe" lists in this book for other possibly sources of hidden gluten. Check your vitamins and all of your medicines to be sure they're gluten-free. Write everything down that you eat, drink, swallow, or touch to your lips. You don't need to be fanatical here, but think about what you're doing. If you're not improving, try to find out the cause. It's usually something simple that you need to change. For example, if you're working with wheat flour and it could get airborne, you may have to consider what you may be breathing and wear a mask while working with it. Or it could be as simple as stop licking envelopes!

I found contamination may happen because some grains may be milled with wheat. The more likely candidates that are milled or grown in the same locations as wheat are corn, millet, teff and buckwheat. (And of course most oats in the U.S. are contaminated and unsafe. See further discussion of oats on the forbidden list.) Some packing-houses package all types of flour, so check that too. To track down the offender, I suggest you don't eat grains (by that I mean flours or cornmeal or snack/cereal items) for just a few days to see if you feel better. Try having some plain, regular rice instead of bread for a few days. Then add foods back one by one as you improve and see if you react. You could possibly have allergies as well as celiac disease and an elimination diet may help you figure out if you need to see an allergist.

Regarding kissing — it's not a good idea to kiss someone while they have a gluten in their mouth, especially if you want a French kiss. It is fine to kiss someone once they've finished eating and swallowed it. I usually drink some water to wash it down and wipe my mouth before kissing my husband, and that is the conservative approach. I also choose lipsticks/lip balms that don't contain gluten. (Most brands are safe, but beware of those with wheat germ oil.) I have asked doctors and have been told that kissing is fine, so there is no need to be fanatical about that either.

### You may be a slow healer.
About 70 percent of people see improvement of their symptoms after the first two weeks on the diet. That leaves 30 percent who don't and it may take longer for you. Don't give up! For slow healers it may take up to 6 months for the villi to completely heal. For many people it's 2 to 3 months, but for others it's longer. Some elderly patients may take 1 to 2 years to fully heal.

If you have lactose intolerance caused by celiac disease, you may be able to use this symptom as an indication of the time it takes your gut to heal. The lactose digesting bacteria live on the villi. If the villi are damaged, you won't have the right environment for these bacteria to survive. As the villi heal, the lactose digesting bacteria may return to digest lactose again.

If you are a slow healer, continue to stick with the diet, and more importantly — make sure you are not getting hidden gluten from somewhere. Most people see gradual improvement if they're following the diet properly. Also, if your lactose intolerance disappears, and then at some point mysteriously returns, that may be a sign that you've ingested hidden gluten and need to be more careful with your diet so you heal again.

Note: See your doctor right away if you are experiencing chronic diarrhea or blood in the stool. These symptoms could possibly be from a serious condition. If you're still not improving, work with your doctor and continue to check for hidden gluten. Get blood work done to see if the antibodies to gluten are gone and you are "normal" again. Choose a simple diet and add new foods when you feel fine. Don't try eating out until your symptoms improve. Eating out is always risky, and it is important to get your body healthy before attempting to take that risk.

A simple menu to start might be the following — for breakfast: eggs, plain yogurt and fruit; for lunch and dinner: grilled meat or fish, baked potato or rice, vegetables, salad with oil and vinegar and fresh fruit. Carefully check the ingredients used to create this menu. Check for added solutions in the meat. It may get boring, but just try it for a few of days and see if it helps you. Then add on recipes from this book as you go. Do basic things first and add items with flours or packaged foods later. If you have chronic diarrhea, you may need electrolytes and minerals like potassium, so ask your doctor about that too.

### You could possibly have a bacterial imbalance.
If you've been very careful with your diet, you have no gluten antibodies in your blood, and still have irritable bowel type symptoms (bloating, nausea, abdominal pain, and constipation or diarrhea symptoms); you may have a bacterial imbalance or small intestinal bacterial overgrowth. A recent study showed that "small intestinal bacterial overgrowth affects most celiacs with persistence of gastrointestinal symptoms after gluten withdrawal."[105]

I personally experienced a bacterial imbalance from taking an antibiotic, and the suggestions here are from my personal experience. These may or may not be helpful to you. If you think this is possible, see your doctor. Your doctor may want to do some breath tests or blood tests. The first test may be a lactulose breath test to check for small bowel bacterial overgrowth. The second test may be the tTG blood test for gluten-antibodies to check for hidden gluten in your diet. Or, your doctor could do a Sorbitol H2-breath test (a newer test), which a recent study shows may be better than antiendomysial antibody blood test to see if you have ingested hidden gluten. (Your doctor may choose the blood test instead because only one breath test may be done during a visit, and the test is so new not all doctors are using it yet.) Your doctor may also want to do a third breath test for lactose to see if lactose intolerance is still a problem. Or your doctor may just want you to experiment and see if lactose bothers you.

If you have a bacterial overgrowth, your doctor may prescribe an appropriate antibiotic. There are several medicines that your doctor may prescribe, depending on the overgrowth. Or your doctor may suggest you try a probiotic that is gluten-free. Probiotics are beneficial bacteria that some people believe may help balance the bacteria in the gut. Some studies from Europe claim they resolve bacterial overgrowths and are an alternative to using antibiotics in this application.

Ask your doctor about using probiotics before you try them. Although I list a few products that could possibly be helpful, you need to make an informed decision that considers your entire medical condition before you begin any treatment. I am not a physician and therefore I highly recommend that you ask your doctor before trying any of these probiotics. What worked for me may not work for you.

Florastor® (www.florastor.com) is called a probiotic, but it is actually a non-pathogenic yeast which may normalize the bacterial flora. It doesn't cause yeast infections; in fact they claim it helps eliminate Candida and restores the bacterial balance in the small bowel. Some physicians claim it may also help those with Crohn's disease. It is gluten-free as of this writing. This product was recommended to me by my doctor to help with irritable bowel symptoms after I took a strong antibiotic that ruined my digestion. I found that it relieved my irritable bowel symptoms and worked better than anything else. It is the only product I ever tried that reduced bloating. Since they claim it normalizes the gut flora, it may correct either diarrhea or constipation. According to their webpage, it has also been clinically studied and used worldwide for 50 years. Journal article links are available on their web page. It may also be taken concurrently with antibiotics, as well as acidophilus probiotics if desired. Florastor® is now available for children.

Culturelle® (www.culturelle.com) is another probiotic that has been clinically studied. It may be used concurrently with antibiotics, and is gluten-free as of this writing. Some people claim it helps to ease their irritable bowel symptoms and their research is available on their web page. It is made by ConAgra® Foods, whose research shows it eliminates diarrhea, and their website has journal article links to support that claim.

Digestive Advantage® (www.digestiveadvantage.com) is a probiotic that is gluten-free as of this writing and claims to ease irritable bowel symptoms. They also have a version to help with lactose intolerance. It is currently available at Wal-Mart® and other stores.

Another probiotic to consider is Reuteri®. This may possibly be helpful to those with celiac disease. The manufacturer claims that Reuteri® improves the crypts of the villi in the small intestine, creating lengthened and deeper folds to better absorb nutrients. (Flat villi without folds do not absorb nutrients.) Note: this product is not a substitute for the gluten-free diet in any way, but it may possibly help to improve the condition of the villi and may possibly help with the healing process. The literature from manufacturers of Reuteri® discussed general intestinal health and did not specifically mention celiac disease. The Reuteri® strain is in products made by several different companies, so check the gluten-free status before you try it. It has also been added to some plain yogurts like Stonyfield®.

A new probiotic from Proctor & Gamble® called Align® is supposed to relieve IBS symptoms. It is gluten-free as of this writing. The web page is www.aligngi.com or call 1-800-208-0112.

Some yogurts like CascadeFresh® (www.cascadefresh.com) contain many strains of probiotic/good bacteria that may be helpful. It is gluten-free as of this writing (gluten-free is on the label), and there are many flavored yogurts that are safe. Breyers® yogurt (www.breyersyogurt.com) also has a probiotic yogurt that some people find helpful, and as of this writing they say their yogurts are gluten-free. Your doctor may want you to eat yogurt while taking an antibiotic. Some of the probiotic products I suggested say in their instructions or on their web pages that you may eat yogurt while using them.

Some yogurts and probiotics contain inulin or FOS. Inulin/FOS is a fiber that also acts as a sugar/food for good bacteria. It is broken down in the large intestine. Some people with IBS, or a bacterial imbalance, or sensitive digestive tracks may experience nausea and bloating from it. Others may find it beneficial and helpful to promote good intestinal bacteria. It may be a good way to get fiber. Some claim that it also may help with calcium absorption. I personally cannot tolerate inulin/FOS. It gives me terrible nausea and abdominal bloating, so I avoid it. Some celiac patients have mistaken a reaction to inulin as a reaction to gluten, so this is something to keep in mind. You may want to start consuming products with inulin slowly to see how you react. Many people can tolerate it once their body adjusts to it. (Stonyfield® plain yogurt uses inulin from chicory and is gluten-free as of this writing. Other companies use inulin from Jerusalem artichoke.)

I suggest that if you try any of these products that you start <u>very slowly</u> perhaps using the children's dosage to see how you will react. Products like Culturelle® say that patients may experience some nausea, bloating, or constipation until you adjust. They have a new version without FOS that contains methylcellulose. For those with diarrhea symptoms this product may be helpful. The Florastor® does not contain inulin/FOS and may be helpful for those with a bacterial imbalance. Some report that you could get a headache or constipation during the initial dose, so they suggest you drink water to avoid that possible side effect. I did not experience this. I started with one tablet daily and increased it to one in the morning and one in the evening after a few days. I started experiencing relief of my irritable bowel symptoms within a week.

You may <u>not</u> be experiencing a bacterial imbalance as discussed here, but lactose intolerance. See food sensitivities below. You should check for that first before trying these products.

Or, you may possibly have a problem with pancreatic enzyme insufficiency, and you should check with your doctor to see if digestive enzymes are needed instead of products for a bacterial imbalance. If needed, there are some over-the-counter brands of digestive enzymes that are available, but be sure to use a brand that is gluten-free.

Be an informed consumer regarding probiotics/nutritionals, and check them out for yourself. Some products may contain dead bacteria or strains not tested. Some say gluten-free but may contain barley grasses that could have contamination. *Probiotics are nutritionals that do not need FDA approval.* Use them at your own risk. You can read about the studies through PubMed, a free government run search engine for medical journal articles. (To find PubMed, either go to http://nihlibrary.nih.gov/ and click on PubMed or see http://www.ncbi.nlm.nih.gov, click on PubMed.) I check PubMed frequently for the new journal articles and research on celiac disease too.

*Note: If you have irritable bowel syndrome and your symptoms do not improve over time, see your doctor for other possible treatment options, in addition to the suggestions noted above.*

## You may have other food sensitivities/medical problem(s) in addition to celiac disease.

Some people may still have problems because they have trouble digesting other foods. The more common problem foods are soy proteins and eggs, or possibly some kinds of meats[106, 107]. You can use alternative bean flours and egg substitutes in most of my recipes, if that is the case. In main dishes you usually can substitute meats. You may need to work with your doctor to see if other food sensitivities exist. Food sensitivities may feel like a gluten-reaction to some people, when they are not.

Some other foods that may cause a reaction are: acidic foods, sorbitol, olestra, guar gum, antibiotics, lactose, bean and nut flours, food allergens: (such as milk, soy, nuts, eggs, corn, fish), fructose intolerance, foods high in salicylates and amines.[6]

Lactose intolerance also may be a problem for many with celiac disease until they heal completely. For most patients they <u>will</u> be able to digest lactose again because once the small intestine completely heals, the right environment returns for the lactose digesting bacteria to flourish. As mentioned earlier, the first sign that many people have that tells them their villi are damaged is lactose intolerance.

You may want to be tested for lactose intolerance, or you may want to try DairyCare® (www.dairycare.com) or DigestiveAdvantage® (www.digestiveadvantage.com), a once-a-day acidophilus that enables you to eat dairy all day without lactose intolerance symptoms. Or you can use Lactaid® Ultra (some other strengths are not gluten-free so be careful), but lactase pills must be taken throughout the day before you consume any dairy products.

I have personally used DairyCare® and found that it worked well for me. I took it concurrently for 3 months with the Florastor® (see above) and it got rid of my lactose intolerance which developed after I took an antibiotic for a sinus infection. My husband took DairyCare® initially as he was healing on the diet and found it very helpful. After about 6 months, he found that he no longer needed it at all. He loved dairy foods and by using this product he didn't have to give them up during the healing process. Many gluten-free products contain milk or lactose, so being able to eat dairy foods opened up more possible food choices. Since many celiacs have osteoporosis, this product enables you to have dairy products which provide calcium in your diet.

You may have to eliminate some foods until you completely heal. Then once healed, you may be able to try them again in small amounts and see if you may be able tolerate them. There is a possibility that you cannot tolerate them because of the damage to your villi. If you had an allergic reaction instead of intolerance, you may have to continue to strictly avoid those foods. Check with your doctor. (An allergic response could be hives or rash, whereas an intolerance response could be gas, bloating or diarrhea. The intolerance response would result from not being able to break down the sugars properly.)

According to an article by Dr. Peter Green, the most common causes for the diet not working are gluten ingestion, lactose intolerance, pancreatic insufficiency, and microscopic colitis. Less common reasons are: the wrong diagnosis, bacterial overgrowth, other food intolerances (fructose, milk, soy), collagenous colitis, inflammatory bowel disease, collagenous sprue, ulcerative jejunitis, enteropathy associated T-cell lymphoma, autoimmune enteropathy and refractory sprue (+/- clonal T cell populations).[108] You may have one of these problems, or a different medical problem that needs to be treated in order for you to feel better. In a previous chapter there is a list of complications and other problems associated with celiac disease, and your doctor may have to find out if there is something else that needs to be treated.

In the next section are some suggested medical tests that your doctor may want to perform.  Dr. Green mentioned several conditions above that could possibly be looked into.  These are not the only ones that I suggest.  Some other medical conditions such as an untreated thyroid problem, or a gallbladder problem, or liver or pancreatic insufficiency, could possibly give you symptoms that may make it seem like you are not getting better on the diet.  For example, if your pancreas is not working properly you may need to take pancreatic enzymes/digestive enzymes to help break down foods.  It is important to have your doctor check you for possible co-existing conditions, so that you can get the right treatment.  Even though you will find digestive enzymes, ox bile, and other digestive aids in the health food store or drug store, it is a good idea to check with your doctor and get the proper diagnosis before trying any of these things.

**You could have a rare condition called refractory sprue.**
If you're still not getting better, you **must** see your doctor.  You could possibly have refractory sprue.  In individuals with refractory sprue, the intestines are so damaged that they are beyond healing properly and returning to completely normal.  It may happen from too many years of not being on the gluten-free diet.  It is similar to what happens in Barrett's esophagus only it's in the intestines.  The tissue actually changes and doesn't return to normal because of so much damage.  The good news is that refractory sprue is rare.  One study suggests that 95% of people that are diagnosed with celiac disease and remain on the diet improve.  (Many doctors find that most thought to have refractory sprue are cheating on the diet or getting hidden gluten.)  The bad news is that the medicines for refractory sprue have many bad side effects.  For example, often steroids are given and they may make your bones weaker and create other problems[106].  Other medications are immunosuppressants which can make you more susceptible to infections.  At Columbia University some of the medications being studied for use in refractory sprue are budeonide, azathioprine and prednisone[109].

People with refractory sprue may have to be checked more frequently and treated for additional complications from malabsorption issues due to intestinal damage.  Some may need intravenous feedings and hospitalizations.  This is another reason to not cheat on your diet so you may be able to avoid this complication.

Most physicians agree that failing to follow the diet properly is the reason for this problem[110].  However, some suggest that your doctor check you for hyperthyroidism and collagenous colitis, as they could coexist with celiac disease, and make it appear you have refractory sprue[108].

One woman I know thought she had refractory sprue but her problem was really from hidden gluten.  (A recent study by the Mayo Clinic suggests that only 18% of non-responding/non-healing celiacs have refractory sprue and the rest are eating hidden gluten.  Half of the people who were not responding in their study were eating items with gluten contamination.)[111]  In the case of my friend, it turned out that she was taking communion.  (Communion wafers contain gluten.)  Once she eliminated that, she still had a problem.  Then she checked her vitamins to find out they contained gluten, and changed brands.  It took several weeks to resolve, but it worked!  Now this lady feels great and is relieved that her gastrointestinal symptoms are gone.  With celiac disease sometimes it's the little things that make a difference!

**Finally, what do to next?**   Get a check up!  See suggestions in the next section.

## Suggested Medical Check Ups

Especially initially, check-ups are very important to maintaining your health.

After your initial diagnosis, it is important to follow the diet and get a check-up after 6 months. Your physician can do blood work to see if you still have antibodies to gluten in your blood, so you know if your diet is working or not. Most likely your doctor will use the new tTG (tissue Transglutaminase) blood test to check for this. Your doctor could possibly give you a Sorbitol H2-breath test[112, 113], which new studies show may also be effective. Hopefully the antibodies will be gone and you will be normal. (Some people have no apparent symptoms that tell them they ingested gluten, so this is a way to track their progress. For example, their only symptom might be that their bones are weakening.) You may also want to ask your doctor to do blood work to check your thyroid and your iron levels. You will get great satisfaction when you compare your results every 6 months to a year and see improvements!

After your initial diagnosis, I suggest you get a Bone Mineral Density or DEXA scan as a baseline. If your density is low, in six months to a year get another scan. This will show you if your bone density levels are improving. This testing is very important to keep your bones strong, especially for those diagnosed as a teenager or adult. (For those diagnosed as an infant or very young child, this test may not be needed until they are older, depending on their doctor's recommendation.)

For adults, if your bone density is low your doctor may prescribe a bone-building medicine, along with calcium, vitamin D, and magnesium which are needed for bone building. Of course, make sure any supplements are gluten-free. Fosamax® and Miacalcin® nasal spray are gluten-free as of this writing. If you are prone to Barrett's esophagus, Fosamax® may irritate this condition, so check with your doctor if any irritation develops. You should be monitored by your doctor at least annually if you are on any bone-building medication. Also, some doctors do <u>not</u> recommend that you go on bone-building medication until your villi heal so that both the drug <u>and</u> the needed nutrients are absorbed properly. Check with your doctor. The Columbia University Celiac Disease Center suggests waiting a year for the villi to completely heal[114].

Another new bone building medication that just came on the market is Forteo® which is a form of parathyroid hormone or PTH. Some doctors have been waiting to prescribe it because it is so new. The Columbia Celiac Disease Center recommends that blood levels of calcium, PTH and vitamin D should be normal, in addition to urinary excretion of calcium being normal before using this drug. Any hyperparathyroidism must be checked and corrected before taking this medication. Also, as with Fosamax®, they suggest waiting until the villi completely heal before starting this medication.[114]

Strictly following the diet may greatly improve your bone density, and there is a chance that some people may not need medication to build bone, especially if osteoporosis is not severe. In some cases the body may restore it on its own. After 6 months to a year you should evaluate your situation with your doctor, and if medication is needed decide together what is best for you.

For other people with very severe osteoporosis, your doctor may feel that waiting may not be an option. As discussed in previous sections of this book, bone fractures from osteoporosis can be serious and painful, so you should try to avoid that complication. If your bone density is extremely low, you may have to start some bone building right away to avoid any bone breakage, depending on your physician's advice. Check with your doctor to find out what is best for you.

Also, check with your doctor about vitamin/mineral supplements. Your doctor may test your vitamin levels in your blood to see if additional supplements are needed. In some cases additional vitamins are only needed for a short time, because as your body heals they will be absorbed more normally. If your doctor believes that you may have problems with your spleen, Dr. Peter Green recommends that you get a pneumovax (inoculation for pneumonia). Patients with spleen dysfunction are more susceptible to pneumonia.[114] (More information may be found on the Columbia University Celiac Disease Center website: www.celiacdiseasecenter.columbia.edu). Note: you may get pneumonia-like symptoms for a few days after the inoculation. You may want to schedule the shot during a time when you know you are able to get proper rest and can deal with this possible reaction.

After your first year on the diet, annual check-ups are important to maintain health. This is to make sure your bones are continuing to get stronger and that your body is absorbing nutrients properly. Annual blood testing for antibodies to gluten may be a good idea to help make sure you are following the diet correctly.

Depending on your age, you may also want to have your gastroenterologist do an initial colonoscopy to have a baseline to check for polyps (which may be a pre-cancerous condition). Polyps are not related to celiac disease, but this test is a part of intestinal health. People usually wait until they are about 50 years old for their first colonoscopy. You may want to get a baseline earlier (in your 40s), especially if you have had intestinal problems or family members with colon cancer. It is possible to have the colonoscopy done at the same time as an endoscopy. The endoscopy looks at the small intestine and the colonoscopy looks at the large intestine.

If you did not have an endoscopy to get your initial celiac diagnosis, your doctor may recommend one to check the health of your small intestine. It is a good idea to obtain a baseline to check against any pre-cancerous condition, since intestinal cancer is a possible complication of celiac disease.

**Note: The endoscopy/small bowel biopsy can only be positive for celiac disease if you are eating gluten.** For this reason, some doctors recommend what they call a gluten-challenge before the test. (Usually this is 4 slices of bread a day for 1 to 3 months before biopsy.) Just be warned that some people may react more severely to gluten after being off it, so a challenge may be difficult. Putting yourself back on gluten for several months is not good for your health if you have celiac disease, but it may be necessary to be sure you are getting the right diagnosis. That is why the <u>preferred</u> method of diagnosis is to get tested <u>before</u> you start the diet.

Some people started the diet because they believed they had celiac disease, received testing but did not go on a gluten-challenge prior to testing, and then falsely believed they no longer had celiac disease. You will have celiac disease your entire life until they find a cure. It is not something you outgrow. If you <u>are</u> following the gluten-free diet, your endoscopy will <u>not</u> show you have celiac disease. You will be normal! <u>A negative test for a person following the diet just shows that you are following the diet correctly.</u>

In a nutshell, here is the "doctoring" I suggest, from what I've learned. Your doctor is your best source for information and care. Use my suggestions as a starting place to begin a conversation with your doctor. If you are having other symptoms that I failed to list, be sure to get them checked.

You may want to make notes from these pages to bring with you to your doctor's appointment.

## Suggested Medical Check-ups[+]

For diagnosis:

1. Blood work for gluten antibodies. The new blood tests are Anti-Tissue Transglutaminase (tTGA) also called tTG (Tissue Transglutaminase), Immunoglobulin A (IgA), and IgA anti-endomysium antibodies (AEA). (In some books you may read that the blood test antibody names are anti-gliadin (AGA), anti-endomysium (EMA), and anti-reticulin (ARA). These are the tests previously used. The older EMA test required the use of monkey esophagus tissue. The tTG test replaced that test so now this tissue does not have to be used.)

2. Small bowel biopsy to confirm the diagnosis of celiac disease, since the blood test is not 100% accurate. Note: Do not go on the gluten-free diet until after your test, or your test will not show whether or not you have celiac disease.

3. Some doctors may do some of the blood tests listed below (points number 1 and 2) before diagnosis, instead of immediately after positive diagnosis.

Immediately after positive diagnosis:

1. Blood work for:

   - vitamin/mineral supplementation needs. Especially for folic acid, calcium, phosphate, iron, magnesium, zinc, vitamins A, $B_{12}$, D, E and K. (Note: an overdose of vitamins A and D may cause liver damage, so you should work with a physician before taking extra vitamins. Liver enzymes should be checked first.)

   - complete metabolic panel (CMP) to check for electrolytes, protein and calcium levels.[115] For patients with diarrhea, potassium and electrolytes should be checked.

   - blood clotting time (Prothrombin time or PT) which may be prolonged due to malabsorption of vitamin K.

   - complete blood cell count (CBC) because many celiac patients are anemic.

   - a platelet count is recommended. (Some celiac patients may have too many blood platelets, and that is something that should be monitored.)[116]

   - blood test for low albumin (protein stores) and abnormally low cholesterol to check for malnutrition.[116]

   - some doctors may check for inflammation. The erythrocyte sedimentation rate (ESR) and a C-Reactive protein (CRP) tests may help evaluate if your symptoms are severe.[115]

   - blood work to check for thyroid dysfunction/parathyroid hormone levels. (This is very important. Some people who seem like they not getting better on the diet may also have thyroid problems that need to be corrected.)

   You may want to ask them to use a "butterfly" needle to make this blood draw easier. It is a thinner needle and they change the tubes on what looks like a long wire away from the arm, instead of at the needle base.

2. Bone Mineral Density/DEXA scan to check for Osteoporosis; preferably the spine and hip. This is very important as studies suggest 90-100% of celiac patients have some bone loss.[18] This is a painless test – a low level type of x-ray. (Note: I do not recommend you have any chiropractic treatments unless you know your bones are strong, in order to avoid bone breakage.)

3. Pneumovax (inoculation for pneumonia) if doctor suspects spleen dysfunction or if you are elderly.

4. A rectal exam. A stool test should be done to check for blood in the stool. Some physicians recommend adults get a colonoscopy to be used as a baseline check for colon cancer, although colon cancer is not a complication of celiac disease.

5. Other tests as recommended, if there are symptoms or complications that need to be monitored.

6. If diarrhea is a problem, discuss whether electrolytes, potassium supplementation, or medication are needed as you heal on the diet.

7. A blood test may be needed to assess liver function[++]. A blood test showing alkaline phosphatase may be prescribed to check bone health and liver function. Kidney function may also need to be checked.

8. A physical exam to check your overall health. Your doctor may check your abdomen for bloated stomach/distention, evidence of weight loss and evidence of muscle atrophy from loss of muscle mass. Blood pressure – including orthostatic hypotension which is a decrease in blood pressure going from seated to standing. A check for a collection of fluids in the arms and legs (peripheral edema). Examine your body for bruising and also dermatitis herpetiformis (rash caused by celiac disease). Check the mouth for glossitis (inflammation of the tongue/mouth ulcers) and cheilosis (reddened cracked lips most often in the corners of the mouth). Evidence of hypocalcemia by tapping an area on the face (Chvostek's sign) and when checking blood pressure if a spasm is seen (Trousseau's sign).[116]

One to Several months after diagnosis

1. Talk to your family about getting tested, as celiac disease runs in families. Recent studies suggest 1 in 22 first degree relatives and 1 in 39 second degree relatives have celiac disease[2]. Family members may also want to consider the gene test. It is more expensive, but if they have the gene for celiac disease they may get it sometime in their lifetime (Usually after an event like puberty, surgery, illness, pregnancy, menopause, etc.) If they don't have the gene, they will never get celiac disease.

2. If diarrhea persists, be monitored by your doctor. It may take time to clear up, but it may cause dehydration which can be serious. If it is not getting better you may need to be checked for pancreatic insufficiency as that may cause diarrhea or steatorrhea (malabsorption of fat).

3. If irritated bowel symptoms persist, get a breath test for possible bacterial overgrowth. Your doctor may want to wait to do this test until your intestines are healing.

4. If you are taking medications such as those for thyroid, hormones, seizures, or drugs that depend on absorption or weight, you may need to be monitored by your doctor. As you heal, your absorption will change. This may need to be ongoing the first year you are on the diet. Many people have found that their doses were reduced because as they healed they absorbed the medications better. Other people have found that some medications were no longer needed once they completely healed.

5. If high-level vitamins were prescribed, these may have to be adjusted/lowered as you are healing. The malabsorption issues should resolve as your intestines heal on the diet, so you most likely will not be taking high levels of vitamins for a long-term.

Six months to a year after diagnosis:

1. Blood work for gluten antibodies to make sure you're following the diet properly. Most doctors prescribe another tTG blood test. If you have other autoimmune conditions like Type 1 Diabetes or Hashimoto's thyroiditis, your doctor may also order an Anti-gliadin IgA (AGA-IgA) test along with the tTG. This is because sometimes the

coinciding autoimmune disorder may cause a false positive in the tTG and they want to be sure you're following the diet properly.

2. Follow-up on those with medications in which dosages may need to be changed because of better intestinal absorption. This may be ongoing the first year. (See point #4 above.)

3. Bone Mineral Density/DEXA scan to ensure bone-building, especially if it was low after diagnosis.

4. If taking bone building medication, check for any possible side-effects. Do not wait to see your doctor if burning of the esophagus is a problem. (Note: some physicians do <u>not</u> recommend starting bone building medication until your intestines are healed on the diet. See section on malabsorption/osteoporosis. Many experts suggest waiting a year, so that the body can absorb the medication and nutrients properly.)

5. Blood work to make sure vitamin/mineral absorption is normal again and to adjust vitamins if necessary.

6. For children, growth development should be checked periodically.

<u>Thereafter: Annual Check-ups</u>

1. Many physicians suggest annual blood work to check for gluten antibodies. This is to make sure that you are staying on the diet and no other complications result.

2. Follow-up on bone building, and Bone Mineral Density/DEXA testing as needed. Some physicians recommend annual bone density tests until bone returns to normal. For patients with normal bone, testing every few years is recommended. Check for possible side-effects to any bone-building medication that you may be taking.

3. Some physicians suggest a cholesterol blood screening. Celiac patients may have cholesterol levels that are too low before starting the diet. After being on the diet the levels usually become normal. But for some patients cholesterol levels could possibly become high, so it is a good idea to have them checked. If it is high, some doctors are recommending time-released niacin (vitamin B) to help lower cholesterol levels. You may want to discuss this with your doctor to see if niacin will lower your levels enough so cholesterol-reducing medications are not needed.

4. Depending on results of colonoscopy, if polyps are found and removed, usually another colonoscopy every 3 to 5 years is recommended by your doctor. Colon polyps are <u>not</u> related to celiac disease but this check is part of good intestinal health.

5. Some doctors recommend <u>one</u> follow-up small bowel biopsy to confirm response and normal digestion. If your small bowel was very damaged at diagnosis, this may be a good idea to see how it is healing. Many doctors do not redo the biopsy if you are doing well on the diet and other tests are normal.

6. Some doctors recommend a good physical exam every year.

As you can see, the other good news is that you will need less and less "doctoring" if you stick with the diet. Following the diet not only can make you feel better, but also can give you more energy and a normal life span. It is worth it!

+Note: I am not a physician and these are suggestions only. I created this list to be used to facilitate conversations with your doctor, regarding the care you need. Because symptoms may vary, the care you may need may vary. Also, you may have other problems concurrently with celiac disease, and appropriate care for those situations will not be listed here.

++Be aware that a test for long term alcohol abuse called Carbohydrate-deficient transferrin (CDT) may be elevated if you have untreated celiac disease. Doctors in Italy found that elevated tTG values were associated with increased CDT levels, and CDT tests should not be used in celiacs patients to authorize the return of a driver's license. [117] Note: Heavy drinking can be much more dangerous for celiacs. Many have elevated liver enzymes and liver problems than those in the general population.

# Final Thoughts – Possible Weight Loss or Weight Gain

The diet is working and you feel great. You've got more energy than you've ever had in your life. Your bones are getting stronger. Maybe you had hair loss and that's stopped. Maybe you experienced gastrointestinal symptoms and now they're gone. You feel better. You're glad that you're gaining weight for the first time in your life. You look better. You're adjusting to the changes you've made in your diet, but there is one more adjustment that maybe you didn't think about.

You're normal now. Yes, you're normal! You will have a normal life span. You've lowered your cancer risk by staying on the diet for life. But now you're normal in another way. You may be gaining weight and you don't know how to stop... This doesn't happen to all celiac patients, but it may happen to some. You may be one of those people who were painfully thin and never "dieted" before in your life to lose weight. Maybe you're used to eating anything and everything, and maybe in amounts larger than most people would eat. So being normal may mean this has changed too.

Your body probably believed it was in "starvation mode" for years, and it may be still trying to grab all of the calories it can from every ounce of food that you eat. It may take some time for your body to adjust to your new healthy gut, and so be patient. If you find that you are gaining weight, don't be tempted to cheat on your diet thinking that this will help you lose weight. You will damage your body and suffer the consequences. Cheating may also make your body think it is in starvation mode again and make it to store up more reserves in the body, which would not help you to maintain a healthy weight. Instead, readjust you thinking so that you will eat normal portion sizes. Keep in mind that normal portion sizes are not "super-sized" portions of the typical fast-food diet. Normal portions are small in comparison (check out the standard-sized portions on the U.S. Food Pyramid chart on the internet, if you need guidance).

> *Important Note: Some people with celiac disease are painfully thin before diagnosis, but others are <u>not</u> thin at all. Most doctors believe that celiac disease is a disease of thin people, but that is not always the case. In fact, some undiagnosed celiac patients are overweight[118] Many overweight celiac patients lose weight on the gluten-free diet, especially those with Hashimoto's thyroiditis and hypoglycemia. These two conditions usually improve with the diet. For other overweight people, malabsorption causes them to crave foods as their body signals them to overeat in an attempt to try to get those missing nutrients. Once they remain gluten-free their body no longer craves the nutrients because they are being absorbed normally. Other overweight people who get diagnosed but cheat on the gluten-free diet don't lose weight until after they stop cheating. This is because constantly going from "starvation mode" to "healing mode" creates the yo-yo diet effect where your body stores every calorie it can, so that it can survive the "starvation" periods. As they remain gluten-free the body realizes it is no longer starving and adjusts, and many overweight people are able to lose weight for the first time in their lives.*

<u>My Husband's Experience:</u>
My husband experienced this transition from "starvation mode" to normal when he first started the diet. Before he started the gluten-free diet, he was very thin and could eat everything in sight without gaining an ounce. However after starting the diet, he was thrilled to discover that he began to gain weight. He had tried to gain weight his whole life and now it was happening! He also found that he had a lot more energy and he wasn't tired as much as before – he felt that this was great! He gained 15 pounds and he looked so much better...but the weight gain didn't stop there. Before he knew it, he gained another 15 pounds. He looked even better, and was happy

with his weight – he felt good. He finally was at a healthier normal weight! I loved the way he looked too. But to his surprise, he didn't stop gaining weight and gained another 15 pounds. Panic nearly set in as he realized he was "normal" and was gaining weight like everyone else. He didn't know what to do, since this was something totally new for him.

Other than the fact that the food was gluten-free, he felt like he was eating normal portion sizes – but in reality, he was eating "super-sized" portions of food. His body was used to eating large quantities of food to get the nutrition it needed with a damaged gut. For example, before diagnosis, for a brunch on Saturday morning my husband would sometimes eat <u>eight</u> pieces of French toast with butter and syrup because he liked it so much! He finally came to the realization that his body was different now. There were some great benefits to the diet, including his new found energy. But he decided to try to lose the last 15 pounds and needed to find a sensible way to do it that could become part of his everyday lifestyle. Since he never ever tried to lose weight in his life, he was at a loss as to what to do and where to start. This was something that he really wanted to do, but how? Where to begin?

He eventually succeeded, but first, he had to learn to cut his portion sizes. He used to eat several cups of cooked rice and fill up his entire plate with it in a large mound and then top it with the main course. His plate looked like it was for a family of four. He had to re-adjust his thinking back to what a normal portion size was. He now eats a satisfying meal, but he realizes that he doesn't have to feel like he can't eat another bite before he stops – his body gets the proper nutrition from a normal size portion. He also learned that he doesn't need to "graze" during the day; he just eats three good meals a day and he is satisfied. He also realized that the Fosamax® he was taking for a brief amount of time was causing burning in his esophagus and made him overeat to ease the pain. His doctor stopped that medication and the irritation went away. In his case, by carefully following the diet, his bone density became normal without using Fosamax® or any other prescription medications.

Next, he cut down on the high calorie gluten-free breads and switched to lower calorie ones. He learned to make better choices, because some (not all) gluten-free substitutes are very fattening, especially those made with a lot of high-calorie potato starch in them. Some brands of gluten-free products are very high in fat, and have more calories than their gluten counterparts.

Initially, my husband ate 2 to 3 slices of bread at every meal. Now he varies his diet more, and doesn't eat as much bread at each meal. He does enjoy the bread and other mixes I developed for GFN Foods™/Gluten-Free Naturals™, as well as the baked goods I developed for this book, but he takes care not to overdo it. He also doesn't eat the high calorie rice breads that we initially tried.

So, in the end my husband lost that last 15 pounds without really adding another diet on top of his gluten-free diet. He simply learned to re-adjust his approach to mealtimes and eat normally. This was a practical approach to losing the excess weight that he could continue his whole life. The weight came off slowly and he naturally leveled off at his ideal weight. I'm sure that most people would agree that this is the best approach to weight loss and you may need to do something similar as your body adapts to becoming normal and healthy now that you are on the gluten-free diet.

<u>More Suggestions for Healthy Weight Loss:</u>
Other suggestions that helped my husband reach and maintain a healthy weight are described below:

- For breakfast, instead of two slices of toast in the morning, perhaps try 1 slice and add a protein like cheese or peanut butter. Or try a sliced apple with a little peanut butter or cheese with your coffee and juice instead of bread. Have a plain yogurt with jam and fruit mixed in. Have some eggs. Have a bowl of cooked grits instead of rice bread.

- Instead of eating a lot of white rice at meals, try brown rice which contains more fiber and will metabolize more slowly than white rice and not cause sugar levels to spike as quickly. The fiber also makes it more filling and satisfying.

- Try Gluten-Free Naturals™ Multigrain bread or Sandwich Bread, which has fiber so you won't be hungry as quickly … and the fiber is not irritating to most people, unlike bean flours and some other breads containing fiber. The breads I developed are delicious and not as high in calories like some of the other loaves of bread, and especially those found in other books. Here's why they are lower in calories:

    - A normal loaf of bread would have 3 to 4 cups of flour at 455 calories per cup. You'd get at least 15 slices out of a 3-cup loaf or at least 20 out of a 4-cup loaf. For many of the breads I developed in this book, this is the case. The same is true for the breads I developed for GFN Foods™ which yields 16 to 22 slices per loaf. However, for many of the gluten-free rice yeast breads (especially those in other cookbooks), they contain even more flour and in some cases you can't cut the slices very thinly because rice is more grainy and crumbly. If it contains dense potato starch you've added over 900 calories per cup, which is why I don't use very much in any of my recipes. Rice flour is also higher in calories at 560 per cup, adding an extra 105 calories per cup of flour in the recipe.
    - A wheat bread may not contain eggs but if it does, it would probably be one or two eggs. Gluten-free breads usually contain three eggs or more to hold them together. (You can use egg whites or fewer eggs to lower calories.)
    - Some recipes in other cookbooks call for whole milk powder, which adds even more calories. Some use baby formula powder which is even higher calories than whole milk powder. Many recipes use a cup of milk powder, which equals three cups of milk! A third cup of milk powder equals one cup of milk. I use a third cup skim milk powder or I use low fat milk or water in the recipe.
    - A wheat bread would have about 2 Tablespoons of fat per loaf. Some gluten-free bread recipes contain a lot more to try to keep them moist. Many recipes have double or triple that amount.
    - The white rice breads are low fiber and low in protein, which causes hunger to return quickly. So you tend to eat more of them.

- For a change of pace, try some of my quick breads. Just remember that they have calories too and "normal" people would eat one muffin or maybe two, instead of three or four. Just don't overdo it. Instead of having several muffins, try a muffin with a boiled egg for an on-the-go breakfast.

- Watch your desserts. Most "normal" people who are not overweight watch their dessert intake. My husband would eat a small loaf of my banana bread (one third of a full-sized loaf) or several muffins for breakfast. Later he would eat cookies for dessert at lunch and dessert at dinner, and maybe eat a snack of candy during the day. Most "normal" people can't do that every day. You can do it sometimes but as you see your weight rise, cut back on the desserts the next few days so your weight goes back down. Use a 3-

pound weight-gain limit as a warning sign to cut back and skip having so many desserts for a few days. Try one dessert or sweet a day instead of three or more sweets. Have what you like and enjoy it, but don't go overboard. If you want the banana bread in the morning that's fine but have an amount that would be about one or two slices. If your weight is rising too much, don't have dessert at every meal.

- Try adding walking to your schedule. One summer I did a 20-minute walk 5 days a week, I didn't change my eating habits and I lost 5 pounds in 2 months. Walking is the best exercise to build your bones (they call it weight bearing exercise), and you'll stay in shape. My husband's doctor recommended at least 20 minutes a day, 5 days a week to help keep bones strong.

  *Note: Always see your doctor before starting an exercise program. Your doctor knows what is best for your situation. For those with weak bones, more strenuous exercises like jogging, weight lifting, or even some bending exercises could potentially break bones. Falls could be an issue until you heal and your bones strengthen. Your doctor may recommend a book such as "Walk Tall, an exercise program for the prevention and treatment of osteoporosis" by Sara Meeks, PT, GCS. This book helps you learn the proper exercises that you may be able to do if your bone mineral density is low. We located this book in our local library, and found it very helpful.*

- For my husband, by eliminating the bread in the morning and replacing it with an apple, and by adding a 20-minute walk 5 days a week, he lost the 15 pounds in a few months. He says it was easy. He still has some desserts and still enjoys a good size lunch and dinner. On weekends he enjoys snacks and special breakfasts (like a ½ of batch of Gluten-Free Naturals™ pancakes for breakfast, or for a snack maybe a bowl of popcorn, or some desserts in the evening), and then during the week he follows this routine and it works for him. His doctor is happy with his weight and how his bones have gotten stronger. He's healthier, he looks great, and most of all he feels great. You can do it too!

- Lastly, try my recipes. Unlike a lot of cookbooks with main courses with lots of extra cheese, extra butter, lots of cans of soup (which are high in calories and sodium), and lots of prepared things that are high in calories and fats, my recipes were created to be good for you, delicious and easy to make. One day I sat down and calculated the calories of some of my recipes and compared them to wheat-filled mixes. Mine were lower in calories than the wheat-filled boxed kind, and I think they are so much more delicious. What can be better than real homemade? Many of my recipes are just as easy as many gluten-filled box mixes. Also, most gluten-filled mixes already include fats in the mix, and then you add additional oil, and my recipes don't have extra hidden fats. Products like Bisquick® not only contain gluten but are particularly high in calories and fat. A cup is over 1,000 calories!

  *Note: If you want the convenience of a mix, I suggest trying the GFN Foods™ mixes. They are not higher calories than their wheat counterparts, like some other brands, and I think they taste better too. The gluten taste testers preferred GFN® Foods' brownies to Duncan-Hines® and Pillsbury® brands! GFN Foods' brownies also do not contain all of the chemicals and added fats found in these brands. They are a way to enjoy an easy to prepare, delicious dessert. Also, unlike some other mixes they are lower in fat and have no trans-fats.*

- Another way to watch your weight is to bring your own food to restaurants. Most restaurant foods have so much unnecessary added butter or cream. (For example, cream sauces in restaurants are made from whole cream, not milk and gluten-free flour.) Recently for a wedding, I prepared some gluten-free meals for my husband and another guest. I called ahead and got the menu, so their meals looked the same as everyone else's, but with three big differences. Their meals were gluten-free, better tasting, and less fattening than the restaurant meals. Many restaurants use frozen items for banquets and they are loaded with extra calories to keep them fresh tasting. Everyone at our table wanted my husband's meal and some teenagers sitting near my husband were hoping to get his leftovers!

*Note: Many restaurants will heat your gluten-free food for you. At the wedding reception, I explained to the manager what was needed. He set up their plates and covered them with plastic wrap. They heated the food in the microwave, and brought them to the table covered with wrap to ensure no contamination or mix-ups. They uncovered the food at the table and their food was the perfect temperature.*

Even if you just ordered a broiled steak in a restaurant, keep this example in mind. A family friend used to own a restaurant and told us how he prepared a juicy steak for his customers. When a person placed their order, he would remove the steak from the freezer and put it in a deep fryer to thaw it. Then he broiled it. Can you imagine how many calories were added with the deep-frying? It had to be a lot, and would be something you'd never do at home. Restaurants may use cheaper, less healthful fats too. Fats make things taste good and keep foods juicy and moist, but I think restaurants often go overboard. In my opinion, higher calorie restaurant food is probably a major reason why Americans are getting heavier than ever before.

This deep fryer example is also another reason to be cautious at restaurants. You can get gluten-contamination from frying in fat where gluten-containing items were fried. You also have to be cautious about other additives to meats like tenderizers, marinades, and fats. I have had a restaurant hamburger where they put a large piece of gluten-containing margarine with herbs and spices in the middle of the patty to make it juicy before frying. This is something to beware of for both the gluten-free and the casein-free diet. Bringing your own is not only safer but less fattening.

So try my recipes. You won't be deprived and you won't be denied. You'll eat better, feel healthier and you won't have all the added unhealthful extra fats in your diet. What to try first? Pick a favorite, and if you find more than one recipe listed for it in this book, I suggest you try the first one I've listed. Usually the first one listed is our favorite; maybe it will be yours too.

---

*Enjoy all of the good food waiting for you in the pages that follow...*

*Now you know all about celiac disease, so let's get to the recipes!*

## Appetizers, Pickles, and Relishes

### Antipasto – Authentic Italian Style

The antipasto of my great-grandmother, grandmother and my mother consisted of many dishes including cheese, meats, fish and vegetables. I've listed the typical foods they would serve. I've revised the list to make it gluten-free. See list at the back of this book for some safe brands to use.

1. One or two thinly sliced meats like gluten-free ham* or gluten-free pepperoni*.
2. A wedge of well aged provolone cheese. (Most are gluten-free, but check ingredients.)
3. A can of white, firm gluten-free tuna*, centered on a round platter and surrounded with Italian tomato salad (see index for recipe).
4. Stuffed celery. Wash tender stalks of celery. Soften some gluten-free cream cheese* and add some chopped chives to taste. Blend well and stuff celery.
5. Deviled eggs (see index for recipe). If desired, garnished with anchovy paste or pimiento strips. Roasted red peppers* (see index for recipe), may also be used as a garnish.
6. A bowl of Caponata (see index for recipe).
7. Pickled vegetables like eggplant, red peppers, artichoke hearts or mushrooms (see index). You can marinade canned artichoke hearts packed in water (drained) the same as the pickled mushrooms recipe. Use less salt if they contain salt.
8. Roasted peppers (see index for recipe) topped with anchovies (optional). I often just put out the roasted peppers* you can buy in a jar. Check the labels, most are gluten-free.
9. Black olives* or Kalamata olives* or pimento stuffed Spanish green olives*. Black are my favorite.
10. Stuffed and baked mushrooms (see index for recipe).
11. Gluten-free bread or breadsticks (optional, see index for recipe).

### Artichoke Heart Dip

This recipe is from my sister. She brought it to a party and everyone devoured it.

| | |
|---|---|
| 1 can artichoke hearts in water (Be sure to check labels) | 1 cup gluten-free mayonnaise* |
| 2 to 3 minced jalapeno peppers or gluten-free ones from a jar (optional) | 1 cup grated gluten-free Swiss cheese (Most are gluten-free, check labels) |
| | 1 cup Parmesan cheese* |

Drain artichokes and chop in a food processor or blender (I use a food processor.) Add 2 to 3 minced jalapeno peppers or gluten-free ones from a jar. (You can also mince the peppers in the food processor.) Remove to a bowl. Add the mayonnaise, the Swiss cheese (grated) and the Parmesan cheese. Blend all and put in a small shallow baking dish. Bake at 350°F for 15 to 20 minutes.

My sister puts it together the night before and refrigerates it, and bakes it the day of the party. Serve with gluten-free rice crackers* or regular gluten-free potato chips*.

*see gluten-free products list at the end of the book

## Bean Dip (Easy)

This recipe is from my friend.  Makes a hot dip that is nice served at parties.

1 recipe refried black beans (see index) or one can gluten-free refried beans*

1 (8 ounce) package gluten-free cream cheese*, softened

1 cup gluten-free salsa* (or see index for recipe)

1 cup gluten-free grated cheddar cheese

Blend refried beans and cream cheese.  Spread into a bottom of a greased pie plate.  Top with the salsa and the cheddar cheese.  Heat in the microwave until cheese melts or heat in the oven at 350°F for 30 minutes.  Serve with gluten-free tortilla chips* (or see index for recipe).

*Variation*:  This dip can be made without the refried beans, and it is also delicious.

## Breadless Sandwiches

My mother came up with this idea for people on the Atkins® diet, and it's good for celiac patients too.

Wash, clean, and dry some Napa Cabbage.  Use the inner, tender leaves.  Cut with a kitchen scissors to make a top and bottom in the size for mini sandwiches.  Fill with a filling of your choice.  It adds crunch to your filling, so no lettuce is needed.  It holds up well too.  This cabbage is also good raw in salads.  It's good for full-size sandwiches by using a whole leaf for each slice of bread.  It is low calorie and gluten-free.

## Buffalo Wings

This recipe comes from Frank's® Red Hot, which is gluten-free as of this writing.  For wings that are less hot and spicy, use ½ cup gluten-free margarine* and ⅓ cup of the hot sauce* instead of what is listed below.

2 ½ to 3 pounds chicken wings
½ cup of Frank's® Red Hot Sauce*
⅓ cup gluten-free margarine*

Gluten-free blue cheese salad dressing (see index) or gluten-free ranch dressing* (see index)
Celery sticks

Split the chicken wings and discard the tips.  Bake wings for 20 minutes at 425°F.  Turn them over and bake them about 25 minutes more until they are fully cooked and crispy.

Or, instead of baking the wings, deep fry them for about 12 minutes at 400°F in a fryer until crispy.  Drain on paper towels.  (Frying makes them more delicious, but adds fat which is why I bake them.)

Melt the margarine in a pot or in the microwave using the defrost cycle.  Blend in the hot sauce.  Dip the wings in the hot sauce and completely coat them.  Serve them with the dressing and celery sticks.

*see gluten-free products list at the end of the book

## Caponata

I like to make this in the summer when eggplants are plentiful at the farmer's market. I use it as part of an Antipasto (see index). This is an authentic Italian recipe from my mother. (Note: one time I peeled the eggplant and it wasn't as good, so I don't recommend peeling the eggplant for this recipe.) This does make a lot of food, so you may want to make half of the recipe.

1 ½ lbs. unpeeled eggplant
3 stalks celery
1 large onion
1 clove garlic, peeled
1 (16 oz.) can gluten-free tomato sauce*
1 cup water (½ can water)
½ cup oil, divided (I use olive oil)
1 ½ teaspoons salt

⅛ teaspoon ground black pepper
½ of a (5 ¼ oz.) jar of pimento stuffed
    Spanish olives*
½ cup wine vinegar
¼ cup sugar
2 Tablespoons rinsed capers* (optional, I
    don't use)

Wash, dry, and dice unpeeled eggplant into a ¾ inch dice. Heat large skillet, and add 6 tablespoons oil and heat. Add cubed eggplant to skillet and fry at medium heat, stirring from time to time until eggplant softens a little and oil is all absorbed. Set aside.

In a saucepan, heat the remaining 2 tablespoons of oil and sauté garlic until lightly browned. Turn off heat, cool. Press the garlic with a fork to release its flavor, then remove garlic from the pan and discard. Chop the onion, wash and remove the strings from the celery with a potato peeler. Slice the celery into ⅓ inch slices. Now add onions to pan and sauté a few minutes. Add celery, tomato sauce, water, salt and pepper and simmer covered for 10 minutes. Remove cover and add the eggplant, vinegar and sugar and simmer slowly until mixture thickens and vegetables are tender. Remove from heat and add the olives and capers (if using them).

Mix all together and place in narrow mouthed jars. Pack the Caponata down into the jars leaving no air spaces and pour a little oil on top to seal. This will help preserve the relish for up to 2 weeks. Cool and refrigerate. (Or vacuum package in a canning jar with a FoodSaver® and refrigerate. Put it in the coldest part of your refrigerator and it will keep another week or so. If you plan to give it as gifts, just be sure to tell people you didn't follow procedures to can it so it must be refrigerated and it must be used soon.)

When ready to serve, pour off the excess oil and save the oil to pour back on top again if needed. Makes 8 cups. This is delicious as part of an antipasto salad or as a relish with carne alla pizziola (see index).

*see gluten-free products list at the end of the book

## Chex® Party Mix

Now that Rice Chex® and Corn Chex® are gluten-free, here is a way to have Chex® Party Mix again. Since gluten-free pretzels are very expensive and only come in a small bag, this is a way to stretch them further and enjoy them longer as a snack. I added the rice crackers to take the place of the bagel chips in the original recipe, but they are not necessary.

6 Tablespoons butter or gluten-free margarine*

2 Tablespoons gluten-free Worcestershire sauce*

1 ½ teaspoons seasoned salt* (I use Season-All® which is gluten-free as of this writing)

¾ teaspoon garlic powder

½ teaspoon onion powder

9 cups Rice Chex® cereal (or use half Rice Chex® and half Corn Chex®)

1 cup mixed nuts

1 cup gluten-free pretzels* (optional)

1 cup gluten-free rice crackers*, broken into 1 inch pieces (optional; gluten-free plain or sesame or other flavors may be used.)

In a small microwave safe bowl, microwave the butter or margarine on high for 40 to 50 seconds until melted. Or use the defrost cycle and microwave for about 1 minute. Stir in the seasonings.

In a large microwave safe bowl, blend together the cereal, nuts, gluten-free pretzels and gluten-free rice crackers. Drizzle the butter mixture over them and blend in. Microwave it for 5 to 6 minutes, stirring after every 2 minutes. Spread on paper towels to cool. Once completely cooled, store in an airtight container so that the cereal stays crisp.

*Variation:* I often make this with just the cereal and nuts. Sprinkle it on salads instead of croutons. It is crunchy and flavorful.

## Chicken Nugget Appetizer

See index and prepare the "Chicken Nuggets" recipe in the Main Dish section. Serve with the Easy Apricot Sauce recipe (see index) or with some warm barbecue sauce (see Barbecue sauce recipe). You can make the nuggets and the sauce ahead of time. Reheat the chicken in a 350°F oven for 5-8 minutes just before serving.

*see gluten-free products list at the end of the book

## Chicken Wings or Chicken Strips Mandarin

You can coat and fry the wings ahead of time, and the next day prepare the sauce and bake. For a crispy chicken main dish, fry chicken strips, drain on paper towels, dip in the sauce and serve with remaining sauce.

15 to 18 chicken wings or 1 ½ to 2
   pounds skinless boneless chicken
   breasts sliced into strips
1 cup cornstarch
2 eggs, well beaten
Generous sprinkling of salt, MSG*
   (optional), and garlic powder
Dash or two of milk (or milk substitute)
   to make the batter the right consistency

¾ cup sugar
½ cup cider or wine vinegar
Several drops of gluten-free soy sauce*
¼ to ½ teaspoon gluten-free ketchup*
¼ cup water
1 Tablespoon cornstarch

Cut wings into 3 sections at joint. Discard the wing tips. Push the meat to one end of each of the bones. They should look like small drumsticks. If using boneless skinless chicken breasts, cut into strips using poultry scissors or a sharp knife. Now mix together the cornstarch, eggs and seasonings. Add enough milk to make a batter of medium consistency. Coat the wings and fry in deep hot oil. Drain well on paper towels.

When ready to serve, combine the sugar, vinegar, soy sauce and ketchup. Mix the water and the cornstarch and blend in. Cook the mixture over medium heat until it comes to a boil. Dip the fried wings in the sauce and place on an oblong pan. Pour remaining sauce over the top of them. Bake in a 350°F oven for 30 minutes for chicken wings. Baste and turn frequently. Good for an appetizer or a main dish.

For chicken strips, dip them in the sauce and serve with rice. Pour remaining sauce over-top or use as a dipping sauce. It's just like General's chicken that you get in restaurants. If you wanted to bake with sauce as above for an appetizer, bake only for 10 minutes or your chicken will dry out and be tough.

*Variation*: The chicken strips are very crunchy, but don't have much flavor without the sauce. For variation, add additional spices or add some Season-All®* or Adobo®* to the batter. Serve with a dip below or use honey as a dip.

Apricot Dipping Sauce – Blend together the following:
   ½ cup gluten-free Apricot jam       1 Tablespoon lemon or orange juice

Hot Mustard Dipping Sauce – Blend together the following:
   3 Tablespoons gluten-free dry mustard*    1 Tablespoon wine vinegar
   2 Tablespoons water

Sweet and Sour Plum Sauce – Blend together the following:
   ½ cup gluten-free plum jelly or jam     1 Tablespoon wine vinegar
   1 Tablespoon gluten-free ketchup*

*see gluten-free products list at the end of the book

## Chili Dip (Easy)

This is an easy recipe from Philadelphia® Brand Cream Cheese, which is gluten-free as of this writing.

1 package gluten-free cream cheese*
1 can Hormel® chili* with beans (it is gluten-free as of this writing. Note: check labels because Hormel® chili without beans contains gluten as of this writing.)
Grated cheddar cheese*
Tortilla chips* (or see index for recipe)

Unwrap the package of cream cheese. Place cream cheese in a microwave safe dish. If desired, spread it to cover the bottom of the dish. Open can of Hormel® chili. Pour chili over cream cheese to cover. Top with grated cheddar cheese. Microwave until cheddar cheese is melted and dip is hot. Serve with tortilla chips.

## Chutney – Nectarine or Peach Version

This is my mother's recipe, and was always gluten-free. There are some brands of gluten-free chutney available in jars that are also good (see list at the end of this book). I enjoy this recipe and make it in the summer when fresh fruit is available from the farmer's market. Just be sure not to use over-ripe fruit or it won't turn out.

1 cup firmly packed light brown sugar
½ cup cider vinegar
4-5 pitted diced unpeeled nectarines (this should measure 2 ½ to 3 cups) or use 2 ½ to 3 cups of peaches. (Note: make sure the peaches are not over-ripe or it won't turn out properly).
1 cup raisins
1 clove garlic, minced
½ lemon, unpeeled and sliced thinly, remove seeds and cut into small pieces
½ teaspoon salt
⅛ teaspoon cayenne pepper
2 ½ Tablespoons finely chopped crystallized ginger, softened in a little hot water to make cutting easier.

If using the peaches, remove the skins first by placing whole peach in hot water and then cold water so the skins will slip off. Peel and dice peaches. Discard pits and skins.

Boil sugar and vinegar in a large pot. Add the diced fruit and all remaining ingredients. Simmer until fruit is cooked and mixture thickens. Cool to room temperature and refrigerate. Serve at room temperature. You can use this chutney in the curried chicken salad. It is also nice served as a condiment with grilled chicken or fish. Chutney can be used as an appetizer. Pour some over a block cream cheese in a dish and serve with gluten-free rice crackers*. Or use leftover chutney in the Chutney Chicken recipe (see index).

## Chutney – Red Pepper and Apricot Version

For best results, dice the pepper and dried apricots into small pieces, about ¼ inch in size. This recipe uses dried fruit instead of fresh so I find it easier to make. Leftover chutney can be used in the Chutney Chicken recipe (see index).

1 large red pepper, diced
1 (6 ounce) package gluten-free dried apricots, diced
½ cup raisins
1 Tablespoon dried minced onion
½ teaspoon garlic powder
½ teaspoon ground ginger
¾ teaspoon salt

½ teaspoon crushed red pepper flakes
¼ to ½ teaspoon cumin (I use ¼ teaspoon)
¼ teaspoon gluten-free dry mustard*
½ cup sugar
6 Tablespoons red wine vinegar

Wash, seed pepper and chop into a ¼ inch dice or chop in a food processor. (Be careful not to over-process if using a food processor.) Chop the dried apricots with a sharp knife on a cutting board. You may find it easier to use poultry scissors. Place all ingredients in a pot. Simmer until fruit is cooked and mixture thickens, about 30 minutes.

Cool to room temperature and refrigerate in a jar. Serve at room temperature. This is nice served as a condiment with grilled chicken or fish. It may also be used as an appetizer by putting some chutney on a block of cream cheese in a dish, and serving it with gluten-free rice crackers.* Or see other suggestions for use in the previous recipe.

## Corn Relish

I like this served at a cookout with hamburgers. This is nice gift to give when you attend a cookout.

1 large onion, chopped
Water
1 cup cider vinegar
10 Tablespoons sugar
¼ teaspoon chili powder
½ to 1 teaspoon gluten-free curry powder*

½ teaspoon turmeric
2 teaspoons celery seed
1 can "niblets" corn (12 oz. size)
2 tender inner stalks of celery
1 red pepper, chopped
1 ½ Tablespoons cornstarch

Chop onion, place in a saucepan and cover with water. Bring to a boil and drain. Place the onion back in the saucepan along with the chopped celery and red pepper. Drain the water from the can of corn and reserve. Add corn and all the other ingredients except the cornstarch and reserved corn liquid. Mix the cornstarch and liquid together and set aside. Cook mixture 10 minutes. Then blend in the cornstarch mixture while stirring until it all comes to a boil and boil a few minutes. Makes 4 cups.

This keeps a long time in the refrigerator, however, if you are planning to give it away as gifts, use sterilized jars and lids and process 10 minutes. This is best served at room temperature.

*see gluten-free products list at the end of the book

## Crab Dip
This is an easy dip to make.

2 (6 ounce) cans gluten-free crabmeat*, drained

1 teaspoon gluten-free mustard*

¼ cup white wine

¾ cup gluten-free mayonnaise*

3 (8 ounce) packages gluten-free cream cheese, softened*

Dash of salt and ground black pepper to taste

Soften cream cheese. Add the rest of the ingredients. Blend with an electric mixer or blend well using a sturdy spoon. Put in an ovenproof dish and bake at 350°F for 15 minutes. Serve warm with fresh vegetables or gluten-free rice crackers.

## Crab or Shrimp Dip (Easy)
I always enjoyed this easy to make dip, even before we ever learned about the gluten-free diet.

1 package gluten-free cream cheese*, softened

1 to 2 cans gluten-free crabmeat* or tiny canned shrimp*, drained

1 bottle gluten-free cocktail sauce*

Spread cream cheese on the bottom of a small attractive bowl. Drain canned fish and pour evenly on top. Top with some of the cocktail sauce. Serve with gluten-free rice crackers* or gluten-free tortilla chips*.

I have also had this dip where you just put a block of the cream cheese on the plate, topped it with the crabmeat, and topped it with the sauce. It's a little messier looking but still delicious.

## Curry Dip
This is my mother's recipe and our favorite vegetable dip. I use leftover dip as a spread on gluten-free chicken breast sandwiches. Even people who say they don't like curry have told me that they really like this.

1 pint (2 cups) gluten-free mayonnaise*

3 Tablespoons gluten-free ketchup*

3 Tablespoons honey

1 ¼ teaspoons gluten-free curry powder*

1 Tablespoon lemon juice

1 Tablespoon grated onion (or use onion flakes moistened with water)

A few dashes of gluten-free hot sauce* or sprinkling of cayenne pepper to taste

Mix all together and serve with raw vegetables. It keeps for several weeks in the refrigerator.

*Variation*: Use up any leftover dip by thinning with a little water and use it as a salad dressing. I like it on a tossed salad containing fresh mushrooms. It is also really good on tomatoes.

Note: I use a little less curry powder when I open a brand-new jar. My mom's favorite type of curry powder is the Madras variety because the flavor is slightly sweet. Curry powder is a blend of spices.  See index for recipe if you want to make your own.  Most brands are gluten-free, but check ingredients to be sure no wheat flour was added to make it free-flowing.  (McCormick® is now gluten-free.)

## Deviled Eggs

These are my mother's recipe and a family favorite.  If you bring them to a party, don't expect to bring home any leftovers.  For a fancy look, fill eggs using a cake decorating bag and large fluted tip.

6 eggs
⅓ cup gluten-free mayonnaise*
Salt and ground black pepper to taste
1 teaspoon grated onion or ¼ teaspoon
   granulated onion powder

1 teaspoon prepared gluten-free mustard*
   or ¼ teaspoon gluten-free dry mustard*
Paprika*
Pimiento strips or tiny shrimp for garnish
   (optional, I don't use)

The secret to making hard boiled eggs that are easy to shell is that you don't use the freshest eggs.  They are still within the selling date, but buy them a week before you plan to boil them.

Place room temperature eggs in a pot and add enough water to cover.  Bring to a boil.  Reduce heat and simmer gently for 20 minutes.  Pour off hot water immediately and add cold water to the pot, shaking the pot to crack the eggs.  Continue pouring in cold tap water until eggs are cool.  Shell eggs.  (Alternatively, you can use the recipe for "Boiled eggs" for another method of cooking your eggs.  That is a good method to use if you find that your yolks have green edges caused by overcooking them.)

Slice in half lengthwise.  Remove yolks and put them in a bowl.  Add the mayonnaise, salt, pepper, onion and mustard to the yolks and blend well.  Fill the egg white hollows and sprinkle with paprika.  Garnish if desired by placing a pimiento strip or shrimp on top.  Small pieces of roasted red pepper may also be used as a garnish.  (Dry your garnish on paper towels before adding.)

## Enchilada Appetizer

This is easy but I think it is a little bit fattening with all of the added sour cream and cheese, so I suggest serving small portions.

1 bag gluten-free tortilla chips* (or see
   index for chip recipe)
1 onion grated (optional) or 1 Tablespoon
   dried minced onion flakes moistened
   with hot water (optional)
1 can Hormel® Chili with beans* (it is
   gluten-free as of this writing.  Note:
   check labels because Hormel® chili

without beans contains gluten as of this
   writing.)
1 (15 ounce) can gluten-free tomato
   sauce* or 2 (8 ounce) cans*
Generous sprinkling chili powder, garlic
   powder and cumin (optional)
1 to 1 ¼ cups gluten-free sour cream*
1 ½ cups gluten-free grated cheddar
   cheese*

Remove ⅓ of the bag of chips and set aside.  Crush the rest of the chips in the bag.  Line the bottom of a rectangular casserole dish with the chips.  Open can of chili and top with that.

*see gluten-free products list at the end of the book

Top with tomato sauce. If you want more of a zing, sprinkle on the spices. Top with ½ cup of cheese. Bake at 375 for 20 minutes. Remove from oven. Top with sour cream and spread to cover. Top with remaining chips and cheese. Bake 5 minutes more. You have to serve this on plates using forks to eat it. Otherwise it's too messy to eat.

## Egg Rolls

I developed this gluten-free Chinese Style egg roll wrap. They are crispy just like the ones at the restaurant on the day you make them. Refrigerate leftovers and reheat them in a toaster oven so that they will be crispy the next day. You don't need any special gluten-free flours to make this. You can use your own egg roll filling or the one I have below.

Pancake Wraps (makes 8):
   4 eggs
   1 ½ cups water

2 Tablespoons oil
½ teaspoon salt
1 ½ cups cornstarch

Blend with a hand blender. Heat a 10 inch iron skillet. (Make sure it is one that is well-seasoned so that they won't stick to the pan.) Use medium high/medium heat. Lightly grease and pour batter into pan until it is covered. Cook until dry on that side and flip with a spatula to cook the other side. When done, remove and stack on a plate until ready to fill.

Chinese Egg Roll Filling:
   ½ cup minced or chopped celery
   1 cup finely shredded cabbage
   2 Tablespoons oil
   ½ cup diced cooked pork, ham or beef
   ½ cup diced cooked or canned shrimp
   ½ cup drained and chopped canned
      bamboo shoots (optional)

½ cup drained and chopped canned water
   chestnuts (optional)
2 scallions, chopped
1 teaspoon salt
½ teaspoon pepper
3 Tablespoons soy sauce*

Put the shredded cabbage and celery in a pot with about ½ cup of boiling water. Cover and cook until it steams and cook for several minutes. Drain in a colander and then put the cabbage/celery mixture in a clean towel and remove the excess moisture.

Heat a fry pan a minute and add the oil. If meat is uncooked, be sure to cook it until done. Add the cabbage and the rest of the filling ingredients. Cook and stir until the mixture is golden color. By using a large fry plan, excess moisture evaporates so the filling will not be too wet. Allow the mixture to cool completely. The secret to this working is to have cool filling.

Place about 4 Tablespoons of the filling (about 1/8th of the filling you made) in the middle of a pancake. Fold in the 2 sides and then roll in into an egg roll and secure it with a toothpick. The toothpick keeps the egg rolls from opening up while frying.

Fry in a deep fryer at about 390°F and fry until golden, which will take about 5 minutes. Or fry in a 10 inch deep skillet with about 2 inches of oil, until golden on all sides. Remove from oil and drain on paper towels. Remove toothpick. Serve with hot mustard or plum sauce or apricot sauce. (See chicken wings appetizer recipe for sauce recipes).

*see gluten-free products list at the end of the book

## Filled New Potatoes
My mother would make these as an appetizer, even before we knew about the gluten-free diet.

Small red new potatoes
Gluten-free sour cream*
Gluten-free bacon*

Boil potatoes until tender. Since they are small they cook more quickly than large potatoes. Drain and cool. Meanwhile, cook bacon until crisp and drain. (I cook bacon in the microwave.) Break bacon into pieces, approximately 1 inch. (I use poultry scissors and cut it.)

Cut potatoes in half and take a tiny slice off the rounded side of each half so that potatoes will be steady when placed into the serving dish. Use a melon baller to scoop out a rounded hole in the center of each potato half. Fill hole with sour cream and top with a piece of bacon. These are colorful and easy to make.

## Herbed Cheese Spread
This reminds me of the herb cheese spreads you can purchase in the gourmet cheese section of your grocery store. Some of those are gluten-free, but this is less expensive and easy to make.

1 to 2 cloves garlic minced (I substitute ⅛ teaspoon garlic powder per clove.)
2 Tablespoons grated Pecorino Romano or Parmesan cheese
1 ½ teaspoons crushed dried basil

¼ teaspoon salt (I use less, since grated cheese can be salty)
Sprinkling of black pepper
1 (8 ounce) package of cream cheese*, softened

If using fresh garlic, mince it in the food processor with the grated cheese and herbs first. Add the cream cheese and whip all ingredients together in a food processor. Add a little less salt and the pepper and whip it in. Taste to see if more salt is needed. Let it whip a few minutes to get some air in the cream cheese and make it a nice consistency.

If using garlic powder instead of fresh garlic, just put all the ingredients in the food processor and whip it together. Let it whip a few minutes to get it a nice consistency.

Spoon the cheese mixture into an attractive crock or bowl. Cover with plastic wrap. This is best made a day ahead of time so that the flavors mellow. Serve it with gluten-free rice crackers.

*Variation*: Try it with 2 to 3 teaspoons dried chopped chives instead of the basil. We use it to make stuffed celery for an appetizer. (Wash and dry tender celery, and then fill with the cheese mixture. Spread it smooth in the celery with a knife.) I use less garlic in the cheese spread when I use it for stuffed celery.

*see gluten-free products list at the end of the book

## Hot Dog Tortilla Wraps

We like hot dogs wrapped in corn tortillas. These are good for an appetizer or for lunch. For the traditional "pigs in a blanket" see index for recipes.

1 package gluten-free hot dogs*
10 gluten-free corn tortillas* (or the amount needed for the hot dogs you have). *Note: Use a fresh package of tortillas. Old tortillas will fall apart.*

American cheese slices* (check ingredients since some cheese foods are not gluten-free)
Gluten-free mustard*

Heat hot dogs in boiling water. Drain the water when they are hot.

Meanwhile, place corn tortillas on a microwave safe plate. Cover with a damp paper towel and microwave for 1 minute on high. This makes corn tortillas pliable.

Place cheese slice on top of each tortilla. Top each with a hot dog. Roll the tortilla and place edge side down on a plate. Complete until all hot dogs are done. For appetizer, carefully cut into small pieces using a sharp knife. Insert a toothpick in each piece, and place on a serving plate. Serve with mustard for dipping. For lunch, serve the hot dogs whole.

*Variation:* Use gluten-free Masa Harina flour to make your own tortillas. Place the hot dogs and cheese inside each tortilla and seal. Fry in a deep fryer until golden. Drain on paper towels. Allow to cool a little because they will be very hot. Serve with gluten-free mustard for dipping.

*Note:* Some brands of paper towels may possibly use a glue containing gluten to seal the ends of the rolls. Do not use the first or last sheets of paper towels on foods. Whether gluten-free or not, you don't want glue on your food.

## Hummus

Most brands of hummus are gluten-free, but here is a way to make your own.

1 (15 ounce) can chickpeas (garbanzo beans) rinsed and drained
½ to 1 teaspoon garlic powder (I use about ¾ tsp.)
½ to 1 teaspoon cumin (I use ½ tsp.)
2 Tablespoons extra virgin olive oil

1 to 2 Tablespoon warm water
2 Tablespoons lemon juice (or to taste)
¼ cup gluten-free tahini, which is ground sesame seed paste
Sprinkling of salt to taste

Blend all in a food processor using the cutting blade. Start with the lower levels of spices and water. Adjust the seasonings and consistency according to your taste and preferences. Process the mixture until smooth. Refrigerate. Serve with corn chips or rice crackers. I also like it as a dip with baby carrots.

*Variation:* Add ¼ of a roasted red pepper before processing, for a different flavor. I use less water when I add some roasted red pepper.

*see gluten-free products list at the end of the book*

*Variation 2*: Sometimes I make my own tahini. Carefully brown sesame seeds by putting them in a pan with a little oil. I heat the pan on medium heat and add the oil. I swirl it around and add the seeds. As soon as the seeds start to sizzle, immediately remove from heat. They will keep cooking in the pan and they will get browner as they cool. Be careful not to overheat, as the seeds burn easily and they cook quickly. Once cool, I put them in a mini food processor and turn them into a paste. I add a little sesame oil to make it a nice consistency and process until smooth.

## Mini-Quiche Appetizers

This makes 24 tiny quiches. You need a non-stick mini muffin pan and a food processor to make this. These are easy to make since you press the dough into the pan. They can be made ahead of time and reheated in a toaster oven.

1 ½ cups Gluten-Free Naturals™ All Purpose Flour or Gluten-Free Naturals™ Sandwich Bread Flour (do not substitute other blends)

Pinch of salt
½ cup butter
2 to 3 Tablespoons cold water

Filling:
1 egg
½ cup chopped ham
½ cup shredded cheese

½ cup milk
⅛ to ¼ teaspoon salt (depending on how salty the ham is)
Additional cheese for top, if desired

Make pie crust by putting the flour, salt and butter in a food processor. Pulse until butter is cut into the flour. Do not over-mix. Add water through the feed tube with processor on and process until the dough balls up and goes to one side. Immediately turn off processor. Divide dough into 24 pieces and press each piece of dough into the bottom and sides of each mini muffin pan cup. (You do not have to grease the pan.)

In the same food processor, add ham, cheese, egg, milk and salt. Pulse until the ham is finely chopped and mixture is well combined. Carefully spoon the mixture into the mini crusts. If desired, top with a little additional cheese. Bake at 350°F for 30 minutes.

## Mushrooms Stuffed with Bread Crumbs

This is my mother's recipe that I converted to make it gluten-free.

12 large mushroom caps
⅔ cup dry bread crumbs made with Gluten-Free Naturals™ Bread, plus seasonings (see index for recipe)
2 Tablespoons Parmesan Cheese

A few dashes of garlic powder or 1 small clove of garlic, minced
3 to 4 Tablespoons oil (preferably olive oil)

Line a baking pan with aluminum foil. Pour a little oil on the foil and spread it over the bottom. (Or use Reynolds® Ready Release foil to save this step). Wash and dry the mushrooms and remove the stem. Cut the stems up into small pieces. Set aside. Mix the bread crumbs, cut up stems, garlic powder and cheese together. Using a fork, add the oil to the crumb mixture a Tablespoon at a time, until all crumbs are thoroughly moistened. Fill the caps generously and place into your prepared pan.  Place the pan on a lower shelf in a pre-heated 350°F oven and bake for 12-15 minutes, or until crumbs are nicely browned.  (By placing the pan on the lower shelf in the oven, the bottom center of your mushrooms cook properly and the crumbs don't get too browned and overdone.)

*Variation*:  I sometimes add some dried parsley to the bread crumb mixture.

## Mushrooms Stuffed with Crabmeat

These are gourmet tasting.  Use caution in purchasing crabmeat; be sure imitation crabmeat was not added to supplement it.  Pure crabmeat is gluten-free, but most imitation crabmeat contains gluten.  For this recipe I use canned crabmeat because I know it is safe.  My husband prefers medium sized mushrooms for this recipe to get more crabmeat taste per bite.

1 pound fresh mushrooms, cleaned
1 can crabmeat* well drained
2 Tablespoons gluten-free mayonnaise*
1 teaspoon egg white powder
½ teaspoon lemon juice
Dash of gluten-free hot sauce* (optional)
Dash of cayenne pepper (optional)
1 Tablespoon fine white rice flour

⅛ teaspoon Old Bay® seasoning (gluten-free as of this writing)
1 ½ teaspoons finely chopped parsley or ½ to 1 teaspoon dried parsley flakes
Sprinkling of salt
¼ cup or more grated mozzarella cheese (optional)

Rinse mushrooms to remove any dirt and dry.  Remove the stems by breaking them off using your fingers.  This creates the hole for the filling.

Drain crabmeat well.  (I clean the lid of the can, open the can, and press the lid firmly into the meat doing it over the sink and drain.  Press in the middle of the lid so as not to cut yourself.)  Put the crabmeat in a small bowl and combine with all the rest of the ingredients and blend.  If you are not using the mozzarella cheese, sprinkle in some additional salt.

Fill mushroom caps with mixture using a spoon.  Place in a 12"x 9"x 2" inch baking pan.  (I prefer a non-stick baking pan.)  Bake mushrooms at 350°F for 20 minutes or until cooked through.

## Mushrooms Stuffed with Sausage

This is a tasty gourmet appetizer.  We prefer using large size mushrooms for this recipe.  Many brands of sausage are gluten-free but if you can't find one, you can make your own bulk sausage using the recipe in this book (see index).

1 pound of gluten-free sweet Italian sausage with casing removed* or bulk sausage* (see list at end of book) or substitute ground pork adding spices like garlic powder, onion powder, salt, ground black pepper, oregano, basil, fennel seed, sage, and chili powder.
1 lb. fresh mushrooms (I choose large ones because they're easier to stuff)

1 clove of garlic, minced or ¼ teaspoon granulated garlic
2 Tablespoons chopped parsley
1 ½ cups (6 oz.) of shredded cheddar cheese or gluten-free mozzarella cheese*
Chopped pimiento or roasted red pepper* (optional, I don't use)

*see gluten-free products list at the end of the book

Rinse mushrooms to remove any dirt and dry. Remove stems and chop them fine. Combine stems, sausage, garlic, and parsley in a skillet. Cook until sausage is browned, stirring frequently. Drain pan drippings. Stir in cheese, mixing well. Fill mushroom caps with sausage mixture. Place in a 12 x 9 x 2 inch baking pan. (I prefer the non-stick type baking pan.) Bake at 350°F for 20 minutes. Garnish with pimiento or roasted red pepper if desired.

## Mushrooms Stuffed with Spinach (also called Stuffed Mushrooms Florentine)
This is another gourmet appetizer.

1 lb. fresh mushrooms (choose large mushrooms)
1 Tablespoon dried minced onion, soaked in a little water to soften
1 clove garlic, minced or ¼ teaspoon granulated garlic or garlic powder
1 package of frozen spinach, thawed
1 roasted red pepper*, chopped (see index or use the kind in the jar) or use a fresh red pepper, and chop and sauté it

¼ teaspoon lemon juice
Salt and ground black pepper to taste
Sprinkling of cayenne pepper (optional)
2 Tablespoons grated Parmesan* or Pecorino Romano cheese
Grated gluten-free mozzarella cheese* (optional)

Rinse mushrooms to remove any dirt and dry. Remove stems using your fingers. Chop the stems. Combine the stems, onion, garlic, spinach and red pepper. Squeeze out excess water from the vegetables, especially the spinach.

(Alternatively, if using fresh red pepper, combine vegetables in a saucepan and sauté a few minutes to remove some of the water and drain well. Allow to cool so you won't burn yourself when filling the mushrooms.)

Add the lemon juice, spices and grated cheese. Fill mushroom caps with mixture. Top with mozzarella if desired. Place in a 12 x 9 x 2 inch baking pan. (I prefer the non-stick type baking pan.) Bake at 350°F for 20 minutes.

## Onion Dip (and Onion Soup Mix Substitute for Dip)
We've always enjoyed onion dip. Some store brands of onion soup mix are gluten-free and others are not. As of 2008 Lipton® Onion Soup mix says it is manufactured in a facility that processes wheat products, so I don't use it. [Now in 2010 I understand that they starting adding barley to it and that means it is definitely not gluten-free!] By making your own, you can also make half the recipe if you wish.

1 (16 ounce) carton of gluten-free sour cream*

1 envelope gluten-free onion soup mix* or onion soup mix substitute (see below)

Blend all and chill before serving so flavors blend. Serve with gluten-free potato chips* or fresh vegetables.

*see gluten-free products list at the end of the book*

Onion Soup Mix Substitute:

2 to 3 Herb-Ox® beef bouillon cubes
  soaked in 2 teaspoons hot water (so
  the cubes dissolve) or 3 to 4 Packets
  Herb-Ox® from Hormel® sodium
  free beef bouillon packets (both
  products are labeled gluten-free)

¼ cup to 6 Tablespoons dried minced
  onion flakes (I use less)
2 teaspoons onion powder
¼ teaspoon sugar (optional; if using
  sodium-free bouillon, no need to add
  sugar)

Soak the cubes in the hot water. Allow them to cool and then they break easily and will dissolve into the sour cream. Add the rest of the ingredients and blend. If using the sodium free bouillon, you may want to add about ¼ teaspoon salt or salt substitute to taste.

Note: I don't like things too salty so I use less bouillon. I suggest you start with 2 cubes dissolved in 1 teaspoon hot water, and then prepare the dip and taste it. If you think it needs the extra bouillon added, dissolve the bouillon cube in the remaining 1 teaspoon water and add it.

## Panelle – Sicilian Fried Chickpea "Bread"

My parents were given this recipe when the traveled in Sicily. Many street vendors sell Panelle, and this recipe just so happens to be gluten-free! They are best served warm after they are fried. I purchase chickpea flour from an Italian market. When you purchase it, check to be sure it has no wheat contamination. Often bean flours are not milled with wheat, but they may become contaminated if packaged in a facility with wheat, or repackaged by the market. This recipe may be doubled or tripled. Note: some recipes for Panelle do contain wheat, so check if you want to eat it in Sicily.

1 ¼ cups chickpea flour
¼ teaspoon salt
½ teaspoon baking powder*

⅛ to ¼ teaspoon ground black pepper
1 ½ cups water
Oil for frying the Panelle

Grease a cookie sheet with cooking spray or oil. Or, you can use several flat dessert plates, to make small pie shaped wedges of panelle. If the dishes have a nice shiny glaze on them, you don't need to grease them. Set aside.

Put the chickpea flour and salt in a saucepan. I prefer a non-stick pan. Add the water slowly, stirring with a whisk as you add the water to avoid getting any lumps. Be sure to mix in any chickpea flour in the corners of the pot. Put the pot on the stove and cook the mixture over medium heat, stirring constantly with the whisk. Do not use high heat or it can burn. You will need to cook it until pulls away from the side of the pan and is very thick. Remove from heat.

Spread the mixture in the cookie sheet or plates, using a rubber spatula, until it is about ¼ inch thick or even a little thinner. I like them thin and crunchy, so I make them between ¼ and ⅛ inch thick. Don't go too thin or you won't be able to slice them. If you choose the full ¼ inch they will be crispy on the outside and creamy on the inside.

Allow it to cool. Once cooled, cut into rectangles that are about 1 ½ inches by 2 ½ inches in size for the ¼ inch thick panelle. I cut them smaller and make them about 1 inch by 1 inch

*see gluten-free products list at the end of the book

for the thinner panelle.  If using plates, cut them in small pie shaped wedges, about 1 inch in width at the outer edge.

Fry the panelle in hot oil, using either a fry pan or a deep fryer.  If your fry pan has a setting, set it to about 375°F.  Whichever you use to fry them, do not overcrowd them.  Turn until both sides are browned.  Drain well on paper towels.  Serve them while they are still warm.  They are nice served as an appetizer, or with a salad.

*Variation*:  If desired, add ¼ to ½ teaspoon dried parsley flakes to add color and flavor.  Dried basil or oregano may also be used.  Or, add one Tablespoon minced fresh parsley instead of the dried.  This gives it a different flavor and some color.

## Pickled Chinese Vegetables
This is my mother's recipe, and was always gluten-free.

4 Tablespoons salt
2 Tablespoons peppercorns
4 dried chili peppers
1 cup boiling water
7 cups cold water
6 quarter size pieces of fresh ginger, peeled and sliced
2 Tablespoons gluten-free vodka*
1 (½ pound) green cabbage

3 to 4 carrots, quartered lengthwise
1 (1 ½ pound) white turnip, cut into wedges
½ to 1 pound green beans, with ends cut off
4 to 8 small fresh cucumbers (gherkins), 3 inches long
2 to 4 broccoli stems cut in half

Make a brine of salt, peppercorns, chili peppers, and hot water.  Blend well and dissolve the salt.  Add the cold water, ginger and vodka.  Place in a gallon jar or 4 smaller ones.

Add the vegetables.  They all must be covered in the brine.  Leave 4 days for tender cabbage, gherkins, broccoli and green beans.  The other vegetables are ready in 6 to 7 days.

## Pickled or Marinated Mushrooms
This is my mother's recipe and they are delicious.  I like them on a salad.  I think these are much better than any jar version I have tried, and you know these are gluten-free.

1 lb. fresh button size mushrooms, cleaned
Boiling water
1 teaspoon salt, added to boiling water
⅔ cup oil
2 Tablespoons lemon juice

2 Tablespoons wine vinegar
1 clove garlic, split or ⅛ teaspoon garlic powder
1 Tablespoon finely chopped parsley
1 teaspoon salt

Clean mushrooms and cut off the stems to make them uniform.  Place mushrooms into salted boiling water a minute and drain.  Place in a jar (I use a clean pickle jar) and make the dressing with the rest of the ingredients.  Pour the dressing over the mushrooms and marinate at least overnight or longer.  Shake the jar to move the mushrooms around so all get the marinade flavor since it will separate.  These are delicious as either an appetizer or served on salads.

*Variation*:  You can use this dressing for pickling some roasted red peppers (see index) or some well-drained cans of water-packed artichoke hearts.  Marinade for several days in the refrigerator.

## Pickled Peaches
Nice served with ham, lamb or poultry.

1 large can (29 oz.) peach halves, draining the juice into a saucepan
¾ cup brown sugar*
½ cup wine vinegar or apple cider vinegar

2 (3 inch) sticks of cinnamon
1 teaspoon whole cloves
1 teaspoon ground allspice

Drain peaches of juice and place juice and other ingredients into a pot and boil for 5 minutes.  Add the peaches and boil another 5 minutes.  Chill in syrup at least overnight.

## Pickles – Bread and Butter Pickles
Many brands of pickles are gluten-free, but here is a way to make your own.  I like making these in the summer when I can get Kirby pickling cucumbers at the farmer's market.  If you grow your own pickles this is a good use for them.  These pickles are wonderful with hamburgers and are good at cookouts.

3 ¾ to 4 pounds of medium sized Kirby cucumbers, unpeeled, cut into ¼ inch thick slices
2 ½ cups sugar
1 cup water
2 cups cider vinegar (4 to 5% acid content)

1 teaspoon non-iodized salt and 1 teaspoon celery seed, or use 2 teaspoons celery salt
1 ½ Tablespoons whole mixed pickling spices
1 Tablespoon whole mustard seed

Since canning takes time and you need special equipment, you can use the refrigerator method if you plan to eat the pickles right away.  This recipe fills three 1-quart sized jars or you can reuse old pickle jars. Wash the jars in the dishwasher before preparing the pickles as directed below.  Once cooled, store the pickles in the refrigerator and eat them within 3 to 4 weeks.  For best flavor, allow the pickles to sit in the brine in the refrigerator at least one day before eating.  Even if the lids pop using this method, you must refrigerator the pickles.  They will not be shelf-stable.  See the variation below on how to make shelf-stable pickles without a canner.  If you plan to give them as gifts, I suggest you use that method instead of this one.

Wash cucumbers, remove and discard ends (both the flower and stem ends), and cut into ¼ inch slices.  Set aside.  In a 5-quart size pot, combine the sugar, water, vinegar, salt, celery seed, pickling spice and whole mustard.  Bring to a boil and stir to dissolve the sugar.  Add the cucumber slices and stir them in the syrup mixture to coat.  Return to a boil and boil for 1 ½ to 3 minutes, and stir to coat.  Remove from heat.  Pour into clean jars.  Cover and cool. Store pickles in the refrigerator.

*see gluten-free products list at the end of the book

*Variation*: For a canning method without using a canner (for this recipe only): You will need a large pot to boil the jars, preferably with a steamer insert in the bottom, or a rack. This helps the water bubble and boil around the jars. You will also need metal canning pliers to safely remove the jars from the boiling water. Use only new canning lids; never re-use them.

Wash 6 pint size canning jars (or use 3 quart sized jars if you have a very large pot with a rack), and immerse jars in boiling water. [I find it easier to put the jars in a large pot, fill with water to cover, and bring it to a boil.] Keep them immersed in boiling water until you are ready to fill them. Immerse new canning lids (not used) in a small pan of boiling water until ready to use too. Prepare pickles as noted above. Remove canning jar from boiling water bath using the canning pliers and pour off any excess water. Be extremely careful; the water is hot! Carefully fill with the boiling hot pickles and the syrup. Fill within ⅛ inch to the rim. Clean rim with a clean damp cloth and top with canning lid. (Carefully remove lids using the canning pliers and place on top of jars.) Screw on ring band. Continue until all jars are filled. Set jars on a folded towel away from drafts to cool. Test seal to be sure it doesn't pop back. Store any unsealed jars in the refrigerator and use within a month. This method makes your pickles shelf stable until you open them. Refrigerate after opening.

## Pickles – Cheap!
A recipe from my mother.

Brine from a jar of gluten-free deli pickles*
Kirby variety of cucumbers or 1 large "burpless" cucumber, sliced
(These varieties of cucumbers are suggested because they have delicate skins that can be eaten.)

Whenever you buy a jar of pickles from the refrigerator section, don't throw away the liquid in the jar when all the pickles are gone. Buy a few fresh Kirby or "burpless" cucumbers and wash them. Slice them as you wish and add to the brine. Refrigerate. In a few days they will be crisp and flavorful. Use within a week of putting it together.

Note: You can only do this one time per jar of pickles.

## Pigs in a Blanket or Cocktail Frankfurters – Biscuit Version
These are covered with a biscuit "blanket" are easy to make. I served them for guests and they thought they were the real thing. This is our favorite version.

1 package gluten-free cocktail
    frankfurters* or regular size gluten-free
    frankfurters*
1 cup Gluten-Free Naturals™ Sandwich
    Bread Flour or Gluten-Free Naturals™
    All Purpose Flour
⅓ cup butter*, cold from refrigerator
Sprinkling of salt

1 teaspoon baking powder
¼ teaspoon baking soda
6 Tablespoons to ½ Cup Gluten-Free
    Plain Yogurt (add slowly as needed so
    dough won't be too wet to roll out)
Water
Gluten-free mustard* (optional)

Prepare biscuits by putting cold butter, gluten-free flour, sprinkling of salt, and baking powder and soda in a food processor. Process until butter is cut in. If you don't have a processor, cut in the butter with a pastry blender. Add the yogurt and process until the dough balls up. If dough is too wet, add 1 to 2 Tablespoons more Sandwich Bread Flour and blend in. You can knead dough to improve blending it. Roll out on waxed paper. You shouldn't need to have to put extra flour on the waxed paper. It should roll out without it. Cut into strips and wrap around the frankfurters. Place on a foil lined pan, or foil lined toaster oven pan. Brush with water so that the dough will absorb it and rise better. If you are not baking them immediately, cover them with plastic wrap so that they don't dry out. If they look a little dry, brush with water again before baking. (Note: If they get too dry they won't rise properly.) Bake for 10 to 15 minutes at 450°F until cooked and lightly browned. Serve on a plate with some gluten-free mustard*. They can be cooked in a toaster oven set to 450°F.

## Pigs in a Blanket or Cocktail Frankfurters – Version 2 using Pie Crust

These are covered with a pie crust "blanket". I prefer the biscuit ones since they rise and are lighter, but these are also good.

1 package gluten-free cocktail frankfurters* or regular size gluten-free frankfurters*
1 cup Gluten-Free Naturals™ Sandwich Bread Flour or Gluten-Free Naturals™ All Purpose Flour

⅓ cup butter*, cold from refrigerator
Sprinkling of salt
1 Tablespoon water
Gluten-free mustard* (optional)

Prepare pie crust by putting cold butter, gluten-free flour and sprinkling of salt in a food processor. Pulse until butter is cut in. Do not over process. Add 1 Tablespoon of water in through the feed tube and process until the dough balls up. If you over processed the dough, refrigerate it to make it easier to roll out. (Or to avoid this, use the traditional method of cutting the butter into the flour, and then adding water.) Roll out on waxed paper. Cut into strips and wrap around the frankfurters. Place on a foil lined pan or toaster oven pan. (I use Reynolds® Release foil on the pan.) Bake for 10 minutes at 450°F until cooked and lightly browned. Serve on a plate with some gluten-free mustard*.

## Pigs in a Blanket or Cocktail Frankfurters – Version 3 using Dough

These are covered with a biscuit type "blanket" and are very tasty but a little bit messy to make and not as attractive as the other versions in appearance. Since they travel pretty well after they are baked, sometimes my husband makes full-size frankfurters with this coating for trips, and then heats them in a microwave.

1 package gluten-free cocktail frankfurters* or regular size gluten-free frankfurters*
1 cup tapioca starch or tapioca flour
¼ cup yellow corn flour or sorghum flour
Sprinkling of salt

1 egg
3 ounces grated cheddar cheese*
2 Tablespoons oil
¼ cup milk, plus some additional milk if needed
Gluten-free mustard* (optional)

*see gluten-free products list at the end of the book

Grease a large pan or cookie sheet or cover with Reynolds® Release foil. Combine the tapioca starch or tapioca flour, corn flour or sorghum flour, and salt in a bowl and blend with a whisk. Add the egg, cheese, oil and milk, mixing it with a spoon. If the dough is too dry, add a very little more milk and if too wet add a little more tapioca starch. The dough should be pliable, a little bit sticky and a little bit stiff. It should not be a thin batter or it won't coat the frankfurters.

With your hands, take some of the dough and surround the frankfurter leaving the ends showing. (If the dough is too sticky you can apply oil to your hands or add a little more tapioca starch to the batter.) Place on the greased baking sheet. If you have any leftover dough you can put that on the baking sheet in the shape of little balls. They will taste like cheese biscuits. Bake for 15 to 20 minutes at 350°F until done. If you used large size frankfurters you can cut them into smaller bite-sized servings. Serve on a plate with some gluten-free mustard*.

## Quesadillas Appetizer
See index for recipe. Slice them into small appetizer pieces.

## Quiche Appetizer
See index for recipes. Slice them into small appetizer pieces. The "Spinach Pie" recipe is also good. Or see Mini-Quiche recipe in this section.

## Red Pepper Relish
This is my mother's recipe.

| | |
|---|---|
| 2 dozen sweet, red peppers | 3 cups sugar |
| 7 medium onions | 2 Tablespoons salt |
| 3 cups wine vinegar | 2 Tablespoons mustard seed |

Wash, seed peppers and coarsely chop by hand or in a food processor. Peel and finely chop onions. You should now have about 2 quarts of chopped peppers and 3 cups onions. Place in a large pot with remaining ingredients and cook, uncovered for 30 minutes.

Seal in sterilized jars. Makes 10 half pint jars of relish that are nice as little gifts. This is delicious on hamburgers and meat loaf (see index).

## Roasted Red Peppers
The secret to great roasted peppers is to buy the thickest, heaviest red peppers you can find. Peppers with thin flesh do not give good results, and only a small yield for all of your effort.

| | |
|---|---|
| Thick large red peppers | Salt and ground black pepper |
| Oil | Black pitted olives or anchovies as a |
| Peeled garlic | garnish |

Wash and dry whole peppers and arrange on a baking sheet. Place the pan directly under the broiling unit (which should be about 3 inches away), and broil until the skin turns black. Turn the peppers onto their opposite sides and broil again to blacken the skin. Now turn the peppers up on end and broil again.  It takes 5 or 6 turns to get every part of the peppers dark black.  When done, the peppers are limp and have some juices running out of them. Let cool enough to handle.  Now peel away and discard the paper thin blackened skin.  As you do this, you will reveal the lovely red flesh underneath.  Cut open the peppers to remove and discard the seeds along with the stem.  Do not wash the peppers to remove any loose seeds as you will lose the natural juice of the peppers.  Cut peppers into strips, sprinkle with salt and pepper and a little oil.  Now cut garlic into halves and tuck them here and there beneath the peppers.  Refrigerate.  When ready to serve, remove and discard the garlic and arrange the peppers on a platter.  Garnish with olives or anchovies.

## Roasted Red Peppers – Easier Version
This recipe comes from my mother.

Cut peppers in half, remove seeds and wash under cold water.  Place peppers (with the rounded part on top) in a roasting pan that is greased with a thin coating of oil.  Drizzle a little oil over the top of the peppers.  Cover with foil and bake at 350°F for a half hour. Remove foil and cook 20 minutes longer until peppers are tender.  Remove the skins carefully so as not to burn yourself.  They will come off easily.  Slice into smaller pieces if desired.  This is a lot easier than the traditional method above.

## Salmon Dip
This dip always goes at parties.  If you want a more smoked salmon flavor, you can add additional liquid smoke.  Just add it a little at a time because it can be strong.  Using the skinless/boneless canned salmon makes this an easy dip to prepare.

1 can (14.75 oz.) Pink Salmon, well drained and bones and skin removed or 2 cans (6 oz.) of skinless boneless canned salmon, well drained
1 package (8 oz.) gluten-free cream cheese*, softened
1 to 2 Tablespoons lemon juice (I use the reconstituted kind in a bottle.)

¾ teaspoons dill weed (I used dried dill and use less)
¾ teaspoon dried chives or 2 Tablespoons thinly sliced green onion (optional)
4 drops gluten-free liquid smoke* or to taste (I use Wright's® brand.  It is double strength so start with 2 drops. Liquid smoke is optional.)

Drain salmon well.  (I wash the lid of the can, open the can and use the lid to squeeze out the juice by pressing it against the salmon over the sink.  Remove lid carefully so you don't cut yourself.)  Remove skin and large bones.  Cream the cream cheese in a bowl and blend in the salmon and all other ingredients.  If you think the dip is too thick, you can add a Tablespoon of milk and blend it in.  I prefer it without the added milk.

Chill several hours before serving to allow flavors to blend.  I make it the night before, and firmly cover the top with plastic wrap, pressing it down on the dip to keep any air from being in contact with it and then I refrigerate it.  Take it out about 15 to 30 minutes before your party so that the cream cheese softens and the chips won't break.  Serve with gluten-free potato chips*.  We also like this dip spread on gluten-free crackers*.   Leftover dip makes a nice sandwich spread.  I am told it also can be added to hot cooked gluten-free pasta or rice to make a creamy sauce, but I have never tried this because we never have much left over!

## Salsa, Mexican Style

There are many brands of salsa you can buy that are gluten-free, and I have listed some brands in the back of this book. However, sometimes you want to make it yourself. This is easier than most recipes because the canned tomatoes are already peeled and diced. Since it is cooked it keeps longer too. If you use fresh, uncooked tomatoes it is best eaten the day you make it.

For an easy way to peel fresh tomatoes: Freeze the tomatoes. When you remove and defrost them from the freezer the peels will come right off. Peel and dice the tomatoes. Add to the recipe as noted and simmer them a few minutes as directed in the recipe. My mother has used this method when she has too many tomatoes from her garden. Freeze them and later make this salsa.

1 Tablespoon olive oil
2 cloves garlic minced or ½ teaspoon garlic powder
1 chopped onion
1 chopped green pepper (optional)
1 small hot pepper, seeded and chopped (see note below), or use 1 large Hungarian hot pepper, or ¼ to ½ teaspoon crushed red pepper flakes. (For "medium" hot, use ¼ teaspoon.)
1 (14.5 oz.) can diced tomatoes or use fresh tomatoes (If using fresh I use Roma or Plum tomatoes; preferably

peeled, but can be left unpeeled).
*Warning: Hunts® tomatoes with green chilies contains gluten as of this writing.*
1 Tablespoon red wine vinegar (or to taste)
1 teaspoon lemon or lime juice (optional)
¾ teaspoon salt (or ½ teaspoon if canned tomatoes are salted)
1 Tablespoon tomato paste (optional)
Generous sprinkling each of oregano, chili powder, and cumin (optional)
Chopped cilantro for color (optional)

Chop onion and peppers and mince garlic. Heat a skillet a little, add oil and add the garlic, onion and peppers and hot pepper flakes if using. (Note, use a skillet so that the juices will evaporate. If you use a pot they will not.) Cook until vegetables are crisp/tender or almost the desired consistency. Add the diced tomatoes and the rest of the ingredients and simmer for about 3 to 5 minutes uncovered to allow the juice from the tomatoes to boil off a little. If juices are too thin, add about a Tablespoon or so of tomato paste.

Allow to cool. Taste and adjust seasonings. Serve with restaurant style tortilla chips. Store the salsa in a jar in the refrigerator. It keeps at least a week or so in the refrigerator.

*Variation:* You may substitute frozen green pepper and onion for the fresh. I freeze hot peppers in my freezer, rinse them and use a poultry scissor to cut them into rings (see note).

*Variation 2:* For black bean salsa, add ½ of a 15 oz. can of black beans, rinsed and drained. Adding black beans will tone down the "heat" if you used too much hot pepper.

Note: I wear rubber gloves when cutting hot peppers. Jalapeno peppers can cause skin irritation. If any of the pepper oil gets under your fingernails, you may feel burning for days. Be careful not to touch your eyes or face. Do not put in contact lenses after you have diced these peppers. Minute amounts of the oil can remain on your skin and cause excessive

*see gluten-free products list at the end of the book

tearing and burning.  This is why I wear gloves.  Wash gloves/hands thoroughly.  For a hotter salsa, do not remove the seeds from the peppers.  Often I use Hungarian Hot peppers which are milder and I use the seeds.  I cut them using a poultry scissors so I don't even have to touch them.  Put the scissors in the dishwasher.  I also find that when frozen, they are not too hard to cut with scissors and their juices are less apt to squirt at me.

## Sausage Dip

This is flavorful and easy to make.  I have had this dip at church suppers.  Serve it with gluten-free tortilla chips.  Leftover dip will taste spicier the next day.  The original recipe used tomatoes with diced green chilies, but since some brands are not gluten-free I use plain diced tomatoes.

1 pound gluten-free bulk sausage* (or see index for recipe)

1 (8 ounce) package gluten-free cream cheese*

1 (14 ounce) can of gluten-free diced tomatoes*

1 small can [or half a can] of gluten-free diced green chilies (optional, I don't use)

1 bag of gluten-free tortilla chips* (or see index for recipe)

Cook sausage in a skillet until no longer pink.  Drain the fat.  Add cream cheese and tomatoes and cook on low-medium heat until it melts.  Once it is hot is ready to serve.  Put in a Crock-Pot® to keep warm at parties.  It will get spicier the longer it is in the crock-pot.  Serve with tortilla chips.

## Shrimp Remoulde

This is a shrimp cocktail with a nice sauce that you can make ahead of time.  My mother served it at a party and we all enjoyed it.

1 pound cooked, cleaned shrimp (I used frozen)

½ cup gluten-free mayonnaise* or ¼ cup gluten-free mayonnaise* and ¼ cup gluten-free sour cream*

2 Tablespoons horseradish* (check ingredients if using the kind from a jar)

1 Tablespoon dried chives

2 teaspoons dried parsley

Dash of salt and pepper

A few drops gluten-free hot sauce*

⅓ of a medium onion chopped finely

1 Tablespoon chopped capers (check ingredients)

Defrost shrimp in a bowl.  Meanwhile, mix rest of ingredients.  After shrimp are defrosted, remove excess water and dry with a paper towel.  Mix the sauce and shrimp together and marinate overnight in the refrigerator.  Serve on a bed of lettuce for a nice presentation.

## Stuffed Celery

This is an easy appetizer that is part of a traditional antipasto.  Some chopped pimiento may be used instead of chives.  Or you can eliminate the chives and just use cream cheese.

Celery

1 (8 ounce) package cream cheese*

1 Tablespoon dried chives

*see gluten-free products list at the end of the book

Wash and dry the celery.  Use the inner more tender stalks.  Blend the cream cheese with the chives.  Stuff the celery in the cavity and smooth with a knife.  If desired, cut into 3 inch pieces.  Serve.

## Sweet and Sour Swedish Meatballs

Follow the recipe for Sweet and Sour Swedish Meatballs found under Main Dishes.  Make the meatballs small in size.  They may be kept warm in a Crock-pot® on a buffet table.

## Tempura

Here is a recipe for those vegetables fried in batter, often served at a Japanese restaurant.  This batter may also be used for other fried foods, such as a coating for chicken.

Raw vegetables of your choice (I use
  mushrooms and zucchini)
1 cup Gluten-Free Naturals™ All Purpose
  Flour
2 eggs
½ teaspoon garlic powder
½ teaspoon onion powder

½ teaspoon salt
Sprinkling of MSG* (optional)
Sprinkling of pepper and paprika
  (optional)
Dash or two of milk (or milk substitute)
  to make the batter the right consistency
Oil for frying

Wash and dry vegetables.  Cut into desired size and set aside.  Mix together the cornstarch, eggs and seasonings.  Add enough milk to make a batter of medium consistency.  Coat the vegetables and fry in deep hot oil.  Drain well on paper towels.  Serve warm.

*Variation:*  In this recipe, cornstarch may be substituted for the Gluten-Free Naturals™ All Purpose Flour.  The batter is a little more difficult to work with and the flavor/texture won't be as good, but it does work.  Use the paprika to give it some color.

## Tortilla Chips

Some brands of tortilla chips look like they would be gluten-free if you read the ingredients on the label, but they are made on the same lines as wheat snacks and are contaminated.  There are some safe brands (see list in the back of this book), but here is a way to make your own if you can't find one.  These are easy to make and much fresher tasting than store bought ones.  This is my mother's recipe.  If you have a convection oven, they turn out even crispier and cook faster than the times listed below.

Gluten-free corn tortillas*                          Salt
Oil or gluten-free cooking spray or water

Cut tortillas into the size of chips by using poultry scissors, and make several pie shaped wedges.  (Or use a large knife and a cutting board to cut them.)  My husband cuts them into quarters and I cut them in sixths, so choose the size you prefer.  Cutting them in eighths is good too.

Cover a baking pan with aluminum foil so that there is no clean-up.  If desired, put a light coat of cooking spray on the foil (optional).  Place the wedges on the baking sheet in a single layer.  Lightly spray with a little cooking spray.  Do not overspray and saturate them, or they will not get crisp.  Lightly sprinkle them with salt.  Using the small amount of cooking spray makes them taste more like the fried chips.  If you are on a low fat or no fat diet, you can

*see gluten-free products list at the end of the book*

sprinkle or spray with a little water instead of cooking spray. Either method helps the salt to stick to the chips. Do not use too much water, or they will be soggy instead of crispy.

Bake at 350°F for 10-12 minutes. Cool slightly before serving. We think the lower temperature and longer baking time works best and produces a crispier chip. A convection oven works even better than a regular oven to make the chips. Bake for 8-10 minutes if using a convection oven. Store chips in an airtight container.

You can purchase tortillas in packages of 100 for a very reasonable price. (They often cost the same as buying 3 of the 12 packs, so you get 64 tortillas for free!) This is a good way to use all of the extra tortillas. I use tortillas in many main dishes in this book (see index). Tortillas also keep a long time if vacuum packaged in bags.

*Variation*: Alternatively, you can bake at 375°F for 8-10 minutes or even 450°F for 5-6 minutes, but at the higher heats watch them carefully as they can burn more quickly. I have scorched them using the 450°F method. If your oven has a window, I suggest you open the oven door to check them as they cook, because you may not be able to see how brown they are through your oven window. (I checked the window and they didn't look done – but in reality they were burning!)

*Variation 2*: Tortilla chips are good under a salad for a taco salad, or topped with cheese for nachos. I have found that when I served these at parties people seem to enjoy these tortilla chips even more than the packaged kind because they are made fresh and they are hot out of the oven. They are not as fattening because they are not deep fried and don't have the trans-fats that some of those products contain. You can also use them in soups instead of crackers.

*Variation 3*: To make nachos, after making the chips top them with grated cheese, sliced chilies and sliced pitted black olives (optional), and return them to the oven until the cheese melts.

*Variation 4*: Instead of salt, sprinkle with Adobo®* seasoning (a blend of salt, garlic, pepper, and turmeric).

*Variation 5*: You can deep fry the tortilla chips instead of baking them, and then drain them on paper towels and sprinkle them with salt. They will be very delicious, but we found this to be messier to make and much higher in fat and calories. Drain well on paper towels or your fingers will get grease on them when you eat them.

*Variation 6*: Cut the tortillas in ¼ inch thin strips, using a knife on a cutting board. Cut them in half or thirds the other way, so that the strips are not too long. Fry them in a fry pan using a ¼ inch of oil. Or fry them in a deep fryer. Drain well on paper towels. Use these chips under Chinese food as Chinese noodles. They are also good used in Egg Drop Soup (see index for recipe) or Hot and Sour Soup (see index for recipe). They can also be used as "crispy-crunchy bits" on a salad.

*see gluten-free products list at the end of the book*

## Soups, Salads, Dressings and Sauces

# SOUPS

Many of these soups are my mother's recipes. Be warned that she likes soups that are a complete meal. One time her grandson asked, "Where's the juice?" when served the Minestrone soup. Regarding her pea soup recipe, when my brother was very young he said, "This soup is as thick as London Fog." Some "soups" seem more like a stew than a soup. I am sure you will enjoy these soups, but you can add more water or broth if soup that resembles canned is more to your liking.

Also, I like to cover the soup as it is cooking and simmer it on low because I use a gas stove. A gas stove is easier to control the heat so it doesn't boil over. My mother, on the other hand, has an electric stove and cooks her soups uncovered because that way they don't boil over and they are more stew-like. If you choose my mother's method, you can add more water if they become too thick.

## Baked Bean Soup

This recipe was given to me by a close friend, and it is a good way to use left-over gluten-free baked beans*. For ease in preparation, I use a hand blender to puree the soup right in the pot. For a variation in flavor, add some gluten-free mustard* or horseradish* to taste.

3 cups cold gluten-free baked beans*
6 cups water
2 slices onion
2 stalks celery with leaves
1 ½ cups gluten-free stewed canned tomatoes*
1 Tablespoon gluten-free ketchup*

1 teaspoon salt
½ teaspoon ground black pepper
1 teaspoon sugar
2 Tablespoons water
2 Tablespoons fine white rice flour or sweet rice flour

Put beans, water, onion, celery, and tomatoes in a pot and boil covered for 30 minutes. Remove from heat and cool so that it is not too hot. (If it is too hot the soup can possibly melt your hand blender or food processor.) Using a hand blender or food processor, puree to desired consistency. If using a food processor, now return the soup to the pot. Add the ketchup, salt, pepper and sugar. Blend the water and the rice flour and add. Cook over medium heat until thickened.

## Bean Soup – My Grandmother's Style

A mild tasting, very plain soup that goes back generations. People tend to like more robust flavors today, so see below for variations.

¾ pound dried beans, use navy, pea or cannelloni
2 quarts water
1 (15 ounce) can gluten-free tomato sauce* or two (8 ounce) cans.
2 cups water
2 cloves garlic, minced
4 ribs celery plus leaves chopped

⅓ cup oil
½ teaspoon oregano
1 teaspoon sugar
1 teaspoon salt
⅛ teaspoon ground black pepper
¼ cup rice

*see gluten-free products list at the end of the book
-145-

The day before making this soup, rinse the beans. Look through them to make sure there are no small stones. Place the beans in a large pot and cover generously with water. Soak beans overnight. (Or, to make this soup the same day, follow the "quick-soak" directions on the package of the beans.)

The next day, pour off the water and add 2 quarts fresh water and 1 teaspoon salt. Cover and bring to a boil. Lower heat and simmer 1 hour. Now add 2 minced cloves of garlic, celery, tomato sauce, 2 cups water, oil, oregano, sugar and pepper. Continue cooking 1 more hour or until beans are tender and soup begins to thicken. Add rice and cook 20 minutes longer. Add more water if soup is too thick and more salt and pepper if needed. This soup is even better the next day.

*Variation*: This is a very mild flavored soup. For more flavor, add some diced ham when you add the tomato sauce. (If ham is salty, use a little less salt.) Or, chili powder may be added to taste. (I usually use 1 teaspoon which adds a nice amount of spice, or a ½ teaspoon may be used to give it some flavor without any heat.) Sometimes I do both of these things and also add a can of diced tomatoes for more tomato flavor and some texture.

## Beef Vegetable Soup – Easy – Stove and Crock-pot Versions

This is my mother's recipe and one of our family favorites. I often make this for company and they always want the recipe. You can also make it in the crock-pot. It's always good the day you make it, but I think the flavors blend and it's even better the next day. I remember making it for a group of college students who not only said it was "yummy" but kept going back for more.

1 lb. lean chopped or ground beef (ground turkey may be used; see variation below)
1 Tablespoon oil
3 chopped onions
3 diced carrots
1 cup peeled and diced potatoes
2 Tablespoons regular rice
1 ½ teaspoons sugar
1 teaspoon salt

1 bay leaf
1 small can corn niblets (optional) or 2 Tablespoons of dried corn (optional)
3 cups water
3 cups tomato juice* (or 1 ½ cups gluten-free tomato sauce* plus 1 ½ cups water)
3 teaspoons gluten-free beef bouillon*

Heat a large kettle. Add oil to pot. Heat oil and swirl around bottom of pot and then add chopped meat. Break up meat as it cooks so that it is in small pieces. Cook until meat loses its red color. If there is a lot of fat, drain it. (I use lean ground beef so there is little fat.) Add all the rest of the ingredients. Cover, bring to a boil, lower heat and simmer for 45 minutes. Remove bay leaf and discard. Makes about 2 quarts of soup.

*Variation*: For a quick "canned" soup: brown meat, add 1 Tablespoon minced dried onion, 2 cans drained mixed vegetables, rice, and sugar. Eliminate salt. Add the rest of the ingredients. Cook 15 to 20 minutes for flavors to blend. Vegetables may be salty, so add salt to taste.

*Variation 2*: Ground turkey can be used in place of beef. Add a ¼ teaspoon garlic powder when using ground turkey to give it better flavor.

*see gluten-free products list at the end of the book

*Variation 3*: See index and use this soup recipe to make "Palpettone Soup".

*Variation 4*: Other vegetables of your choice may be added such as sliced mushrooms or chopped green pepper or shredded zucchini.

*Variation 5*: For crock-pot version, brown the meat and drain fat. Add the meat and the rest of the ingredients into crock-pot using 2 cups water instead of 3. Cover and cook on low for 8 to 10 hours.

## Black Bean Soup – The way my mother makes it

This is a delicious soup from my mother, using dried beans. I have made this on a cold snowy day when I was inside anyway. This is time consuming to make (2 ½ hours cooking time), so I usually make my easier version recipe.

1 ½ cups dried black turtle beans
1 ½ quarts water
1 teaspoon gluten-free chicken soup base*
  or gluten-free bouillon*
1 teaspoon salt
2 Tablespoons oil
1 medium onion, chopped
1 medium potato, peeled and chopped

1 carrot, sliced
2 stalks celery, chopped
2 bay leaves
1 teaspoon oregano
1 clove garlic
½ juice of large lemon (or 1 to 2
  Tablespoons lemon juice)

Sort and wash beans. Add water, salt, chicken base, 1 Tablespoon oil and cook 1 ½ hours. Sauté the vegetables in the remaining oil. Add to soup and cook 1 hour more. Add lemon, garlic and oregano at the end. Remove bay leaves. Serve with rice.

## Black Bean Soup – Easier Version

This is my quick method and we always enjoy it. If you don't have ham, use some leftover gluten-free cooked and crumbled bacon to give it a nice flavor. Often if I have a small amount of leftover ham, I chop it and put it in the freezer in a freezer bag. Then I add it to this soup while still frozen.

1 (16 ounce) can black beans
2 ½ cups water (you can use up to 3 cups)
½ gluten-free ham steak, cubed* (or some
  leftover gluten-free ham)
2-3 carrots, peeled and sliced
1 potato, peeled and diced
1 onion, chopped or 1 Tablespoon
  dehydrated onion flakes

¼ teaspoon garlic powder or ¼ teaspoon
  granulated garlic
1 bay leaf
Sprinkling of celery salt
¼ teaspoon oregano
Gluten-free sour cream* and fresh or
  dried chives as a garnish (optional)

Put all in a pot. Cover, bring to a boil, lower heat and simmer for 1 hour. Remove bay leaf. Remove from heat and let cool a little. Using a hand blender, puree the beans and vegetables. Serve with a dollop of gluten-free sour cream* and chives, if desired.

Variation: This can be made in a crock-pot. Use 2 to 2 ½ cups water. Cover and cook 8 to 10 hours on low or 4 to 6 hours on high.

## Butter Bean Soup

This is a simple tasting soup. You can chop the vegetables in a food processor to make it easier to prepare. My mother says it is a favorite of my Dad's, but my husband doesn't like it because he doesn't like butter beans (lima beans).

1 ½ cups finely chopped celery
1 cup finely chopped carrots
¼ cup chopped onions (I use more)
3 Tablespoons oil
4 cups water
1 (16 ounce) can butter beans

1 (14 ounce) can of gluten-free tomatoes*
1 teaspoon dried basil
½ teaspoon salt
¼ teaspoon pepper
1 to 2 cups leftover diced chicken
   (optional, my mother doesn't add it)

In a pot, sauté the celery, carrots, and onions in about 3 Tablespoons of oil. Add all of the rest of the ingredients into the pot. Simmer for 25 minutes.

*Variation*: For variety, add 1 chopped yellow squash with the vegetables. Or, add a little gluten-free tomato sauce* for color. Some gluten-free pasta or rice may also be added. Some gluten-free grated cheese such as Parmesan or Pecorino Romano may also be added.

## Cabbage and Beans (also called Bean and Vegetable Minestra)

This is an easy soupy dish that Italians would serve as a first course. It is inexpensive and would satisfy you so you would only want a small piece of meat (the expensive part of the meal) afterwards. I enjoy it because I grew up with it, but for some it may be an acquired taste. It is not something that my husband likes. This is also a high fiber dish, which can be good for some celiacs since much of the gluten-free diet may be low fiber, because white rice flour is very low in fiber.

1 to 2 pounds of escarole or savoy
   cabbage or kale
¼ cup oil

2 cloves garlic, peeled
1 large can red or white cannelloni beans
Salt and ground black pepper to taste

Wash and slice the vegetable you chose and cook in a large pot with a little salted water. Cook until tender. Remove the vegetable from the pot. Wipe pot dry and add oil. Sauté the garlic in oil over low heat until garlic is soft and not brown. Remove from heat and cool slightly. Mash garlic with fork to release flavor and then discard the large pieces. Add the can of beans plus liquid to pot. We use white beans with escarole, red beans with kale and either red or white with Savoy cabbage. Add the vegetables to beans and heat a few minutes to blend. Add salt and pepper to taste. Serve in soup bowls.

*see gluten-free products list at the end of the book

## Chicken, Velvet Corn Soup

This is a recipe from my Mother. I use a food processor to easily mince the ham and chicken. This is a good recipe to use up a small amount of leftover ham and chicken.

2 Tablespoons cooked and minced gluten-free ham* or bacon*
1 whole boneless, skinless chicken breast
3 egg whites (add 1 to chicken, and whip the other 2), or substitute egg white powder and water for egg whites)
1 (8 oz.) can of gluten-free creamed corn*

3 cups chicken broth (I use water plus gluten-free chicken base*)
1 cup water
¼ teaspoon salt
2 Tablespoons cornstarch
3 Tablespoons cold water

Mince the ham in a processor, or crumble bacon, and set aside. Then mince the chicken in the processor and place in a large bowl. Add 1 egg white to the chicken, then add the creamed corn and mix well.

In a clean bowl, beat the 2 remaining egg whites to form soft peaks.

Heat broth, salt and 1 cup water to boiling. Now stir in chicken and corn mixture and let cook 2 minutes. Dissolve the cornstarch in 3 Tablespoons cold water (I use the same bowl the chicken was in) and stir into the hot broth to thicken. Reduce the heat and stir in the egg white. Serve in individual bowls and garnish with the minced ham.

*Variation*: I have made this soup using leftover corn cut from the cob. I added a ½ Tablespoon extra cornstarch to the corn mixture, since I did not have the cream sauce from canned corn.

## Chicken Soup

See variation under "Cockaleekie Soup, Easier Version".

## Cockaleekie Soup

This soup is quite a bit of work to prepare, but you'll enjoy it on a cold winter day. If you can get a stewing hen, the soup will be even more flavorful. If not, a regular chicken works just fine. Choose a chicken without added solutions (check ingredients) to be sure it's gluten-free. See list at the end of this book for suggested brands.

1 plump stewing hen or whole chicken*
2 quarts water
2 cloves garlic
1 bay leaf
1 teaspoon salt
Dash or two of ground black pepper
2 ribs of celery

2 carrots, scraped
1 onion
6 cups water
2 Tablespoons gluten-free chicken base*
4 leeks
½ cup rice

Place the chicken, 2 quarts water, garlic, bay leaf, salt, pepper, celery, whole carrots, whole onion in a large pot. Bring to a boil, reduce heat and partially cover. Simmer for 1 ½ hours

*see gluten-free products list at the end of the book

or until the chicken is very tender. Meanwhile place the 6 cups water and chicken base in another pot to cook. Carefully wash the leeks (they can contain gritty sand) and slice thinly using all the white part and a little of the green part. Add to the pot with the 6 cups water. Cover and cook for 45 minutes. Add the rice and cook 15 minutes more. You can take some of the dark tough part of the leeks and add to the chicken pot.

After cooking the chicken remove it and the carrots from the pot and set aside to cool. Pour broth and rest of vegetables through a colander into a large pot. Press the vegetables against the colander with a spoon to squeeze out all the liquid in them. Skim off the fat or cool and refrigerate to lift all the fat off the broth. Remove the chicken from the bones and discard the bones and skin. Cut chicken into bite size chunks. Dice the carrots and add to the broth with the chicken. Now pour the rice and leek mixture into the broth. Heat and serve.

## Cockaleekie Soup – Easier Version
This is my version of my Mother's soup.

1 package cut up chicken* parts (I use often use chicken legs or thighs*)
2 quarts water
1 bay leaf
2 cloves garlic
Dash or 2 of ground black pepper
1 teaspoon salt

¼ cup rice
2 ribs of celery chopped (leafy tops may be used, if desired)
2 carrots, scraped (leave whole)
1 onion chopped
4 leeks washed carefully and sliced thinly
2 Tablespoons gluten-free chicken base*

Wash leeks carefully, since they can sometimes contain gritty sand. Slice thinly using the white part and a little bit of the green. Add all ingredients (except rice) to a large pot and bring to a boil. Cover and simmer a half hour. Add rice, cover and simmer a half hour more. Remove chicken and carrots using a large slotted spoon or tongs. Allow them to cool. Remove the meat from the bone and cut into bite size pieces. Discard the skin and bones. Add the meat back to the soup. Dice carrots and add to the soup (now that they are cooked they are easy to cut). Allow it to cool and refrigerate. It's better made a day ahead of time, so that the flavors blend and you can skim the fat off the top.

*Variation*: This soup is also very good made without the leeks. Follow the recipe as above and eliminate them. You can't call it "Cockaleekie", but it is a very delicious Chicken Soup. I often make it for people when they just get out of the hospital. There were times when people refused to eat anything because they were sick but then they tasted this soup, they finished it, and it made them feel better. If they are on a low salt diet, don't use the chicken base and reduce the salt. Instead I use double the amount chicken to give it flavor. You can remove the extra chicken when the soup is done and use it in other recipes, such as chicken salad or Chinese food. Or, for no-salt diets, Herb-Ox® sodium-free/gluten-free bouillon can be used to add some flavor.

## Corn or Salmon Chowder
Some people tolerate evaporated milk better than milk, which is why I included directions for both. Others can tolerate Lactaid® milk* better, which works well with this soup since the corn has a sweet flavor. Use whatever milk is best for you. I often make this soup when I have leftover bacon.

3 ounces or 2 to 3 slices of salt pork or bacon
½ cup minced onion
1 cup diced potatoes
½ chopped green pepper (optional)
½ teaspoon salt
2 to 3 dashes ground black pepper
1 ½ cups water

12 ounce can evaporated milk or 1 ½ cups milk plus 1 Tablespoon fine white rice flour
1 (16 ounce) can gluten-free creamed corn* or 1 large can salmon (about 14.75 ounce) with skin and bones removed (or 2 small cans skinless/boneless salmon)

Cut salt pork into a small dice and put into a medium saucepan. If using bacon, I dice it small using poultry scissors. Heat slowly until some fat melts. Add the minced onion and sauté a few minutes. Add the water, salt, (green pepper if using) and potatoes and bring to a boil. Cook 10-15 minutes until potatoes are tender. Add the can of milk (or milk mixed with rice flour) and the can of creamed corn. Add dashes of pepper. Heat through. Let stand one hour to blend flavors. Reheat slowly to serve so milk does not curdle. Add salt if needed.

To make salmon chowder, just add a can of drained salmon in place of the canned corn. Be sure to remove bones and skin of the fish before adding to the soup, or use 2 small cans of the skinless/boneless salmon.

## Cream of Anything Soup
This is my mother's recipe and a nice, satisfying, mild tasting soup.

3 Tablespoons butter
½ cup chopped leeks (white part)
½ cup chopped onion
¼ cup diced celery
3 Tablespoons fine white rice flour
2 cans (13.75 ounce) gluten-free chicken broth or 3 ½ cups water and gluten-free bouillon* or chicken base*
1 cup gluten-free light cream*

Pinch of oregano
Salt and pepper to taste
2 Tablespoons Madera wine
1 cup of any one of these vegetables of your choice: mushrooms, broccoli, zucchini, Brussels sprouts, carrots, asparagus or spinach, cauliflower

Sauté leeks, onion, and celery in butter. Add the rice flour to the broth and slowly mix until smooth. Heat until the broth comes to a boil, stirring occasionally. Add the vegetables of your choice, the oregano, the salt and the pepper. Simmer 20 minutes or until the vegetables are tender. Cool just until the soup is easy to handle and then puree in a blender. After blending it, return the soup to the pot. Or let the soup cool down and puree using a hand blender in the pot.

*see gluten-free products list at the end of the book

Add wine and heat. When hot, add the cream and serve. Be sure not to boil the soup after the cream is added or it will curdle.

You can make an economical cauliflower soup by using the green leaves and only 2 flowerets.

*Variation*: Whole evaporated milk may be used instead of light cream. This soup may be made without the wine, but add ¼ cup gluten-free cheese for flavor.

## Cream of Broccoli Soup

I like this so much better than the canned version. By using a hand blender, this soup is easy to make. If you don't want to use evaporated milk, use 1 ½ cups milk plus 1 Tablespoon fine white rice flour.

| | |
|---|---|
| 1 lb. broccoli, fresh or frozen | 1 teaspoon gluten-free bouillon* (I use |
| 1 Tablespoon instant onion flakes | chicken or mushroom flavor) |
| 1 teaspoon salt | 1 can evaporated milk |
| ¼ teaspoon ground black pepper | 1 Tablespoon fine white rice flour or |
| 1 ⅓ cups water | sweet rice flour |

If using fresh broccoli, wash, trim and cut into small pieces. Place the broccoli in a medium pot or saucepan. Add onion, salt, pepper, water and bouillon. Cover and bring to a boil. Reduce heat and simmer until tender (about 10-15 minutes). Remove lid and allow the soup to cool a little. Using a hand blender, puree the soup in the pot. Add rice flour to the milk and blend. Add the milk mixture to the pot, and simmer until it thickens.

*Variations*: Mushrooms, asparagus or zucchini can be substituted for broccoli. You can also add 1 teaspoon of dried sweet basil for a different flavor.

## Cream of Chicken Soup

This is my mother's version. This involves some time to make, but we enjoy it on a cold winter day. Make the soup a day ahead of time so you can skim the fat off the top and discard it.

| | |
|---|---|
| 1 (4 to 5 lb) stewing hen or chicken* | 1 ½ teaspoons salt |
| 4 ribs of celery | ½ teaspoon ground black pepper |
| 1 small onion | Water |
| 2 carrots | Chicken fat |
| 2 bay leaves | ½ cup fine rice flour or sweet rice flour |
| 1 parsnip (optional) | 2 cups milk |
| 1 clove garlic | |

The day before you want this dish, start the soup. Place the chicken in a large pot and cover with water. Boil 15 minutes to 20 minutes and skim off any foam that floats to the top and discard the foam.

Scrape carrots and parsnip and add to the pot (no need to slice now, slice it later when it's cooked and easier to cut). Add the peeled onion, celery, peeled clove of garlic, bay leaves and seasonings. Simmer covered about 1 ½ hours. Remove chicken and carrots and set

*see gluten-free products list at the end of the book*

aside. When cool, remove skin from chicken and small rib bones that get into soup and discard. Cut chicken into serving pieces and slice carrots. Place a colander over a large bowl and ladle soup into in, keeping soup. Throw away bay leaves. Now instead of throwing the rest of the vegetables away, squeeze all of the liquid out of them through the colander and into the soup. Your soup won't be as clear but it will be more flavorful. Place soup in one container and chicken and carrots in another and cool to room temperature and refrigerate.

The next day, lift the fat off the top of the soup and discard. Put broth into a pot. Blend milk and rice flour together and add to the pot. Add chicken and carrots. Bring to a boil until soup thickens.

## Cream of Chicken Soup – Easier Version
This is my version.

1 large package of chicken legs with backs, cleaned and skinned (4 legs) or backless thighs skinned
Water to cover
2 teaspoons gluten-free chicken base*
1 teaspoon salt
¼ to ⅛ teaspoon garlic powder (depending on your taste)

1 onion, diced
2-4 ribs of celery, chopped
2 or more carrots, sliced
¼ to ½ teaspoon ground black pepper (depending on your taste)
2 cups milk
4 Tablespoons fine white rice flour or sweet rice flour

Put chicken in a large pot and cover with water. Add all other ingredients. Simmer 45 minutes to 1 hour. Remove chicken (I use a slotted spoon or tongs), and set it on a large plate or bowl and allow it to cool. (This is so that you can remove the bones without burning your hands.)

In a measuring cup blend the rice flour and the milk. Add to pot and bring to a boil and stir. Remove from heat and cover to keep it warm while you remove the bones from chicken. Discard bones. Return the chicken to the pot and stir in. Serve.

*Variation*: Put some hot cooked rice in each bowl and add the soup over top of it for a nice presentation.

## Cream of Mushroom Soup
I often use canned mushrooms so it is easier to make, but the fresh are even better.

2 packages sliced mushrooms, or 2 cans mushrooms drained, reserving juice
1 Tablespoon oil
½ teaspoon onion powder (I use granulated onion powder)
½ teaspoon salt
⅛ teaspoon ground black pepper

1 ½ cups water
3 Tablespoons fine white rice flour or sweet rice flour
1 teaspoon gluten-free bouillon* or mushroom soup base*
1 ½ cups milk

*see gluten-free products list at the end of the book

If using fresh mushrooms, wash and slice them. Put oil in the pot and add mushrooms and sauté a little. Mix together water, rice flour and bouillon and add to the pot. Add salt and pepper. Cover and bring to a boil. Remove lid and simmer on medium/low heat for 5 to 10 minutes until mushrooms finish cooking. It will be thick, but when you add the milk it will be the right consistency. Add the milk to the pot, and heat to serving temperature. If you used the canned mushrooms and your soup is a little thick add some of the water from the can.

I like the granulated onion powder better than the regular onion powder. The regular powder tends to clump up in the jar and is difficult to measure and use.

## Cream of Mushroom Soup Substitute for Baked Recipes
Use this only in baked casserole recipes that say to add a can of mushroom soup. I think that the bouillon and mushroom water provide enough salt, but more may be added to taste.

1 cup milk

1 teaspoon gluten-free bouillon* (I use Better than Bouillon® mushroom or chicken flavor, which is gluten-free as of this writing)

1 can of mushrooms, un-drained

3 Tablespoons fine white rice flour or sweet rice flour

½ teaspoon onion powder (optional)

Blend together all ingredients. Pour over casserole. Use in baked casseroles calling for a can of cream of mushroom soup.

## Egg Drop Soup
The Egg Drop Soup often served in Chinese restaurants contains gluten because of the bouillon used. Here is a way to make your own. When I have only small portions of Chinese food leftover, I make this soup to stretch the meal. It is quick and easy to make.

6 cups chicken broth (I use gluten-free chicken base* and water)

Scallions, chopped; or dehydrated chives

½ teaspoon sugar (optional)

½ teaspoon salt (do not use if bouillon is salty)

Dash of pepper

¼ teaspoon gluten-free MSG* (optional)

1 ½ teaspoons cornstarch

¼ cup water

1 egg

Put all in a pot except for the cornstarch, ¼ cup water and the egg. Bring to a boil and simmer 5 minutes. Mix the cornstarch with ¼ cup water and add to the soup. Beat the egg. Take a large spoon and swirl the soup and slowly drizzle the egg in until it cooks. Makes 4 servings.

*Variation*: If desired, serve with fried Tortilla strips/chips (see index for recipe) cut thin as Chinese noodles.

## French Onion Soup

This is my mother's recipe.  The wine gives it a delicious flavor.

2 to 3 Spanish Onions (or large onions)
2 Tablespoons butter
2 cans gluten-free beef broth* or 4 cups
    water plus 4 teaspoons gluten-free
    bouillon*

1 to 2 Tablespoons Madeira wine (do not
    eliminate or it won't taste as good)
Toasted or day-old Gluten-Free
    Naturals™ French bread (optional)
Grated parmesan cheese or sliced
    provolone cheese

Peel and slice onions into rings.  (I slice it in a food processor.)  Melt the butter in pot or saucepan and add the onions.  Cook slowly over low heat, with the cover on the pan.  Check onions and stir from time to time so that they become very tender, but not browned.  When tender, add broth and wine, and heat through.  Pour into individual oven proof bowls.  (Do not make them too full, so you won't spill it putting it into the oven.)  Top with toasted gluten-free bread (if using).  Sprinkle generously with cheese or if using provolone top with slices.  Put bowls on a cookie sheet and place under broiler just to melt cheese.  (I do this in a toaster oven, and I use only the provolone cheese and no bread.  You can also heat it in the microwave, but the cheese won't get brown and bubbly on the top.)  Serve.  Makes 4 to 6 servings.

## French Onion Soup – Easy Crock-pot Version

This is restaurant style soup that is very easy.  It won't be good without the wine, so do not eliminate it.  This is my version.

1 very large onion (Spanish onion), thinly
    sliced (I slice it in a food processor)
4 cups gluten-free beef broth* (I use 4
    cups water plus 4 teaspoons gluten- free
    bouillon*)
¼ cup Marsala wine

Grated Pecorino Romano or Parmesan
    Cheese
Toasted or day-old Gluten-Free
    Naturals™ French bread (optional)
Sliced Provolone Cheese, for presentation

Place sliced onions, broth and wine in the Crock-pot® slow cooker.  Cook 10 hours until onion is tender.  To serve, ladle soup in bowls (not too full) and sprinkle with grated Pecorino Romano cheese.  Top with gluten-free bread (if using) and then with a slice of provolone cheese.  Put it briefly in the microwave or under the broiler to melt.   Be careful not to spill the hot soup.  If you fill your bowls too full, it will spill as you're putting it into the microwave or oven.

## Goulash Soup

This is my mother's recipe and we always enjoy it.

1 pound chuck or round steak, cut into ½
    inch diced pieces (I use poultry scissors
    to cut the meat).
2 Tablespoons butter* or oil
1 ½ quarts water

1 teaspoon salt
2 Tablespoons paprika
Few dashes of ground black pepper
2 medium potatoes, diced
2 green peppers, diced

*see gluten-free products list at the end of the book

Heat a kettle (or I use a large Teflon® pot), add oil or butter and heat a few seconds. Add diced meat and brown. (The browning of the meat gives good color and flavor to the soup.) Add water, salt, pepper and paprika and cook covered for about an hour. Add diced vegetables and continue to cook covered until the meat and vegetables are tender, about a ½ hour longer.

## Hot and Sour Oriental Soup – Crock-pot Version

I make this in a Crock-pot® slow cooker. The vinegar provides the sour, and the black pepper provides the heat. If you want to serve this with mock Chinese noodles, slice some corn tortillas into thin pieces and fry them. Drain them well on paper towels, and serve them with the soup.

4 cups gluten-free chicken broth* (I use gluten-free bouillon* and water)
1 (6 ounce) can of sliced mushrooms, drained or 1 (8 ounce) package of fresh mushrooms, cleaned and sliced
1 (8 ounce) can sliced water chestnuts, drained (I cut them in half)
A few chopped scallions or 1 Tablespoon dried chives
1 rib of celery, sliced
3 Tablespoons quick cooking tapioca
3 Tablespoons wine vinegar

1 Tablespoon gluten-free soy sauce*
1 teaspoon sugar
½ teaspoon ground black pepper
1 or 2 (4.2 ounce) cans of tiny shrimp, drained (I use one)
4 ounces tofu, sliced into small cubes (check labels to be sure it is gluten-free) (optional, I don't use)
1 egg, beaten
2 Tablespoons fresh parsley, minced as a garnish (optional)

Combine the broth, mushrooms, water chestnuts, tapioca, vinegar, soy, sugar, and pepper in a crock-pot. Cover and cook on low for 9 to 11 hours or on high from 3 to 4 hours. Cut tofu in small cubes. Add cubed tofu and drained canned shrimp. Cook a few minutes on high to heat through. Meanwhile, beat egg. Stir soup and while stirring slowly pour egg in to make egg drop. Top with parsley if desired. (This soup is also good without the egg drop).

*Variation:* If you don't like shrimp, cooked ground pork can be used. Add it at the beginning when you add the other ingredients.

## Irish Chowder

We enjoy this soup on cold days. This recipe is from my mother.

1 pound stew meat, diced
¼ cup split peas
¼ cup rice
2 quarts water
2 diced carrots
2 chopped onions

2 ribs celery, chopped including leaves
2 medium potatoes, diced
2 teaspoons gluten-free chicken base* or gluten-free bouillon*
1 teaspoon salt
Ground black pepper

Take all ingredients except the rice and potatoes and put them in a pot. Simmer for 45 minutes. Add potatoes and cover and cook 20 minutes more. Then add rice and simmer 25 minutes more. Check seasonings and add more water if too thick.

## Leftover Soup

My mother frequently makes this recipe and it's always delicious. Just remember that you can never make the same soup twice, since leftovers change! Do not eliminate the chili powder or the flavors won't blend properly. I have made this in the crock-pot with excellent results. I often make this soup the day after having company over, especially if there is leftover tossed salad.

| | |
|---|---|
| 1 large soup bone | 1 large green pepper, chopped |
| 1 teaspoon salt | 1 large can tomatoes*, cut up |
| Few dashes ground black pepper | 1 can kidney beans |
| 1 teaspoon chili powder | 2 quarts water |
| 1 large onion, chopped | Leftovers of your choice |

Place all the ingredients in a large pot and start to cook it. Now clean out your refrigerator of all leftovers and make a most delicious soup. Just be sure to chop everything well. Gluten-free macaroni, cheese, gluten-free gravies, vegetables, coleslaw, salads and their dressings can be chopped and added to the pot. Everything except gelatin and dessert can go into the pot as long as it has not spoiled. Cook for 1 ½ hours. Adjust seasonings to taste. Remove bone and serve with grated Pecorino Romano or Parmesan cheese. This soup is better the next day.

*Variation*: This can be made without the soup bone, but I think it's tastier if you use it. Instead of the soup bone, I use 1 teaspoon gluten-free bouillon* or soup base* in place of the salt. When it is done, taste to see if more salt is needed.

*Variation 2*: This can be made in the crock-pot. Use 1 cup less water. Cook 8 to 10 hours on low.

## Lentil Soup

My mother often made this soup for us when we were children.

| | |
|---|---|
| 1 pound lentils | ½ teaspoon oregano |
| 7 cups water | Ground black pepper |
| ¼ cup oil | Additions: (optional) |
| 2 cloves minced garlic | A little chopped cooked escarole |
| 4 ribs celery and leaves, chopped | ½ package frozen chopped spinach |
| 1 (8 oz.) can gluten-free tomato sauce* | 2 Tablespoons rice |
| 1 teaspoon salt | |

Pour lentils, a little at a time, into a plate and check to see if there are any pebbles present. Discard pebbles. Place lentils into a large pot and wash, then drain. (Or put them in a large sieve, rinse, and then put them in the pot.) Add 7 cups of water, put on the stove and add garlic, celery, oil, salt, pepper and tomato sauce.

*see gluten-free products list at the end of the book*

Cook for 1 hour. If you want to add rice, add it 30 minutes before the end of cooking. Sometimes oregano gives off a bitter taste. Add 1 teaspoon sugar to counteract this.

## Manhattan Clam Chowder
This recipe is from my sister-in-law, and was always gluten-free.

4 strips gluten-free bacon*, chopped
2 medium onions, chopped fine
4 carrots, chopped fine
1 stalk celery, chopped fine (leafy tops may be included)
1 to 2 Tablespoons chopped parsley or 1 to 2 teaspoons dried parsley (optional)
1 large (28 ounce) can tomatoes*, cut up
2 cans minced clams*

2 teaspoons salt
Dash ground black pepper
1 bay leaf
1 ½ teaspoons thyme or oregano (I don't use thyme because its flavor gets stronger in leftovers, so I use oregano.)
3 medium potatoes, chopped fine

Cut bacon into small pieces and fry in a large kettle until almost crisp. Chop peeled onions very fine, toss in with bacon and cook until limp. Next add finely diced carrots, celery and chopped parsley. Cook over a low heat for about 5 minutes, stirring occasionally.

Drain tomatoes and put liquid in a large measuring cup. Drain clams and add clam liquid to tomato liquid. Add enough water to make 1 ½ quarts (6 cups) of liquid. Add the tomatoes to the vegetable mixture. Reserve clams. Pour liquid into kettle and season with salt, pepper, bay leaf and thyme.

Cook to a boil, then reduce heat, cover and cook gently for 45 minutes. At this point add the very finely diced potatoes, and cover and cook 20 minutes longer. Add the chopped clams and cook slowly, this time uncovered for 15 minutes.

Check to see if carrots and potatoes are tender. If not, cover and simmer gently until done.

*Variation*: I have added all of the vegetables, spices, and liquid in the beginning and simmered everything for 50 minutes except the clams. Then I added the clams and simmered 10 minutes more. If the oregano gives a little bitter flavor, add a teaspoon of sugar to counteract this.

## Meatballs (Tiny size) to add to Soups
If you want to make half the recipe, use one egg yolk instead of one whole egg. I usually make a whole batch and use some in soup and put some in tomato sauce. You can make these ahead of time and freeze them. When we were children we always asked my grandmother to make the chicken soup with tiny meatballs for the holidays. Here is my gluten-free version of them.

1 lb. chopped meat
¼ cup grated Parmesan cheese
1 egg
¼ teaspoon salt

Dash of ground black pepper
¼ cup fine white rice flour or brown rice flour
2 teaspoons dried parsley (optional)

*see gluten-free products list at the end of the book

If you plan to put these meatballs in chicken soup, heat a pot of boiling water on the stove. Meanwhile, in a bowl, blend together the egg, salt and pepper, cheese, and rice flour with a whisk. Blend in dried parsley if using. Wash your hands. Add the meat to the egg mixture, and blend together, working it in with your hands. Moisten hands and shape into marble sized meatballs. Place the meatballs into the boiling water. Stir gently to separate meatballs. Cook only a few minutes uncovered. (They will rise to the top.) I remove them with a slotted spoon. Discard this cooking water if adding the meatballs to chicken soup.

If making beef soup, the meatballs could be cooked directly in the soup. Or, the cooking water could be used as part of the water for a pot of beef soup. It will be too cloudy to use for chicken soup.

## Minestra – My Great Grandmother's Version

We don't know if my great-grandmother invented this dish or not. My mother never found it in any recipe book and neither have I. My mother says it is the Italian version of boiled dinner. If you like cooked greens, you will probably like this. I did not like it as a child, but I like it now. This recipe makes a lot of food.

| | |
|---|---|
| 1 chicken* (preferably a stewing hen) | 3 or more varieties of greens; choosing |
| 2 pounds gluten-free Italian sausage* | either escarole, broccoli, spinach, or |
| 2 large cloves of garlic, peeled | Savoy or white cabbage. |
| 1 (8 inch) piece of gluten-free pepperoni* | Salt and ground black pepper to taste |
| (Cut it into 8 pieces after it is cooked.) | Italian spoon bread (see index) |

The day before you plan to serve this, start cooking this dish by placing the meats in a large soup kettle. Cover with water and bring to a boil. Reduce heat and partially cover and cook. It should take about an hour. When meats are cooked, remove and place in a large container reserving all the broth. When cool, cut chicken into large serving pieces, discarding skin and tiny bones and leaving only the thigh and drumstick bones if you wish. Taste broth to see if salt and pepper are needed. Cool broth to room temperature and refrigerate. Refrigerate meat when cool.

Next day, place a little salted water into a pot. Wash and prepare vegetables. Cut cabbage into wedges and remove and discard core, cut broccoli into flowerets. Cut escarole into 2 inch pieces, etc. My mother used a combination of broccoli, Savoy cabbage and escarole but any vegetables you prefer will be good. You should have about 8 cups of cooked vegetables.

Place one variety of greens into boiling water and cook until tender. Remove and place in a bowl and boil the second green in the same water as the first and so on. Discard the water that the greens were cooked in.

Now take the broth from the refrigerator and remove the fat. Discard the fat. Heat broth and meats and add well-drained greens. Don't add the water the greens cooked in as it is bitter and will ruin your soup. Heat all together until hot and serve in deep dishes giving each person an assortment of meats, some greens and a piece of Italian spoon bread (see index). Top it all with broth. Make sure all have soup spoons to get every last drop. Serves 8.

*see gluten-free products list at the end of the book

## Minestrone – My Mother's Version

My mother invented this soup because my brother wouldn't eat soup with beans in it. She overcame this problem by pureeing the beans. He not only ate the soup but loved it and so did the whole family. The pureed beans thicken the soup nicely.

3 Tablespoons oil
1 diced onion
1 teaspoon chopped parsley
1 Tablespoon dried basil
2 cloves garlic, minced
¼ cup gluten-free tomato sauce* or 1 Tablespoon tomato paste (you can freeze the rest of the tomato paste for another use).
1 large can cannelloni white beans
2 quarts water
Few dashes ground black pepper

Grated Italian cheese (we like Pecorino Romano)
3 fresh tomatoes, peeled, seeded and chopped or 1 lb. can gluten-free diced tomatoes*
3 ribs of celery, chopped
2 carrots, scraped and diced
2 medium potatoes, peeled and diced
¼ of a small cabbage, shredded
1 zucchini, grated
1 teaspoon salt
½ cup cooked rice

Place oil in a large pot and add onion, parsley, basil and garlic and sauté a few minutes. Add tomato sauce or tomato paste and a little water and cook 5 minutes. (Note: The secret to bringing out the tomato flavor is adding it to the oil and cooking it in.) Empty a can of cannelloni beans into a blender and puree. (I put them in the cup of my hand blender and puree.) Add this and the water to the pot. Now add all the vegetables, salt and pepper and cook slowly for 1 hour. Add cooked rice and heat through. If you want to use raw rice, add ¼ cup half-way through the cooking time. Adjust the seasonings and serve with grated cheese sprinkled over the top.

*Variation*: This is a soup you can change according to what you have on hand and the amount of time you have to put it together. Sometimes I don't puree the beans and just put them in whole. Sometimes I add ¼ cup brown rice at the beginning, so I don't have to add rice half-way through. Other times I don't add the cabbage or zucchini. Sometimes I add additional vegetables. Or, sometimes I add leftover cooked vegetables at the end so they heat through.

## Mulligatawny Chicken Soup

This soup gets its flavor from curry and apple, for an exotic change from plain chicken soup.

1 stewing hen or gluten-free chicken* (A stewing hen is tougher but it adds more flavor. A good butcher may have them.)
2 to 3 large carrots
2 to 3 stalks celery
1 teaspoon salt
2 quarts water
1 large onion, chopped
¼ cup chicken fat or butter

1 large apple
4 to 5 teaspoons gluten-free curry powder* (or see index for recipe)
1 teaspoon salt to taste
3 Tablespoons fine white rice flour or sweet rice flour
2 ½ cups hot cooked rice (prepare rice [see index] using 1 cup uncooked rice)

The day before, make a chicken soup by combining chicken, carrots, celery, 1 teaspoon salt and 2 quarts water. Cook 1 to 1 ½ hours or until chicken is tender. Pour soup through a colander into a bowl to reserve liquid. When chicken is cool enough to handle, remove meat from bones and dice 3 cups of chicken. Slice carrots and celery and add to chicken and refrigerate. Pour soup into a covered container. Bring to room temperature and refrigerate.

The next day, remove the chicken fat off the top of the soup. Take ½ cup of fat and melt into a large soup kettle. Add onion and sauté over low heat until soft. Add apple and curry powder and continue to cook until apple is soft. Discard the rest of the chicken fat or save for another use. Add the rice flour to the pot and blend, then add 3 cups of chick broth gradually, stirring all the while. Cook until broth comes to a boil and thickens. Now add 3 more cups of broth plus the chicken and vegetables and heat. Serve over cooked rice.

Note: My mother likes to render chicken fat and uses it to brown potatoes, or in pie crusts for meat pies, or for recipes like "Gingerhen" gingerbread. See index for "Chicken Fat" recipe.

## Mushroom Soup, Russian Style
The dried mushrooms make a very flavorful soup. They may be difficult to find, but are worth the effort. I usually find them at ShopRite® grocery stores.

4 ounces dried mushrooms (sold in a
  plastic container)
3 Tablespoons rice
2 chopped onions
2 chopped leeks
2 diced carrots
2 Tablespoons butter*
2 diced potatoes (optional)
2 bay leaves

1 ½ teaspoons salt
Sprinkling ground black pepper
2 quarts water
2 Tablespoons fine white rice flour or
  sweet rice flour
¼ cup milk or 2 Tablespoons gluten-free
  sour cream*

Soak mushrooms in a little hot water to soften. Meanwhile, wash leeks thoroughly and dry and chop only the white part. Prepare onions and carrots. Now remove mushrooms from water and cut into small pieces. (I use a poultry scissors.) Discard the water it soaked in as it often has a little grit in it. Using a large pot, melt butter and then sauté carrots, onions and leeks until lightly browned. Add water and bring to a boil. Add salt, pepper and mushrooms. Cook a half-hour and then add diced potatoes if desired and rice and cook one half-hour more. When vegetables are tender, remove bay leaf and thicken soup with rice flour and milk (which you have blended thoroughly together.) (Or use sour cream in place of the rice flour and milk.) Add to soup while stirring and bring to a boil.

## Noodles – Homemade to add to Soups

There are gluten-free noodles and pastas out there that you can add to soups, but sometimes you just want something different. Here are a few of my mother's recipes converted to gluten-free.

(1) Spaetzle (little dumplings)

This is a favorite of ours. See index for the recipes. The Spaetzle freeze well, so I make the full amount and use what I need and freeze the rest for another time. I store small amounts in small bags in the freezer, so you can just add it to the soup when needed. They may be added frozen to boiling soup. (The rice version freezes a little better than the other version, but both are good.)

Also, unlike wheat noodles the Spaetzle do not continue to absorb liquid after they are added to soups. This is great if you want to make soup ahead of time. Spaetzle also freeze well when <u>in</u> the soup. I often make a full pot of soup and freeze the rest. (Just leave enough space in the top of your freezer container, since soups expand when frozen.)

(2) Pancake Noodles

You can use leftover gluten-free crepes (see index) or use this recipe below:

2 heaping Tablespoons Gluten-Free Naturals™ All Purpose Flour, or cornstarch, or
   defatted soy flour
1 egg
2 Tablespoons milk
1 Tablespoon oil
Pinch of salt

Using a hand blender, blend ingredients and make as in crepes for manicotti (see index). (Soy flour is difficult to blend with liquids, so mix first with a fork and then the blender.) Make crepes. When cooled, cut pancakes as thin as you like. These noodles do not absorb your soup like regular noodles. (Note: Noodles made with cornstarch do not freeze well, so if you plan to freeze your soup use a different gluten-free flour or use one of the other recipes listed in this section.)

(3) Stracciatella

My Mother's original recipe used 2 Tablespoons of semolina [hard wheat] flour which is gluten! I think this version is very close to her original recipe, using ground rice.

2 eggs
2 Tablespoons course grind rice flour (such as Cream of Rice® cereal)
Or 1-2 Tablespoons fine white rice flour
2 Tablespoons grated Parmesan cheese

Mix all together and pour into simmering soup, stirring while it cooks a minute or two. (Cooking times may vary depending on the grind of rice used.) Remove from heat and serve. Makes enough for 1 quart of soup.

*see gluten-free products list at the end of the book*

(4) Fried Corn Tortilla Strips

These are added to Mexican Tortilla Soup. They're also nice to add to other soups as well. They also remind me of Chinese fried noodles when added to Egg Drop Soup, and can also be used under Chinese dishes as you would Chinese noodles.

Corn tortillas
Oil to fry them in

Slice tortillas into thin strips. I cut them in half and then cut them in strips on a cutting board using a sharp knife. Fry in a pan with about 1 inch of oil. Or use a deep fryer. (Be sure no wheat containing items were previously fried in the same oil.) Drain well on paper towels. If desired, they may be salted to make a nice snack.

## Palpettone Soup

My mother gave me this recipe. It like a meatloaf made in a soup. It can be made in a Crock-pot® too.

1 ½ recipe for Italian meatballs or 1 ½ recipe for meat loaf

1 recipe for "beef vegetable soup" (see index) eliminating the chopped meat portion of that recipe, since you are using the meatball recipe instead.

Prepare meatball or meat loaf recipe in a soup kettle. Remove from kettle and shape into one large meatball and place on waxed paper or a plate. (The bottom will get flat.) Now, using the same kettle, add the ingredients in the soup recipe except the chopped meat. Cover; bring to a boil, and lower heat to a simmer. Then carefully lower the Palpettone (large meatball) into the soup. I do this using 1 or 2 large pancake turner/spatulas. Simmer gently 1 ½ hours. Remove Palpettone and place on a clean plate. Cover with another plate to press down a little and cool. Serve soup with thinly sliced, cooled Palpettone and a salad.

## Pea Soup or "Green Soup" and "Green Soup with Pennies"

My mother often made this soup when we were young and made the "easy cheesecake" for dessert. It was one of our favorite meals and we always finished the soup quickly to get that cheesecake. It was also an inexpensive meal that helped her budget. One time my mother didn't have bacon so she used half of a package of brown and serve sausage instead. We liked it so much she made it that way every since. She called them pennies which was a way to get us to try it and eat it.

2 quarts water
1 lb. split green peas
1 chopped onion
2 stalks celery, chopped
1 large chopped carrot
1 large dried bay leaf
2 teaspoons salt (use less if ham is salty)

Some ground black pepper
½ teaspoon oregano
6 slices bacon* (or use some diced ham*) or ½ a package of "Brown and Serve" type sausage sliced (Jones Dairy Farm® is gluten-free as of this writing)

Sort and wash split peas. Combine the rest of the ingredients in a pot. Cook 45 to 50 minutes. (First bring mixture to a boil, then lower heat, partially cover and simmer until peas are tender.)

*see gluten-free products list at the end of the book

Cool and remove bay leaf. (Note: Be sure to remove the bay leaf before you puree the soup! The bay leaf will not puree and will create hard pieces throughout the soup. You should not consume a dried bay leaf; it could scratch your throat or harm your intestines.) Puree the soup with a hand blender, or in a blender, or in a food processor a little at a time.

Prepare the bacon by putting it in the microwave according to the package directions. Drain fat and allow the bacon to cool so you can handle it enough to cut it into small pieces. If using sausage and you think the sausage may be fatty, brown it and drain the fat. Otherwise if using the Jones Dairy Farm® brand I just slice it frozen and add it frozen to the soup.

Crumble the bacon or slice the sausage and add to pureed soup. Cook an additional 10 minutes to blend the flavors. Serves 6-8.

*Variation*: Use a leftover ham bone instead of the bacon. Add the bone when you put in the peas. After cooking, remove and allow it to cool. Puree the soup. Remove any ham on the bone and add it to the soup. I have also made this soup using a leftover smoked turkey carcass and it was delicious. Just be sure you remove all the bones from the soup before you puree it.

## Potato Soup

This soup is a good use for leftover mashed potatoes. Some people with lactose intolerance can tolerate evaporated milk better than regular milk; hence I've provided this substitution.

2 ¼ cups milk or 1 (12 ounce) can evaporated milk plus 1 cup water
1 gluten-free chicken bouillon cube*
1 cup mashed potatoes (can be leftover, and made with butter*, milk, sour cream*)
¼ teaspoon onion powder

¼ teaspoon salt
1 Tablespoon butter*
2 Tablespoons fine white rice flour or sweet rice flour
1 can mixed vegetables, drained

Combine all ingredients and heat through until flour thickens. To make vichyssoise (cold potato soup), do not add the mixed vegetables. Instead, cook the soup and then chill the soup and garnish with chives or parsley.

## Scotch Broth

This is my mother's recipe. It's a good way to use leftover lamb.

1 ½ pounds lamb neck bones or frozen
   New Zealand lamb shanks
2 to 4 carrots
1 Spanish onion (large onion)
2 quarts water
1 bay leaf

½ teaspoon salt
2 to 3 dashes ground black pepper
1 Tablespoon gluten-free chicken base* or
   gluten-free bouillon*
⅓ cup rice

The day before serving, place meat, carrots, onion, bay leaf, salt, pepper, chicken base and water in a pot, and cook 1 hour. (You can do this in a crock-pot on low 10-12 hours.) Remove bay leaf and discard. Pour broth through a large colander into a bowl and squeeze juices out of onion by pressing it with a spoon. Cool the broth and what is left in the colander to room temperature. Cut meat into bite size pieces and dice carrots. The squeezed out onion may be discarded. Refrigerate each in separate containers. (I cover the bowl with plastic wrap and put the vegetables in a small covered container.) The next day, lift off and discard the fat from the broth and place broth into a soup kettle. Add rice, meat and carrots and cook a ½ hour longer. Serve.

*Variation*: Sometimes I chop the onion instead of putting it in whole. I cook the soup as noted above. I remove the bay leaf and skip the step of putting the soup through a colander. I let the soup cool and put the whole pot in the refrigerator. I use a Farberware® metal pot with plastic handles that are designed for extreme temperature changes. The next day I skim the fat, remove the bones and carrots. I dice the meat and carrots. Then I add them back to the soup. Add the rice and cook it a ½ hour as directed. (Use caution as some pots cannot handle extreme temperature changes or refrigeration, so do not do this unless you know yours can. Do not try this with enamel pots.) My mother keeps them separate because it is easier to get the fat off the soup, and you don't lose any vegetables with her method. I sometimes skim off vegetables along with the fat and discard them.

Note: Do not put a hot pot of soup in your refrigerator or you can possibly break your refrigerator and make all of your other food go bad. To cool down a pot of soup that is still too warm to refrigerate, put ice water in your metal kitchen sink. Add the metal pot, being sure that the water is not too high and does not get into the soup. Stir the contents to cool it down. Let it sit there a while until cool. Place a towel on your counter. Remove the pot, place it on the towel and dry the outside of the pot. Now you can put the cooled soup in the refrigerator. Be sure to do this only with a pot that can handle extreme temperature changes.

*see gluten-free products list at the end of the book*

## Tomato Soup – Condensed Style – Easy Stove or Crock-pot Version

Very easy to make and we like it better than the gluten-containing condensed soups. Do not add salt, since there is enough salt in the tomato juice. My mother and I invented this soup. Not only is this cheaper than condensed soup, but I think it is easier to make because the condensed soup can be lumpy due to the difficulty of mixing the water in. This is a favorite version of ours.

1 (46 ounce) can tomato juice*  
3 Tablespoons fine white rice flour

2 Tablespoons sugar  
¾ teaspoon Worcestershire Sauce*

Put the rice flour in a pot or a crock-pot. Slowly mix in the tomato juice using a whisk. Whisk in the sugar and Worcestershire sauce. For stove version, heat until hot and thickened. For the crock-pot version, cover and cook on high for 4 hours or on low for 8 hours.

This is nice served with a gluten-free cheese sandwich. Before going to church I often set up the bread machine with our favorite bread recipe, and set up the crock-pot with this soup. I come home to have warm bread and soup for lunch. (Note: be sure any bread recipe you use in the machine is a tested recipe, so that you know you won't have a problem if you leave the bread machine unattended.) We like a cheese sandwich with this soup.

*Variation:* As of this writing, all varieties of V8® vegetable juice from Campbell's® are gluten-free and can be used instead of the tomato juice. They have a low sodium version for those who want less salt in their diet.

## Tomato Soup – Condensed Style, Version 2

If you have less than a full can of tomato juice, this is also a good version to try. My mother and I invented this recipe.

4 cups gluten-free tomato juice*  
2 Tablespoons fine white rice flour  
4 teaspoons sugar  
½ teaspoon Worcestershire* sauce, or more or less to taste

Sprinkling of MSG* (optional, I don't use)  
Salt to taste (usually not needed, as tomato juice already contains salt)  
Dash of onion juice (optional, I don't use)

Put rice flour in a pot. Mix the rice flour with a little of the tomato juice to blend it in. Add the rest of the juice and mix in the rest of the ingredients. Heat until it thickens and is hot. It will bubble around the edges. Stir and serve. We like this soup served in mugs instead of bowls.

*Variation:* For a cream of tomato soup, use 3 cups juice. Add one cup of milk after it thickens. Do not boil the milk or it will curdle.

*Variation 2:* Top with a little shredded cheddar cheese for garnish.

*Variation 3:* As of this writing, all varieties of V8® vegetable juice from Campbell's® are gluten-free and can be used instead of the tomato juice.

*see gluten-free products list at the end of the book

## Tomato Soup – Creamed Condensed Style
Since many brands of canned tomato soup usually contain wheat, here is an easy way to make your own. This version is good if you have tomato puree on hand.

2 cups gluten-free tomato puree*
4 teaspoons fine white rice flour (use 3 teaspoons if puree is very thick)
1 cup water

2 teaspoons salt (or a little less)
2 dashes of pepper
1 Tablespoon sugar (I use a little more)
3 cups milk

Put tomato puree in a pot. Mix rice flour with water. Add to puree. Add salt, pepper, and sugar. Stir together and heat until thick and bubbly. Remove from heat.

Measure the milk in a microwave safe measuring cup. Heat it on high power for 1 minute in the microwave. Add milk to the soup. Blend. We find this makes the soup the right temperature. If soup needs to be warmer, heat but do not boil or the milk will curdle. Garnish with grated cheddar cheese if desired.

*Variation:* For a stronger tomato flavor, you can use the entire 28 ounce can of puree instead of just two cups. Do not add the 1 cup water. Use a ¼ cup less milk.

## Tomato-Basil Cream Soup
This is a delicious tomato soup with Italian flavor. If you want a creamier soup, use the tomato puree and the onion powder. I like the chunks so I use the whole tomatoes and onion flakes.

1 (28 oz.) can peeled tomatoes, un-drained; or 1 can tomato puree (for a smoother soup)
2 Tablespoons dried minced onion; or 1 Tablespoon onion powder (for a smoother soup)
½ teaspoon garlic powder
Pinch of ground red pepper (optional)

2 Tablespoons chopped fresh basil or 2 teaspoons dried basil
1 teaspoon salt
½ teaspoon sugar
1 Tablespoon fine white rice flour
3 Tablespoons Pecorino Romano Cheese
4 cups milk
Fresh basil leaves for garnish (optional)

Put the canned tomatoes or puree, minced onion or powder, garlic powder, basil, red pepper (if using), salt, sugar, and fine white rice flour in a pot. Using a poultry scissor gently cut the tomatoes into pieces; otherwise you can use clean hands to crush them but be careful as they may squirt. Heat all ingredients together, cover, and simmer for 10 minutes. Remove from heat. Add the milk and Pecorino Romano cheese. Heat until hot but do not boil. Season to taste with additional salt and pepper, if needed. If desired, garnish with some fresh basil leaves. You can also garnish with a sprinkling of grated cheese.

*see gluten-free products list at the end of the book

## Tomato Rice Soup – Stove and Crock-pot Method

Since many brands of canned tomato rice soup contain wheat, here is an easy way to make your own using tomato paste. It also costs less. I think the lemon juice gives it a nice flavor. My husband says this soup tastes like "Spaghetti-o's®".

2 ½ cups water
1 (6 ounce) can tomato paste
1 teaspoon gluten-free chicken bouillon*
2 teaspoons lemon juice (I use reconstituted)
4 teaspoons sugar

½ teaspoon seasoned salt (I use ¼ teaspoon celery salt and ¼ teaspoon salt) or to taste
1 bay leaf
½ cup cooked rice

In a saucepan, mix all ingredients. Cook 10 minutes. The soup will be thick. If you like a thinner soup, thin with additional water. Remove bay leaf and serve.

*Variation*: You can make this soup using uncooked rice by using ¼ cup uncooked rice and adding an additional 1 cup of water. Cook 20 minutes until the rice is cooked. Add additional water or milk before serving, if soup is too thick.

*Variation 2*: This soup can be made in a crock-pot. Use the uncooked rice method noted in the first variation. Put all ingredients in the crock-pot and cook covered on high for 4 hours. If soup is too thick, add additional water or some milk before serving. Tomato soup seems to taste less acidic by cooking it in a crock-pot.

*Variation 3*: Top with some grated cheddar cheese for garnish. The cheese adds a nice flavor.

## Tortilla Soup

Think of this as vegetable soup with Mexican saltine crackers. I use 6 tortillas because I enjoy munching on the leftover tortilla chips.

4 to 6 corn tortillas
½ cup oil
Salt
1 whole skinless/boneless chicken breast, cut up into bite sized pieces
1 large onion, chopped
1 green pepper, chopped (optional)
1 stalk of celery, chopped
2 carrots, peeled and chopped

4 cups gluten-free chicken broth* or 4 cups water and 4 teaspoons gluten-free chicken base* or bouillon*
1 cup tomato sauce, or 1 (8 ounce) can tomato sauce*
½ teaspoon salt
½ teaspoon chili powder
⅛ teaspoon pepper (or a little less)
Grated cheddar cheese as a garnish

Cut up one corn tortilla into very small pieces. Set this one tortilla aside. It will be used to thicken the soup.

Cut the rest of the tortillas into ¼ inch strips going across, using a sharp knife and a cutting board. Cut them into about 1 inch lengths going down the other way. You have noodle-like strips.  Fry these in the ½ cup oil.  Drain them well on paper towels and salt them lightly.  These are your Mexican crackers to add when you serve the soup.

Allow oil to cool.  Meanwhile, cut up the vegetables and the chicken.  (I use a poultry scissors to cut the chicken.)

Drain off all the oil except for about 1 to 2 Tablespoons.  (Do not pour hot oil down the drain of your sink, as hot oil can melt or ruin the pipes.)  Sauté the vegetables, chicken, and the cut up tortilla you set aside in the remaining Tablespoon oil.  Add the chicken broth, tomato sauce, salt, chili powder and spices.  Cover and simmer for 30 minutes.

To serve, ladle soup into bowls, top each bowl with some grated cheddar cheese and the tortilla chips.

*Variation:*  You may substitute 1 zucchini chopped for the celery.  Add it 15 minutes before the end of cooking, since zucchini cooks faster than celery.

*Variation 2:*  Gluten-free tortilla chips* may be substituted, instead of making your own.  Instead of using the one cut up tortilla to thicken the soup, add one Tablespoon of fine white rice flour to the chicken broth.  You may want to use a little less salt in the soup, as some brands of chips may be salty.

*Variation 3:*  Ground pork or diced pork may be substituted for chicken.  If using ground pork, sauté it first so that it loses its pink color, and then add the vegetables.

*Variation 4:*  Diced frozen onion and green pepper may be substituted for the fresh.  Frozen peas may be used instead of celery.  Frozen carrots may also be used.  Using frozen vegetables saves chopping and makes this a quick soup to make.  I prefer adding the frozen carrots and peas in the last 15 minutes of cooking time so that they don't get over-cooked.

## Turkey Carcass Soup
When carving your turkey, do not discard any bones because you will then have the makings for one final turkey treat – a beautiful soup.  Make this recipe only if your turkey had gluten-free stuffing or contained no stuffing. (Note: you should not eat from a turkey that had any wheat stuffing in it. Gluten will contaminate the meat and the gravy.)

| | |
|---|---|
| Turkey carcass | Salt and ground black pepper to taste |
| Any leftover gelatin in roasting pan | Clove of garlic |
| Any leftover gluten-free gravy | Bay leaf |
| 2 carrots | 1 teaspoon sugar |
| 2 ribs of celery | ½ cup cooked rice (optional) |
| 1 parsnip (optional) | |
| 1 onion, peeled | |

Put carcass and any loose bones in a large pot along with leftover gravy and gelatin.  Scrape and clean parsnips, carrots and celery and place whole on top of bones.  Peel onion and place whole in pot also.  Add garlic, bay leaf, salt, pepper and sugar.  Cover all with water.  Cover the pot with the lid and simmer 1 hour.  Cool.

*see gluten-free products list at the end of the book*

Remove carrots, celery and parsnip and dice.  Pour broth through a strainer into a large bowl.  Now remove any meat on bones and dice.  You will be surprised at how much meat you will recover, usually about 2 cups.  Discard bones, turkey skin, onion and garlic clove.  (Or press onion through the strainer to get its juices into the soup.)  Return broth, turkey meat and vegetables to pot.  Add cooked rice and heat through.  Remove from heat and serve.

*Variation*:  My mother discards the onion and garlic.  Instead, I dice the onion before putting it in the pot.  I use ⅛ teaspoon garlic powder instead of a clove of garlic.  I return the diced onion to the soup after straining it to get the bones out.  I skip the step of pressing vegetables through a strainer.  (Sometimes I only use the large turkey bones, and I just remove those and don't strain the soup at all.)

<u>Write your own recipes here</u>:

# SALADS

## Apple Salad or Waldorf Salad
This is a special apple salad that my mother would serve at luncheons.

6 cups unpeeled, diced, yellow Delicious apples
6 oz. gluten-free cream cheese*, softened
½ cup gluten-free mayonnaise*
1 Tablespoon real maple syrup or honey
3 Tablespoons cream sherry

⅛ teaspoon ground nutmeg
4 stalks celery, diced
½ cup dried currants or raisins
½ cup coarsely broken pecans or walnuts

Dice the apples. Remove the strings from the celery and chop it. Add raisins and nuts. Mix all other ingredients well in a bowl and pour over apple mixture. Toss and serve.

## Beet Salad with Eggs (also called Pickled Beets)
I always enjoy this, it's very easy, and it looks nice on a buffet table. It's inexpensive too. This makes those bright colored eggs that you often see in salad bars. It's also a good use for leftover Easter eggs. I like to make this a day or two ahead of time for better flavor.

6 hard boiled eggs, peeled
1 can sliced beets

⅓ cup cider vinegar
⅔ cup sugar

To make boiled eggs that are easy to peel, purchase them a week before you plan to boil them. To boil eggs, place room temperature eggs in a pot and add enough water to cover. Bring to a boil. Reduce heat and simmer gently for 20 minutes. Pour off hot water immediately and add cold water to the pot, shaking the pot to crack the eggs. Continue pouring in cold tap water until eggs are cool. Shell eggs and place in a wide mouth glass jar. (I use an empty pickle jar with a lid for this.)

Open the can of beets and drain all the liquid into a small saucepan. Add the vinegar and sugar to the saucepan. Heat the vinegar, sugar and beet juice until it boils, and stir to make sure all of the sugar is dissolved. Watch carefully because this can boil over quickly if unattended, and make a mess. Once it boils, remove immediately from the heat. Put the beets into the jar over the eggs. Pour the beet juice mixture over the beets and eggs. Gently push the beets with a metal spoon (plastic spoon may stain) so that they are firmly packed, but not so much that you break up the beet slices. You want them covered with the juice as best you can. Allow it to cool and store it covered in the refrigerator. To serve, remove beets and eggs from the juice with a slotted metal spoon. Put on a serving platter. To store leftovers, return to the juice and refrigerate.

Note: I put the eggs on the bottom of the jar because otherwise they sometimes float to the top and not be completely submerged. Then you don't get completely red colored eggs.

## Beet Salad with Sour Cream
An easy to prepare salad that looks nice on a buffet table.

2 cans julienne beets
1 cup gluten-free sour cream*

2 teaspoons gluten-free horseradish*
Salt and ground black pepper

Drain beets well and mix with other ingredients.  Refrigerate.

## Beet Salad over Lettuce
This is good for a light lunch or side-salad.  This recipe comes from my mother.

Lettuce leaves
1 can sliced beets, drained
1 medium sweet onion, sliced in rings (I use Vidalia® onions since they are sweeter.)

Mushrooms, cleaned and sliced
Hard Boiled Egg, chopped
Gluten-Free Ranch salad dressing* (or see index for recipe)

Place lettuce leaf on each plate.  Top with some drained beets.  Top the beets with sliced mushrooms.  Place onion rings attractively on top of each.  Sprinkle with some chopped egg.  Pass dressing.

*Variation*:  Pickled Beets (see recipe on previous page) can be served in this manner, with the "pickled" hard boiled eggs sliced and placed on top of the beets.

## Black Bean and Corn Salad (also called Texas Caviar)
This recipe from my mother is best when made ahead of time.  It is nice as a side salad for lunch.  Or it can be served over lettuce.  It is also good used as a salsa with grilled chicken or steak.  It is easy to put together because it is mostly all drained canned vegetables, and it can be made ahead of time and refrigerated so the flavors improve.

1 (15 ounce) can of black beans*, rinsed and drained
1 (11 ounce or 15 ounce) can of corn or Mexicorn® (corn with red and green peppers), drained
1 (14 ounce) can of diced tomatoes*, drained
1 or 2 green onions, chopped or 1 Tablespoon dried chives

1 Tablespoon dehydrated onion flakes
1 clove garlic, minced or ⅛ to ¼ teaspoon garlic powder
1 teaspoon cumin
1 ½ teaspoons brown sugar
3 Tablespoons oil
3 Tablespoons balsamic vinegar
Salt and pepper to taste

Blend all in a container with a lid.  Cover and refrigerate overnight.  Stir to blend flavors.

## Carrot Raisin Salad

This makes a lot. I either make half of the recipe or use any leftover salad in carrot cake. Or leftover salad can also be added to flavored gelatin* (such as orange or lemon) to make a gelatin mold/salad.

1 pound carrots (I prefer carrots from California), peeled and grated
1 (20 oz.) can crushed pineapple with juice
1 to 2 handfuls of raisin (I prefer sultanas or golden raisins)

1 to 2 handfuls of chopped walnuts
Dash of salt
Enough gluten-free mayonnaise* to moisten

Mix all together and serve.

## Chicken Salad

This is my mother's recipe and a good way to use leftover chicken. It's nice for a luncheon.

2 cups cooked chicken
½ cup chopped celery
½ cup raisins
½ cup chopped almonds or pecans
½ to 1 teaspoon gluten-free curry powder*

2 heaping Tablespoons gluten-free chutney (see index for recipe or purchase gluten-free chutney*)
Dash of salt
Enough gluten-free mayonnaise* to moisten

Mix all together and serve on lettuce leaf or stuff a tomato. Serves four.

*Variation*: This salad is much more flavorful with the chutney, but it can be made without it.

*Variation 2*: For a more traditional chicken salad, make it using only the chicken, celery, salt and mayonnaise.

## Chickpea (or Garbanzo Bean) Salad

An easy salad that is something different.

1 hard cooked egg yolk, mashed
¼ cup olive oil
3 Tablespoons red wine vinegar
1 clove garlic, minced
1 Tablespoon capers* (optional), drained, rinsed and chopped

2 Tablespoons parsley, minced (optional)
1 to 2 Tablespoons onion, chopped fine or 1 teaspoon dried minced onion flakes
1 (15 ½ ounce) can chickpeas (also called garbanzo beans), rinsed and drained
Salt (use only if you don't add capers)

Mash the egg yolk. Add the olive oil. Add the rest of the ingredients and blend. Taste to see if salt is needed, if you didn't use capers. Make the day before. Serve at room temperature. If desired, add diced red pepper (fresh, or the roasted kind in a jar*) for color.

## Chickpea (or Garbanzo Bean) Salad – Version 2
This version from my mother is also very good.

¼ cup olive oil
2 Tablespoons red wine vinegar
1 Tablespoon Balsamic vinegar
1 clove garlic, minced
1 Tablespoon capers*, drained, rinsed and chopped (optional, I don't use)
2 Tablespoons parsley, minced (optional)
1 to 2 Tablespoons onion, chopped fine or 1 teaspoon dried minced onion flakes

1 diced roasted red pepper (I use the kind from a jar)
1 large jar (or can) sliced mushrooms, drained
1 (15 ½ ounce) can chickpeas (also called garbanzo beans), rinsed and drained
1 can medium pitted olives, drained
½ to ¾ teaspoon sugar

Put all ingredients in a jar. Secure lid and shake to blend flavors. Marinate for 2 to 3 days in the refrigerator before serving.

## Coleslaw – Quick and Easy Version
I often quickly put this together for picnics. Add salt (if desired) when you're ready to serve so that it won't get watery. The salt makes the water come out of the cabbage. My favorite Cole Slaw is made with Cole Slaw Dressing (see index), but this method is also good and so easy!

1 bag of coleslaw salad mix
1 Tablespoon sugar

2 Tablespoons cider vinegar
⅓ to ½ cup gluten-free mayonnaise*

In a bowl, blend together sugar, vinegar and ⅓ cup mayonnaise using a whisk. Add in the coleslaw mix using a spoon. Blend well. Add more mayonnaise if needed.

*Variation*: You can use Miracle Whip® instead of mayonnaise (gluten-free as of this writing) and eliminate the vinegar (or use less vinegar). Sometimes I also add ¼ teaspoon of celery seed (or more) for a different flavor.

## Cranberry Eggnog Gelatin Mold
This is nice on a holiday buffet table.

1 package gluten-free vanilla pudding* (not instant)
1 (3 oz.) package lemon gelatin
2 cups water
1 Tablespoon gluten-free rum*
1 (3 oz.) package raspberry gelatin

1 (16 oz.) can whole cranberry sauce
½ cup celery, chopped
¼ cup chopped pecans
1 cup gluten-free heavy cream*, whipped
½ teaspoon ground nutmeg

Combine and boil together the pudding mix, lemon gelatin and water. When cooled, add rum and set aside. Dissolve raspberry gelatin in 1 cup boiling water. Stir in the cranberry sauce, pecans and chopped celery. Chill until it thickens but not set. Add nutmeg to whipped cream and fold into cooled vanilla pudding mixture. Put half of pudding mixture into an oiled 8 x 8 inch pan. Chill. Top with all of the cranberry mixture and chill. Then add the rest of pudding mixture. Chill at least 6 hours or overnight.

*see gluten-free products list at the end of the book

Note: My mother uses an oiled ring mold placing the pudding mixture in first then chilling it. She then pours in the cranberry mixture. This gives 2 layers instead of 3. It looks pretty for a holiday buffet. You can use gluten-free cooking spray to oil the mold. Tupperware® gelatin molds also work well. You do not have grease them because the gelatin is easy to remove with the extra Tupperware® seal on the bottom.

## Cranberry and Evaporated Milk Gelatin Salad
This is a different version, using evaporated milk instead of cream.

1 package (6 oz.) red gelatin
1 can (20 oz.) crushed pineapple (do not use fresh pineapple or it will not gel)
1 package (8 oz) gluten-free cream cheese*, softened

½ cup chopped nuts
1 can whole cranberry sauce
1 can (12 oz) evaporated milk

Combine gelatin and pineapple in a heavy saucepan. Heat over low heat until gelatin is dissolved. Stir in cheese until it is well blended. Stir in nuts and cranberries and milk. Put into a greased 8 cup mold. (I use an un-greased Tupperware® mold for this.) Chill thoroughly for several hours or overnight. Remove from mold and serve on salad greens.

## Cranberry Wine Gelatin Mold
I like this one for the holidays. It has a beautiful red color and tastes delicious. This recipe also works well using the jelled cranberry sauce.

2 (3 ounce) packages raspberry gelatin
1 ¼ cups hot water
1 can whole cranberry sauce
½ cup sweet port wine or ¼ cup Marsala wine

1 cup gluten-free sour cream*
1 can crushed pineapple
1 (3 ounce) package softened gluten-free cream cheese*
½ cup chopped nuts

Put gelatin in a large bowl. Add hot water and stir until gelatin dissolves. Add cranberry sauce, un-drained pineapple and wine. Stir. Pour gelatin mixture into an oiled flat pan and refrigerate until firm. Mix together the softened cream cheese and sour cream. Spread over gelatin and sprinkle with nuts. Or place half of gelatin in an oiled mold. (I use a Tupperware® mold so I don't have to oil it.) Refrigerate until firm. Spread cream cheese mixture and nuts over top. Then top with remaining gelatin and refrigerate until firm.

## Cucumber Salad
This recipe comes from my mother. It is best when made the night before.

2 cucumbers, thinly sliced ½ of a sweet onion (such as Vidalia®), thinly sliced
½ cup sugar (I use less, about ⅓ cup)
½ cup water

¼ cup vinegar
¼ cup oil
¼ teaspoon celery seed

*see gluten-free products list at the end of the book

If cucumbers are un-waxed, score them with a fork to make a nice edge. Otherwise peel them and slice. Thinly slice the onion. Place them in some lightly salted ice water for 1 hour. Meanwhile, put the ½ cup sugar and ½ cup water in a pot. Heat and stir until sugar melts. Let cool.

After the hour, drain and rinse the cucumbers. Put in a jar with a lid. Add the sugar water, the oil, vinegar, and celery seed. Refrigerate overnight. Stir before serving.

## Egg Salad
This is flavorful in a sandwich or on a bed of lettuce.

6 hard boiled eggs
⅓ cup gluten-free mayonnaise*
1 teaspoon grated onion or ¼ teaspoon
   granulated onion powder

1 teaspoon prepared gluten-free mustard*
   or ¼ teaspoon gluten-free dry mustard*
Salt and pepper to taste
1 stalk celery, chopped

Place room temperature eggs in a pot and add enough water to cover. Bring to a boil. Reduce heat and simmer gently for 20 minutes. Pour off hot water immediately and add cold water to the pot, shaking the pot to crack the eggs. Continue pouring in cold tap water until eggs are cool or add ice cubes to help cool them down quickly. Shell and mash the eggs with a fork. I sometimes use my food processor to cut up the eggs using only a quick pulse (do not over-process). Stir in the mayonnaise, salt, pepper, onion and mustard. Add celery. I like it on top of a lettuce salad or as a part of a gluten-free sandwich.

## Frozen Fruit Salad
Unusual, but a hit at my mother's luncheon group meetings during the summer.

2 ripe bananas, mashed
1 (3 oz.) package gluten-free cream
   cheese*, softened
1 small can of crushed pineapple, drained
½ cup chopped pecans

1 small jar gluten-free maraschino
   cherries*, drained and diced
1 cup gluten-free whipped heavy cream*
1 teaspoon sugar

Whip cream with 1 teaspoon sugar and fold in remaining ingredients. Pour into a freezer tray or empty orange juice can. Freeze. When ready to use open the bottom of the can and push contents out. Slice into ½ inch slices and serve on lettuce.

## Fruit Salad for a Party
This recipe is from my sister.

Cut up fresh fruit. Add a can of chunk pineapple in its own juice, reserving the juice. Mix a gluten-free instant vanilla pudding mix* with the pineapple juice from the canned pineapple. Mix the juice mixture in with the fruit before it fully sets. (Pineapple juice keeps diced apples from turning brown, so cut up apples may be used in your fruit salad.)

*Variation*: If you're not sure the pudding you have is gluten-free, instead you can add some sugar and a little vanilla instead. The juice won't be thickened, but your fruit salad will still be delicious.

*Variation 2*: For a fruit salad containing berries, you can eliminate the pudding and pineapple juice and use jam to intensify the berry flavor. Add some gluten-free jam* melted in the microwave or some gluten-free fruit syrup* such as strawberry or raspberry. I usually do this variation for a fruit salad containing a lot of strawberries.

## Grape, Hazelnut, and Cheese Tossed Salad

We went to a restaurant that served this gluten-free salad. We enjoyed it so much that I duplicated it at home. For people with tomato allergies, red grapes can be a substitute for grape tomatoes in a salad. Try it and see. A salad dressing with a little added sweetness compliments the grapes.

Mesclun (tender salad greens)
Whole or chopped hazelnuts (filberts), toasted (almonds can also be used)
Red grapes, washed, dried, and cut in half (I use a small bunch)
Honey

Our favorite Italian dressing made with red wine vinegar, without grated cheese (see index)
Thinly sliced and cubed gluten-free cheese (I use Provolone. The restaurant used thinly sliced Manchego cheese.)

Rinse and dry salad greens (or spin in a salad spinner) and put into a salad bowl. Toast hazelnuts by putting them in a toaster oven at 300°F for 3 to 5 minutes. Watch carefully as they can burn quickly. They should be golden brown, and not too dark. (They continue to brown after you remove them from the oven.) Toasting the nuts brings out their flavor and makes them more delicious. When cool, add to salad greens. Wash grapes, dry, cut in half and add to salad. Drizzle salad with a small amount of honey. Top with salad dressing and provolone cheese. Toss salad well and serve.

*Variation*: Make a tossed salad topping it with "Sweet Pecans" (see index for recipe), sliced grapes, and soft goat cheese, crumbled. Since the nuts have sweetness, you don't need to add the honey to the dressing. Just use our favorite Italian dressing (see index for recipe). This combination is good on the Mesclun greens or Romaine lettuce.

## Green Bean and Bacon Salad

This recipe comes from a good friend of mine. Serve this cold. It's delicious at a picnic.

2 (10 ounce) boxes frozen cut green beans thawed or equivalent fresh beans
½ pound bacon, diced (I use a little less)
1 bunch scallions, chopped
2 teaspoons chopped parsley

⅓ cup olive oil
1 teaspoon lemon juice
2 teaspoons red wine vinegar
Salt and ground black pepper to taste

Blanch the beans in boiling water 1 minute for frozen green beans, or cook until crisp/tender for fresh. Drain and rinse in cold water. Drain. Cook the bacon until almost crisp. (Sometimes if it is too crispy it can be hard to chew in a cold salad). Remove from pan and drain on paper towels. Dice bacon. Combine beans, bacon, scallions and parsley in

*see gluten-free products list at the end of the book

a bowl.  Mix together oil, lemon juice and vinegar.  Add to bean mixture and toss.  Add salt and pepper to taste.  Refrigerate 2 to 3 hours.  Toss salad a couple of times while chilling.  Serves 6 to 8 people.

## Heavenly Ambrosia Salad
A friend gave me this recipe.  It is sweet so it can be used as a salad or as dessert.  This recipe doesn't contain sour cream.  Some people with lactose intolerance find cream very difficult to digest.

1 small package gluten-free pistachio instant pudding*
1 (16 to 20 ounce) can of chunk pineapple (packed in pineapple juice not syrup)
1 (8 ounce) can of crushed pineapple (packed in pineapple juice not syrup)
1 cup shredded coconut*

1 cup walnuts, chopped or in pieces
1 (12 to 16 ounce) thawed container of Cool Whip® (gluten-free as of this writing)
1 cup gluten-free miniature marshmallows*

Combine both cans of pineapple and their juice.  Sprinkle the pudding on top.  Let it stand for 3 minutes.  Add the coconut and walnuts and carefully mix together.  Slowly fold in the whipped topping and marshmallows.  Refrigerate 2 hours before serving.

## Heavenly Hash Fruit Salad
My sister-in-law gave me this recipe.  It has always been gluten-free and is easy to make.

1 pint gluten-free sour cream*
1 cup gluten-free miniature marshmallows*
1 cup shredded coconut
1 cup chunk pineapple

1 cup mandarin oranges
1 cup of any kind of grapes
1 cup chunk sliced peaches
1 cup of any other kind of fruit desired

Combine all ingredients in a large bowl at least one day before you plan to use it and refrigerate.  Stir once after several hours.  Serve as a salad or dessert.

## Hungarian Cabbage Salad
This is a change from regular coleslaw.

1 ½ pounds cabbage
2 tomatoes
1 gluten-free sour or dill pickle*
1 red pepper
1 green pepper
2 Tablespoons cider vinegar

2 Tablespoons olive oil
2 Tablespoons corn oil
2 Tablespoons lemon juice
2 Tablespoons honey
1 teaspoon salt
3 to 4 drops gluten-free hot sauce*

Cut and core cabbage.  Wash and remove seeds from tomatoes and peppers.  Grate all in a food processor.  Make dressing with remaining ingredients, and toss with vegetables.  You can add 3 to 4 drops of hot pepper sauce for added zing to your salad.  This lasts two to three days in the refrigerator.

*see gluten-free products list at the end of the book

## Macaroni Salad

I served this at a picnic, and no one knew it was gluten-free. This is my mother's recipe. I use the tuna in oil and don't drain it. Then I use less mayonnaise. I find the oil gives it more taste. You can also use the water packed tuna but you must drain the water. Use the chunk light because this less expensive tuna has a strong fish taste and works well with the bland macaroni in this salad.

½ pound gluten-free elbow macaroni*
cooked (I use Tinkyada® or Sam
Mills®)
1 can gluten-free tuna fish*, chunk light
oil-packed (undrained) or water-packed
(drained)
½ cup celery, diced

2 Tablespoons cider vinegar
1 Tablespoon sugar
¼ teaspoon ground black pepper
Salt to taste
Gluten-free mayonnaise*
Few frozen green peas for color (optional)

Cook and drain macaroni. (Note: cook it the full amount of time on the package or 2 minutes longer at a full boil. Otherwise they are too hard for a cold pasta salad. For the Tinkyada® brand pasta you can use the "energy saving" method which is boil 2 minutes, cover, let it sit 20 minutes, test for doneness, and then drain. If using Sam Mills® Pasta d'Oro, cook 2 to 4 minutes longer than directed.)

In a large bowl, mix together vinegar, sugar and pepper. Add macaroni, tuna, peas (if using) and just enough mayonnaise to moisten. Taste to see if salt is needed. (Some tuna is more salty than others, so you must judge how much salt to use by taste.)

Note: This salad is best the day you make it. The next day the gluten-free pasta will absorb most of the mayonnaise so it will be drier. You may have to add a little more mayonnaise before you serve it the next day.

## Mango (or Peach) Salad or Dessert

I received a can of mangos as a gift and didn't know what to do with them until my mother gave me this recipe.

3 (3 oz.) packages of lemon gelatin*
1 (8 oz.) package of gluten-free cream
cheese*

3 cups boiling water
1 (28 to 30 oz.) can of mangos with juice
or canned peaches with juice

Dissolve lemon gelatin in boiling water. In a blender or food processor, combine cream cheese, mangos (or peaches) with the juice and blend. Stir into the gelatin and pour into a 2-quart mold that has been sprayed with gluten-free cooking spray*. Refrigerate until set. Serve with sauce (recipe follows) for the salad or whipped cream for the dessert.

Sauce for Mango Salad:
  2 eggs
  1 ½ cups sugar

Juice and rinds of 2 oranges and 2 lemons

Combine in a saucepan. Boil 5-7 minutes to thicken. Remove and strain. Refrigerate. Remove from refrigerator 30 minutes before serving.

*see gluten-free products list at the end of the book

## Marinated Shrimp Antipasto Salad
This is a make-ahead salad. This recipe makes a lot, so you may want to halve the recipe. As you can see from the ingredients list, you can vary this recipe depending on what you prefer, or have on hand.

1 cup oil (I use corn or canola oil)
⅔ cup lemon juice (I use bottled)
2 Tablespoons gluten-free Dijon mustard*
2 teaspoons sugar
1 teaspoon oregano
½ teaspoon marjoram
1 teaspoon salt
1 ½ pounds medium shrimp, cooked, deveined and shelled. (I defrost frozen cooked shrimp and remove the tails)
6 ounces of sliced gluten-free Provolone cheese, cut into cubes

4 ounces sliced gluten-free pepperoni* cut into small pieces. (Other gluten-free meats like salami or ham may be used.)
1 (6 ounce) can of small ripe pitted olives, drained (If using larger olives, slice them)
2 Tablespoons dried minced onion, or ¼ to ½ cup onion chopped fine (I like Vidalia onions), or ¼ to ½ cup sliced green onions or 2 Tablespoons dried chives.
1 large red pepper, seeded and diced, or diced roasted red pepper

Make dressing by whisking together the oil, lemon juice, mustard, sugar, herbs and salt. Add the rest of the ingredients and blend. (I use kitchen scissors to remove shrimp tails and cut the sliced meat and cheese.) Push down ingredients under marinade; cover and store in the refrigerator. This salad is best when you allow it to marinate for 4 to 6 hours or overnight in the refrigerator. (Note: I don't use olive oil in this salad, since it gets very thick when refrigerated. I prefer to be able to serve it right away from the refrigerator rather than having to have the salad sit out until the oil is room temperature.)

Stir salad and serve over a bed of lettuce. Use some of the marinade as dressing on the lettuce. This looks nice on a buffet table.

## Martha's Vineyard Salad
It looks very impressive on a buffet, and it's delicious! This recipe is my mother's. She developed it from tasting it at a restaurant. She has that gift of being able to taste something in a restaurant and then go home and recreate it. Read labels carefully when purchasing blue cheese. Some companies use a bread mold that is grown on wheat bread to make their cheese.

Raspberry Dressing (see recipe under Dressings)
Boston or Romaine lettuce
Red onion, thinly sliced

Toasted pine nuts or almonds
Crumbled gluten-free blue cheese* or gluten-free goat cheese (fromage de chèvre)

In a serving platter, put down a layer of cleaned romaine or Boston lettuce. Top with thinly sliced red onion, toasted pine nuts or almonds, and crumbled goat cheese. Top with dressing and serve.

*Variation*: For a change, top this salad with well-drained canned mandarin oranges or sliced fresh strawberries before adding the dressing.

*see gluten-free products list at the end of the book

## Orange and Green Salad

This is my mother's recipe and a good luncheon salad. Don't make this dressing ahead of time or it will be too hot and spicy. It is best made immediately before serving. Or use Martha's Vineyard Dressing.

1 red onion sliced and placed in cold
   water with 1 teaspoon sugar
3 navel oranges
3 cups salad greens
½ teaspoons gluten-free dry mustard*

¼ teaspoon cumin
2 Tablespoons vinegar
4 Tablespoons oil
Salt and ground black pepper to taste

Slice onion thinly and place in a bowl of cold water in which a teaspoon of sugar has been added. Refrigerate onion. This will make the onion sweeter and remove some of the "bite".) Peel and thinly slice oranges. (I slice them the same way as I would slice an onion when making onion rings. Slice it one end of the orange to the other using a serrated knife. Clean and coarsely tear the greens and place on a salad plate. Arrange orange slices attractively over the top. Drain the onions, wipe dry with a paper towel and sprinkle over oranges. Make dressing with remaining ingredients, shake well and pour over salad. Serves 4.

*Variation*: This goes nicely with grilled chicken breasts.

## Pasta Salad – Italian Style

The bacon adds a lot of flavor. If you prefer to use another smoked meat, try gluten-free pepperoni* or gluten-free cold-cuts like salami*. This eliminates the step of cooking bacon.

1 package of gluten-free tri-colored rice
   spirals/vegetable twists (I use Mrs.
   Leeper's® or Tinkyada®), cooked and
   drained
4 slices of gluten-free bacon, cooked and
   drained

1 package grape tomatoes, washed, dried
   and sliced in half lengthwise
Gluten-free cheese, cubed or grated like
   cheddar or provolone
Italian Salad Dressing (see index)

Cook pasta according to package directions and test. If too firm, cook about 2 to 4 minutes longer so that they won't be too hard in the salad. Drain, rinse and shake out excess water. Place in a bowl. Meanwhile, cook bacon in the microwave on paper towels (I cook for 5-6 minutes). Drain the fat with paper towels, and then crumble. Add to the bowl. Cube cheese (I use Mozzarella, or Munster or Provolone) and add to the bowl. Add tomatoes. Pour some dressing and blend. Taste and add more if needed.

*Variation*: Other vegetables can be added to your salad. My mother marinates vegetables a day or two before adding them so that they will be flavorful. Marinate them in 1 cup water, ¼ cup wine vinegar, 1 Tablespoon sugar and 1 teaspoon seasoned salt* or garlic salt. Store them in the refrigerator. When ready to use, drain and add to your salad.

You can marinate cooked or defrosted frozen vegetables using this method. If using uncooked fresh vegetables I recommend that you blanch them first. (Put then in boiling water a few minutes, and then cold water.) Then add the drained vegetables to the marinade.

## Pasta Salad with Salmon

Many pasta salads have tuna, but the salmon is a nice change. I think this pasta salad is best the day you make it. Since gluten-free pasta tends to absorb liquid, the next day you may have to add some additional mayonnaise. If you don't want to use peas, you can use fresh chopped parsley for color.

1 (12 ounce package) Tinkyada®
 vegetable spirals or Sam Mills® spirals
1 can (14.75 oz) Pink Salmon, drained,
 with large bones and skin removed or 2
 (6 oz.) cans skinless/boneless salmon,
 drained
1 cup celery, diced

¼ cup cider vinegar
2 Tablespoons sugar
¼ to ½ teaspoon ground black pepper
Salt to taste (caution: salmon can be salty)
Gluten-free mayonnaise*
Few frozen green peas for color (optional)

Cook and drain macaroni. (I suggest you cook it the <u>full amount of time</u> on the package at a full boil or even 2 to 4 minutes longer, otherwise they are too hard for a cold pasta salad. For the Sam Mills® pasta, I boil it 2 to 4 minutes more than directed.) In a large bowl, mix together vinegar, sugar and pepper. Add macaroni, salmon, peas (if using) and just enough mayonnaise to moisten. Taste to see if salt is needed.

## Potato Salad – Our Favorite Version

This is flavorful and delicious. At picnics people always ask for the recipe. It was my mother's idea to use the "Old Bay®" seasoning. Her "hot potato" method really makes the salad so flavorful. (Without the hot potato method, your potato salad will be flavorless or watery tasting.)

2 ½ pounds new potatoes
⅓ cup cider vinegar
⅓ cup granulated sugar
1 teaspoon salt
⅓ to ⅔ cup gluten-free mayonnaise*
1 slice of onion, minced

Diced celery (optional – I don't use)
Generous sprinkling of "Old Bay®"
 seasoning*
3 to 4 good shakes of celery salt or seed
 (optional)
Paprika

Boil potatoes in their jackets (skins) until tender. Place the vinegar, sugar and salt in a small saucepan and simmer until sugar dissolves. (You can heat the vinegar mixture in the microwave.)

The next step is the most important of all if you want delicious potato salad. Peel and slice the potatoes while still hot. The best way to do this is to have a clean pair of rubber gloves to wear that are designated for this purpose. You can also keep a bowl of cold water in the sink to submerge your hands from time to time if you feel the heat through the gloves. The job goes quickly as the peels come off easily when the potatoes are hot.

Slice potatoes on a cutting board and place in a covered plastic container. Pour the hot vinegar mixture over the potatoes. Cover tightly and shake gently to moisten all potatoes. Let cool before continuing. When you remove the cover, you will see that the hot potatoes have absorbed all the liquid. This is what seals the flavor into the potatoes. Now sprinkle on the "Old Bay" seasoning, celery salt, the minced onion and ⅓ cup mayonnaise. Toss gently.

*see gluten-free products list at the end of the book

If the salad looks dry, add more mayonnaise. Place in a serving bowl and garnish with paprika.

Note: Never let the cool water get on the hot potatoes, only use it to cool your hands during the peeling step. I always wear heavy Playtex® rubber gloves to avoid burning my hands.

*Variation*: I have made the potatoes ahead of time and cooled them. Slice and store the potatoes in a large microwave safe bowl. Cover and refrigerate. The next day reheat them until hot in the microwave before you add the vinegar. Be careful, the potatoes will get very hot. This method is good, but the best is when you follow the steps above. (Recipes that suggest using cold potatoes yield potato salads that taste watery and flavorless. The heat of the potatoes makes them absorb the vinegar.) I have also tried allowing the potatoes to cool, slice them unpeeled using a food processor with a large feed tube, and then followed the steps reheating the potatoes as above. This also works but it's not as pretty with the skins. I think the best method is the original.

*Variation 2*: It can be made without the "Old Bay" seasoning. One time I forgot to add it. It's still good but is much better with it.

## Potato Salad – Version 2
My mother updated her recipe, for a new variation. Here is her new version.

2 ½ pounds new potatoes, cooked, sliced,
  at room temperature or warm
¼ cup cider vinegar
2 Tablespoons granulated sugar
1 teaspoon salt
½ teaspoon of "Old Bay®"seasoning*

¾ cups gluten-free mayonnaise* (or less)
1 slice of onion, minced
3 to 4 good shakes of celery seed
  (optional)
Paprika (optional)
Diced celery (optional – I don't use)

Boil potatoes in their jackets (skins) until tender. Place the vinegar, sugar, salt and Old Bay in a small saucepan and simmer until sugar dissolves. Do not boil.

Follow directions as above for boiling, peeling, and slicing potatoes. The salad turns out better when potatoes are hot, but with the hot liquid it will also absorb into the potatoes if potatoes are warm or room temperature.

Place potatoes in a covered plastic container that won't melt when hot. Pour the hot vinegar mixture over the potatoes. Either gently mix with a spoon until absorbed or cover tightly and shake gently to moisten all potatoes. Let cool before continuing. When you remove the cover, you will see that the hot potatoes have absorbed all the liquid. This is what seals the flavor into the potatoes. Add minced onion, celery seed (if using), celery (if using) and mayonnaise. Toss gently. If the salad looks dry, add more mayonnaise. Place in a serving bowl and garnish with paprika.

*Variation:* Onion powder may be used in place of onion. Add a generous sprinkling to the vinegar before you heat it.

*\*see gluten-free products list at the end of the book*

## Potato Salad (No Mayonnaise version)

This is a delicious and slightly tart tasting salad because of the vinegar. It keeps well because it has no mayonnaise in it. We always enjoy it. If you don't have the gluten-free hot sauce, it's good without it — or you can add a little cayenne pepper, to taste, if you want that "zing".

3 pounds small or new potatoes
   (California or Red Bliss) boiled, peeled
   and sliced
1 cup chopped celery
1 cup chopped onion
1 cup chopped parsley
¾ cup cider vinegar

¼ cup water
2 teaspoons sugar
2 teaspoons salt
¼ teaspoon ground black pepper
8 drops gluten-free hot sauce* (optional)
¾ cup light olive oil

Potatoes should still be warm. If not, warm them in the microwave before starting.

Place the potatoes, celery, onions and parsley in a large Tupperware® type bowl. Mix water, vinegar, sugar, salt and pepper and hot pepper sauce together and add. Cover and shake bowl to blend and let stand ½ hour. Add oil and mix carefully, shaking and rotating the bowl so as not to break the potato slices too much. Taste and add more salt or sugar if needed.

## Potato Salad, Hot German Style

This is flavorful, without mayonnaise. Don't eliminate the bacon or it won't taste right.

6 medium sized potatoes
6 slices of bacon
¾ cup chopped or thinly sliced onion
2 Tablespoons sweet rice or fine white
   rice flour
2 ½ Tablespoons sugar

1 ½ teaspoons salt
½ teaspoon celery seed
Dash of ground black pepper
¾ cup water
½ cup wine or cider vinegar

In a pot, boil the potatoes in their skins until tender. Meanwhile in a fry-pan, fry the bacon slices until crisp. Remove from the fat and set the bacon aside. Keep the bacon fat. (There is usually about ⅓ cup. If there is more than that, I discard the excess.) When potatoes are tender, peel and thinly slice them into a bowl. When bacon has cooled, break into pieces.

Cook the onion in the bacon fat that you kept. Turn off the heat. Mix in the rice flour, sugar, salt, celery seed and pepper. Then gradually stir in the water and vinegar. Be careful because the hot fat could spatter on you when you add the liquid.

Turn the heat back on, and cook and stir until the mixture boils. Boil 1 minute. Pour over the hot potatoes. Add the crisp bacon. Gently toss without breaking potatoes. Cover and let stand until ready to serve. If making ahead of time, when cool store in the refrigerator. Heat it in the microwave, so that it will be hot potato salad.

*see gluten-free products list at the end of the book*

## Sea Foam Gelatin Salad
This is nice on a buffet table.

1 package lime gelatin*  
1 medium can diced pears in juice

1 cup gluten-free heavy cream*  
1 (8 ounce) package cream cheese

Drain pears reserving liquid. Heat 1 cup of pear juice. Pour hot pear juice over lime gelatin and blend. Whip cream cheese into gelatin mixture. Cool. Add diced pears and fold in one cup whipped cream.

Spray a 1 ½ quart mold with gluten-free cooking spray*. Fill with mixture. Refrigerate until firm. This makes a nice accompaniment with baked ham or roast turkey or a buffet of cold meats.

## Shrimp Salad
Shrimp is gluten-free. However, some with dermatitis herpetiformis get rash flares from excessive iodine. If this is a problem for you, take a multivitamin with less iodine on the days you eat shrimp.

1 bag medium or small frozen cooked  
  shrimp, thawed, tails removed  
Gluten-free mayonnaise*  
Celery, diced or defrosted frozen peas

Salt and ground black pepper to taste  
Few dashes gluten-free hot pepper sauce*  
  (I use Frank's Red Hot® which is  
  gluten-free as of this writing)

Thaw the shrimp in cold water. Remove the shell on the tails. Cut the shrimp into pieces, if desired. (I use a poultry scissors to cut them.) Add some diced celery (or peas) and enough mayonnaise to moisten. Add a few dashes of hot pepper sauce and some salt and pepper. Mix well. Taste and adjust seasonings. This is good on top of a lettuce salad.

## Three Bean Salad
My mother developed this recipe. Some we had tried had too much sugar or too much dressing. This has just the right amount and the right taste. It's also easy to make and keeps a long time in the refrigerator. It always goes over well at our barbecues.

1 can French cut green beans  
1 can wax beans  
1 can kidney beans  
1 onion (we prefer red onion), thinly  
  sliced (I use a food processor to slice it)  
¼ teaspoon ground black pepper

few dashes salt  
⅓ cup oil  
⅓ cup wine vinegar or cider vinegar  
⅓ cup sugar

Drain beans well and combine with onions in a container. Mix all other ingredients together and pour over vegetables. (I measure and mix in a large measuring cup.) Push down the vegetables in the liquid. Cover and refrigerate overnight to marinate.

## Tomato Salad or Caprese Salad

This is a favorite when we get tomatoes fresh from the garden. We also grow fresh basil to use it in this salad. This salad is easy to make and looks nice on a buffet table. (Caprese means Capri Style.)

Ripe tomatoes
Oil (I use olive oil)
Salt
Ground black pepper
Garlic powder

Basil and/or oregano (dried or minced fresh)
Mozzarella cheese, preferably "fresh" such as Belgioioso® brand which is gluten-free as of this writing (optional)

Slice the tomatoes and arrange attractively on a platter. Drizzle some olive oil over the top. Then sprinkle with salt, pepper and garlic powder. Then take a good pinch of basil and/or oregano and scatter over the top. (Or use some fresh basil leaves. Wash and dry the leaves and then cut them into small pieces.) Top each tomato with a small slice of fresh mozzarella cheese. Grated mozzarella may also be used.

Another method is to alternate the slices of tomato, cheese and basil, around the plate in a circle. Overlap them, so you see about half of each slice of tomato and cheese. Add the basil. Drizzle with olive oil, sprinkle with salt, pepper and garlic powder.

## Tomato Salad using Cherry or Grape Tomatoes

My husband grows grape tomatoes and basil in our garden every year, so I make this easy salad.

Ripe grape or cherry tomatoes
4 or more leaves of fresh basil
Balsamic vinegar
Olive oil

Salt
Ground black pepper
Garlic powder
Pecorino Romano or Parmesan cheese

Wash tomatoes and cut in half and put in bowl. Wash basil leaves and cut into small pieces with scissors and add. Drizzle some balsamic vinegar and olive oil over top. Then sprinkle with salt, pepper, garlic powder, and cheese. Mix and serve.

## Unusual Gelatin Salad

This is nice on a buffet table. This recipe from my mother tastes better than the recipe sounds.

1 (3 ounce) package raspberry gelatin*
½ cup hot water
1 can (1 lb. size) gluten-free stewed tomatoes*
2 drops gluten-free hot pepper sauce*

⅔ gluten-free sour cream*
1 teaspoon gluten-free horseradish*
Dash of salt
¼ teaspoon sugar

Mix gelatin with hot water and stir to dissolve. Open can of tomatoes and crush them a little with a fork. Add pepper sauce and combine with gelatin. Pour into a lightly oiled mold. Refrigerate to set. Serve with sauce made with remaining ingredients.

*see gluten-free products list at the end of the book

# SALAD DRESSINGS

## Blue Cheese Dressing
This is a very rich dressing.  Be sure to use a brand of blue cheese that is safe.  Some manufacturers grow the blue mold on wheat bread.

2 ounces gluten-free blue cheese*
½ cup sour cream*
¼ cup mayonnaise*
1 teaspoon apple cider vinegar

¼ teaspoon salt (or less if cheese is very salty)
1 to 2 tablespoons milk or water

Crumble the blue cheese in a bowl.  Add the sour cream, mayonnaise, vinegar and salt and blend in.  Add enough the milk or water to make the dressing a consistency that you like.

*Variation*:  Use less water if you want to serve this as a dip with vegetables or Buffalo wings.

## Coleslaw Dressing
Every time I brought coleslaw made with this dressing to barbecues, people asked me for the recipe.

5 Tablespoons sugar
1 Tablespoon plus 1 teaspoon fine white rice flour or sweet rice flour
1 teaspoon gluten-free dry mustard*
Pinch of salt
1 egg, beaten

¼ cup apple cider vinegar
¾ cup water
Butter, a piece about the size of a walnut
1 cup gluten-free mayonnaise*

Combine the vinegar, water and butter in a pan.  Bring to a boil.  Turn off heat.

Combine the sugar, rice flour, dry mustard, salt and egg in a bowl.  While beating, pour the hot vinegar mixture into the egg mixture.  (Do not do it the other way around or the egg will cook and this recipe will not work.)

Return the mixture to the pot and bring to a boil.  Remove from heat and cool.  Beat well and add the 1 cup mayonnaise.

Mix with shredded cabbage and carrots.  This dressing can be made ahead of time, and blended with the cabbage and carrots right before serving.

## Grandmother's Salad Dressing
This is the authentic way that Italians made salad dressing.

The "old timers" never had bottled salad dressings around.  Each salad had its dressing made especially for it just before serving.  After cutting up enough vegetables to serve your family, dribble about 1 Tablespoon of oil per person over top.  Then add half as much wine or balsamic vinegar.  Now add some salt, pepper and garlic powder. Then scrub your hands, roll up your sleeves and toss. The bare warm hands seem to help distribute the dressings evenly.  Taste a small piece of salad; correct the seasonings and serve.

*see gluten-free products list at the end of the book

*Variations*: You can add grated Parmesan or Pecorino Romano cheese and some crushed dried basil or oregano.  Or add crumbled feta cheese or gluten-free goat cheese (fromage de chèvre) or gluten-free blue cheese* to vary your dressing.  If you use feta, use less salt.

## Herb Dressing
In the summer we like to grow herbs, and this is a delicious use for them.  You can also substitute dried herbs if you don't have the fresh.  One teaspoon dried herbs equal one Tablespoon fresh herbs.

½ cup oil (use part or all olive oil)
5 Tablespoons wine vinegar
1 teaspoon sugar
½ to ¾ teaspoon salt
½ teaspoon ground black pepper
¼ teaspoon garlic powder (optional)

1 Tablespoon Dijonnaise® mustard* (gluten-free as of this writing) or other gluten-free mustard
Generous Tablespoon each of fresh chopped parsley, chives, and basil (best when picked before they flower) or 1 teaspoon each of dried

Put all in a blender.  It's delicious on tomatoes.

## Honey Mustard Dressing
I prefer this to the bottled dressings I've tried.  The original recipe came from a local restaurant, but I adapted it so that it is gluten-free and easier to make.

½ cup gluten-free mayonnaise*
1 teaspoon onion powder
2 Tablespoons gluten-free mustard*
¼ cup honey

2 Tablespoons cider vinegar
½ teaspoon parsley flakes
¼ teaspoon salt
3 Tablespoons oil

Blend all with a whisk until smooth.  Refrigerate.  Makes 1 cup of dressing.  I like to store this in a squeeze bottle for easy pouring.  (I reuse the squeeze mustard containers and label it.)

I prefer spicy mustard for this dressing, but yellow mustard is good too.  French's ® and Hellman's Dijonnaise® are gluten-free as of this writing, and are very good in this recipe.

## Italian Salad Dressing – Our Favorite
My mother invented this recipe for salad dressing, and it is our favorite.  Every time I make it, people ask where they can get it.  My addition to the recipe is the Pecorino Romano cheese.  We love it on salads, and it's also good as a marinade.  People like it so much that I have seen them dip bread it in, use it on baked potatoes or rice, and put it on everything on their plate and not just their salad!  It doesn't have added gums or thickeners, so shake it before you use it.

¾ cup oil (I use olive oil; either regular or extra virgin or ½ and ½)
⅓ cup wine vinegar
1 teaspoon salt
1 teaspoon sugar

½ teaspoon garlic powder
¼ teaspoon gluten-free dry mustard
⅛ teaspoon black pepper
3 Tablespoons grated Pecorino Romano cheese (optional)

*see gluten-free products list at the end of the book

Place all in a covered jar and blend well. This keeps well and I don't refrigerate it if I don't use the cheese.

If using the cheese, be sure to refrigerate the dressing. If you used olive oil the dressing will look cloudy and thick when you take it out of the refrigerator. It will liquefy in about 20 minutes, so take it out as you are preparing your meal. This is normal for olive oil.

*Variation*: For Balsamic Dressing, use ¼ cup wine vinegar and 1 Tablespoon balsamic vinegar instead of the vinegar listed above.

*Variation 2*: For Tarragon Vinegar Dressing using the homemade vinegar in this book, Use 1 to 2 Tablespoons of tarragon vinegar and for the balance use wine vinegar.

## Ranch Dressing

Some brands of ranch dressing contain gluten as of this writing, so here is a way to make your own.

½ cup gluten-free mayonnaise*
1 teaspoon dried parsley (or 1 Tablespoon
   fresh parsley, finely chopped)
¼ teaspoon onion powder
⅛ teaspoon garlic powder

¼ teaspoon salt, or to taste
¼ teaspoon ground black pepper
¼ teaspoon dry mustard*
¾ cup gluten-free buttermilk*

Mix all ingredients together with a whisk. Chill at least 30 minutes before serving. Store covered in the refrigerator, for up to about a week or so.

## Raspberry Vinaigrette Salad Dressing

My mother invented this dressing. It's just as delicious as those with the expensive raspberry vinegar. Also, sometimes flavored vinegars are made with cheaper vinegars that could contain gluten.

¼ cup gluten-free raspberry syrup*
¼ cup oil (not olive oil)
¼ cup wine vinegar

¼ teaspoon gluten-free dry mustard*
½ teaspoon salt
Dash of ground black pepper

Blend all. This dressing is delicious on the Martha's Vineyard Salad (see index).

## Raspberry Vinaigrette Salad Dressing, Version 2

My mother invented this dressing as well. If you like things less sweet, you may prefer this version.

2 Tablespoons gluten-free raspberry
   syrup*
⅔ cup vegetable oil (not olive oil)
¼ cup wine vinegar

¼ teaspoon gluten-free dry mustard*
½ teaspoon salt

Blend all. This dressing is delicious on the Martha's Vineyard Salad (see index).

*see gluten-free products list at the end of the book

## Red French Dressing

For best results make this a day ahead of time. It's a tangy dressing that is a little sweet. If you want it for the same day, soak the onion flakes in hot water a few minutes, drain and add to the dressing. It is similar to the "Sweet Salad Dressing" (see index) but this contains more ketchup.

½ cup oil
⅓ cup wine vinegar
2 ½ teaspoons sugar
½ teaspoon salt
¼ teaspoon gluten-free dry mustard*
¼ teaspoon paprika

⅛ teaspoon garlic powder
1 ½ teaspoons onion flakes
⅛ teaspoon ground black pepper
6 Tablespoons gluten-free ketchup*
½ teaspoon lemon juice

Mix all together in a jar and blend. Blend before serving.

## Sherry French Dressing

I prefer this dressing as a marinade, but it is also very good on greens and tomatoes. The original recipe called for 1 egg yolk, but I prefer the egg powder because I don't like using uncooked raw egg in a salad dressing. (I don't worry about it in a marinade because the meat will be cooked.) If you want to use the raw egg yolk, choose a brand like Eggland's Best® because their eggs have a reduced risk of salmonella. You can call them at 1-800-922-EGGS to verify this.

¼ cup wine vinegar
1 small clove of garlic
Egg powder or egg white powder*
   equivalent to ½ an egg or 1 egg yolk
1 teaspoon salt
2 teaspoon sugar

Some freshly ground black pepper
½ teaspoon celery seed
1 ¼ cups salad oil
½ cup olive oil
¼ cup cream sherry

Place all ingredients in the cup of your hand blender and blend well. If using a regular blender, put everything except the oils in and blend. Add the oils in a thin stream with the blender on, and do the same with the sherry.

## Sweet Salad Dressing

I like this dressing on a spinach salad with crumbled bacon. This is my mother's recipe. I prefer this one over the "Red French Dressing" recipe. This is also easier to make.

1 cup oil
⅓ cup vinegar
½ teaspoon salt
¼ cup sugar

2 Tablespoons gluten-free ketchup*
2 Tablespoons minced onion or 1
   Tablespoon dehydrated onion flakes
⅛ teaspoon ground black pepper

Blend all. This is delicious on spinach salad or tossed salad.

*see gluten-free products list at the end of the book

## Thousand Island Dressing

This is easy to make. I make it by taste so it is slightly different every time, but always good.

Blend together some gluten-free mayonnaise*, gluten-free ketchup*, and gluten-free pickle relish*. I start out with some mayonnaise. Add some ketchup until I have the color I like, and then I add a small amount of relish until it looks like those bottled versions. If it's too thick you can add a little water or a little relish "juice" or pickle "juice" (i.e. liquid from a jar of gluten-free relish* or pickles*).

It's delicious on a chef's salad made with some leftover gluten-free ham, chicken or turkey, gluten-free cheese, and hard boiled eggs.

*Variation*: To make tartar sauce, do the same procedure using only mayonnaise and relish.

*Variation 2*: You can add some chopped hard-boiled egg to the Thousand Island Dressing, if desired. I don't because I like to put sliced egg in the salad.

## Write your own recipes here:

# SAUCES – Marinades, Barbecue and Dipping

## Apricot Sauce
Use this with the chicken nuggets for dipping.  It can also be used as a glaze on grilled chicken.

1 jar of apricot jam
1 Tablespoon gluten-free soy sauce*

2 cloves garlic, minced
1 to 2 dashes of gluten-free hot sauce*

Heat all in a saucepan until it is melted and blended.

## Barbecue Sauce – Our Favorite Version
I did a lot of experimenting and this is our favorite barbecue sauce.  It's easy to make and keeps a long time in the refrigerator.  We prefer it to any brand we've ever tried.  I prefer to use the light color corn syrup that does <u>not</u> contain vanilla.

2 cups boiling water
½ cup light corn syrup* (If you like a
   sweeter barbeque sauce, add an
   additional 2 to 3 Tablespoons)
1 small can (12 oz.) tomato paste
½ cup wine vinegar
2 Tablespoons molasses
3 Tablespoons brown sugar

1 teaspoon liquid smoke (I use Haddon
   House® brand or a ½ teaspoon
   Wrights® brand)
½ teaspoon salt
¼ teaspoon onion powder
¼ to ⅛ teaspoon garlic powder,
   depending on your taste
¼ teaspoon ground black pepper
⅛ teaspoon paprika

Combine all ingredients in a pot.  Whisk until smooth.  Simmer on the stove about 45 minutes until thick.  For extra thick sauce, cook it an hour.  Cool and store in a covered container in the refrigerator.  It's delicious on chicken, pork, and ribs and also as a dipping sauce with chicken nuggets.  This keeps a long time in the refrigerator.

*Variation*:  If you are allergic to corn or don't have any corn syrup, you can substitute ½ cup sugar and 2 Tablespoons of water for the corn syrup.  (It works but I prefer the results using the corn syrup.)

## Barbecue Sauce
This was given to me by a college friend.

4 Tablespoons cider vinegar
4 Tablespoons sugar
⅓ cup water
1 Tablespoon gluten-free mustard*
¼ teaspoon ground black pepper
½ teaspoon salt
2 teaspoons lemon juice

1 or 2 Tablespoons instant onion,
   depending on your taste
2 Tablespoons butter
1 Tablespoon gluten-free Worcestershire
   sauce*
½ cup gluten-free ketchup*

*see gluten-free products list at the end of the book*

Mix together vinegar, sugar, water, mustard, pepper, salt, lemon juice, onion and butter in a pan. Simmer for 10 to 15 minutes. Add the Worcestershire sauce and ketchup. Simmer uncovered for about 30 minutes until desired thickness is reached. Be careful, as this barbecue sauce burns easily.

## Barbecue Marinade Sauce (Uncooked)
This is great to put together ahead of time for a barbeque. It is perfect for the grill.

6 Tablespoons packed brown sugar
¼ cup gluten-free ketchup*
2 Tablespoons molasses
2 Tablespoons cider vinegar
2 Tablespoons oil
1 ½ Tablespoons gluten-free mustard*
1 or 2 large cloves garlic

1 teaspoon gluten-free Worcestershire Sauce*
¼ teaspoon salt
¼ teaspoon cayenne pepper
⅛ teaspoon ground black pepper

Combine all ingredients with a whisk or use a hand blender in a bowl. Blend until smooth. If making this sauce ahead of time, refrigerate until use.

Pour the sauce over 1 to 2 pounds of meat (beef, chicken or pork) and marinate for at least 2 hours or overnight in the refrigerator before cooking.

Since chicken doesn't seem to absorb flavors as quickly as beef, I suggest you marinate chicken overnight or even for 2 days in the refrigerator.

Recently, I have used this marinade on pork chops. I soaked them in it for 2 days in the refrigerator, grilled them, and they were delicious. People at my cookout all wanted the recipe. I liked that I could do it ahead of time and it turned out so moist and tasty. I purchased the whole pork tenderloin and had the butcher cut them into thick chops so that they would remain juicy on the grill. Cook the first side for 5 minutes, turn, and cook until done. Do not overcook. Cut and check inside that they are fully cooked through.

Note: Just be sure to check the date on your meat so that the number of days in the marinade in the refrigerator will be within the time that the meat is still fresh. Also, always discard any leftover marinade used on raw meat.

## Chicken Marinade
This recipe comes from my sister. She says that it is her children's favorite. Chicken prepared this way is good in gluten-free sandwiches or in salads.

5 Tablespoons lemon juice or orange juice
3 Tablespoons gluten-free soy sauce*
2 cloves of chopped garlic or ¼ teaspoon garlic powder

1 teaspoon dried basil or dried oregano
½ teaspoon ground pepper

Place a Ziploc® bag in a bowl. (I put it in a bowl to stabilize the bag, so it doesn't spill.) Add marinade ingredients inside the bag and blend. Add chicken, seal bag, adjust bag to get

*see gluten-free products list at the end of the book

marinade on all of the chicken. Marinate for an hour. Grill on a clean grill. Always discard leftover marinade that you used on raw meat.

## Chicken Marinade – Brine/Barbeque

This recipe is for 2 to 3 whole chickens, so you may want to half the recipe. Chicken parts also require less marinade. This is slow cooked on the grill and served at church suppers.

2 cups cider vinegar
2 cups water
1 cup oil
⅓ cup kosher salt
2 Tablespoons Worcestershire sauce
2 Tablespoons lemon juice

2 teaspoons hot sauce*
2 to 3 broiler chickens. These are the small chickens that have less meat on the breasts than fryers. You can split these in half and serve one-half per person. Or chicken parts may be used.

Mix in a large pot that will hold the chickens. Marinate for 2-4 hours. Barbeque on a low flame on the grill. Using tongs periodically lift the chicken and dip in the marinade to add more, or spoon or brush it on instead. Barbeque until done.

## Cocktail Sauce

There are several brands that are gluten-free, but here is a way to make your own. Use this as a dipping sauce for cooked cocktail shrimp.

1 cup gluten-free ketchup* or gluten-free chili sauce* (Heinz® is gluten-free as of this writing)
2 Tablespoons horseradish (or more or less to taste)

1 teaspoon lemon juice
1 teaspoon Worcestershire sauce*
1 Tablespoon gluten-free mustard* (I like Hellman's® Dijonnaise™ which is gluten-free as of this writing)

Blend together in a bowl. Serve with shrimp or other seafood.

## Honey Mustard Marinade

This makes a lot, so you will have enough to use for several times. It doesn't taste like much after you blend it, but the subtle flavors come out in the meat after you grill it. I especially like it on chicken and found that the meat was moist and juicy. I prefer it made with the gluten-free Dijon mustard*.

¾ cup oil
⅓ cup wine vinegar
6 Tablespoons honey
¼ teaspoon garlic powder

¾ teaspoon salt
¼ cup gluten-free Dijon mustard* or 4 teaspoons gluten-free dry mustard*
½ teaspoon dill weed

Blend all together. If making ahead of time, keep refrigerated until use.

Marinate meat overnight in the refrigerator, using enough to cover both sides. (I pour a little in a pie plate or large bowl, add skinless boneless chicken breasts, and pour more on top. Cover with plastic wrap and refrigerate.) Grill on a clean grill. Baste with additional marinade if desired, although I have found this is not necessary. Always discard any leftover marinade you used on raw meat.

*see gluten-free products list at the end of the book*

You can also marinate skinless boneless chicken breasts for several days and they will turn out very good. I recently put this together 2 days before a cookout, and it was delicious. Just be sure to check the date on the meat to be sure that it will still be fresh after the 2 days in the refrigerator.

Note: You can also put frozen chicken in the refrigerator in a large bowl to defrost. Cover with marinade. It will start absorbing the flavors as it defrosts.

## Italian Salad Dressing Marinade

Use our favorite Italian Salad Dressing (see index) as a marinade. I particularly like it on boneless skinless chicken breasts. Put chicken (or whatever meat you choose) in a pan with deep sides, cover with dressing. Turn meat over and get it on all sides of the meat. Marinate for at least a ½ hour. An hour is even better. Or cover the pan with plastic wrap and refrigerate for up to 24 hours. The next day, you're ready to grill it. The meat will be juicy and delicious. Sometimes when I want to defrost meat, I put it in the refrigerator and add the marinade at that time and that works well too. Just be sure the pan is deep enough to hold the chicken and marinade once it defrosts. You can also use this marinade on other meats like London Broil. You can marinate it at least a half-hour, or a few hours, or overnight as above.

Note: Instead of using olive oil for the dressing, I use corn oil or canola oil because it doesn't thicken like olive oil in the refrigerator. However, if you want to use olive oil, it will work too. It looks really strange when you remove it from the refrigerator because of the thick oil.

## Meat Marinade Sauce – Our Favorite Version
This is a quick and easy recipe from my Mother. It also doesn't waste a lot of marinade. This recipe is for up to 2 steaks so double it if you're making more.

| | |
|---|---|
| 1 Tablespoon gluten-free soy sauce* | 2 teaspoons gluten-free Worcestershire sauce* |
| 1 Tablespoon oil | Sprinkling of garlic powder(optional) |
| 1 Tablespoon honey | |

Blend all ingredients. This is enough marinade for one or two steaks. Marinade a half-hour or so. You can also add 1 Tablespoon of wine, so that it can help tenderize the meat, if you prefer.

## Spicy French Marinade

This recipe was given to me as a salad dressing, but I prefer it as a marinade. It's especially good for chicken. It makes a large amount which is enough for several times.

14 Tablespoons (or ¾ cup plus 2 Tablespoons) of cider vinegar
1 cup olive oil or substitute another oil
2 teaspoons gluten-free dry mustard*
3 teaspoons ground black pepper (I use less, either 1 or 2 teaspoons)
2 teaspoons gluten-free Worcestershire sauce*

1 clove garlic, minced (I use ¼ teaspoon garlic powder)
2 teaspoons salt
Juice of 1 lemon (or I use 2 to 3 Tablespoons bottled lemon juice)
Dash of gluten-free hot sauce* or sprinkling of red pepper flakes (optional – I don't use)

Blend all ingredients in a jar. Marinate meat for several hours.

## Tastes Like Marinade

My brother-in-law likes to grill, but sometimes forgets to marinate the meat before dinner time. Here is an alternative way he developed to flavor your meat.

Oil
Garlic Powder
Salt and Pepper

Dried Oregano
Boneless Chicken Breasts or other meat

Brush or dip meat in a little oil, or spray with gluten-free cooking spray. Generously sprinkle with garlic powder, salt, pepper and oregano. Grill until meat is cooked through, but not over-cooked. We think the oregano makes it taste like it was marinated.

## Teriyaki Marinade Sauce – My Favorite Version

Most commercial teriyaki marinades contain gluten, because most soy sauces contain gluten. It's easy to make your own, and less expensive too.

¼ cup gluten-free soy sauce*
¼ cup water
¼ cup brown sugar
2 Tablespoons lemon juice

⅛ teaspoon ground ginger or 1 teaspoon fresh ground ginger
¼ teaspoon garlic powder or 2 cloves garlic minced

Combine all ingredients, blend well. Let meat marinade for 2 hours up to no more than 24 hours in the refrigerator. Make half the recipe for 2 steaks.

This marinade is also very good on salmon steaks. Let it marinate for at least 2 hours.

*see gluten-free products list at the end of the book

## Teriyaki Marinade Sauce – Version 2

This version contains wine, which can help tenderize the meat. This is also good, but I prefer the previous recipe.

¼ cup dry sherry
1 Tablespoon sugar
6 Tablespoons gluten-free soy sauce*

1 clove garlic, crushed or ⅛ teaspoon garlic powder
1 Tablespoon gluten-free Worcestershire sauce*

Combine all ingredients. Marinate fish 30-40 minutes and chicken or beef longer. The wine can help to tenderize the meat.

## Write your own recipes here:

## SAUCES – for Pasta or Rice

### Calamari Sauce

This is an acquired taste, because calamari is squid.  Since I ate calamari when I was young, I enjoy it.  I especially like to have it prepared like this for Christmas or New Years day.  Today you can purchase squid already cleaned and frozen.  I remember spending hours helping my Mom clean them when I was a little girl.  Serve this fish sauce over gluten-free pasta or rice.

2 to 3 Tablespoons oil
2 cloves garlic
1 large can gluten-free tomato puree*
Large pinch of oregano
Salt and ground black pepper to taste

1 ½ lbs. cleaned calamari (squid) cut into rings.  (You can purchase them frozen.  Be sure they say they are already cleaned.)

Sauté the garlic in the oil until it is golden in color on all sides.  (Be careful not to burn it or you will ruin this dish.)  Remove from heat, cool a minute and mash with a fork.  Discard large pieces.  Add tomato puree, oregano, salt and pepper.  Cook about 15 minutes then add squid and cook about a half-hour longer, or as directed on the calamari package.

Test squid with a cake tester.  If tester pierces the flesh easily, it is done.  Don't overcook as the squid will fall apart. Overcooking can also make it too chewy like rubber bands.  When cooked properly it is delicious and tender.  Serve over gluten-free spaghetti, gluten-free linguini or rice.

### Chinese Stir Fry Sauce

When I have small amounts of leftover meat, I put together a stir-fry.  I stir-fry some fresh or frozen vegetables, add my leftover meat and then add this sauce.

1 cup water
1 teaspoon gluten-free chicken* or beef base* (depending on type of meat used)

1 Tablespoon soy sauce
1 Tablespoon corn starch
1 teaspoon dry sherry (optional)

Blend together.  When vegetables and meat are cooked, add sauce and bring to a boil.  Serve over rice.

### Mushroom Sauce – Bianca (white) for Gluten-Free Pasta or Brown Rice

This is my mother's recipe.  This sauce is delicious over gluten-free spaghetti (we like Tinkyada® or Sam Mills® brand), or over brown rice (see variation below).  It is also easy to make.

¼ cup oil (I use olive oil)
1 to 1 ½ pounds sliced mushrooms, rinsed
½ cup coarsely chopped parsley or 2 Tablespoons dry parsley flakes
1 teaspoon salt
½ teaspoon ground black pepper

¼ teaspoon garlic powder or granulated garlic powder
1 pound gluten-free spaghetti* or 2 cups brown rice (prepared as below for Variation 2)
Generous sprinkling of Pecorino Romano or Parmesan cheese

*see gluten-free products list at the end of the book*

In a saucepan, add the oil, sliced mushrooms, parsley, salt, pepper and garlic powder into a pan. Stir to blend. Cover and cook a few minutes until mushrooms are cooked. Do not overcook the mushrooms. Pour over the cooked gluten-free spaghetti* or rice. Blend. Top with generous sprinklings of cheese.

(Note: Do not eliminate the oil in this recipe. The oil not only provides flavor but also prevents your pasta or rice from becoming waterlogged. It is enough sauce for a large quantity of food, so you really are not getting much oil per serving.)

*Variation*: You can substitute 2-3 cans of mushrooms for the fresh. The results are very good and it's easier to make, but I prefer the fresh.

*Variation 2*: We enjoy this sauce over brown rice. In a pot bring 5 cups water to a boil. Add 2 Tablespoons dehydrated onion flakes. Add 1 teaspoon salt. Add 2 cups brown rice. Cover and bring to a boil. Lower and simmer for 45 to 50 minutes. While that is cooking, prepare this sauce.

> Note: If you want to shorten the cooking time of the brown rice, the night before put cool water and rice in a pot and cover. (Same method used to soak dry beans.) The next day, add salt and put the pot on the stove, add onion flakes if desired, bring to a boil, cover and cook about 30 minutes. Soaking the rice not only softens it for faster cooking, but also germinates the rice which provides health benefits. "Researchers found that a compound that helps rice seed grow, springs back into action when brown rice is placed in water overnight before cooking, significantly reducing the nerve and vascular damage that often results from diabetes... The germ layer activated by soaking brown rice contains many vitamins and minerals in addition to the bioactive ingredient that would be beneficial to everyone."[119] Germinated brown rice improved fasting glucose, good homocysteine levels, and good cholesterol levels.[119-122]

*Variation 3*: Add some leftover diced ham* or turkey salami* to the sauce and heat through for a more complete meal, and a delicious change. This sauce with the ham is delicious over Rizopia® wild rice raditorre (little radiators) pasta. Frozen peas may also be added with the ham if desired.

## Pesto Sauce

This pesto sauce is my mother's recipe and is very good. Use only a few Tablespoons at a time as it is flavorful and it is best when used sparingly. My mother and I make it in the summer or early fall, freeze it, and enjoy it during the winter.

1 bunch parsley
Fresh basil
1 (8 ounce) package softened gluten-free
  cream cheese*
½ cup oil, use some olive oil
2 cloves garlic

½ cup Parmesan cheese, grated
1 cup gluten-free heavy cream*
½ teaspoon ground black pepper
2 Tablespoons pine nuts
Salt to taste

*see gluten-free products list at the end of the book*

Pack washed parsley leaves and basil leaves together to equal 2 cups. Add all ingredients to a blender or food processor and blend until smooth. This makes enough to use many times. You can use this sauce on cooked rice or cooked gluten-free pasta. It is also good on gluten-free spinach spaghetti.

I pour it into ice cube trays, freeze, and then put the cubes into a freezer bag. When I want to use it, I just grab a few cubes, heat it, and blend it into my cooked and drained gluten-free pasta. (It heats well in the microwave). Another method is to freeze the sauce in Tupperware® hamburger storage containers. Once frozen you can remove them from the containers and put them in a freezer bags. Each hamburger size disk is good for 1 pound of pasta. If packaged in heavy duty freezer bags, this sauce keeps a long time. I have kept it longer than a year and it was still good.

*Variation*: Use this sauce on top of a fresh tomato pizza. Use a Gluten-Free Naturals™ pizza crust mix. After baking as directed, top with fresh tomato slices. On top of each tomato slice, put a dab of this pesto sauce. Top with mozzarella cheese and bake 4 to 5 minutes more. It is delicious and "very gourmet."

*Variation 2*: This sauce can be used in making lasagna, instead of using tomato sauce. I use it with the Lasagna Northern Style (see index). I have a friend who is allergic to tomatoes and she enjoyed the lasagna made with this sauce. I also have made the Northern Style Lasagna with pesto sauce for patients on chemotherapy, since chemotherapy drugs can make acidic foods like tomato sauce taste like metal.

*Variation 3*: If you want to use Pecorino Romano cheese instead of Parmesan, use less cheese. Pecorino Romano has a much stronger flavor. I use about ⅓ cup.

## Tomato Sauce with Meat, Authentic Italian Version
This is my mother's recipe and an authentic Italian sauce. It's my favorite sauce. Her grandmother's secret to a delicious sauce was to add some pork, which is why she adds the sausage. See her recipe "Meats to add to Tomato sauce" below for variations.

¼ cup oil
3 to 4 cloves garlic
2 (28 oz.) cans of gluten-free tomato
   puree*
1 (28 oz.) can of gluten-free crushed
   tomatoes*
1 (12 oz.) can Italian style tomato paste
1 cup water or white wine
1 recipe meatballs (see index) optional

1 ⅓ lbs. gluten-free Italian sausage*
2 teaspoons salt
2 teaspoons oregano or 4 (6 inch) sprigs
   of fresh
1 Tablespoon basil or 12 fresh leaves
1 to 2 teaspoons sugar
Sprinkling of ground black pepper
½ cup grated Pecorino Romano cheese

Place oil in a pot. Sauté the cloves of garlic until light brown on all sides. Remove pot from heat to cool. Mash garlic with a fork and discard only the large pieces. Empty all cans into pot and clean out any residue left in the cans with a little wine or water and add it to the pot. Add meat and remaining ingredients. (See the next recipe for other meats that may be added.) Cover pot and simmer for 1 hour. Stir sauce a few times during cooking to prevent

*see gluten-free products list at the end of the book

burning. (Sauce tends to burn more easily when cooking on an electric stove, so stir more frequently if using one.) Add the cheese and stir in.

Follow the directions below for meats to add to tomato sauce.

## Tomato Sauce Additions – Meats to add to Italian Version Above

Use any one or any assortments of the following meats to add flavor to your tomato sauce. (Add the meats at the beginning of the cooking time for your sauce as noted in the recipe above.) My mother and grandmother always liked to add a little pork to their sauces because they felt it made it more delicious. My mother likes to put more than one type of meat so that she had a different type of meat each time she served pasta.

Meatballs (see index for recipe)

Sausages – cut sweet gluten-free Italian sausages* into serving pieces and place in a skillet with ¼ inch of water. Cover and simmer until the fat of the sausages melts out and the sausages start to fry in their own fat. Remove cover and brown on all sides. Drain fat and add the meat to the sauce. One or two links of gluten-free hot sausage* can also be used if you like a spicy sauce.

Braciole – buy two thin round steaks. Chop ⅓ bunch of fresh Italian parsley and add 2 minced cloves of garlic, a little salt and pepper, ⅓ cup Pecorino Romano cheese and a few pine nuts. Cut steaks in half, spread with parsley filling and roll like a jelly-roll. Tie in 3 places with thread or butcher's string. Brown in the same pot you are to cook your sauce. (After they are browned, cook them in the sauce.) Once cooked, remove the string, slice and serve. This is a delicious gluten-free alternative to sausage.

Boneless pork – my mother always said that the best sauces contain pork. Add a small pork roast or pork chops and cook it along with your sauce. It's an easy way to cook the pork and you get an extra meal. I like to serve the pork chops with mashed potatoes with some of the sauce on them. If using a roast, just be sure it's cooked through.

Ground pork, beef, or turkey, (or a combination) – browned, drained of fat, and broken up into small pieces is also good. You can also use "meatloaf mix" which from my butcher is a combination of ground pork, beef and veal without any bread filler.

## Tomato Sauce – Vegetable Version from my Mother

This is a nice vegetable filled sauce. I use it to make vegetable lasagna. You can substitute frozen carrots, peppers and onions to speed up the preparation time, but fresh are better.

¼ cup oil
1 clove garlic, minced or ⅛ teaspoon garlic powder or granulated garlic
1 cup chopped onion
½ cup chopped carrots
½ cup chopped green peppers
¼ cup chopped celery
⅓ cup chopped mushrooms (optional)
1 teaspoon sugar

1 teaspoon salt
¼ teaspoon chili powder
¼ teaspoon ground nutmeg
1 lb. lean ground meat (beef, turkey or pork)
1 lb. 9 oz. container of gluten-free Italian strained or crushed tomatoes*
1 cup dry white wine
2 large pinches oregano

Heat oil and sauté vegetables a few minutes, add ground meat and cook until it loses its red color. Add spices and wine and cook 10 minutes over low heat. Add tomatoes and oregano. Cover pot and cook for 30-40 minutes more until vegetables are tender.

## Tomato Sauce with Ground Meat, American Version for Spaghetti

This is more of an American version of spaghetti sauce from my father's aunt.

¼ cup olive oil
1 cup chopped onions
1 to 2 cloves garlic, minced (or more if desired)
1 lb. chopped beef or pork
Salt to taste

Ground black pepper to taste
3 (29 ounce) cans gluten-free tomato puree*
Sprinkling dry oregano
Sprinkling dry basil
Dash of cayenne pepper

In a large open fry pan (I use chicken fryer size) heat the oil. Add the onions and garlic and sauté until tender and lightly browned. Add the chopped meat and continue cooking and stirring until beef is lightly browned and separated and somewhat dry. Add salt and pepper.

Stir in the three cans of tomato puree, mixing well and sprinkling with a covering of oregano and basil and a few dashes of cayenne pepper.

Simmer uncovered on low heat for 2 hours until thickened as desired, stirring occasionally. Make sure heat is not too high or the bottom will burn. Also, if the heat is too high the sauce will spatter all over your stove.

*see gluten-free products list at the end of the book

# Main Dishes – Beef, Poultry, Seafood, Pork, Lamb, Crock-pot

## BEEF

### Austrian Rostbraten
This is a nice company dish. Most brands of regular bacon (not flavored bacon) are gluten-free.

2 lbs. sirloin steak
4 Tbsp. butter
4 Tbsp. oil
2 large Spanish onions, sliced in rings

Salt and ground black pepper
Gluten-free meat tenderizer*
6 slices of bacon* fried crisp and
    crumbled

Microwave bacon (for garnish) following package directions. Meanwhile, cut steak into 4 serving pieces. Pound each piece with a meat mallet. Sprinkle on some gluten-free meat tenderizer and pound until the meat is ¼ inch thick and will cover half a dinner plate. Using 2 frying pans or skillets, use half butter and oil in one and sauté the onions slowly. Sprinkle with salt and pepper and cover a while. Then remove cover and stir. Do not brown the onions. They should be yellow and very limp. Heat the second skillet. When hot add the other half of the oil and butter and heat a minute. Now fry steaks only one to two minutes per side. To serve, make a bed of onions on a plate, top with one steak and then the crumbled bacon.

### Barbecued Beef Chicken Steaks or Ribs of Beef
Chicken steaks are a cut of beef that resembles the shape of a chicken breast. They are usually inexpensive because they are a tough cut of meat. This is a delicious way to have them. I love the aroma when this is cooking. My husband also likes this recipe made using ribs.

2 lbs. beef chicken steaks or 3 lbs. beef
    ribs
2 teaspoons salt
¼ teaspoon ground black pepper
1 teaspoon gluten-free dry mustard* (or 4
    teaspoons gluten-free prepared
    mustard*)
1 Tablespoon gluten-free Worcestershire
    sauce*

1 Tablespoon sugar
½ cup gluten-free ketchup*
¼ cup water
½ cup minced onion (or 1 Tablespoon
    dry minced onion)
1 clove garlic, minced (or ¼ teaspoon
    powdered garlic or granulated garlic)
Oil

Heat a heavy pan and add 3 Tablespoons oil. Brown the meat well. Then mix all the other ingredients together and pour over the top. Cook it on low heat for 1 ½ hours, or until meat is nice and tender.

Slice into thin slices and top with the sauce. Serve with mashed potatoes.

## Beef Rouladen

As a child I liked this dish so much, that I would choose it for my birthday dinner. My mother changed the recipe and eliminated the pickles of the original version, and we prefer it this way.

3 round steaks cut about ¼ inch thick
3 slices bacon*
Prepared mustard
1 large onion, chopped fine
Salt and ground black pepper

Oil
1 cup water
Wooden uncolored toothpicks (Use natural wooden toothpicks, not the kind that have different colors.)

Cut steaks in half to make 6 almost square pieces of meat. Spread generously with mustard, place one sixth of the onion over the mustard and then a half slice of bacon. Roll like a jelly-roll and secure with a toothpick. Heat skillet and add oil. Heat a few moments and add rolls. Brown it on all sides. Remove from heat and add the water. Return to heat and cover and simmer 45 minutes or until a fork easily goes through a roll. Test pan while cooking to be sure it doesn't go dry and burn the rolls. Add more water if needed. When completely cooked, taste pan juices. Add salt and pepper if needed. Put rolls on serving dish. Remove toothpicks and pour juices over top. Serves 3.

## Beef Stew

This is the stew you remember. The fine white rice flour browns well and makes a nice gravy.

1 lb. stew meat
Fine white rice flour for dredging
1 tsp. salt
Few dashes of ground black pepper
1 bay leaf

1 large chopped onion
2 large carrots
6 medium potatoes
2 Tablespoons oil for frying

Cut large cubes of meat so that pieces are uniform in size. Place a piece of waxed paper next to the stove and place about a ½ cup of rice flour on it. Roll each piece of meat in flour. Heat your pot a few minutes. (I prefer using a Teflon® pot, but do not overheat.) Add the oil and heat another minute, then add a few pieces of floured meat at a time and brown on all sides. The browner the meat, the better your gravy will be. Just be sure you don't burn it, so cook it over medium heat. Remove the meat as it browns and add a few more floured pieces until all the meat is browned. Add more oil to the pot if needed and place the onions in the pot. Cook them until lightly brown. Now place all the meat back into the pot and cover with water. Add 1 teaspoon salt, few dashes of pepper and bay leaf. Bring to a boil, reduce heat, cover and simmer 1 hour. Check pot every 20 minutes or so, stir and add more water if needed. Scrape carrots, cut into chunks and add to the pot. Peel potatoes, cut into chunks and also add to the pot. Add additional water if needed and simmer another ½ hour. Stew is done when meat and vegetables are tender. Check seasonings. If gravy is too thick add a little water. If gravy is too thin, remove cover and cook a little longer to evaporate some of the liquid. Remove bay leaf and serve.

*Variation:* You can add some frozen peas right after you add the potatoes.

*see gluten-free products list at the end of the book

*Variation 2*: Sometimes London Broil is on sale and cheaper than stew meat. It is a much more tender meat. If using London Broil, cut it in chunks and brown it as instructed above. Then add the vegetables, water, and seasonings. I also add some garlic powder since London Broil can be less flavorful. Cook it about 30 minutes or so until the meat and vegetables are tender. Using this cut of meat makes it faster and easier to prepare.

## Beef Stroganoff
This is a delicious company dish. I make it for special occasions.

1 ½ lbs. beef tenderloin (filet mignon), sliced very thin
1 whole large Spanish onion, diced
4 oz. butter
2 oz. tomato paste
2 Tablespoons fine white rice flour or sweet rice flour

Tiny pinch of thyme (optional)
¼ teaspoon oregano
1 bay leaf
2 cups chicken broth, heated
1 cup gluten-free sour cream*
½ cup sautéed sliced mushrooms
Salt and ground black pepper

Melt the butter in the pan and smother the onions by cooking on low heat until translucent, not browned. Add tomato paste and seasonings and cook a few minutes longer. Add the rice flour and mix well, then add the hot chicken broth while stirring. (I use 2 cups of hot water plus 2 teaspoons gluten-free chicken base*.) Cook for 30 minutes. If too thick, add a little more broth. Meanwhile, sauté mushrooms in another skillet and set aside.

When sauce is nearly completed, sauté beef 3 to 4 minutes. Strain sauce, blend in the sour cream and add mushrooms, salt and pepper. Pour over meat and mix lightly. Serve with rice.

*Variation*: To make this an easier dish to make, you can eliminate the step of straining the sauce by substituting 1 Tablespoon onion powder for the diced onion, and making sure you remove the bay leaf. You can also substitute a drained can of mushrooms. I prefer the original version, but this is easier to make and good too.

## Carne Alla Pizzaiola
This is "Meat the way the pizza man makes it". This is one of those passed-down recipes from my mother's family. The amount of vegetables used is not exact. I use a couple of large potatoes, a green pepper, and a package of mushrooms, but you can use what you have on-hand.

3 lbs. boneless chuck steak
1 (15 oz.) can gluten-free tomato sauce* (or two 8 oz. cans)
2 Tablespoons oil
1 teaspoon oregano

Pinch of sugar
Salt and ground black pepper
Cubed potatoes (optional)
Sliced green peppers
Sliced mushrooms (optional)

Cut meat into serving pieces and remove all visible fat. Heat a large skilled a few minutes. Add oil and heat one minute more. Place a few pieces of steak in a pan and brown on each side. Repeat until all meat is browned. Remove pan from heat and then add the tomato sauce. Return pot to heat and add a sprinkle of salt and pepper, pinch of sugar and oregano.

*see gluten-free products list at the end of the book

Put heat on low, cover pot and cook 1 ½ hours. Check pot once in a while to be sure there is enough liquid. When meat is almost tender, you can add potatoes and cook 15 minutes more, then add peppers and mushrooms and cook 10 minutes more or until potatoes are tender. Gravy should be just the right thickness and a rich red color, but if it is dry just add a little water. My grandmother never added the vegetables to this dish but rather served it with mashed potatoes. My mother added the vegetables sometimes to make it a one-pot meal. The sauce can be served over gluten-free spaghetti*. I like it served over the potatoes.

## Cheesy Burger 'Roni'

This is like Hamburger-Helper®, and is a one-pot skillet meal. No need for a separate pot to boil the macaroni. We like the recipe as written, but you can eliminate the herbs or vegetables if preparing this for children, so that it will be milder in flavor. You can make this in about 30 minutes. I use 1 cup of cheese instead of 2 to cut the calories, so if you use less you may have to add a little extra salt.

1 pound ground beef or turkey* or pork
1 chopped green pepper (or ½ cup frozen chopped green pepper.)
1 to 2 Tablespoons dried minced onion flakes (or 1 medium onion chopped or ½ cup frozen chopped onion or ½ teaspoon onion powder)
2 cups boiling water (use 2 ¼ to 2 ½ cups water if using Sam Mills®)
6 ounces (1 ½ cups) gluten-free elbow macaroni (I use Tinkyada® or Sam Mills®)
2 (8 ounce) cans gluten-free tomato sauce* or 1 (15 ounce) can

1 (4 ounce) can of mushrooms, drained (optional)
1 (14 ounce) can of diced tomatoes, undrained (optional)
¼ teaspoon each of garlic powder and dried basil
½ teaspoon each of salt, dried oregano or dried marjoram
1 teaspoon chili powder
⅛ teaspoon dried sage (optional)
2 teaspoons Worcestershire sauce*
1 to 2 cups grated gluten-free cheese* (I use either American or Cheddar. Mozzarella can also be used.)

Brown ground meat in a 12 inch or 10 inch skillet with a lid. Drain any excess fat from meat. While meat is browning, boil water in tea kettle or in the microwave.

Add the rest of the ingredients to the meat mixture, except the cheese. Simmer covered for 10 minutes, stir mixture and check if a little additional water is needed. (If it is too thick, the bottom could burn.)

If using a different brand of macaroni, check it for doneness at 10 minutes since some brands cook up faster than others. If not done or if using Tinkyada® brand, cover and simmer 10 minutes more. (Note: If you have too much liquid, you can simmer it uncovered instead of covered at this point. Watch it carefully because if too much liquid evaporates it can burn.)

Check the macaroni for doneness. If macaroni is done, turn off the heat, stir in the grated cheese, cover and let it sit for 5 minutes. This melts in the cheese and allows the macaroni to absorb a little more liquid. It also makes it the right temperature for serving. Taste and add more salt if needed, since some cheeses are saltier than others.

*see gluten-free products list at the end of the book

*Variation*: If using a ½ package of Sam Mills® pasta (8 ounces instead of 6 ounces), use 2 ½ to 2 ¾ cups water instead of 2 cups. I also add the (14 ounce) can of diced tomatoes. Other varieties of pasta may be used instead of elbows such as shells or lasagna corte.

## Chili con Carne (Chili with Meat)

This is my mother's recipe. This chili isn't very spicy, because our family didn't like spicy food. You may want to add more chili powder, a Jalapeno pepper or some gluten-free hot sauce* if you like spicy chili. I especially like to use this chili to make a stuffed potato with cheese. It's also good over rice.

2 Tablespoons oil
1 ¼ pound lean chopped meat (either ground beef, turkey or pork)
½ cup chopped onion
¼ cup chopped green pepper
¾ teaspoon salt
1 teaspoon cumin, ground
2 teaspoons chili powder
¼ teaspoon oregano

1 clove garlic, minced or ¼ teaspoon garlic powder or granulated garlic
2 cups or 1 (15 oz.) can or 2 (8 oz.) cans gluten-free tomato sauce*
1 (16 oz.) can pinto beans (or kidney beans)
1 cup water

Heat a pan a minute, add oil, and allow the oil to heat a minute and then add meat. Cook meat until it loses its red color. Drain off any fat. Add the rest of ingredients, bring to a boil, lower heat partially cover pan and simmer 45 minutes. Makes almost 2 quarts. Serve over polenta (see index), rice, or baked potatoes.

*Variation*: See index for Crock-pot method.

## Corned Beef Hash

I have served this at brunches. It's also good for a light lunch or supper.

3 medium potatoes
1 medium chopped onion
1 can gluten-free corn beef*

Salt and ground black pepper
Butter

Peel potatoes and cut into chunks. Peel onion and chop coarsely. Place in a saucepan, cover with water and boil until tender. Drain well. Mash with a potato masher and while still very hot, add the can of corn beef and blend well. Add a few dashes of black pepper and taste to see if salt is needed. Add salt to taste. Blend well and put into a shallow, buttered baking dish. Dot the top with butter or spray it with gluten-free cooking spray*. Bake it at 350°F for 30 minutes or until top is crispy and lightly browned.

Or you can cool the mixture after blending all together and then make hamburger size cakes. Fry in a little butter or oil until crisp. Either way, it is good served with ketchup or a fried sunny side up egg on top.

## Enchiladas and Enchilada Casserole

Mexican dishes using corn or corn tortillas are perfect for the gluten-free diet. We always enjoy this recipe. See variation for enchilada casserole.

1 lb. ground meat (ground turkey, ground pork or ground beef or a combination)
1 onion, diced (fresh or frozen)
1 green pepper, diced (fresh or frozen)
⅛ teaspoon garlic powder or 1 clove minced
2 cups gluten-free tomato sauce* (I use 2 small cans)
1 small can corn drained (optional)

¼ cup sliced pitted black olives
½ teaspoon salt or a little less if using olives
2 teaspoons chili powder
⅛ teaspoon cumin (optional)
¾ cup grated cheddar cheese (or more or less to taste)
Corn Tortillas* (I use 12)

Put meat in a large skillet. Break up and cook until it loses its red color. Drain any excess fat. Add onions and green paper. Cook until onions start to get translucent. Add 1 cup of tomato sauce, corn, olives, salt, chili powder and cumin. Simmer a few minutes to get flavors to blend. Remove from heat. Allow the filling to cool to a temperature you can handle, so you do not burn yourself when filling the enchiladas.

Open second can of sauce. Pour half into a large rectangular pan or casserole. Set aside. Take the corn tortillas, put on a plate, cover them with a damp paper towel, and microwave one minute to make them flexible. Take them one at a time and put filling down the center, roll and place seam side down into the sauce. When finished, top with remaining sauce to cover. Top with the grated cheese. If desired you can add a few sliced olives per enchilada for garnish. Bake 30 minutes at 350°F until heated through and the cheese melts.

Note: Instead of heating tortillas in the microwave, some people prefer to warm up some of the sauce, dip the tortillas in the sauce and then fill them. I find it too messy and prefer my microwave method.

*Variation:* Instead of using a rectangular pan, you can use individual casserole dishes that are oven safe. I have ones that hold 2 enchiladas per casserole. It makes a nice presentation for company.

*Variation 2:* You can use this filling for tacos. Use only 1 can of sauce. Cook the filling a little longer until vegetables are cooked to the desired consistency since you will not be baking the filling. Or, instead of tomato sauce, fresh diced tomatoes may be used in the taco filling.

*Variation 3:* Instead of rolling your tortillas, you can layer it using this recipe and call it enchilada casserole. Cover the bottom of a small casserole with half the sauce. Then layer with one third of the tortillas. Top with half the meat. Repeat. Top with the remaining tortillas and the sauce. Top with cheese and bake as directed above.

*Variation 4:* Unbaked version (for microwave meals). Cook the meat mixture a little longer until vegetables are the desired consistency since you will not be baking it. Follow the

*see gluten-free products list at the end of the book

procedure in Variation 3, but instead divide it among four or more microwave containers. (I use a size container where each layer is one tortilla.) Top with cheese. Refrigerate it once cooled and reheat it in the microwave when ready to serve.

The layering method in Variation 3 and 4 works well if your tortillas are not as pliable as they could be and do not roll easily. (Sometimes tortillas are not as pliable when they get close to the expiration date, and this is a good way to use them.)

## Falso Magro (False Lean)

This is an old family recipe of my mother's. It's a lot of work, but if you're willing to go through all of the trouble it looks nice on a buffet table. You serve it at room temperature. I think enjoying this is an acquired taste. If you are Italian and remember having this, it will bring back memories for you.

1 large round steak
1 lb. lean chopped beef
2 eggs
2 yolks
4 Tablespoons Pecorino Romano Cheese, grated (such as Locatelli® Romano)
¼ cup chopped parsley
Salt, ground black pepper, little grated nutmeg
Pinch or 2 of oregano

4 thin slices gluten-free Mozzarella* or Provolone cheese
2 hard boiled eggs, coarsely chopped
1 (8 inch) long piece of gluten-free Italian sausage*
Butcher's string
Oil
2 chopped onions
⅔ cup red wine
Gluten-free tomato sauce*

Have your butcher cut you a large round steak about ⅓ inch thick and measuring about 8 inches by 10 inches, or buy a ½ inch thick steak and pound it to the desired size. Mix chopped meat with eggs, egg yolks (save whites in the freezer for future use), Pecorino Romano cheese, parsley and a little salt, pepper and nutmeg. Place this mixture on top of the steak, leaving about 1 inch of steak uncovered at either end of the short (8 inch) sides. Place cheese on top of the chopped meat mixture. Then put chopped egg down the center. Cook sausage briefly in a little water to remove excess fat. Drain and place on top of the egg being sure at least 1 inch of egg is showing on either side of the sausage.

Now roll the meat around the filling having the steak wrapped completely around the outside of filling, overlapping a little. Do not roll as a jelly roll. It should be a large roll, one circle around and not a spiral. Tie roll in 2 or 3 places with butcher's string. Heat a large pot, and then add a little oil and heat. Add chopped onions and sauté. Push onions aside and place roll in pot. Brown all around then add wine, little salt and pepper and simmer 1 ½ hours adding a little water from time to time if needed. Test to be sure meat is tender. Remove, cool and refrigerate. Save the pan juices in a separate container in the refrigerator.

On the day you are to serve it, remove the meat from the refrigerator early in the day, remove the strings and slice into ¼ inch slices. Place on a round platter leaving room in the center for a bowl. Leave at room temperature. Heat some tomato sauce to very hot, and add pan juices the meat was cooked in. (Skim off any fat from the top of the juices before adding.) Put into a bowl and serve.

## Flank Steak, marinated
Very easy and delicious.  This is also delicious cooked on an outdoor grill.

1 ½ lb. flank steak
¼ cup gluten-free soy sauce*
¼ cup red or white wine

Sprinkling of salt, ground black pepper,
   garlic and onion powder

Marinate for 1 hour.  Broil 5 minutes per side for medium rare.

## Goulash or Gulyus
This recipe is my mother's and we always enjoy it.  I converted it to be gluten-free.

2 lbs. stew meat
Fine white rice flour
3 Tablespoons oil
2 sliced onions
1 teaspoon salt

Few dashes ground black pepper
1 Tablespoon gluten-free paprika*
   (Hungarian paprika has good flavor, but
   read labels to make sure it's gluten-free)

Dredge meat cubes in the rice flour.  Heat a 2 ½ quart saucepan a minute, add oil and heat another minute.  Add a few cubes of meat and brown on all sides.  Remove from pan and add a few more pieces of meat until all are browned.  Remove meat from pan.  Now add the onions to the pot and cook until lightly browned.  Return meat to pot and add the rest of the ingredients.  Mix together.  Add enough water to the pot to just cover the meat.  Bring to a boil.  Lower heat, cover and simmer over low heat for 1 ½ to 2 hours or until meat is very tender.  Just be sure to check the pot a few times during cooking and add additional water if needed.  This is good over rice or gluten-free noodles*.

*Variation*:  In the summer I often find that London Broil cut of meat is cheaper than stew meat.  I cut it up into chunks and cook this dish for 20 to 30 minutes instead of 1 ½ to 2 hours.  It's delicious, tender and a time-saver.

## Meatballs – My Favorite Version
Since I always have rice flour on hand, I tend to make this version the most.  It's easy and delicious.
The pine nuts are for an authentic Italian version (my mother always put them in when I was a child),
but they are delicious without them too.

¼ cup fine brown or white rice flour
1 lb. lean chopped meat
1 teaspoon salt
3 Tablespoons grated Pecorino Romano
   cheese

¼ cup chopped parsley (optional)
2 to 3 Tablespoons pine nuts (optional)
2 cloves of minced garlic
Dash or two of ground black pepper
2 eggs

Blend all ingredients, except meat, with a whisk.  Add meat and incorporate with egg mixture using your hands.  Shape into 12 meatballs.  Fry until all sides are brown, and then add to sauce.  (See recipe for tomato sauce, or add to gluten-free tomato sauce* from a jar and finish cooking meatballs in the sauce).  If you don't care to fry, place them on a foil lined baking sheet and broil a few minutes on each side.

*see gluten-free products list at the end of the book*

Also, sometimes I take 2 meatballs per person, flatten them to be like hamburgers and pan fry them until cooked through. Serve with a tossed green salad. They are very flavorful.

## Meatballs – Version 2

I have found that the gluten-free rice bread is grainy when added to meatballs. Using tapioca is very goopy to work with, but they brown really well and it helps thicken your sauce. The cornflakes also work well, but you will see yellow specks even after they are finely crushed.

4 Tablespoons quick cooking tapioca soaked in 6 Tablespoons of milk, until milk is absorbed or ⅓ to ½ cup gluten-free cornflakes*
1 lb. lean chopped meat
1 teaspoon salt
3 Tablespoons grated Pecorino Romano cheese

¼ cup chopped parsley (optional)
2 to 3 Tablespoons pine nuts (optional)
2 cloves of minced garlic
Dash or two of ground black pepper
2 eggs
Additional sprinkling of rice flour if too wet

Mix the tapioca and milk in a bowl. Set aside about a ½ hour or put it together the night before and keep it in the refrigerator. If using cornflakes, put in a food processor with all of the ingredients except the meat and pine nuts. Place the meat into bowl. Add the tapioca (if using) or cornflake mixture (if using) and the rest of the ingredients and mix well. Shape into 12 meatballs. Fry in a skillet with some oil, drain, and add to sauce. If you don't like to fry, place them on a foil lined baking sheet and broil a few minutes on each side.

Also, sometimes I take 2 meatballs per person, flatten them to be like hamburgers and fry. They are very flavorful. Serve with a tossed green salad.

## Meatballs – Porcupine Style

Easy to put together and no eggs or bread crumbs are used. These bake in the oven so no frying is needed.

1 pound lean ground beef (I use ground round)
½ cup uncooked white rice
½ cup cool water
1 small chopped onion or 1 Tablespoon dried onion flakes
¼ teaspoon garlic powder

½ teaspoon salt
¼ teaspoon black pepper
¼ teaspoon dried basil
1 cup water
1 (8 ounce) can gluten-free tomato sauce*
1 Tablespoon gluten-free Worcestershire sauce*

Mix together the rice, water, onion, salt, pepper and basil in a bowl. Add the ground meat and work the rice mixture into the meat using your hands. Do not overwork or the meat can get tough. Form into about 12 meatballs and place either in a non-stick 7" x 11" pan or a casserole dish with a cover. (I use an oval Corningware® casserole dish with a lid.)

Use the same bowl and mix together the water, tomato sauce and Worcestershire sauce. Pour over the meatballs. Cover and bake at 375°F for 40 minutes or until the rice is tender. Uncover and bake 5 to 10 minutes more until the sauce thickens.

*Variation:* Lean ground turkey may be used instead of ground beef. I add an additional ¼ teaspoon garlic powder if I am using turkey. This gives the meat a much better flavor.

## Meatballs with Sun Dried Tomatoes
**The sauce is very flavorful, and is nice served over rice.**

¼ cup sun-dried tomatoes
1 cup hot water, plus additional water
1 diced onion
1 stalk of celery, diced
¾ teaspoon dried basil
¾ teaspoon dried oregano
1 Tablespoon gluten-free Worcestershire Sauce* (optional)
1 teaspoon gluten-free beef bouillon*
¼ teaspoon salt (optional)
⅛ teaspoon ground black pepper
1 pound lean ground beef

¼ cup fine white rice flour or brown rice flour
2-3 Tablespoons Pecorino Romano cheese
1 teaspoon dried parsley
¼ teaspoon salt
¼ teaspoon garlic powder (optional)
1 egg
2-3 Tablespoons fine white rice flour or cornstarch
¼ cup cold water

Soak the sun-dried tomatoes in hot water for a minute or so to make them easy to dice. (Some brands are pliable enough that you can dice using a poultry scissor and skip this step.) Drain tomato water into a measuring cup and add enough water to make 1 ½ cups. (Or use just water). Put the water in your pot. Allow tomatoes to cool enough to handle and dice. Add the tomatoes, onion, celery, basil, oregano, Worcestershire, bouillon, salt and pepper. Cover and bring to a boil.

Meanwhile, in a bowl combine the meat with the rice flour, cheese, parsley, garlic powder, salt and egg. Mix well and form into small sized meatballs.

Turn off the heat under the pot and carefully add the meatballs to the tomato mixture. Return the pot to heat. Simmer covered for 1 hour. After cooking about 30 minutes, check to be sure there is enough water in the pot; add more water if necessary so that it doesn't burn.

If your sauce is thin, add the 2 to 3 Tablespoons of rice flour to the ¼ cup water. Add to pot and cook until it thickens.

*Variation:* This dish can be made in a crock-pot. Use ½ cup less water. Cook 4 to 6 hours on high or 8 to 10 hours on low. Turn crock to high at the end of cooking; add the rice flour or cornstarch and water. Allow the sauce to thicken before serving.

*see gluten-free products list at the end of the book*

## Meatballs – Swedish/Norwegian Style
My husband says that these remind him of the meatballs his Norwegian Grandmother used to make.

2 Tablespoons fine white rice flour,
  brown rice flour or sweet rice flour
1 Tablespoon dehydrated onion flakes
1 teaspoon salt
2 eggs
Few dashes of ground black pepper

1 pound lean chopped meat (I use beef,
  ground round)
1 cup water
1 ½ Tablespoons sweet or fine white rice
  flour

Whisk together all ingredients except the ground meat, water and 1 ½ Tablespoons rice flour. Add the meat and blend with your hands. Do not overwork. If it is too wet you can add another Tablespoon or so of rice flour. Form into small meatballs. Heat a skillet and brown the meatballs well on all sides. Drain fat. Add 1 cup hot water and 1 ½ Tablespoons sweet or fine white rice flour. Add and cook until meatballs are cooked through and the sauce is thick. If you brown the meatballs well (do not burn), you will have a nice brown gravy.

## Meatcake A La Lindstrom
If you like beets, you will like this. It's a good way to use leftover pickled beet salad (see index).

1 ½ lbs. lean chopped meat
4 oz. cold minced potatoes
4 oz. pickled beets, minced (see index for
  pickled beet salad recipe)
2 egg yolks (you can freeze egg whites for
  another use)

1 ½ teaspoons salt
Ground black pepper
2 Tablespoons grated onion
2 Tablespoons chopped capers* (optional)

Work all ingredients until well blended and make 12 cakes about ¾ inch thick. Heat fry pan and then add one or two Tablespoons of oil and some butter. Fry cakes on low heat until nicely browned. Pour drippings over cakes and garnish with pickled beets. Serves 6.

## Meat Loaf
This is a family favorite of ours. I usually make this rice flour version because it's easier, but the cornflake version (see variation) is good too. If you use the gluten-free cornflakes you will see yellow specks in your meatloaf. This meatloaf freezes well, so I often double the recipe.

1 lb. lean chopped meat or meat loaf
  combination of beef, pork and veal (I
  often use ½ ground beef and ½ ground
  turkey, which is good too)
2 eggs
¼ cup fine white rice flour or brown rice
  flour (or see variations below)

1 Tablespoon dehydrated onion flakes (or
  1 onion grated)
1 teaspoon salt
Few dashes of ground black pepper

In a small bowl mix the rice flour, eggs, dehydrated onion, salt and pepper with a whisk. If it's too wet, add a little more rice flour.

*see gluten-free products list at the end of the book

Wash your hands.  Put the meat in a large bowl.  Pour the rice flour mixture into the meat. Using your hands, blend thoroughly until mixed.  You want to thoroughly mix it to incorporate it into the meat, but not over mixed or the meat will get tough.  Place in a loaf pan and bake for 1 hour at 350°F.  I like it served with ketchup on it, but it's delicious without.  Finish the meal with a baked potato and a salad.

*Variation*: Use 1 cup gluten-free cornflakes* (either regular or honey flavor) in place of rice flour.  Add 1 Tablespoon gluten-free ketchup* (optional) if desired.  I like to use the ketchup when I use the cornflakes.  When using cornflakes, put the cornflakes, ketchup, eggs, salt and pepper in your food processor.  Pulse until flakes are pulverized, and blended into the eggs.

*Variation 2*: Gluten-free cracker crumbs may be used in place of the rice flour.  The crackers may be crushed in a heavy duty plastic bag using a rolling pin.  If your crackers are salted, use less salt in the meat loaf.

*Variation 3*: Cream of Rice® may be substituted for the rice flour.  However, I prefer the results with the rice flour because the texture is better and the egg mixes in better.

*Variation 4*: Gluten-Free Naturals™ bread can be used instead of rice flour.  Pulverize bread in a food processor and use about 6 to 8 Tablespoons of fresh bread crumbs.  Or use ¼ cup of dried gluten-free bread crumbs.

*Variation 5*: Chopped parsley may be added to the egg mixture, if desired.

## Mexican Lasagna
**This is easier to make than traditional lasagna.**

1 lb. ground meat (either beef, pork or turkey)
1 onion, chopped or 2 Tablespoons dried minced onion flakes
1 green pepper, chopped (optional)
1 or 2 Hungarian hot peppers with seeds, chopped (optional)
¾ teaspoon salt
1 teaspoon gluten-free chili powder*

¼ teaspoon garlic powder
¼ teaspoon oregano
2 (8 ounce) cans tomato sauce* or 2 cups gluten-free tomato sauce*
2 cups gluten-free cottage cheese*
1 cup grated mozzarella cheese*
¼ cup sliced olives for garnish
1 cup gluten-free sour cream* (optional)
1 package of 12 corn tortillas*

Cook meat in a skillet and drain excess fat.  Add onions, pepper, hot pepper and cook until soft.  Add spices and 1 can (1 cup) of tomato sauce.

Open second can of tomato sauce.  Pour half into a 9 x 9 inch square pan.  Layer 4 tortillas on the sauce.  (I break the tortillas in half, but if you want a neater presentation, cut each tortilla into strips.)  Add half the meat mixture.  Top with half the cottage cheese.  Do another layer of 4 tortillas.  Top with the remaining meat and cottage cheese.  Top with 4

*see gluten-free products list at the end of the book

tortillas.  Pour on the remaining sauce.  Top with mozzarella cheese and olives.  Bake at 350°F for 30 minutes until cheese melts and lasagna is hot.

If hot peppers were used, serve with sour cream if desired.

*Variation*:  A small can of gluten-free diced chopped chilies may be used instead of the hot peppers.

## Mexican Skillet

This is a favorite easy and quick dish to make in one pot.  Be sure you have enough liquid, or the rice will not cook properly.  I like this because it's a complete meal in less than 30 minutes.

1 lb. ground beef or ground turkey
½ cup chopped onion (fresh or frozen)
½ cup chopped green pepper (fresh or frozen)
¼ teaspoon garlic powder (add a little extra garlic powder if using ground turkey)
1 (16 ounce) can peeled tomatoes, mashed a little, or 1 can diced tomatoes*

1 cup uncooked rice
2 ½ cups liquid (juice from the can of tomatoes plus water)
2 teaspoons chili powder
½ teaspoon salt
½ teaspoon cumin (optional)
½ cup grated Parmesan cheese or ½ cup grated cheddar cheese

Heat a skillet a minute.  Add 2 Tablespoons of oil and heat another minute then add the meat.  Stir and cook until meat has lost its red color and has separated.  Drain off any fat.  Add onion and green pepper and sauté a few minutes longer.  Add all other ingredients except cheese.  Cover and simmer on low heat 20 minutes.  Sprinkle cheese on top and stir in to melt.  Serve.  I frequently make this and a salad for dinner.  Leftovers are good for lunches.  It reheats well in the microwave.

*Variation*:  Add a (14 oz.) can of drained and rinsed black beans or kidney beans when you add the other ingredients to make a one dish chili with rice.  For a spicier chili, add an additional teaspoon of chili powder.  I prefer cheddar cheese if adding the beans.

## Pepper Steak – Chinese Style

When my mother first made this dish, she used fresh ginger that was called for in the recipe. When she didn't have the fresh, she substituted the candied ginger. We liked it so much better that our family has made it that way ever since.

1 ½ to 2 pounds green peppers
1 large Spanish onion (or two medium onions)
1 pound top round or sirloin steak
2 Tablespoons cornstarch
2 Tablespoons gluten-free soy sauce*
4 Tablespoons water
½ teaspoon gluten-free MSG/monosodium glutamate* (optional, I don't use)

2 cloves minced garlic
1 piece candied ginger, about the size of a quarter
Salt and ground black pepper
2 Tablespoons oil
1 ½ cups hot water
1 heaping teaspoon gluten-free chicken base* or gluten-free chicken bouillon cube*

Partially freeze the steak so you can cut it into thin slices. Wash, seed and cut green peppers into bite size pieces. Peel and slice onion. Cut candied ginger into tiny pieces. Heat water and add chicken base or chicken cube. Make sauce by combining cornstarch, cold water, soy sauce, MSG and minced garlic. Heat wok, add oil then add meat and cook until each thin slice has lost its red color. Remove from pan. Add a little more oil if needed then put vegetables into the wok and stir-fry 3 minutes. Sprinkle with a little salt and pepper and cut up candied ginger. Pour in the hot water into which you have dissolved the chicken base or cube. Cover and cook 6 minutes. Check to see if peppers are cooked to the crisp tender stage. If so, return meat to wok and add sauce, being sure the cornstarch is thoroughly blended. Stir and cook until sauce is thickened. Serve with Rice.

## Salisbury Steak

This is easy and requires no eggs.

1 pound ground beef
⅓ cup finely chopped onion
2 Tablespoons fine white rice flour or brown rice flour
¾ teaspoon salt
⅛ teaspoon pepper
1 onion, thinly sliced into rings

1 can mushrooms, drained (optional)
1 ½ teaspoons gluten-free bouillon*
1 ½ cups water or 1 (14.5 ounce) can of gluten-free beef broth may be used
2 Tablespoons Worcestershire sauce*
1 to 2 Tablespoons fine white rice flour

Combine beef, finely chopped onion, 2 Tablespoons rice flour, salt and pepper. Form into 4 or 5 patties.

Heat a skillet a minute, spray with gluten-free cooking spray and add patties. Cook over medium heat for about 5 minutes one side. Turn patties over, add sliced onions and cook about 5 minutes more. Add the rest of the ingredients. Sprinkle the rice flour over the top and mix it in. Cover and cook for 10 to 15 minutes until meat is done. Remove lid. If sauce is not thick enough, sprinkle a little more rice flour in (about 1 Tablespoon), mix it in and let the sauce bubble. This is nice served with mashed potatoes.

*see gluten-free products list at the end of the book

*Variation*: Use 2 Tablespoons Madeira wine and 1 ½ teaspoons Worcestershire (instead of the 2 Tablespoons Worcestershire) for a different flavor.

## Sauerbraten

This is delicious German dish.  The meat is tender and the gravy is delicious.  You need to put this together 2 to 3 days ahead of time.

| | |
|---|---|
| 3 lbs. rump roast | ¼ cup sugar |
| Salt and ground black pepper | 2 Tablespoons oil |
| Sprinkling of ground nutmeg | 2 Tablespoons fine white rice flour or |
| 1 medium onion, sliced |    sweet rice flour |
| 1 bay leaf | ¼ cup milk |
| ¾ cup water | |
| ¾ cup cider or wine vinegar | |

About 2 or 3 days before cooking the roast, you must start to marinate the meat.  Sprinkle the roast with salt, pepper, and nutmeg and rub into the meat.  Place in a glass or stainless steel bowl along with the sliced onion and bay leaf.  (Sometimes I use a large glass loaf pan for this.)  Heat the sugar, vinegar and water to boiling and stir to dissolve sugar.  Pour over meat.  Allow to cool.  Cover and refrigerate.  After 24 hours, turn the meat over to be sure to marinate it evenly.

When ready to cook, remove the meat from marinade and dry with a paper towel.  Keep marinade.  Place a large pot on the stove and heat a minute.  Add oil and swirl it around and let heat another minute.  This will prevent the meat from sticking.  Place the meat into the pot and brown it on all sides.  Add marinade and bring to a boil.  Reduce heat, cover and cook 2 to 3 hours until tender.  Test meat with a cake tester.  If it passes through the meat easily, it has cooked long enough.  Remove meat to a hot platter while making the gravy.  Mix the rice flour and milk together and slowly add to the pan liquid.  Stir until gravy thickens and comes to a boil.  Don't worry if there are lumps as you must pass the gravy through a strainer to remove the onions and bay leaf anyway.  (I strain it by putting a large sieve over a 4-cup measuring bowl and pouring in the gravy.)  Strain and put the gravy back into the pot to keep warm while slicing meat.  Place the meat on a platter and pour a little gravy over the top.  Pass the rest of the gravy in a gravy boat.  Serve with mashed potatoes and red cabbage (see index).  Or, serve with red cabbage (see index) and spaetzle (see index) for an authentic meal.

Note:  The right cut of meat is important for this to turn out properly.  Using too tough a cut will yield stringy meat.

*Variation*:  My mother cuts the 3-pound roast into three 1-pound pieces.  That way the roast absorbs more of the marinade and flavor.  She also says by having the roast in 3 pieces you don't have to cook it as long for the center to be done.  This enables you to cut the meat into nicer slices, since it is cooked more evenly.

## Sauerbraten Short Ribs

This recipe is very tangy with a strong flavor.  The sauce is nice on mashed potatoes, rice or gluten-free noodles* or spaetzle (see index).  You can substitute chuck or stewing beef for the short ribs.  The original recipe from my father's aunt called for ginger snap cookies to thicken and flavor the sauce, but this turns out just as well if not better.

3 to 4 pounds short ribs (check labels, some have added solutions that may not be gluten-free)
1 cup gluten-free ketchup*
1 cup water
2 Tablespoons sugar
2 Tablespoons cider vinegar
1 Tablespoon gluten-free horseradish*
1 Tablespoon gluten-free Worcestershire sauce*

1 Tablespoon gluten-free dry mustard*
½ teaspoon ground black pepper
½ teaspoon ground allspice
¼ teaspoon ground ginger
1 teaspoon sugar
2 onions, chopped
1 teaspoon salt
1 bay leaf
2 Tablespoons fine white rice flour or sweet rice flour

Stir together ketchup, water, sugar, cider vinegar, horseradish, mustard, Worcestershire sauce, pepper, allspice, ginger, sugar, onion and salt.  Pour into a heavy plastic bag that is resting in a large bowl.  Add the short ribs and bay leaf.  Toss to coat meat with marinade.  Seal the bag and refrigerate overnight.  Place marinated ribs and marinade in a pot, cover and simmer 2 ½ to 3 hours or until tender.  Stir often while it is cooking.  Thicken gravy with the rice flour blended with a little water.  If you want a thicker sauce, add a little more rice flour and simmer a few minutes more.  Remove bay leaf.

*Variation*: I have made this in the crock-pot by eliminating the water.  Put all ingredients (except the rice flour) in a removable crock and marinate overnight in the refrigerator.  The next day, put it in your crock-pot and cook it for 10-12 hours on low.  Turn the crock-pot on high.  Add the rice flour by sprinkling it in and stirring it so no lumps form.  Let it thicken the sauce before serving.

## Sirloin Tip Roast – Easy

Get a Sirloin Tip Roast that is not too thick (or have butcher cut it to the thickness of London Broil).  Bake at 450°F for 15 minutes per pound.  Slice thinly and serve.  It is an easy way to make a roast beef for use in salads, sandwiches, etc.

## "Souper" Burgers

There is no need to purchase expensive dry onion soup mix that may contain gluten.

2 gluten-free beef bouillon cubes* (I use Hormel® which are labeled gluten-free)
2 Tablespoons dehydrated onion flakes or dried minced onion
¼ cup water

Sprinklings of garlic and onion powder
2 teaspoons dried parsley flakes (optional)
2 pounds of ground beef (I use 90% lean/10% fat)

*see gluten-free products list at the end of the book

Use warm water and place bouillon cubes and dried onion to soak for a few minutes. Crush cubes and blend in. (After the cubes absorb water they are easy to crush.) Add the rest of the spices and the beef, and blend together by hand. Form into quarter pound burger patties. For best flavor, grill on a gas or charcoal grill. For additional flavor, soak some mesquite wood chips (about ¼ to ½ cup) in water and put them on the coals. Cook burgers until done. Because these burgers are flavorful, sometimes I serve them without rolls.

## Stir Fry with Beef

This is an easy way to make stir fry, using chopped frozen vegetables. I prefer real sliced beef, but you can use those frozen sandwich steaks that are all beef with nothing added. This recipe does not contain bouillon, and the flavor is very good without it.

½ pound thin sliced steak, cut into slices approximately 1" by 2 ½" or 1 (8 to 12 ounce) package of frozen all beef sandwich steaks
2 teaspoons gluten-free soy sauce*
2 teaspoons cornstarch
1 teaspoon sugar
1 Tablespoon oil
1 green or red pepper, sliced or chopped (or use a handful of chopped frozen green pepper)

1 medium onion, sliced or chopped (or use a handful of chopped frozen onion)
1 (16 ounce) bag of frozen stir fry mixed vegetables (or 1 pound package of frozen vegetables of your choice)
1 cup water
1 Tablespoon cornstarch
2 Tablespoons gluten-free soy sauce* (or less, to taste)
2 Tablespoons gluten-free ketchup*
1 teaspoon sugar

Slice the beef, and marinade it by mixing with the 2 teaspoons soy sauce, 2 teaspoons cornstarch and the 1 teaspoon sugar. (If using frozen sandwich steaks, put them in the pan on low to defrost and break apart into slices with a spatula. Turn off heat. Add the marinade, blend, and then turn the heat back on and cook. Remove from pan and set aside.)

Heat a wok or large skillet, and then add the oil. Stir fry the meat until cooked, and remove. (I return it to the same dish I used for the marinade, because the meat will be cooked again.) Drain any beef fat. Stir fry the pepper and onions in a little oil. Then add the frozen vegetables. (If using all frozen vegetables, add them all at once.) Stir fry until crisp tender. Add a little more oil if needed.

Mix the sauce by combining the rest of the ingredients. Add that to the vegetables. Return the meat, stir, and heat until the sauce thickens. Serve over rice.

## Stuffed Cabbage

This is my grandmother's recipe and a favorite of ours.  She added chopped onion and substituted Savoy cabbage because this cabbage is more tender and delicate in flavor. (When you look for it at the grocery store, it is the cabbage with curly looking leaves.)  You also don't have to pre-boil it for this recipe, as would if using white cabbage.  We've made it this way ever since.

1 pound ground beef
2 cups chopped onion
½ cup rice, cooked according to package
   directions
½ teaspoon salt
Few dashes ground black pepper
8 Savoy cabbage leaves

½ teaspoon salt
Dash of ground black pepper
1 ½ Tablespoons sugar
⅓ cup lemon juice
15 oz. can gluten-free tomato sauce*or
   two 8 oz. cans.

Buy a medium head of Savoy cabbage. (This is a green cabbage with curly edges on the leaves.)  Core it and carefully remove the 8 outer leaves.  It is usually quite easy to remove the leaves of Savoy cabbage, as it is not as tight a head of cabbage as the regular white variety of cabbages.

The regular variety of cabbage or white variety always needs to be pre-boiled.  However, if you do find it difficult to remove the leaves of the Savoy cabbage without tearing them, place the whole head of cabbage in a pot of boiling water and cook for 5 minutes.  Remove from pot, cool enough to handle and then remove leaves needed.

Place each leaf rough side up.  Slice away the top of the large center rib of each leaf <u>without</u> cutting through the leaves.  In other words, cut off the top part of the rib and make that part of the leaf flat like the rest of the leaf.  Discard what is cut away.  This removal of the tough part of rib makes for easier rolling.  Mix meat with cooked rice, ½ teaspoon salt and a little pepper.  Chop onions.  Using a covered skillet, place 1 to 2 Tablespoons oil in it and sauté the onions until limp.  Take out half of the onions and place into the meat mixture and mix well.

Now make your meat into eight equal size elongated meatballs.  Place one portion of meat in the center of a cabbage leaf (which you have rough side up).  Fold sides of leaf over filling and roll from the bottom up into a tight little package.  Place in skillet, seam side down, on top of the onions.  Continue in this fashion until all meat and leaves are used and rolls are neatly placed in a single layer in the skillet.  You can now place the rest of the cabbage cut in wedges on top or save it to make "cabbage sauté side dish" or "cabbage and beans" or "Minestra soup" (see index).  Now top the rolls with the sauce ingredients, sugar, salt, pepper, tomato sauce, and lemon juice.  Bring to a boil, reduce heat to simmer, cover skillet and cook 45 minutes.

I like this dish served with mashed potatoes.  I like the sauce on top of the potatoes.

*see gluten-free products list at the end of the book*

## Stuffed Green Peppers

This is my mother's original recipe and is one of our favorites. Sometimes I use "meatloaf mix" a combination of ground beef, pork and veal to make this recipe.

4 large green peppers
1 large chopped onion
1 pound chopped meat (beef, turkey or
   pork)
1 teaspoon salt
Ground black pepper
Sprinkling of MSG (optional)

2 to 3 Tablespoons oil
½ cup raw rice
1 egg
2 to 3 Tablespoons fine white rice flour
1 ½ cups to 2 cups tomato sauce* (I use
   canned sauce)

Wash peppers and cut in half, cutting through the stem. Remove seeds and stem and wash again. Boil some water and cook peppers about 8 minutes until crisp tender. Drain and cool while making filling. In the same pot cook your rice according to package directions. Using a skillet, heat oil and sauté chopped onion gently on low heat then add meat and cook and stir until meat loses its red color and is in tiny pieces. Drain fat. Remove from heat and add salt and pepper, MSG if using, and a few tablespoons of tomato sauce. Drain cooked rice and add to meat along with the eggs and just enough rice flour to absorb any liquid. Mix well and fill shells. Place in a baking dish and pour rest of sauce on top. Bake at 350°F for 30 minutes.

*Variation 1*: Add ½ cup of grated cheddar or mozzarella cheese to the meat before you fill the pepper shells.

*Variation 2*: I make the rice in the microwave and start that first before I boil the peppers so that it can be completed faster. In a deep microwave safe container, combine 1 cup boiling water, ½ cup rice and ¼ teaspoon salt. Blend, and microwave <u>uncovered</u> 15 minutes until done. (If using cold water instead of boiling, microwave an extra 5 minutes.) Do not cover or it will boil over and make a mess of your microwave.

## Stuffed Green Peppers – Easy One Pot Skillet Version – My Favorite

These are quick and can be made in about 30 minutes in one pot. My mother created this recipe and I adapted it. I find that I make this one most frequently because it is the easiest. No flour or egg is needed. No extra pot is needed to boil the peppers. On those hot summer days when peppers are plentiful, this is a way to make stuffed peppers without the extra heat from the oven in the kitchen.

1 Tablespoon oil
4 large peppers
2 large onions, chopped
¾ pound to 1 pound lean chopped beef
   or ground turkey or ground pork
¼ to ½ teaspoon garlic powder or use
   fresh garlic that has been minced
   through a garlic press
½ cup rice

1 small can (12 ounce) tomato paste
2 ½ cups hot water
1 ½ teaspoons salt
1 teaspoon chili powder
1 teaspoon cumin (optional – I don't use
   since my chili powder contains cumin.)
Sprinkling or two of ground black pepper
Pinch of oregano
Grated gluten-free cheddar cheese*
   (optional)

*see gluten-free products list at the end of the book

Use a very large 12" skillet (fry pan) with a cover. Set cover aside. Heat skillet a minute, add the 1 Tablespoon oil and sauté the chopped meat and 2 chopped onions over medium high heat. Sprinkle meat with garlic powder. Stir once in a while, until meat is browned and onions are cooked. (I use lean meat, but if your meat is fatty, drain the fat.)

While meat and onions cook, wash the green peppers and dry. Cut them in half going the long way (through the stem). Remove the stem and discard the seeds. Set aside. You will have 8 pepper halves.

Now that the meat is no longer red, add ½ cup rice, 2 ½ cups hot water, tomato paste, 1 ½ teaspoons salt, the cumin (optional), chili powder, black pepper and oregano to the pot. Stir mixture, bring to a boil, reduce heat, cover tightly and simmer 10 minutes.

Remove cover and lay the 8 pepper cups on top of the mixture, open side of the peppers up. Cover and cook 10 minutes more. Remove from heat and check peppers for doneness. If you want the peppers cooked more, let them sit in the pot with the cover on for 5 more minutes or so.

Remove cover and carefully take out the pepper cups with tongs as they will have water in them. Drain the water in the sink and place pepper cups on a plate. (Or put them in individual microwave containers.) The filling should be thick with all liquid absorbed and the rice should be tender. There should be approximately 4 ½ cups filling. Stuff the peppers using all the filling. Press down on the filling so it all holds together. Top with grated cheese if desired.

*Variation*: Use 3 Tablespoons tomato paste in with the meat instead of the whole can. Follow directions as above. Fill the peppers. Since your sauce won't have as much tomato flavor, top each pepper with some tomato sauce. To do this, open 1 (8 ounce) gluten-free can of tomato sauce* and put it in your pan. Put in a pinch of sugar, salt and black pepper and stir to heat. Top the peppers with the sauce. (You can add a drained canned of green beans to the sauce to heat through. Remove the beans and serve on the side. Top the peppers with the sauce.)

*Variation 2*: Other vegetables like drained canned corn, drained mushrooms, and even frozen peas may be added to the meat. I call this variation "Fiesta Pepper Boats".

*Variation 3*: My mother sometimes prefers to make these as 4 whole peppers instead of 8 pepper halves. To do this, choose large peppers that are short and wide. Cut the stems off the peppers instead of cutting them in half. Remove seeds. Follow directions above, and push the four pepper cups down into the mixture, so that they will fit in the pot with the lid on.

*see gluten-free products list at the end of the book

## Stuffed Filet Mignon
This is a good company dish.

Filet mignon steaks, each cut 1 ½ inches
   thick
½ Tablespoon butter or olive oil per steak
2 Tablespoons minced green onion per
   steak

4 mushrooms per steak
1 slice of bacon per steak
1 Tablespoon Madeira wine per steak
Dash of salt and ground black pepper

Slice each steak lengthwise in half but not all the way through. Wash, dry and chop mushrooms. Melt the ½ Tablespoon butter per steak in a fry pan. Sauté the green onion on low heat a few minutes. Then add mushrooms, salt and pepper. Cook about 5 minutes until moisture disappears. Stir in wine and continue to cook and stir to evaporate most of the liquid. Take off the heat and let cool. Stuff each steak with the mushroom mixture then wrap a piece of bacon around steak to cover the slit and stuffing and secure with a toothpick. Broil for 5 minutes per side. Serve with a baked potato or Viennese rice (see index) and a salad.

## Stuffed Potato with Chili (easy)
I like these better than the ones at Wendy's®. They're easy to make, and they're inexpensive too.

1 can Hormel® Chili with beans (gluten-
   free as of this writing, caution, chili with
   no beans contains gluten) <u>or</u> leftover
   homemade chili (see index)

4 large potatoes, washed
Gluten-free grated cheddar cheese* or
   sliced cheddar cheese
Gluten-free sour cream* (optional)

Wash potatoes and bake in the microwave until fork tender. (For my microwave oven it's usually 7 minutes.) Remove from oven and slice in half lengthwise. Open can of chili and put some on top of each potato half. If using leftover chili, which would be refrigerated, I suggest heating it in the microwave first to warm it before putting it on the potato. (Canned chili would be room temperature so you can skip that step.)

Top each with cheddar cheese. Microwave until chili is heated and cheese melts. Serve with a dollop of sour cream if desired. This is great for a quick lunch. If I make these for dinner I serve with a salad.

*Variation*: You can use gluten-free Monterey Jack or other cheese instead of cheddar.

*Variation 2*: For a meatless dish, top potatoes with vegetables and cheese instead of chili. (I like drained canned mushrooms.)

*Variation 3*: Leftover ham cubes with vegetables and cheese is also very good.

Note: I find that instead of using a vegetable brush to wash potatoes, a nail brush works much better. The bristles are designed to be gentler to surface skin, and the bristles clean better and last longer. I used one by Fuller Brush® and it is manufactured in the USA.

*\*see gluten-free products list at the end of the book*

## Suki Yaki
A tasty Japanese Dish.  This is my mother's recipe.

Oil
4 minute steaks (I prefer the ones from
  the fresh meat counter)
2 stalks celery, sliced thinly or sliced on an
  angle
2 large onions, sliced
12 scallions, washed well and sliced
1 small can sliced mushrooms or 8 fresh

1 package leaf spinach, partially thawed
1 can bamboo shoots (check ingredients)
¼ cup gluten-free soy sauce*
½ cup gluten-free beef broth* or ½
  teaspoon gluten-free soup base* and ½
  cup water
1 Tablespoon sugar

Wash and remove strings from celery with a potato peeler.  Lay celery, rounded side up on a cutting board.  Slice away from you, holding the knife parallel to the board to cut thin yet large slices.  Peel and slice onion.  Clean and cut the white part of scallions into 1 inch pieces.  Partially thaw spinach by taking it out of the freezer an hour or so before cooking time.  Open can of bamboo shoots and mushrooms and drain.  Heat a skillet a minute.  Add a couple of Tablespoons oil and swirl around let it heat a minute.  Brown thin steaks and remove from pan.  Add scallions, celery and onion to skillet and sauté 5 minutes.

Meanwhile, slice meat into strips.  Now add the soy sauce, beef broth, sugar and vegetables to pan, cover and cook at low heat 10 minutes.  Remove cover, add meat and heat another minute or 2.  Serve over rice.  Makes 2 generous servings.

## Sweet and Sour Brisket
This is good for company.  I like it served with mashed potatoes.

2 to 3 pounds brisket
2 Tablespoons oil
2 carrots
1 onion
2 stalks of celery

¼ cup cider vinegar
3 Tablespoons sugar
Salt and ground black pepper

Scrape and dice carrots.  Dice onions.  Wash, dry and remove strings and dice celery.  Take a covered skillet and heat one minute on the stove.  Add the oil, swirl it around the bottom of the skillet and heat one minute.  Wipe meat with paper towel and place carefully into heated oil.  If pot and oil are heated in this fashion, the meat will not stick.  Brown brisket on both sides, then add vegetables and sauté a few minutes.  Add rest of ingredients, lower heat to simmer and cover.  Cook on low about 2 hours.  Test with a cake tester.  If it passes through easily, it is done.  When ready to serve, remove the meat from the pan and slice into thin slices cutting across the grain.

Arrange on a platter, top with vegetables and moisten with a little of the pan juices.  Pass the rest of the gravy in a gravy boat.  This is delicious and is an easy dish for company.  Serves 6.

## Sweet and Sour Swedish Meatballs

These are delicious as a main course or as an appetizer.  The first time I had this, I had no idea that there was cranberry sauce in it, since it becomes meatballs in a brown sauce.  The meatballs are very tender because of the added vegetables.  This recipe is from a good friend and neighbor.

2 pounds lean chopped beef
6 Tablespoons fine white rice flour or brown rice flour (add 2 Tablespoons more if it seems too wet)
1 teaspoon salt (the original recipe did not have the salt, but I think it needs it)
4 large eggs
1 large scraped and carrot sliced very small or chopped finely in a food processor

1 medium onion, chopped finely or chopped in a food processor, or 1 Tablespoon dehydrated onion flakes
2 cloves garlic, minced or chopped finely in a food processor
1 (15 oz) jar gluten-free Marinara (meatless) tomato sauce*
1 can whole cranberry sauce
Additional chopped onion and sliced carrots

Chop onion, carrot and garlic fine, either by hand or in a food processor or blender.  Add rice flour, salt, and eggs and blend thoroughly, by adding to the food processor or blender, or by mixing by hand.  Put meat in a bowl and pour out the egg mixture and add to the meat.  Blend well to fully incorporate but do not overwork, or the meat will get tough.  Shape into meatballs (large if for a main course or small for an appetizer) with moistened hands and place on a foil lined baking sheet.  Broil 3 minutes, turn balls over and broil an additional 3 minutes just to firm up the meat.  (Or you can brown the meatballs in a fry pan on the stove.)  Now place meatballs in a large pot.  Add some sliced carrots, chopped onion, the Marinara sauce and cranberry sauce.  Simmer on low heat 1 ¼ hours.  These meatballs freeze well.  These are nice served with rice or gluten-free noodles* for a main dish.

## Osso Buco

This is a gourmet, Italian restaurant style dish.

6 Veal Shanks (rounded steaks with bone)
Fine white rice flour
Olive oil
½ cup dry white wine
1 (14 oz.) can of peeled tomatoes, cut up
Salt and ground black pepper

⅛ teaspoon garlic powder
Grated rind of ½ lemon
2 teaspoons anchovy paste (about 1 ½ to 2 inches of paste)

Dredge shanks in rice flour.  Brown the meat in olive oil.  Add the white wine and cook for 15 minutes.  Now add the tomatoes and salt and pepper.  Cover and cook until tender.  (This can be cooked in a crock-pot).

Blend together the garlic, lemon rind and anchovy paste.  Before serving, put over the meat and turn once or twice to distribute the flavor.

Serve with Rice Milanese, which is rice cooked with chicken broth, minced onion, wine, and Parmesan cheese.  Also delicious with plain rice that has some butter and Parmesan cheese added.  Or try the Viennese Rice (see index).

*see gluten-free products list at the end of the book

## Tamale Pie

We enjoy this dish and it's very easy to make. I've made this in 30 minutes. Traditional tamales are cornmeal pockets filled with meat and steamed in corn husks. This dish has the same flavor without the work. (My friend who doesn't have celiac disease tried it and liked it so much that she buys the Gluten-Free Naturals® Corn Bread Mix to make it. She tried all of the other regular brands in this recipe and says she likes the gluten-free version much better.)

1 pound ground meat (ground turkey, pork or beef may be used)
1 to 1 ½ cups gluten-free salsa*
⅛ teaspoon garlic powder (I use ¼ teaspoon if using ground turkey)
½ teaspoon salt

2 teaspoons chili powder
¾ cups grated cheddar cheese (more or less to taste)
1 Gluten-Free Naturals™ Corn Muffin/Corn Bread Mix, prepared according to package directions

Put meat in a large skillet. Break up and cook until it loses its red color. Drain any excess fat. Add the salsa, garlic powder, salt, chili powder and blend well and heat until hot. Put the meat mixture into a 9 x 9 inch square non-stick pan. Top with the grated cheese.

Meanwhile, prepare corn muffin mix as directed. (The cornbread will rise a little higher if you blend it with an electric mixer.) Pour over meat/cheese mixture and spread the cornbread mixture to cover.

Bake for about 25 minutes at 400°F. The top should be lightly browned. Remove from oven and run a knife along the edge of the pan to loosen the cornbread. Cut into large squares and serve using a large spatula. The meat and cheese will be in the bottom of the cornbread, so it is easy to serve. A salad completes the meal. Refrigerate any leftovers. Tamale pie reheats well in the microwave.

## Tamale Pie – Version 2

This makes a lot of food for a crowd and uses polenta instead of cornbread on top.

2 lbs. ground meat (I like a combination of either ground turkey, pork or beef)
2 onions, diced (fresh or frozen)
2 green peppers, diced (fresh or frozen)
¼ teaspoon garlic powder or 2 cloves minced
3 cups gluten-free tomato sauce*
1 small can corn drained (optional)
½ cup sliced pitted black olives

1 teaspoon salt (add extra ¼ to ½ teaspoon if you don't add olives)
4 teaspoons chili powder
¼ teaspoon cumin (optional)
1 ½ cups grated cheddar cheese (or more or less to taste)

Polenta:       ¾ cup cornmeal
              4 cups water
              1 teaspoon salt

Put meat in a large pan. Break up and cook until it loses its red color. Drain any excess fat. Add onions and green pepper. Cook until onions start to get translucent. Add the tomato sauce, add the corn if using, olives, and the 1 ¼ teaspoons salt (I use 1 teaspoon), chili powder and cumin.

*see gluten-free products list at the end of the book

Meanwhile, put 4 cups boiling water into a large microwave safe pan. (I use a deep Corningware® casserole dish). Add cornmeal and salt and stir. Microwave 6 minutes and stir with a whisk. Stir the polenta gently at first until blended (to avoid getting hot water on you), and then more vigorously once it's blended. Cook an additional 2 minutes and stir again. It will be creamy and thick. Microwave temperatures may vary. If needed cook another 4 minutes.

Put the meat mixture into a large rectangular pan, about 9" x 11". Top with the grated-cheese. Then top with the polenta mixture. Spread to fully cover the pan. To make the polenta get browner on the top, spray it with gluten-free cooking spray*. Bake 30 minutes at 350°F until the polenta is set. Cut into large squares with a knife and serve using a large spatula. The meat mixture and polenta will remain separate, so spoon some of the meat mixture on top of the polenta when you serve it. A salad completes the meal.

## Tamale Pie – Mexican Version
This version has a pie crust made from Masa Harina. Do not substitute regular corn flour or it will not work. The combination of the corn crust and the creamed corn give this a nice corn flavor. The original recipe did not have the canned tomatoes, but we like them so I add them. Or, you can add some diced red pepper for another variation. Or, Taco filling can be used in this pie crust.

Crust:
- 1 ¼ cup Masa Harina (corn flour treated with lime, used to make tortillas) as of this writing Maseca® brand is gluten-free
- ⅔ cup water
- 2 tablespoons oil
- 1 to 2 teaspoons chili powder (I use 1)
- ¾ teaspoon salt (I use a little less)

Filling:
- 1 to 1 ½ pounds ground beef or pork, cooked and drained
- 1 clove of garlic, minced
- 1 onion, chopped
- 1 green pepper, chopped or 1 (4 ounce) can of mild diced green chilies well drained
- 1 diced and seeded jalapeno pepper (optional, I don't use)
- 1 teaspoon salt
- ⅛ teaspoon pepper
- ½ teaspoon oregano
- 1 (14 or 15 ounce) can of gluten-free creamed corn*
- 1 small can of sliced black olives, well-drained
- 1 can of diced tomatoes, well-drained (optional)
- 1 cup of shredded cheddar cheese*

Mix Masa Harina with the water, oil, chili powder and salt until well blended. Grease a 1 ½ quart casserole well with butter. Press the Masa mixture the casserole dish to form a crust on the sides and bottom. Use your hands, and press it to make the crust thickness even.

Cook ground beef or pork in a skillet until no longer pink. Drain any excess fat. Add the garlic, onion, green pepper and jalapeno pepper. Cook until vegetables are tender. Blend together the rest of the ingredients, except the cheese. Heat the mixture 2 to 3 minutes. Fill the prepared crust. Top with shredded cheese.

*see gluten-free products list at the end of the book

Bake at 350°F for 35 to 40 minutes.  Or if you are in a rush you can bake it at 375°F for about 20 minutes.

*Variation*:  Use 2 to 2 ½ cups cooked chicken instead of beef or pork.  (If you prefer the flavor of thyme, substitute it for the oregano.)  Blend the chicken in with the cooked onion and follow the rest of the directions.

*Variation 2*:  Use this crust to thinly line greased, oven-safe single-serving bowls.  Fill with chili (see index for recipe. I prepare it using less tomato sauce so it will not make the crust soggy.  Or, use several cans of gluten-free chili with beans*).  Top with cheese and bake until the crust is set, and the chili is heated through and cheese is melted.

# CHICKEN AND TURKEY

## Arroz con Pollo – Cuban Style Chicken and Rice

My Aunt has a Cuban friend who gave this recipe and says it is very authentic. I prefer this dish the day I make it. Leftovers won't have any sauce on the rice because the rice absorbs all the liquid. If I'm not making this for a crowd, then I make half the recipe for this reason.

1 frying chicken (about 2 ½ lbs.) cut up in approximately 8 pieces (I use backless thighs and skin them first to make it a less fatty dish)
1 cup long grain rice
1 green pepper, chopped
1 large onion, chopped
2 cloves garlic

3 cups chicken broth (or 3 cups water and 3 teaspoons gluten-free soup base*)
2 (8 oz.) cans tomato sauce, divided
1 tsp. salt (or to taste)
½ tsp. ground black pepper (or to taste)
½ can of pitted black olives, sliced
2-3 Tbsp. cooking oil (I use olive oil)

In a Dutch oven or large deep fry pan, brown the chicken pieces in oil. They should be golden in color. Remove chicken and set aside. Place chopped onion, diced pepper and minced garlic into the same oil and sauté over low heat until soft and golden. Add raw rice and sauté a minute or so, or until the rice is translucent. Now place the chicken pieces on top of the rice mixture. Add salt and pepper, the chicken broth and one can of tomato sauce. Lower the heat and simmer, covered until the liquid is absorbed and the chicken and rice are tender, about 20 minutes or so. Add the other can of tomato sauce and black olives and allow them to heat through a minute or so. Place chicken pieces on one side of the serving platter and mound the rice on the other side. Serves 4.

## Artichoke and Mushroom Chicken

Use thick skinless boneless chicken thighs or breasts to make this stove-top dish. If using thinner meat, shorten the cooking time or it will be overcooked.

6 thick boneless, skinless chicken thighs or breasts
Fine white rice flour to dip chicken in
Salt, Pepper and Garlic Powder
2 to 3 Tablespoons of oil (I use olive oil)
1 small can of mushrooms, drained or 1 (8 to 10 ounce) package of sliced fresh mushrooms, rinsed

1 (12 to 14 ounce) can or jar of artichoke hearts, drained (check ingredients)
2 to 4 Tablespoons dry Marsala wine
1 to 2 Tablespoons lemon juice (I use bottled)
Thin sliced gluten-free Swiss cheese
1 Tablespoon fine white rice flour to thicken sauce

Dip the chicken in the rice flour. Sprinkle with salt, pepper and garlic. Heat a large skillet with a lid a minute. Add the oil and swirl it around. Add the chicken and brown it on one side, about 3 minutes or so. Turn it over. Brown the chicken about 3 minutes. Add the rest of the ingredients. I like a stronger flavored sauce, so I use 4 Tablespoons Marsala and 2 Tablespoons lemon juice. Cover and simmer for 10 to 15 minutes until chicken is done. I cut a piece of chicken to check that it is no longer pink inside.

If the sauce is too thin, sprinkle some rice flour into the sauce and stir in. I use about 1 Tablespoon. Allow it to bubble and thicken. Top each chicken piece with a thin slice of cheese. Put the lid on the pot. Remove from heat. Allow to sit a minute or two until the cheese melts.

This is nice served with rice or mashed potatoes.

## Barbecue Chicken
I microwave chicken before grilling it so that it not only cooks faster, but so that the center is done.

Our favorite way to cook chicken is on the grill. Take cleaned chicken parts (with bones) and put them in a microwave safe dish. (I use a deep-dish pie pan or deep/flat casserole for this.) Microwave it on high power for 10 minutes. This will ensure that your chicken gets cooked near the bone. Now bring them out to your barbecue grill (be careful of any hot meat juices in pan), and grill on high heat. Brush with our favorite barbecue sauce (see index). Grill until done. Delicious!

## Baked Chicken
This is my Mom's recipe that I converted to gluten-free. It is a family favorite.

Chicken pieces with bones and skin (the thighs are my favorite, but drumsticks and breasts are good this way too.)
Garlic powder

Salt and Pepper
Gluten-Free Naturals™ All Purpose Flour
Gluten-Free Cooking Spray

Sprinkle garlic powder, salt and pepper on chicken. Dip chicken into the Flour to coat it on both sides. (I put the Flour on a piece of waxed paper, so there is no dish to clean.)

Line a pan (at least 1 inch deep) with aluminum foil for easy clean-up. (I use a glass or aluminum pan.) Spray foil with a little cooking spray. Place chicken pieces skin-side up in pan. Spray tops of chicken with a little cooking spray so that the tops are no longer powdery. Bake at 350°F for 1 hour. If desired, put some washed and pierced potatoes in the oven on the rack at the same time, so you will have hot chicken and baked potatoes. Both need to cook 1 hour. I serve this with a green vegetable for a complete meal.

*Variation*: If desired, you can make a nice gravy from the pan juices. Pour the juices into a measuring cup that separates the fat from the broth. Put a little rice flour (I use about a Tablespoon) in a pot. Pour in the juices (not the fat) and mix the rice flour in using a whisk. Cook on medium heat until it bubbles and thickens, stirring occasionally to make sure it doesn't stick at the bottom. Your gravy will have nice flavor from the chicken and the spices sprinkled on it. I find you don't need to add anything to it.

*Variation 2*: For crispier skin on the chicken, put the chicken under the broiler to brown it first. Watch carefully so it doesn't burn. Then bake the chicken for about 45 minutes at 350°F, until done.

## Barbecue Fruited Chicken
**This is my Grandmother's recipe. For smaller quantities of chicken, make half the recipe.**

5 to 6 lbs. chicken pieces
6 Tablespoons gluten-free barbecue sauce
  (see index for recipe)

6 Tablespoons peach or apricot preserves
  or orange marmalade

Place chicken in a single layer on a baking dish. Bake 45 minutes in a 350°F oven. Remove from oven and pour off drippings and save to use in soup. Melt preserve and barbecue sauce together and mix well. Spoon some sauce over each piece of chicken being sure to cover completely. Bake an additional 15-20 minutes or until glazed.

## Chicken A La King
**This is my Mother's recipe, which I adapted to make it gluten-free.**

3 Tablespoons chicken fat or butter
¼ lb. sliced fresh mushrooms
⅓ green pepper, cut into thin strips
3 to 4 Tablespoons fine white rice flour or
  sweet rice flour (depending how thick
  you like your sauce)
1 ⅓ cup half and half or evaporated milk

1 ⅓ cup chicken broth
2 cups diced cooked chicken
½ cup pimiento or roasted red pepper, cut
  into strips (optional)
Salt and ground black pepper to taste

Melt the fat in a saucepan and add mushrooms and green pepper strips. Cover and simmer over low heat 5 minutes. Remove vegetables and set aside. Turn off heat. Pour in ⅓ cup of the milk and add the rice flour and blend. Add the rest of the milk and whisk together. Add the broth. Return to heat and cook while stirring until sauce thickens. Add the chicken and all of the vegetables; reduce the heat and cook only until chicken is nice and hot. Now add the salt and pepper to taste. Serve over rice or gluten-free waffles (see index).

## Chicken A La King – Easier version
**This is my version. It is easier to make and doesn't use cream.**

2 cups plus ⅔ cups milk
3 to 4 Tablespoons fine white rice flour or
  sweet rice flour (depending how thick
  you like your sauce)
1 teaspoon gluten-free chicken base* or
  gluten-free bouillon cube*
2 cups diced cooked chicken

½ cup pimiento or roasted red pepper, cut
  into strips (optional)
⅓ to ½ cup frozen peas
1 can mushrooms, drained but liquid set
  aside
Salt and ground black pepper to taste

Pour in ⅓ cup of the milk and add the rice flour and blend using a whisk. Add the rest of the milk and whisk together. Add the chicken base. Return to heat and cook while stirring until sauce thickens. Add the frozen peas and heat until they thaw. Add the chicken and mushrooms, reduce heat and cook only until chicken is nice and hot. If sauce is too thick, add some of the mushroom water. Now add the salt and pepper to taste. Serve over rice or gluten-free waffles (see index).

*see gluten-free products list at the end of the book

## Chicken Cacciatore

I find this easy to make. You can change the flavor according to your preferences. You can leave the skin on the chicken, but it will be a fattier dish. Or, you can purchase the chicken without the skin.

1 large package chicken thighs with bone,
 skin removed
Rice flour
Salt and ground black pepper
Garlic powder
Oil
1 large Spanish onion, diced, (optional)
Sliced black olives (optional)
1 can mushrooms drained (optional)

1 jar gluten-free tomato sauce (I use
 Classico® four cheese tomato sauce or
 Francesco Rinaldi® three cheese tomato
 sauce, which are both gluten-free as of
 this writing)
½ cup dry wine (I use dry Vermouth) or
 water – add more if sauce is too thick

Remove skin from chicken and dip in rice flour. Sprinkle with salt, pepper and garlic powder. Heat a small amount oil for a moment in a large 12" fryer pan. Add chicken and brown it on 1 side. Turn chicken over. Brown it a few moments on the other side. Add diced onions and mushrooms if desired. Add tomato sauce and wine. Cover, reduce heat and let simmer 20 minutes until chicken is done. Serve with gluten-free spaghetti or rice.

*Variation*: Frozen peas or diced green peppers may be added with the other vegetables.

*Variation 2*: If using boneless chicken thighs, shorten the cooking time. They may cook as quickly as 10 or 15 minutes. Check for doneness.

*Variation 3*: Oven method with brown rice. Prepare 1 cup brown rice according to package directions (2 cups cooked) or use leftover rice. Grease casserole. Mix onions, olives and mushrooms into rice. Line the bottom of casserole with rice mixture. Top with raw chicken. Pour sauce mixed with wine over all. Bake 1 hour. Check after 30 minutes and if top of chicken is getting too dry cover pan with foil.

## Chicken and Carrots

My grandmother invented this dish, and I converted it to be gluten-free. It's a chicken stew that is faster to make than a of beef stew.

6 Tablespoons fine white rice flour
Garlic powder, salt and ground black
 pepper
4 chicken breasts with bone (remove small
 bones)
Oil

1 ¾ cups water
Salt and ground black pepper
4 or 5 carrots, scraped (peeled) and
 chopped
Frozen peas (optional)

Dredge the chicken in the rice flour. Sprinkle with garlic powder, salt and pepper. Brown them in the oil on both sides. Mix the flour you didn't use in with the water and add. Add the salt and pepper and the carrots. Cover and cook 20 minutes. If you want to add the peas, add them 5 minutes before the end of cooking time. Serve over rice.

*\*see gluten-free products list at the end of the book*

*Variation 1*: Frozen sliced carrots may be used instead of raw carrots. Add them according to package directions cooking time.

*Variation 2*: If your chicken is not very flavorful, a little bouillon may be added, but use it sparingly as it can make the dish too salty.

## Chicken Livers with Vinegar

My mother grew up during the Depression and didn't believe in throwing away food. She would save the chicken livers (they often come in the neck cavity of a whole chicken) and freeze them until she had enough to make this dish. For some people, chicken livers may be an acquired taste.

½ lb. chicken livers
1 large Spanish onion
¼ cup cider vinegar

Salt and ground black pepper
Oil

Slice the onion and sauté in a little oil. Add livers and sauté just until they firm up a little. Pour the vinegar over top and sprinkle with salt and pepper. Cover and simmer a few minutes or until the vinegar almost evaporates and the livers are thoroughly cooked.

Whenever you buy chickens, take the livers and place in a jar that will hold enough for a meal for your family and freeze. When the jar is full, thaw and prepare. It's like getting a free meal. My mother also liked chicken livers threaded on a skewer with a slice of bacon intertwined with them, then broiled a few minutes on each side.

## Chicken Marsala

This is a wonderful company dish. I like this version better than what I've ordered in a restaurant. My brother-in-law gave us the original recipe and my mother helped me convert it. My husband often prepares this dish to bring to weddings, parties, and work-related dinners when he knows he needs to bring a gluten-free entree. It reheats well in the microwave.

¼ cup butter or olive oil
2 cloves of garlic, chopped or garlic
  powder
1 lb. chicken breast, boneless
Tapioca starch or tapioca flour or fine
  white rice flour for dusting chicken
Salt and pepper

¼ lb. Swiss cheese (I use gluten-free,
  packaged pre-sliced cheese to avoid
  possible contamination from the deli-
  slicing machine.)
1 cup canned mushrooms (or I use 1
  package sliced fresh mushrooms)
Dash of parsley
1 cup Marsala wine

Pound the chicken breasts flat (about ¼ inch thick). Dredge in tapioca starch or rice flour. Sprinkle with salt and pepper. Melt the butter in a sauté pan (or use olive oil) and add the garlic. (If you do not have garlic, sprinkle the chicken with garlic powder.) Add the chicken breasts and brown on both sides over medium heat. Add the mushrooms and Marsala. Raise the heat to high and reduce the Marsala until slightly thickened. (If sauce is too thin, sprinkle in a little rice flour in the sauce, mix in, and allow the sauce to bubble and thicken.)

Put a slice of Swiss cheese over each chicken breast. Cover pan just long enough to melt the cheese. Remove from heat and sprinkle breasts with parsley. Serves 2 to 3. Good served with rice.

Note: Tapioca starch makes the chicken seem more tender in texture. However, it does not freeze well so if you plan to freeze this dish use the rice flour. Rice flour also works well and thickens the sauce a little better than the tapioca starch. The choice is yours.

*Variation*: If you don't have Marsala wine you can substitute dry Vermouth. It's good but with a different flavor. When I'm serving a crowd, I double or triple the recipe and cut the chicken into bite size pieces before cooking them. They cook faster that way. Then I complete the recipe except for adding the cheese. Then I put the meat and sauce in a large oval or oblong casserole dish. I cover with cheese, and cover the casserole dish. You can reheat it in the oven and have a gourmet make-ahead company dish.

## Chicken Nuggets
I make these frequently. I often serve them for company and everyone enjoys them.

4 chicken breasts
½ cup corn flour
2 teaspoons McCormick's Season-All® Seasoned Salt (as of this writing it is gluten-free)

½ teaspoon dry oregano
Generous sprinkling of garlic powder (optional)
Milk
Oil for pan frying

On a piece of waxed paper, mix together the flour, Season-All® and oregano. Cut the chicken into bite-sized pieces using a poultry scissor or a sharp knife. Dip the chicken nuggets in milk and then coat them in the dry mixture. In a wok or 12" fry pan, heat the pan with some oil. Add the chicken and brown it, turning it to brown all sides. Make sure it is cooked through. Drain on paper towels to remove any excess oil. Serve.

*Variation*: Try dipping the cooked nuggets in some of our favorite barbecue sauce (see index), honey or gluten-free salad dressing of your choice (but they are also good plain!) Children like the bite-sized nuggets. You may want to use half the Season-All® for very young children if they like bland flavors. The 10 and 12-year olds I served it to liked it as written. So did the adults.

*Variation* 2: Gluten-Free Naturals™ All Purpose Flour or Gluten-Free Naturals™ Cookie Flour Blend may be used in place of the corn flour. No need to dip the nuggets in milk, since it adheres to the chicken better than the corn flour.

## Chicken Parmesan – Oven Method with Cheese Coating

This is quick and easy, and can be made in 20 minutes. The cheese gives a delicious, flavorful gluten-free coating that keeps the chicken moist. If your cheese is extra salty, use less salt.

½ cup gluten-free grated Parmesan cheese*

½ to 1 teaspoon salt (I use less salt if breasts are thin and more if they are thick)

1 teaspoon sugar

1 teaspoon garlic powder

1 teaspoon dried basil

1 teaspoon oregano

¼ teaspoon gluten-free dried mustard*

⅛ teaspoon pepper

2 teaspoons egg white powder (optional)

2 pounds of boneless chicken breasts (about 6 chicken breast halves)

Milk or water to dip cutlets

On a large piece of waxed paper, blend cheese, spices, and egg white powder.

Use chicken breast halves. Dip in milk or water and dip in cheese mixture. Press evenly to coat. Place in a shallow ungreased baking pan. Bake at 400°F for 20 to 25 minutes.

*Variation*: Use this coating for tilapia fish. Rinse fish and dip in the cheese mixture. Place on a non-stick pan. Bake at 375°F for 15 minutes.

Note: My mother always took the leftover egg and poured in the leftover crumbs and mixed them together. She formed what she called "Patty Cakes". If you have a lot of egg, then add more crumbs to form one or two patties. They were about 1 ½ to 2 inches wide by ½ inch high. Bake the Patty Cakes in the same pan along with the chicken. They will be flavorful because of the crumbs and cheese. As children we all wanted to eat them and some of my siblings liked them better than the chicken! I still make them and enjoy them. Since this was just a way to use the leftover ingredients up, Mom would cut them and we'd share them so we'd each get a piece.

## Chicken Parmesan – Oven Method with Crumbs

This is quick and easy, and can be made in 20 minutes. I often use a glass pan and can reduce the oven temperature by 5 degrees. This has a lot less fat than the stove type version, and it keeps your stove clean. I often like to just sprinkle in spices to make the bread crumb mixture, but if you prefer an exact recipe to make bread crumbs using crackers and cheese, see index.

1 to 1 ½ pounds of chicken cutlets

1 to 2 eggs

1 to 2 Tablespoons olive oil

8 Tablespoons dried bread crumbs made with Gluten-Free Naturals™ Bread or crushed gluten-free crackers (I use 3 Ener-G® low protein crackers [like saltines] and pulverize them in the food processor)

Generous sprinklings of spices like garlic, oregano, basil, salt and ground black

pepper. (Do not use too much salt if using crackers since crackers are salty.) Or see recipe for Italian bread crumbs (see index)

3 Tablespoons grated Parmesan or Pecorino Romano cheese (I prefer Romano or combination)

3 ounces shredded gluten-free mozzarella cheese (optional)

Gluten-free tomato sauce (optional)

*see gluten-free products list at the end of the book

In a food processor, pulverize the crackers.  On a piece of waxed paper, combine the gluten-free cracker crumbs, spices, and cheese.

With a fork, whip the egg and oil in a shallow plate or pie pan.  I usually find 1 egg and 1 Tablespoon oil enough to cover all the cutlets, but sometimes with smaller cutlets you may need more since there is more surface area to cover.  I suggest starting with one egg and making more only if needed.

Separate the cutlets.  Dip the cutlets in the egg mixture and then coat with the crumb mixture.  Arrange on a shallow non-stick baking dish or cookie sheet.  Bake at 450°F for 20 minutes.

(If using tomato sauce and/or mozzarella cheese, bake chicken 15 minutes, top with sauce and/or mozzarella cheese and bake for 5 minutes more or until cheese melts.)

*Variation:*  Cornflake crumbs may be used instead of crackers.  Add the spices and a sprinkling of salt since the cornflakes are not salty like the crackers.

## Chicken or Veal Parmesan – Stovetop method
This is more like traditional chicken/veal parmesan in its preparation.

Boneless, skinless chicken breasts or veal cutlets (if cutlets are too thick I pound them to make them thinner)
Gluten-Free Naturals™ Cake Blend or Cookie Blend mixed with spices (see recipe for bread crumbs) or dried bread crumbs made with Gluten-Free Naturals™ bread
1 egg plus 1 Tablespoon water
2 to 4 Tablespoons oil (I use olive oil)
Gluten-free tomato sauce
Sliced gluten-free Mozzarella cheese

Place a sheet of waxed paper on the counter.  Put a little of the Gluten-Free Naturals™ Cookie Blend mixture with the spices on the waxed paper.  Take a shallow bowl or pie pan and blend the egg and water in the pan.  Dip chicken in egg mixture on both sides.  Drip off the excess and then dip in the flour mixture and completely cover both sides.  I set aside the coated pieces on another piece of waxed paper.  When all pieces are coated, heat a skillet, add oil and heat a little longer.  Fry meat until golden brown.  Meat should be cooked through.  Place meat on a lightly sauced baking pan.  Place a little tomato sauce over each cutlet and then top with a slice of mozzarella cheese.  Place in a 350°F oven for 15 minutes or until meat is heated through and the cheese melts.

Note:  This flour blend works well when pan fried, but not for Chicken Parmesan Oven-Method.

*Variation:*  Gluten-free cracker crumbs may also be used.  See recipe for bread crumbs using crackers.

*Variation 2:*  To avoid the baking step, I heat the sauce in the microwave.  Place chicken on a plate or microwave safe container.  Top the chicken with the sauce, top with cheese, and

*see gluten-free products list at the end of the book

microwave only until cheese melts. It may be 20 seconds since chicken is hot. Do not overcook. This saves 15 minutes of baking time. I do this when I am in a hurry to get dinner on the table, or to avoid using the oven on a hot day. The baking method is better if you have the time.

## Chicken, Peas and Mushrooms

I think my grandmother may have invented the original recipe. I converted it to gluten-free and added the Season-All® seasoning instead of salt. I like the fact that you can make it in one pot.

4 boneless, skinless chicken breasts
½ cup Gluten-Free Naturals™ All
   Purpose Flour
1 to 2 teaspoons Season-All® Salt* or
   sprinklings of salt, ground black pepper,
   garlic powder and gluten-free spices of
   your choice, or see recipe for bread
   crumbs

¼ teaspoon oregano
Milk
1 medium Spanish onion, sliced
1 can green peas
¼ pound mushrooms, sliced (or you may
   substitute a can, drained)

Cut each chicken breast into 4 or 5 pieces. (I use a poultry scissors to do this.) Place one sheet of waxed paper on the counter. Mix the Flour, seasoned salt, and oregano on the waxed paper. Pour a little bit of milk into a pie pan. Dip the chicken in the milk and then the flour mixture and evenly coat the chicken. Heat a skillet, add a little oil and heat another minute. Then sauté the chicken until it is golden brown on all sides. Remove and drain on paper towels. Wipe out the skillet with a paper towel to remove any flour that may have settled on the bottom. Add a little more oil to the skillet and cook the onions until golden yellow and soft. Add the sliced mushrooms and cook a few minutes. Drain all but ¼ cup of liquid from peas. Add the peas plus the ¼ cup liquid to the pan. Top with chicken, cover and cook just until all is heated through. Check seasonings; adding a little salt and pepper, toss and serve. It is very nice served with mashed potatoes.

*Variations*: You may add garlic with the onions, if you like garlic. You may also top the chicken with grated mozzarella cheese if desired. It will melt when you heat it through. If you have some leftover ham or crumbled bacon, you can add that in with the peas.

*Variation 2*: Make chicken as directed in the chicken parmesan recipe. Meanwhile, in a skillet, cook the onions, peas and mushrooms. Set aside. When chicken parmesan comes out of the oven, place cutlets on warmed vegetables, bring to the table and serve.

## Chicken Pizzaiola

This gives off the aroma of pizza baking in the oven. This is my grandmother's recipe.

1 cut up fryer, cut into 8 pieces
4 medium potatoes, cut into eighths
2 medium onions, cut into chunks
1 large can peeled tomatoes*, most are
   gluten-free but check labels

Salt
Ground black pepper
Garlic powder
Oregano
Oil

*see gluten-free products list at the end of the book

Pour a few Tablespoons of oil in a baking dish.  Roll the chicken in the oil to cover all pieces.  Placing the chicken skin side down, sprinkle with salt, pepper and garlic powder.  Turn chicken skin side up and tuck chunks of onion and potatoes between pieces of chicken.  Sprinkle all with more salt, pepper and garlic powder.  Drizzle more oil over vegetables and roast in a 350°F oven for ½ hour.  Remove from oven and turn potatoes over to cook evenly, then open can of tomatoes.  Crush the tomatoes slightly by hand and pour over whole dish.  Sprinkle generously with oregano using about 4 pinches.  Return to oven and cook another ½ hour longer or until the potatoes are cooked and part of chicken and potatoes are dark brown.  A simple salad or green vegetable rounds out the meal.  Serves 4.

## Chicken Ravello

The combination of flavors works well together.  Do not eliminate the salt pork or this will not taste good.  You can substitute bacon for the salt pork.

6 whole chicken legs without backbones
1 ½ to 2 oz. gluten-free salt pork,
    chopped (or gluten-free bacon*)
2 Tablespoons olive oil
Dash or 2 of ground black pepper

½ cup Marsala wine
30 button mushrooms
10 oz. package frozen peas
2 medium onions, chopped

Skin the chicken legs and set aside.  Heat skillet, add oil, then salt pork and onions. Sauté slowly until lightly browned.  Push onions and pork aside and add legs to skillet, browning them on both sides.  Distribute the onion mixture over chicken; add the black pepper and wine.  Cover and simmer over low heat 20 minutes.  Add the mushrooms and peas to the skillet.  Cook covered another 10 minutes then only partially cover pot while simmering a little longer to reduce sauce.  Serve with mashed or baked potatoes and a tomato salad.

## Chicken with Wild Rice Stuffing

This is a gourmet stuffing with dried cranberries.  This stuffing is also nice in roasted chicken.

1 cup brown rice
½ cup wild rice, rinsed
2 Tablespoons dried minced onion
¼ cup dried cranberries (Ocean Spray® is
    gluten-free as of this writing)
½ teaspoon salt

3 ½ cups hot water
6 boneless, skinless chicken breast halves,
    use thick chicken breasts
1 egg white (or beaten whole egg may be
    used)
Chopped Pecans

Put brown rice, rinsed wild rice, minced onion, dried cranberries, salt and water in a pot.  Bring to a boil.  Cover and simmer for 45 minutes.  All of the water should be absorbed.  Uncover and stir.

Carefully cut chicken breasts horizontally in the thick part of the meat, to create a pocket for the stuffing.  Do not cut all the way through the meat.  Dip one side in the egg white and then the pecans.  Set chicken breasts in a greased baking pan with the pecan side on top.  Carefully lift the top of each piece of chicken and fill with stuffing.  Put any remaining

*see gluten-free products list at the end of the book

stuffing around the chicken pieces. Top chicken with additional pecans, if desired. Bake at 350°F for 30 minutes or until chicken is done.

*Variation*: To save time, don't stuff the breasts. Instead put the rice mixture in the greased pan. Coat chicken with chopped pecans and place over rice. Bake at 375°F for 15 to 20 minutes until done. I think the chicken turns out a little moister at the lower temperature, but this is much faster to put together.

*Variation 2*: You can use dried apricots instead of cranberries. Just be sure they are gluten-free.

*Variation 3*: To make this nut free, eliminate pecans. Coat the chicken with fresh bread crumbs by taking 2 slices of Gluten-Free Naturals™ bread and putting in a food processor until pulverized. Coat the chicken in egg and crumbs.

## Chinese Chicken and Broccoli
Chinese food is excellent on the gluten-free diet. Just make sure you use gluten-free soy sauce. Most Chinese and Japanese restaurants use soy sauce that contains wheat.

2 whole skinless, boneless chicken breasts, sliced in ⅛ inch slices
1 Tablespoon gluten-free soy sauce*
1 Tablespoon sherry
1 Tablespoon cornstarch
Oil, for stir frying
Generous dash of garlic powder
1 cup chopped onions (optional) or use chopped frozen onion

1 20 ounce package of frozen broccoli (chopped or spears may be used)
1 cup chopped celery (optional)
1 cup gluten-free chicken broth* (or 1 cup water plus 1 teaspoon gluten-free chicken base*)
2 Tablespoons cornstarch (or 1 Tablespoon for a thinner sauce)
1 Tablespoon gluten-free soy sauce*

Slice chicken breasts. (I use poultry scissors.) Mix first 5 ingredients together in a small bowl and marinate the meat several minutes. Meanwhile, cook all of the vegetables in a wok in 1 Tablespoon oil until crisp-tender. Sprinkle with garlic powder. Remove vegetables from the pan. Cook chicken mixture adding additional oil as needed. When done, mix the chicken with the vegetables in the wok. Mix chicken broth, 1 Tablespoon soy sauce and cornstarch in a bowl or liquid measuring cup. Add to pan and cook until the cornstarch mixture bubbles and thickens. Serve over rice. Makes 4 large servings.

*Variation*: You can add a can of drained mushrooms when you add the sauce ingredients.

## Chinese Chicken with Cashews, Microwave Version

*An easy recipe from my sister, that works best in a microwave that has medium power. If you have a high wattage microwave, I recommend you follow my stove version directions below. In some microwaves the oil can get too hot and spatter on you, so use caution and don't risk it if you're not sure about your microwave. (Note: In some high wattage microwaves you may want to cook the chicken breasts whole and then cut them into cubes after cooking. This helps prevent overcooking the meat.)*

3 Tablespoons oil
2 large skinless, boneless chicken breasts
   cut into ¾ inch cubes
¼ teaspoon garlic powder
2 Tablespoons gluten-free soy sauce*
1 Tablespoon sherry
1 Tablespoon cornstarch
¼ teaspoon ground ginger

¼ teaspoon salt (I eliminate if using salted
   nuts)
1 green pepper cut into ¾ inch cubes
1 onion diced (optional)
⅔ cup cashews, halved (or peanuts may be
   used)

Pour oil into a 4 ½ or 5 inch deep casserole dish (one that has a cover). Heat the oil uncovered in the microwave for 4 minutes on medium. Meanwhile, combine the chicken breasts, garlic, soy sauce, sherry, cornstarch, ginger and salt to marinade them. Carefully add to oil (caution it may spatter). Cook covered for 4 minutes in the microwave and stir twice. Cut pepper and onion while chicken is cooking. Add green pepper, onion, cashews and any remaining marinade. Cook covered for 4 to 5 minutes, stirring twice. Let stand 2-3 minutes. Check to be sure that the chicken is cooked through. If not, cook it longer a minute at a time and stir. This is nice served over rice.

*Variation*: For a stovetop version: Combine chicken breasts, garlic, soy sauce, sherry, cornstarch, ginger and salt. Let chicken marinate about 5 minutes. Heat a skillet for a minute or two. Pour oil into skillet. Heat the oil a few minutes only, and do not make it too hot. (Heating the oil first helps prevent the meat from sticking, especially if you have a pan without a non-stick coating.) Carefully add the chicken and stir fry until chicken is almost done. Add the green pepper, onion, cashews, and any leftover marinade. Stir fry about 5 minutes or so more until chicken is done and vegetables are cooked.

## Chinese Chicken with Peanuts

*Another delicious Chinese dish.*

2 whole skinless, boneless chicken breasts,
   sliced in ⅛ inch slices
1 Tablespoon gluten-free soy sauce*
1 Tablespoon sherry
1 Tablespoon cornstarch
Oil, for stir frying
Generous dash of garlic powder
1 cup chopped onions or use chopped
   frozen onions
Chopped scallions (optional)
1 package of frozen snow peas, thawed

1 cup chopped celery (optional)
½ cup orange juice
1 cup gluten-free chicken broth* (or ½
   cup water plus ½ teaspoon gluten-free
   chicken base*)
1 Tablespoon gluten-free soy sauce* (use
   less if peanuts are salted.)
¼ teaspoon ground ginger
2 Tablespoons cornstarch (or 1
   Tablespoon for a thinner sauce)
½ cup peanuts (not dry roasted)

*\*see gluten-free products list at the end of the book*

Slice chicken breasts. (I use poultry scissors.) Mix first 5 ingredients together in a small bowl and marinate the meat several minutes. Meanwhile, cook all of the vegetables in a wok in 1 Tablespoon oil until crisp-tender. Sprinkle with garlic powder. Remove vegetables from the pan. Cook chicken mixture adding additional oil as needed. When done, mix the chicken with the vegetables in the wok. Mix the orange juice, chicken broth, 1 Tablespoon soy sauce, ginger and cornstarch. Add to pan and cook until the cornstarch mixture bubbles and thickens. Add the peanuts. Serve over rice. Makes 4 large servings.

*Variation*: You can add a can of drained mushrooms when you add the sauce ingredients.

*Variation 2*: For a spicy dish, add a sprinkling of cayenne pepper or red pepper flakes when browning the chicken.

## Chinese Pepper Chicken and Walnuts
This is a very spicy recipe from my aunt. I use a pinch of crushed red pepper and use only ¼ teaspoon ginger for a milder taste.

3 Tablespoons gluten-free soy sauce*
1 Tablespoon cornstarch
2 large chicken breasts (skinned, boned and cut into about ½ inch cubes)
2 teaspoons sugar
1 teaspoon wine vinegar
¼ cup oil

1 teaspoon crushed red pepper (I use a pinch or ¼ teaspoon at most)
⅓ cup sliced scallions or chopped onions
½ teaspoon ground ginger (I use ¼ teaspoon or less)
½ cup walnut halves (or more if desired)

Blend 1 Tablespoon of the soy sauce and cornstarch in a bowl. Mix in the chicken cubes and set aside. Combine the remaining 2 Tablespoons of soy sauce, the sugar and the vinegar in a small bowl. Set aside.

In a wok or a chicken fryer, heat oil over moderately high heat. Add the red pepper and cook until it darkens (turns black). Add chicken and stir fry 2 minutes. Remove chicken with slotted spoon and set aside. In the same oil, stir-fry the scallions 1 minute (or longer if using onions). Return chicken to pan and cook 2 minutes more, stirring constantly. Add soy mixture, mix in walnuts and heat thoroughly.

Serve with hot cooked rice and a stir-fried green vegetable such as broccoli. Serves 2 to 3.

It's easier and faster to get neat chicken cubes if the breasts are cut while partially frozen. I also find that using a pair of poultry shears is a big timesaver.

## Chutney Chicken

If you have made the chutney recipe (see index), this is a good recipe to use it up.  This is nice served over brown rice.

4 boneless, skinless chicken breast halves (about ¼ pound each)
Fine white rice flour or tapioca starch or tapioca flour
2 Tablespoons oil (I use olive oil)
¾ cups gluten-free chutney (see index for recipes for Nectarine/Peach Chutney or Red Pepper Chutney)
½ cup dry white wine or chicken broth*

¼ cup water (or use a little less if your Peach Chutney has a lot of juice)
2 cloves garlic, minced or ¼ teaspoon garlic powder
½ teaspoon salt
½ teaspoon gluten-free curry powder*
Chopped or slivered almonds for garnish (optional)

Coat chicken lightly with the fine white rice flour or tapioca starch.  (I prefer the tapioca starch in this recipe.)  Heat the oil in a skillet.  Add the chicken and cook on each side until lightly browned (or golden in color if using tapioca starch).  Turn chicken over.  Combine the rest of the ingredients (except almonds) and pour over the chicken.  Cover, reduce heat to simmer and cook for about 20 minutes, stirring occasionally, until chicken is about done.  If sauce is thin, you can sprinkle in a little more fine white rice flour or tapioca starch to the sauce and mix it in.  Allow to boil and thicken.  Remove from heat.  Check to be sure that the chicken is done and no longer pink.  Garnish with almonds, if desired.  Serve over rice with the sauce.

## Cornflake Crumb Baked Chicken or Potato Chip Baked Chicken

This recipe makes a wonderful coating for chicken or pork chops.  We like it better than the "Shake 'n Bake®" type mixes that contain gluten.  If you don't want a dipping sauce, make half of the mayonnaise, mustard and Parmesan cheese mixture.

4 chicken breast cutlets
½ cup gluten-free mayonnaise*
1 ½ Tablespoons prepared gluten-free mustard*

¼ cup grated Parmesan cheese
1 cup gluten-free cornflakes*, crushed into crumbs

Make cornflake crumbs by putting the cornflakes in a heavy-duty freezer bag, remove air and seal.  Crush with a rolling pin.  (My local grocery store carries gluten-free cornflake crumbs so I can eliminate this step.)

Make the sauce by combining mayonnaise, mustard and Parmesan cheese.  Set half of this mixture aside.  (I remove half of the mixture to another bowl, to be sure not to contaminate it with raw chicken, since it will be used later as a dipping sauce.)

Brush both sides of chicken with the other half of sauce mixture.  (I sometimes dip the chicken in it and use my hands to coat.)  Then coat the chicken well with the cornflake crumbs.  Place in a lightly greased baking dish and bake at 400°F for approximately 20-25 minutes or until golden brown.  Use the remaining mayonnaise sauce you set aside for dipping.

*see gluten-free products list at the end of the book*

*Variation*: The cornflake crumbs are wonderful on Pork Chops. Make half the mayonnaise mixture, and eliminate the dipping sauce. It's very good without the extra sauce. Baking times can vary depending how thick the pork chops are. Test for doneness by cutting with a knife to be sure cutlets are no longer pink inside.

*Variation 2*: My mother prepares a mixture of ½ cup gluten-free mayonnaise*, ⅓ cup grated cheese and ½ teaspoon garlic powder instead of the mixture above. She spreads it on boneless/skinless chicken breasts with a knife. Then she either dips it in gluten-free cornflake crumbs* or other gluten-free crumbs (see index for bread crumb recipe). Her method is to spread the mixture on one side and dip it in the crumbs, and then spread the mixture on the other side and turn it over in the crumbs. She bakes at 350°F for 30 minutes because the cutlets she uses are not too thick. Test for doneness by cutting with a knife to be sure cutlets are no longer pink inside.

*Variation 3*: Crushed gluten-free potato chips* may be used instead of cornflake crumbs. For Honey Mustard/Potato Chip chicken: use ½ cup mayonnaise, 1 Tablespoon of Dijon mustard*, and 2 Tablespoons of honey. Use the same method as above but dip them in crushed potato chips. If you cut the chicken into strips first, you can bake it at 425°F for about 10-12 minutes. You may need to make additional mayonnaise mixture and crumbs if making chicken strips. I prefer the chicken with the first recipe and the cornflake crumbs, but this is nice for a change. Don't use the parmesan cheese mixture with the potato chips or it will be too salty.

*Variation 4*: Corn Chex® recently became gluten-free. You can pulverize them to use as crumbs, but we think the cornflakes are better in this recipe.

## Country Captain
This is one of my favorite dishes. It's good with or without the raisins and almonds.

8 pieces of chicken, skinned (we prefer chicken thighs without the backs)
Salt and ground black pepper
Gluten-free flour such fine white rice flour, tapioca starch or tapioca flour, cornstarch or brown rice flour
1 chopped onion
1 seeded and chopped green pepper
1 minced clove of garlic or ¼ teaspoon granulated garlic
Oil

½ teaspoon salt
Ground black pepper
1 teaspoon gluten-free curry powder* (or see index for curry powder recipe)
1 (15 oz) can gluten-free tomato sauce* or 2 (8 oz.) cans
Tiny pinch of oregano (optional)
¼ cup raisins (optional)
¼ cup slivered almonds (optional)

Sprinkle chicken with salt and pepper. Roll the chicken in the gluten-free flour to coat. Heat a large skillet a few minutes. (Use a skillet that has a cover.) Add 1 to 2 Tablespoons of oil and heat a minute. (This prevents the chicken from sticking.) Add floured chicken and brown it on one side. Turn chicken over and add vegetables. Continue to sauté until second side of chicken has browned lightly. Add curry to pan and blend into oil and remove

*see gluten-free products list at the end of the book*

from heat. (Adding the curry to the oil will better release its flavor.) Add tomato sauce, salt and a few dashes of black pepper. The oregano, raisins and almonds can be added at this time. Bring sauce to a boil, reduce heat, cover and simmer 20-30 minutes. Serve with rice.

*Variation:* As children, my siblings didn't like the oregano, raisins and nuts in this dish, so my mother eliminated those ingredients. Sometimes she would make a rice pilaf by cooking the rice in gluten-free chicken broth* and adding the raisins and nuts to the rice.

*Variation 2:* Skinless boneless chicken thighs may be used. Cook about 10-15 minutes instead of 20-30 minutes. Check the center for doneness. Some skinless boneless thighs are thicker than others and times may vary.

## Fried Chicken
This is our favorite version, dipped in a batter. You will need a fryer and a baking pan with a rack to make this. (A cooling rack on top of a baking sheet will work.)

1 package of Chicken fryer parts (chicken with bones. I prefer legs and thighs but choose your favorites)
Sprinkling of salt, ground black pepper, and celery salt on chicken
Gluten-Free Naturals™ All Purpose Flour to dip chicken in
Batter:

1 cup Gluten-Free Naturals™ All Purpose Flour
1 teaspoon baking powder
1 teaspoon salt
½ cup milk
2 eggs
1 Tablespoon oil
Oil for frying

Sprinkle chicken with salt, pepper, and celery salt (if desired). Dip in flour. Make the batter with the gluten-free flour, baking powder, salt, milk, eggs and 1 Tablespoon oil.

Heat oil in a fryer until it gets to the right temperature for frying. I use a 12 inch frying pan with deep sides or a Fry Daddy® Fryer. For chicken, the oil temperature should be 375°F. Fry until golden brown on both sides.

Take a large pan. I use a 9 x 13 inch baking pan, or you can use a jelly roll pan. Line it with foil. Place a cooling rack over top. Take the chicken and place it on the rack. When you have all of your chicken cooked put it in the oven and bake it at 250°F for 2 ½ to 3 hours, until cooked through. The oil will drain from the chicken onto the foil. (Alternatively, you can bake at 350°F for 45 minutes to an hour. We prefer the slow cooking method but if you're in a rush the faster cooking works well.)

*see gluten-free products list at the end of the book

## Fried Chicken – Version 2

You will need a deep fryer and a baking pan with a rack to make this dish. We prefer the first version but this one is also good. You can eliminate the buttermilk and just coat the chicken in the flour mixture and fry it.

1 package of Chicken fryer parts (chicken with bones)
Gluten-Free Buttermilk* or gluten-free plain yogurt*
⅔ cup Gluten-Free Naturals™ All Purpose Flour
1 ½ teaspoons garlic powder

1 ½ teaspoons onion powder
1 teaspoon salt
Sprinkling of ground black pepper
Paprika
Oil

Heat oil in a fryer until it gets to the right temperature for frying. For chicken that would be 375°F. (I use a Fry Daddy® fryer.) Be careful that it does not overheat. Meanwhile combine the flour and spices on a piece of waxed paper. Dip the chicken in the buttermilk or yogurt and then coat them in the flour on the waxed paper. (Yogurt will yield a thicker coating. I prefer the buttermilk.) Fry until golden and drain on paper towels. Take a large pan and put a piece of foil on it. Take a rack and place it in a pan. Cook in the oven at 250°F for 2 ½ to 3 hours, until cooked through. The oil will drain from the chicken onto the foil. (Alternatively, you can bake at 350°F for 45 minutes to an hour. We prefer the slow cooking method but if you're in a rush the faster cooking works too.)

*Variation*: You can use skinless boneless chicken breasts, and eliminate the need to bake it afterwards. Since there are no bones, the chicken will cook through. Drain on paper towels to remove excess oil before serving. If you blot the chicken with paper towels, blot carefully because the oil is hot and can easily burn you.

*Variation 2*: Use the tempura recipe (see index) to coat chicken in a batter and fry. If using chicken parts that have bones, bake in the oven after you fry it the same method as above. If using skinless boneless chicken breasts or thighs, you will not have to bake it.

*Variation 3*: Use the batter fried fish recipe (see index) to coat chicken in a batter and fry. If using chicken parts that have bones, bake in the oven after you fry it the same method as above. If using skinless boneless chicken breasts or thighs, you will not have to bake it.

*Variation 4*: Gluten-Free Naturals™ Cookie Flour Blend may be used in place of Gluten-Free Naturals™ All Purpose Flour.

## Grilled Lime Cilantro Chicken

This recipe works well using either a stove top grill pan indoors or outside on a barbeque grill. Leftover chicken is good on a tossed salad. I like it served with or without the sauce.

4 to 6 boneless chicken breast halves
2 Tablespoons corn or canola oil
4 Tablespoons lime juice (preferably fresh)
2 teaspoons dried cilantro
Generous sprinklings of granulated garlic, salt and pepper

Sauce:
4 Tablespoons mayonnaise*
Sprinkling of hot pepper flakes
2 Tablespoons lime juice
Salt and pepper

Blend together the oil, 4 Tablespoons lime juice, and dried cilantro in a bowl. Add the chicken and coat on both sides with this mixture. Generously sprinkle with the garlic, salt and pepper. Marinate for an hour.

Blend sauce ingredients and refrigerate until ready to serve. Grill chicken until no longer pink in the center. When chicken is done, serve and pour some sauce over the top of each piece.

## Hawaiian Chicken

This recipe is from a Mother-Daughter Luncheon my mother and I attended when I was very young.

6-8 pieces of chicken
4 Tablespoons gluten-free soy sauce*
1 Tablespoon sugar
1 Tablespoon sherry*
½ teaspoon salt
½ teaspoon dried garlic or granulated garlic

1 teaspoon ground ginger
1 small can pineapple slices, un-drained and cut into pieces
1 cup liquid (chicken pan juices plus water to equal 1 cup)
1 Tablespoon cornstarch

Wash chicken and place in a foil lined pan. Bake in the oven at 350°F for 1 hour. When done, pour pan juices into a measuring cup and add enough water to make 1 cup of liquid. Keep chicken warm. Mix liquid and the rest of the ingredients together in a large saucepan. Bring to a boil. Add the chicken and simmer a few minutes.

*Variation*: Add cooked vegetables like carrots, celery, or green beans to make a more complete meal.

## Honey Baked Fruited Chicken

This makes a nice glazed coating. It is good the day you make it, because the chicken has a crispy skin. Leftovers are best reheated in the oven or the coating will be soggy. This dish can be made without the fruit.

3 lbs. chicken, cut up
2 to 3 Tablespoons butter or gluten-free
    margarine* or oil can be used
⅓ cup honey
2 Tablespoons gluten-free mustard*

1 teaspoon salt
1 teaspoon gluten-free curry powder*
Canned peaches or canned mangos
Hot cooked rice

Put chicken in a baking pan. Place it in heated a 350°F oven and set timer for 30 minutes. Meanwhile, combine the butter, honey, salt, mustard and curry. Heat on the stove until butter melts. Blend well. When timer sounds, baste chicken with one-third of this mixture. Set time for 15 minutes and baste again when timer sounds. Remove from oven and tuck the fruit around chicken and baste one last time. Set timer and bake 15 minutes more. (Total baking time is 1 hour and 15 minutes) Serve with rice.

## Nut Coated Chicken

I prefer the Parmesan coated chicken recipe, but this is nice for a change, especially if you like almonds. It is also casein-free. Using slivered almonds makes this dish look fancy for company.

4 skinless, boneless chicken breast halves
(about 1 pound)
1 teaspoon gluten-free Dijon mustard*
1 teaspoon water

2 Tablespoons gluten-free mayonnaise*
Slivered almonds or Almond meal may
also be used
¼ (or more) cup apricot preserves, melted

Heat the oven to 425°F. Place some almonds on a piece of waxed paper, trying to keep them in a single layer. Blend the mustard, water and mayonnaise together in a shallow plate or pie plate. Dip chicken breasts in the mayonnaise mixture to get a light coating on them. Take and coat them in the nuts, moving around the waxed paper to get a single layer of nuts on the chicken. Place the chicken in the baking dish. Bake uncovered for 25 to 30 minutes until chicken is no longer pink and juices run clear. Drizzle with melted apricot preserves, and serve extra as a dipping sauce.

*Variation*: Instead of apricot preserves, Honey Mustard Salad Dressing (see index) makes a nice dipping sauce. Or, drizzle some of our favorite Italian Dressing (see index) over the cutlets before serving.

*Variation 2*: For very thick chicken cutlets, marinate them first in our favorite Italian salad dressing (see index for recipe). Dry with paper towels. Dip in egg and coat in nuts or nut meal. This makes the chicken more flavorful.

## Paella

I had this dish during our trip in Spain. I modified it to make it easier to prepare using long grain rice. I also use less oil. The original Spanish recipe used a ½ cup and we found this to be too much oil.

4 Tablespoons oil (preferably olive oil)
8 pieces of chicken, about 2 ½ pounds (I use drumsticks or thighs)
Sprinkling of salt, pepper, garlic powder (or use Adobo® Seasoning)*
2 cups of rice (I use long grain rice)
1 clove of garlic, minced
1 green pepper or yellow pepper, diced
1 red pepper, diced

1 onion, diced
1 (14.5 ounce) can of diced tomatoes*
Pinch of saffron or ½ teaspoon turmeric (or both)
4 ¾ cups of hot chicken stock (I use water and gluten-free chicken soup base*)
Fresh parsley (or defrosted frozen peas may be used for color)
Salt to taste

Heat a large 12 inch fryer. Add some oil and brown the chicken on all sides. Sprinkle chicken with salt, pepper and garlic powder as you are browning it. Remove it from the pan.

In the same pan, add a little more oil if needed. Add the rice and vegetables and sauté about 5 minutes. Heat chicken stock and add turmeric and saffron to it. Stir the chicken stock and tomatoes into rice mixture. Top it with the chicken. Cover and cook for about 20 minutes. Remove cover. Add the parsley (or peas if using). Let it rest for 5 minutes before serving.

## Potato Flake Coated Baked Chicken, Version 1

This is the recipe we use for church suppers. It is easy to make and contains no eggs. When you use potato flakes, don't make the coating too thick or it will turn into a layer of mashed potatoes on the outside of your chicken instead of a coating.

¾ cups Potato Buds®* or potato flakes*
¼ cup grated Parmesan cheese
1 teaspoon oregano

Oil
2 ½ to 3 pounds broiler fryer chicken pieces

On a piece of waxed paper, mix together potato flakes, parmesan cheese and oregano. Dip chicken in oil, then in the potato flake mixture. Grease a 13 x 9 x 2 inch pan generously with oil or gluten-free cooking spray. Put the chicken in the pan, and bake at 350°F for 1 hour. (Chicken is done when the juice is no longer pink when the center of the thickest part is cut.)

## Potato Flake Coated Baked Chicken, Version 2

The original recipe came from Betty Crocker®. I actually prefer it using potato flour (not starch) instead of the potato flakes. If you use potato flakes, don't make the coating too thick or it will turn into a layer of mashed potatoes on the outside of your chicken instead of a coating.

2 to 3 Tablespoons oil
1 ¼ cups Potato Buds®* or potato flakes* (or potato flour may be used but use half as much)
¼ cup grated Parmesan cheese

½ teaspoon salt
¼ teaspoon ground black pepper
2 ½ to 3 pounds broiler fryer chicken pieces
1 egg, beaten

*see gluten-free products list at the end of the book

Grease a 13 x 9 x 2 inch pan generously with oil or gluten-free cooking spray. On waxed paper, mix together the potato flakes, cheese, salt and pepper. Beat egg in a pie plate. Dip chicken into egg, then into potato mixture. Shake off excess and put it into the baking pan, placing skin side up. If using potato flour instead of flakes, spray the chicken with some non-stick cooking spray. This will help to make a better coating and not leave dry flour patches after baking. Bake uncovered at 425°F for 50 minutes or until done. (Chicken is done when the juice is no longer pink when the center of the thickest part is cut.)

## Sweet and Sour Chicken

This is my mother's recipe, and it is a nice "sweet and sour" without pineapple. You can use chicken with or without the skin on it, depending on your preference. I use backless thighs, because my husband prefers it without the skin, and they are the easiest parts of chicken to skin. See variation below for using skinless/boneless chicken thighs.

4 quarters of chicken (or 8 to 10 backless thighs)
Fine white rice flour (optional – I use only if chicken is skinless)
1 large onion, chopped or use equivalent frozen chopped onion

2 Tablespoons oil
½ (10 oz.) package French cut frozen green beans, slightly thawed
2 carrots, scraped and sliced or use equivalent frozen sliced carrots

Sweet and Sour Sauce:
3 Tablespoons gluten-free soy sauce*
1 Tablespoon cornstarch (or use a little less if you coated the chicken in rice flour)
¼ cup light brown sugar

2 tablespoons wine or cider vinegar
1 Tablespoon orange juice
1 Tablespoon ketchup
⅔ cup water

Rinse chicken and wipe dry with a paper towel. If you decide to remove the skin, dip chicken in some fine rice flour to coat. If chicken has the skin, this step is not necessary.

Heat skillet, then add oil and heat a minute. Add chicken to skillet and brown nicely on one side. Then turn chicken over and add chopped onions. While chicken is browning, combine the sauce ingredients. When chicken is nicely browned, remove from pan and add sauce and sliced carrots. Heat and stir until sauce bubbles and thickens. Return chicken to pan, top with green beans, cover and bring to a boil, then lower heat and simmer 10 minutes. Serve chicken with rice and serve sauce spooned over top. Serves 4.

*Variation:* Skinless/boneless thighs may be used. If using, coat chicken in fine white rice flour first, so they brown well. Less cooking time may be needed since the chicken is boneless. Instead of flattening the meat, I keep them rounded in the shape of the thigh while cooking. You may also use a little less cornstarch in the sauce if you coated the chicken in rice flour, since the rice flour will help thicken the sauce.

## Tarragon Grilled Chicken

This is nice on the grill. I use the tarragon vinegar made from the recipe in this book (see index). Caution with some store-bought brands of tarragon vinegar, since they may contain gluten.

4 skinless, boneless chicken breast halves (usually one package)
¼ teaspoon garlic powder
1 Tablespoon gluten-free Dijon mustard*
1 Tablespoon gluten-free tarragon vinegar (see index for recipe) or wine vinegar may be used

¼ cup oil (I use olive oil)
1 Tablespoon fresh minced tarragon or 1 teaspoon dried tarragon
¼ to ½ teaspoon salt (or to taste)
⅛ to ¼ teaspoon pepper (or to taste)

Place chicken in a pan with sides for the marinade. Mix dressing ingredients. Pour over chicken and coat on all sides. Marinate for a ½ hour or more. Grill or broil or pan-fry. It's best grilled. On my grill it takes about 8 minutes per side but grill temperatures may vary.

## Tender Turkey Meatballs

I often make these meatballs, but don't usually make the curry sauce. See variations below.

2 lbs. ground turkey
1 clove garlic or ½ teaspoon garlic powder
3 to 4 Tablespoons of fine white rice flour or sweet rice flour
2 teaspoons gluten-free beef bouillon*
¼ cup milk or gluten-free milk substitute*

1 Tablespoon gluten-free soy sauce*
1 egg
1 teaspoon chopped parsley or sprinkling of parsley flakes
1 medium onion, chopped or 1 Tablespoon dehydrated onion flakes

Combine all ingredients. If too dry, add a little milk. If too wet, add a little more rice flour. Shape into about 20 meatballs the size of a walnut. Put in a pan with a cover. Add a little water and steam to cook through, about 15 to 20 minutes.

*Variation*: You can add these to a tomato sauce or add to soups. They are also good with the sauce in the Country Captain recipe (see index). You can also serve them in this spicy curry sauce recipe (although my husband prefers the other sauces):

Curry Sauce:
2 to 3 Tablespoons olive oil
1 medium onion chopped
2 stalks celery
1 to 2 teaspoons gluten-free curry powder* (depending on your taste)
1 teaspoon oregano

1 teaspoon ground cinnamon
½ teaspoon gluten-free chicken bouillon*
2 Tablespoons cornstarch
1 cup water
½ cup raisins (optional)

Sauté onion and celery in oil. Add the spices and the bouillon. Mix the cornstarch in the water and add to the onion mixture. Add the raw meatballs from the recipe above. Add the raisins, if using. Cover and simmer 15 to 20 minutes and serve over rice.

*see gluten-free products list at the end of the book

## Teriyaki Barbeque Chicken
This is easy to put together, and has no corn sweeteners for those allergic to corn.

12 chicken thighs (bone-in)
¼ cup gluten-free soy sauce*
3 Tablespoons honey
½ teaspoon garlic powder
½ teaspoon onion powder (optional)

2 Tablespoons tomato paste *(You can freeze the remainder for another use. Store it in a plastic freezer bag, not in the can.)*
¼ teaspoon gluten-free liquid smoke* (optional)

Preheat oven to 350°F. Line a baking pan with Reynolds® Release foil for easy clean up. Put the chicken in the pan and bake for 45 minutes. Blend together the rest of the ingredients. Brush on chicken. Bake another 15 minutes until chicken is cooked through and no longer pink.

## Turkey Meatloaf
Easy to make and the ground turkey can be more tender than beef. My husband never liked turkey burgers, but likes this meatloaf and thought it was ground beef. If you can't find gluten-free onion soup mix, substitute gluten-free beef bouillon* and dried onion minced onion.

2 pounds gluten-free ground turkey* (I prefer the 93% lean. Some brands of turkey add skin which increases the fat content.) You can also use half ground turkey and half ground beef.
1 envelope of gluten-free onion soup mix (or see "onion dip" recipe for a substitute)

2 eggs
½ to ¾ cup of brown rice flour or fine white rice flour or gluten-free bread crumbs
1 to 2 Tablespoons dried onion flakes or dried minced onion (optional)

Mix all ingredients together in a bowl. Put in two glass loaf pans and shape. Bake at 350°F for 1 hour, or until center is no longer pink. I usually put some washed potatoes in the oven with the meatloaf since potatoes also cook in 1 hour. (Be sure to prick potatoes with a fork to let out steam or they can explode in the oven.) I serve with the potatoes and a green vegetable for a complete meal. This meatloaf freezes well, so you can freeze the second meatloaf for another time. Leftovers reheat well in the microwave oven.

## Turkey – Roasted
Here are my detailed instructions to roast a turkey, and they've always turned out delicious.

Purchase a turkey* that is minimally processed and gluten-free. Remove the turkey parts in the cavities (large opening and neck opening) and rinse the turkey with cool water. Clean out any entrails. (By this I mean rinse out any of the goopy red stuff inside the bottom of the large cavity.) Place the turkey in a pan with high sides and one that fits the turkey. If it's too large you won't get much gravy because it will all evaporate. If it's too small and the turkey is hanging over the edge, the juices will get all over your oven and make a mess.

*see gluten-free products list at the end of the book

Oil the skin of the turkey. (I use my hands to rub some oil on it. I like olive oil, but any kind may be used.) Next, sprinkle the turkey skin with salt, pepper, and garlic powder. Also sprinkle with onion powder if desired.

If you plan to stuff the bird (see index for recipe), stuff the bird with thoroughly <u>cooled</u> stuffing. I make gluten-free bread stuffing (see index) or rice stuffing (see index) a day ahead of time and refrigerate. Hot stuffing can cause bad bacteria to grow inside the bird.

Bake according to the directions on the package the turkey came in. It will need to bake longer if stuffed. Before putting it in the oven, cover with foil (make a tent of foil so it won't stick to the skin.) Remove the foil before the last hour of baking, to make the turkey skin get nice and brown. You can baste it half-way through if desired, by using a baster and pouring the juices on top of the turkey skin. (I usually don't do this.)

If the turkey doesn't come with a pop-up timer, I suggest you use a meat thermometer so you know when it's done. The temperature should be about 180°F deep in the thigh, and juices should run clear. Remove from oven, and set aside for 10 minutes before carving so it will be easier to slice.

Since the pan juices don't usually make enough gravy, use some of the turkey parts from inside the bird to make additional pan juices. Take the turkey parts from the cavity from when you cleaned the turkey. Remove and discard the bag the parts came in. I use the neck, the heart, and the gizzard. I do not use the liver and discard or freeze it for another use. (The liver is goopy and the other parts are firm.) Rinse the neck, heart and gizzard and put them in a small pot. Cover the turkey parts with water. Let it boil a few minutes and skim off any foam that may rise to the top. Discard the foam. Add gluten-free bouillon if desired, or add some salt, pepper and garlic or onion powder. Cover and cook until done on low. (I cook about an hour and check midway that there is enough liquid. It's done when the meat comes off the turkey neck easily.) Set aside. Remove the neck and parts, cool them and remove the bits of meat and add to the gravy if desired.

When your turkey is done, remove from the oven. Remove the juices with a turkey baster. I use a gravy measuring cup that separates the fat from the broth. If you don't have one, put it in a glass liquid measuring cup, take the baster and remove the broth on the bottom and transfer it to your pot that you cooked the turkey neck broth. Try not to put too much fat.

Take a small amount of water or broth and some fine white rice flour or sweet rice flour (a Tablespoon or two depending on the amount of broth) and blend it and add it to the pot that you removed the neck, etc. Cook to thicken, while stirring. If you need it thicker, sprinkle in more rice flour, stir well and boil. If it's too thick add more water. Adjust seasonings to taste.

*Variation*: If you want brown colored gravy, you can de-glaze the pan using the method described under the pork roast recipe. This only works if you have brown particles stuck to the pan. You would remove the turkey and the juices from the pan. (Put the juices in a measuring cup or gravy boat that separates the juices from the fat.) De-glaze the pan with some hot water to get the brown particles to dissolve. Add the juices (but not all the fat) back to the pan. Add some rice flour as above. (If you have a gas stove like I do, I put the

Corningware® pan I used to cook the turkey on the burner. If you have an electric stove, put all juices in a saucepan.) Bring to a boil. Adjust seasonings and thickness of gravy as mentioned above.

*Variation 2*: To use one of those Reynolds® Brown-n-Bags, use 1 Tablespoon of rice flour, shake it in the bag, and follow the directions. I recommend putting one sliced onion under your turkey. Then rub the turkey with some oil and sprinkle it with garlic powder, salt and pepper. Close the bag, use the twist tie it comes with, put the slits recommended on the top and follow the directions. When I make the gravy, I take the well cooked onions that were under the turkey and puree them in a food processor. I then add them back into the gravy. It makes the gravy more flavorful. Then I take all the meat juices, and skim off the fat using a special measuring cup that removes the fat. I put some rice flour in a pot, add some of the juices to mix the flour in, add the rest of the juices, stir and bring it to a boil. This method makes the gravy have a nice brown color because of the onions and the browning in the bag.

## Vermouth Chicken

This is an easy Italian recipe. This is one recipe where you don't have an exact measurement for the herbs and spices. Sprinkle them on according to your preferences. My husband likes that the chicken just falls off the bone, and the vermouth soaks in the meat so it is not dry.

| | |
|---|---|
| 3 pounds of chicken parts (with bones) | 1 cup sweet vermouth |
| Olive oil | 6 potatoes, washed, cut and quartered |
| Garlic powder | 1 large sliced onion |
| Salt, pepper, dried basil, dried oregano | 1 can peas, drained |

Put chicken in a large pan with sides. Put potatoes and onion in the pan. Everything should be in a single layer. Sprinkle everything with some garlic powder, salt, pepper, basil and oregano. Cover with aluminum foil. Bake at 400°F for 45 minutes. Remove foil. Add 1 cup of drained canned peas. Put them around the chicken. Add the vermouth and bake for 45 minutes more.

Serve with a salad to make a complete meal.

## Vineyard Chicken or Chicken with Grapes and Wine

My husband likes this for something different. This is a good use for leftover grapes.

| | |
|---|---|
| 1 cup seedless red grapes, washed and cut in half | ¼ teaspoon garlic powder |
| 2 ½ pounds of skinless, boneless chicken breasts, cut into bite sized cubes | 3 Tablespoons fine white rice flour |
| 1 teaspoon dried parsley flakes | 2 Tablespoons oil (or a little more) |
| ½ teaspoon dried basil flakes | ⅓ cup dry white wine, or for variation I use Marsala wine or dry Vermouth |
| ¼ teaspoon dried tarragon, crumbled | ⅔ cup chicken broth (or I use water plus gluten-free chicken base*) |
| ¼ teaspoon paprika | 1 teaspoon lemon juice (I use bottled) |
| ½ teaspoon salt (or a little more to taste) | |
| ⅛ teaspoon pepper | |

*see gluten-free products list at the end of the book

Rinse grapes and cut in half.  Set aside.  Cut chicken breasts into cubes.  (I use poultry scissors.)

Put herbs/spices and rice flour on to a piece of waxed paper (so you don't dirty a bowl) and blend together.  Coat chicken cubes in this mixture.

Heat a non-stick skillet a minute and then add the oil.  Add the coated chicken cubes and cook until lightly browned on all sides.

Add wine, chicken broth and lemon juice.  Simmer for 5 minutes.  If sauce is too thin, add some of the leftover spice/rice flour mixture and simmer a minute or two more to thicken.  Add the grapes and stir them in.  Serve.

# FISH AND SEAFOOD

## Baked Flounder with Cheese Sauce

Because you cook the fish in milk, it's very moist and not dried out like some baked fish. This recipe is from my sister-in-law, and I adapted it to make it gluten-free.

2 lbs. Flounder fillets
2 Tablespoons butter
Dash of salt and ground black pepper
1 ¼ cups milk (divided)
3 Tablespoons fine white rice flour or
   sweet rice flour

1 cup grated cheddar cheese
3 Tablespoons sherry (I use good sherry, not cooking sherry. The sherry strongly flavors this dish, so make sure you like the taste.)
Dash paprika

Wash fish and dry on paper towels. Brush with 2 Tablespoons butter, sprinkle with salt and pepper. Roll up and put in baking dish. Add ½ cup milk and bake uncovered 30 minutes at 350°F.

Add a small amount of the ¾ cups milk into a pot. Add the rice flour and blend. Add the rest of the milk. Bring to a boil. Add cheese, melt, and then add the sherry. Drain the liquid from the baked fish and add to the cheese sauce. Add only as much as needed to make the sauce creamy. Pour over the fish, sprinkle with paprika and place under the broiler for 4 minutes until brown.

*Variations*: Tilapia fish may be used instead of flounder. Diced red pepper can be added over the fish before putting it in the oven, to add color and flavor. Some frozen peas may also be added to the milk when making the cheese sauce. I often add both the red pepper and peas, and serve the fish over rice for a complete meal.

## Broiled Fish

This is very easy.

2 fillets (4-5 oz. each)
Juice of 1 lemon (or 2 to 3 Tablespoons
   lemon juice)

Old Bay® seasoning*

Place fish on a lightly greased broiler pan. Liberally sprinkle fish lemon juice and with Old Bay®. Broil fish 2-4 minutes. Turn fish over. Sprinkle with more lemon juice and Old Bay. Broil 3-4 minutes or until fish flakes easily. Makes two servings. Do not overcook the fish.

*Variation*: If you don't have Old Bay seasoning, you can use a combination of celery salt, paprika, and some ground black pepper to season the fish.

## Batter Fried Fish

You need to whip up the egg whites to make this. It makes a puffy coating. It will be crispy the day you make it, but leftovers will not be crisp.

2 Egg whites or 4 teaspoons egg white powder and 2 Tablespoons water
⅓ cup cornstarch
½ teaspoon paprika (coating will not brown without it)
¼ cup fine white rice flour

½ teaspoon or sprinkling of salt or 1 teaspoon gluten-free seasoned salt (I use Old Bay® or Season-All®)
1 pound white fish (I use whiting, but any fish like haddock or sole may be used)
Oil for frying

Whip egg whites until stiff. Fold in cornstarch and paprika and set aside. On a piece of waxed paper, place the rice flour. If using seasoning, mix it into the flour. Rinse fish and gently pat it dry with a paper towel so it's not sopping wet. Sprinkle it with salt if not using seasoning. Place the fish in the rice flour mixture and coat it evenly.

Heat the oil in a fryer pan or a deep fryer. Do not let the oil overheat. (If using a thermometer and deep fryer, the oil would be about 350°F. Alternatively, use a ¼ inch of oil in a large skillet fry pan and heat until a small bit of batter starts to sizzle.) Dredge the fish in the egg white/cornstarch mixture and coat. Cover with as much batter as possible. Immediately put into the oil to fry.

Fry for about 3 minutes per side. The coating should be puffy and crisp. The fish should be tender. Drain on paper towels to get rid of any excess oil. Serve hot. My husband likes these served with French fries and coleslaw for a fish-n-chips dinner. (Don't serve with malt vinegar as malt contains gluten. We like this fish "as-is", but it's also good with gluten-free ketchup* or gluten-free tartar sauce* or Balsamic white vinegar. I find that Balsamic white vinegar is a good substitute for malt vinegar.)

*Variation*: Instead of this batter, you can use the batter recipe listed under fried chicken.

## Cod and Peas in Mushroom Sauce

We like this recipe better than the original recipe that contained gluten-filled condensed soup.

1 Tablespoon chopped green onion
1 clove chopped garlic or ¼ teaspoon garlic powder or granulated garlic
⅓ cup diced red pepper
1 Tablespoon butter
2 cups milk
2 Tablespoons fine white rice flour or sweet rice flour

¼ teaspoon ground black pepper
1 Tablespoon lemon juice
1 can of mushrooms, drained
1 package (16 oz.) frozen cod fish, partially thawed
1 cup frozen peas
Red pepper strips for garnish

In a saucepan, briefly sauté onion, garlic and diced red pepper in the butter. Blend the rice flour into the milk and add to the pan. Add the pepper and bring to a boil. Remove from heat. Place fish in a lightly greased shallow baking dish. Stir lemon, peas and mushrooms into sauce and pour over fish. Cover and bake in a preheated 400°F oven for 25 minutes.

*see gluten-free products list at the end of the book

Uncover and bake 10 minutes more or until fish flakes easily when tested with a fork. Garnish with pepper strips or pimiento.

*Variation*: Other thick fish fillets can be used such as halibut, red snapper and salmon. If using unfrozen fish, turn oven off after 20 minutes and bake 5 minutes longer. Remove and place on a rack for a short while before serving.

## Crab Cakes

Use caution when purchasing crabmeat. Crabmeat by itself is gluten-free. Most imitation crabmeat contains gluten. Only purchase fresh lump crabmeat from a trusted seafood market, to be sure they have not supplemented it with some imitation crabmeat. Or purchase the live crabs and steam them yourself. Or use canned crabmeat. Do not order crab salad or cakes in a restaurant because restaurants are permitted to use a percentage of imitation crabmeat in those items. I use canned crabmeat because they would have to list the imitation crabmeat or fillers on their ingredients list. Use the same caution with lobster cakes or salad. There is imitation lobster meat that also contains gluten.

½ pound lump gluten-free crabmeat* (I use high quality canned lump crabmeat, or use 2 cans well drained)
2 Tablespoons to ¼ cup gluten-free mayonnaise*
2 teaspoons egg white powder or 1 egg white, lightly beaten
1 teaspoon lemon juice

Dash of gluten-free hot sauce* or to taste
Dash of cayenne pepper, or to taste
¼ teaspoon Old Bay® seasoning
1 Tablespoon finely chopped parsley or powdered flakes
2 Tablespoons fine white rice flour or a little more if too wet

Pick through the crabmeat with your fingers and discard pieces of cartilage. If using canned crabmeat, drain very well and have as little liquid as possible. Combine all the ingredients except the crabmeat and blend. Add the crabmeat and mix well. If too wet, add a little more rice flour. Take ¼th of the mixture and form into a thick patty and place in a non-stick fry pan. It should make 4 patties. Place in a fry pan with a little oil and brown on both sides. Delicious served with the sour cream sauce for Salmon Cakes (see index), or serve with gluten-free tartar sauce. Tartar sauce can be made by blending some gluten-free mayonnaise*, gluten-free pickle relish*, and a little lemon juice (optional).

*Variation*: One time we didn't drain the canned crabmeat too well. After adding 2 more tablespoons of rice flour, we decided to make crab pancakes out of the mixture in a small non-stick skillet. They were about ¼ inch in height and about 6 inches in diameter. They had the same flavor and were also good.

## Fish Parmesan

This is quick and easy. Use the variation under the Chicken Parmesan – Oven Method with Cheese Coating. Rinse fish (I use Tilapia), coat with cheese mixture, bake on a non-stick pan for 15 minutes at 375°F.

## Fish Tacos

I had Fish Tacos in San Diego. They are a good way to use leftover gluten-free fried fish and coleslaw. Heat some gluten-free corn tortillas. (I put the desired amount on a microwave safe plate. Cover with a damp paper towel and heat 1 minute.) On each tortilla put some warmed fried fish (see index for recipe) and some coleslaw (see index for recipe, or use packaged coleslaw mix with some gluten-free Ranch dressing*). Top them with some cheese and gluten-free salsa*, if desired. Some lemon juice or gluten-free hot sauce* can also be put on the fish to add even more flavor.

## Fried Fish

This is a favorite of ours. If using cornmeal or corn flour be sure to use a brand that is gluten-free. Some can have gluten contamination.

½ cup Gluten-Free Naturals™ All Purpose Flour or corn flour or corn meal

3 teaspoons Old Bay® seasoning (as of this writing it is gluten-free)

1 ½ pounds of fish (I use whiting fillets or tilapia fillets)

Oil for frying

Mix the flour and seasoning together on a piece of waxed paper. Rinse the fish and get rid of excess moisture on paper towels. Dip fish in flour and coat on both sides. Heat oil and fry about 3 minutes per side until fish is golden brown and cooked through. (I pan fry the fish, but you could also deep fry the fish.) Serve with gluten-free ketchup* or gluten-free tartar sauce*. (You can make your own tartar sauce by mixing gluten-free mayonnaise* and gluten-free relish*.)

*Variation:* Deep fry the fish and drain well on paper towels. For an authentic fish 'n' chips dinner, serve with some fried potatoes. I fry the potatoes first and drain them well on paper towels. I place the potatoes on a pan and keep them warm in the oven while I fry the fish.

## Fried Fish – Oven Style

My mother invented this recipe because my brother likes fried fish, but she didn't like to fry. This recipe must be followed exactly without substitutions in order for it to work.

2 pounds of fish fillet or steaks

½ cup milk

1 ½ teaspoons salt

2 cups dry bread crumbs made from Gluten-Free Naturals™ bread

2 Tablespoons oil

Mix the milk and the salt. Put the bread crumbs on a piece of waxed paper (so as not to dirty another dish). Dip the fish in the milk, then in the bread crumbs, coating the fish completely. Put your oven on using its hottest temperature, 500°F to 600°F. Oil your baking pan well. Place the fish on top and dribble the rest of the oil on top of the fish. Place in preheated oven and bake for 10 minutes.

## Grilled Fish
Make sure you have a clean grill.  A grill previously used to cook bread, meats with gluten-containing soy sauce or barbecue sauce will transfer gluten to your food if not thoroughly cleaned off.  You can carefully try to cook over a clean piece of aluminum foil, but the results won't be quite the same.

| | |
|---|---|
| Fish | Salt and ground black pepper |
| Gluten-free Mayonnaise* | Parsley Flakes |
| Garlic Powder | Paprika |

Cover the fish with a very thin coating of the mayonnaise.  Rub it in with your fingers.  This will keep the fish moist.  (If you don't rub it in it will look like a white egg coating on it when cooked.)  Be sure not to dip a spoon back into the mayonnaise that has touched raw fish.  (I use the squeeze bottle of mayonnaise so I know it's never contaminated.)  Sprinkle generously with spices and grill about 3-4 minutes per side.  Remove from grill and check with a fork to see if fish flakes and is done.  Return to grill if needed but do not overcook.

## Mussels
This is my mother's recipe and I think these are better than the mussels served in fine Italian restaurants.  Make sure mussels are fresh.  When you clean mussels, they should close.  As soon as I touch them they close their shells tightly, and that is what you want so you know they are safe to eat. They may sometimes close a little slowly, but the key is that they shut tight.  If they stay open before you cook them they are no longer alive and must be discarded because they are unsafe to eat.

| | |
|---|---|
| 2 dozen mussels in shells | ½ teaspoon salt |
| 2 Tablespoons oil | ½ inch piece of hot dried red pepper |
| 2 cloves garlic | Sprinkle of oregano |
| 1 (8 oz) can of gluten-free tomato sauce* | |

Heat the oil in a large saucepan.  Sauté garlic on low heat to soften.  Mash garlic with fork and discard any large pieces.  Cool a few minutes then add tomato sauce, piece of hot pepper, salt and a little oregano.  Scrub mussels being sure to remove all seaweed caught in them.  Heat sauce and place mussels in pot and cook over high heat until all mussels are open.  Serve in soup bowls.  Mussels can be served over rice.  Be sure to remove hot pepper. Serves 4.

## Salmon Cakes
We enjoy this for a light and quick supper with a salad.  I came up with the idea of using potato flakes and we like it better than salmon cakes made with bread crumbs.  This dish is quick to make and inexpensive.  I usually keep a can of salmon on-hand for a quick meal.  Canned salmon is also high in calcium.  Since many celiacs have osteoporosis, it may be a good idea to eat foods high in calcium.

| | |
|---|---|
| 1 egg, slightly beaten | ½ teaspoon dried rosemary, crushed (I |
| ¼ cup dehydrated onion flakes | use a little less or use fresh) |
| ¼ cup Potato Buds®* or potato flakes* | ⅛ teaspoon ground black pepper |
| 1 Tablespoon lemon juice | 1 can (14.75 oz) Pink Salmon or 2 (6 oz.) |
| | cans skinless/boneless salmon |

Blend the egg, onion, potato buds, lemon juice, rosemary and pepper in a bowl.

*see gluten-free products list at the end of the book

Drain the salmon, discarding the water. Remove large bones and skin and discard. Add the salmon to the egg mixture. Flake the salmon and blend well. (I use my hands.) Form into 4 or 5 patties. Pan-fry in a small amount of oil until lightly browned on both sides. (I prefer making these in a Teflon® fry-pan.) Serves 2.

Top the cakes with the sour cream dressing in the recipe below or gluten-free ranch dressing (see index). For a lighter dressing, top the salmon cakes with a mixture of yogurt with a dash of garlic powder, dried dill weed, onion powder and salt. Some people with lactose intolerance can tolerate yogurt better than sour cream.

Sour Cream Dressing:
1 ½ Tablespoons dehydrated chives
½ teaspoon gluten-free Dijon mustard*
2 Tablespoons wine vinegar
1 Tablespoon water
⅛ teaspoon salt

⅛ teaspoon ground black pepper
Generous sprinkling onion powder
½ cup gluten-free sour cream*

## Salmon Cakes – Version 2
**A heartier version using dry breadcrumbs made from Gluten-Free Naturals™ bread.**

2 eggs, slightly beaten
½ cup gluten-free dry breadcrumbs
2 to 4 Tablespoons dehydrated onion
    flakes
2 teaspoons lemon juice (bottled is fine)

1 Tablespoon chopped fresh parsley or 1
    teaspoon dried parsley flakes
2 Tablespoon gluten-free mayonnaise*
¼ teaspoon garlic salt
1 can (14.75 oz) Pink Salmon or 2 (6 oz.)
    cans skinless/boneless salmon

Blend all ingredients except the salmon in a bowl. Drain the salmon, discarding the water. Remove large bones and skin and discard. Add the salmon to the egg mixture. Flake the salmon and blend well. (I use my hands.) Form into 6 or 8 patties. Pan-fry in a small amount of oil until lightly browned on both sides. (I prefer making these in a Teflon® fry-pan.) If desired serve on gluten-free rolls with lettuce and tomato slices and gluten-free tartar sauce* for Salmon burgers.

*see gluten-free products list at the end of the book

*Joyfully Gluten-Free*　　　　　　　　　　　　　　　　　　*Fish and Seafood*

## Salmon Cakes – using fresh salmon

If you prefer fresh salmon, here is another way to make salmon cakes. This is easy to make in a food processor and they cook very quickly.

1 pound fresh salmon, skin and bones removed

¾ teaspoon salt

¼ pound Nova style smoked salmon*, flaked (check ingredients that it's just smoked and contains no gluten) or eliminate and add a dash of gluten-free liquid smoke* (optional)

1 Tablespoon dried minced onion flakes (or 1 teaspoon onion powder may be used)

¼ cup red pepper, minced (optional)

1 teaspoon gluten-free horseradish* (optional, I don't use)

2 Tablespoons gluten-free mayonnaise*

½ teaspoon ground black pepper

½ cup Potato Buds®* or potato flakes*

A Tablespoon or so of oil for frying (I find this is not needed if you use a Teflon® pan)

Put all ingredients, except oil, in a food processor and blend 2 minutes until combined. Form into 12 cakes (or I make 7 or 8 larger ones) and sauté until lightly browned, about 3 minutes per side. I use a Teflon® pan so I do not need to add oil. Do not overcook. They can brown quickly.

Serve with Sour Cream Dressing (see previous recipe, at the top of this page), or gluten-free ranch dressing (see index).

## Salmon Steaks – Grilled or Skillet Method

Quick, easy and delicious! This is a favorite of ours.

4 (4 ounce) salmon steaks or a large salmon fillet (thawed if frozen)

1 Tablespoon soy sauce*

⅛ teaspoon garlic powder

1 Tablespoon butter or gluten-free margarine* (for skillet method only)

Lemon slices as garnish (optional)

Sprinkle soy sauce and garlic on fish. If using salmon steaks, put fish on a hot barbecue grill. Cook 3-4 minutes and turn over. Cook 3-4 minutes more until done.

If you don't have salmon steaks but instead have fillets, put the non-skin side down first. You always want to cook the skin side last; otherwise, your entire fillet will fall into the coals. The skin keeps it together.

Note: The grill must be thoroughly cleaned if anyone has previously grilled wheat bread or anything with gluten soy sauce, etc. on it. Gluten will transfer to your food. If your grill is not clean, you can carefully cook it over a clean piece of aluminum foil on the grill or see below as to how to make it on the stove.

For the stove method, put 1 Tablespoon butter in the pan and melt it. Either sprinkle the soy sauce and garlic on the fish or alternatively, add the soy sauce and garlic powder to the pan. Add the fish to the pan.

*see gluten-free products list at the end of the book*

-261-

Cook on one side from 1 to 5 minutes, then turn it over and cook another 4 to 5 minutes until the fish flakes easily with a fork. You can also make it under the broiler using the grill method. However you prepare it, it's delicious!

## Shrimp Cantonese (Shrimp with Lobster Sauce)
This is very authentic and delicious. This is my mother's recipe.

½ cup ground raw pork (or see variation 2 of this recipe to make your own)
2 lbs. uncooked shelled and de-veined large shrimp
1 teaspoon sugar
2 Tablespoons cornstarch
1 ½ teaspoons gluten-free MSG or monosodium glutamate powder* (optional)

3 Tablespoons gluten-free soy sauce*
¼ cup cold water
4 Tablespoons oil
2 cloves garlic, crushed or minced
½ teaspoon ground ginger
Salt and ground black pepper
1 ½ cups gluten-free stock or bouillon*
3 finely chopped scallions
2 well beaten eggs

Cut shrimp down the middle but not all the way through. Mix cornstarch, sugar, MSG, soy sauce and cold water together and set aside.

Place oil and ginger in skillet or wok. Add ground pork and shrimp and sauté 3 minutes. Sprinkle on salt, pepper, crushed garlic and mix in. Add 1 ½ cups broth, cover and cook 10 minutes. Add starch mixture while stirring until smooth and thick. Stir in well beaten eggs and scallions and shut off the heat immediately. Stir well and serve with rice. Serves 4 to 6.

*Variation*: Small shrimp may be used but reduce cooking time or they will be overdone and ruined. Or, cooked thawed shrimp may also be used and added with the scallions. However, we prefer this dish using the uncooked shrimp and prepared as above.

*Variation 2*: One time I didn't have the ground pork, but I had some boneless pork chops. I put them in the food processor and used the mincing blade to make my own ground pork. The meat was tender, not fatty, and we enjoyed it. It's not the same as ground pork from the butcher, but we liked it better because it was so tender and lean.

## Shrimp Cocktail
My mother usually prepares shrimp cocktail the day before a party. This is the best method to cook fresh shrimp, and keep them moist and tender. If you would rather not do the work, you can buy frozen cooked shrimp instead and thaw them. Most brands are gluten-free, but check ingredients. In the back of the book I have listed some safe brands of cocktail sauce to serve with your shrimp or see index for cocktail sauce recipe.

Wash the shrimp and drop them into salted boiling water. As soon as the shrimp turn pink and begin to curl, remove them from the boiling water (using a large slotted spoon) and plunge them into cold water so as to stop the cooking. Reserve the lightly salted water the shrimp cooked in.

*see gluten-free products list at the end of the book

Shell and de-vein the shrimp.  After the water they cooked in has cooled, put the water in a container and place the shrimp in the water.  Storing the shrimp in this water will keep them tender and moist.  Cover and refrigerate until ready to serve.

Remove the shrimp from the water before serving.  For a fancy dinner first course, serve them in champagne glasses filled with some shredded lettuce and some gluten-free cocktail sauce in the middle.  (Or see index for recipe for cocktail sauce.)  Place shrimp on top of the lettuce, around the inside edge of the glass.

## Shrimp Rockefeller

This recipe comes from my father's cousin.  It makes a fancy dish for company.  You can put it together earlier in the day and then bake it when your guests arrive.

2 pounds shrimp, cooked, shelled and deveined.  (Or purchase cooked frozen shrimp, defrost and remove the tails)
½ pound fresh spinach
½ cup plus 3 Tablespoons butter
1 Tablespoon plus ¼ teaspoon gluten-free Worcestershire Sauce*
2 teaspoons anchovy paste
2 ¼ teaspoon salt
Few drops of gluten-free hot pepper sauce*
6 scallions, chopped fine
2 cups chopped lettuce
1 ½ stalks of celery, chopped fine
1 clove of garlic, minced

½ cup fresh parsley, minced
½ cup soft gluten-free bread crumbs (Use day-old gluten-free bread and pulverize it in a food processor)
Cream Sauce:
3 Tablespoons rice flour
1 ½ cup milk
⅛ teaspoon black pepper
3 Tablespoons grated Parmesan Cheese*
Topping:
3 Tablespoons gluten-free cracker* crumbs or gluten-free dried bread crumbs (optional, I don't use)

If shrimp is frozen, defrost and remove tails.  Set aside.

Wash, drain and chop spinach.  Or buy the pre-washed package and chop it.  Heat together the ½ cup butter (1 stick), 1 Tablespoon Worcestershire Sauce, anchovy paste, 1 ½ teaspoons salt, and the dash of hot pepper sauce.  Add the chopped spinach, scallions, lettuce, celery, garlic and parsley.  Simmer for 10 minutes until the vegetables are tender. Add the fresh bread crumbs and taste for seasoning.  Spread the mixture over the bottom of a shallow baking dish or 6 individual scallop shells dishes for baking.  Cover the mixture with the shrimp.

Make a medium cream sauce by putting 3 Tablespoons rice flour in a pot.  Blend in the 1 ½ cup milk using a whisk.  Cook until thick over medium heat, stirring the mixture.  Melt in the 3 Tablespoons butter and add ¼ teaspoon Worcestershire sauce, the Parmesan cheese and ¾ teaspoon of salt, and the sprinkling of black pepper.  Pour over the shrimp.  If desired, top with some crushed gluten-free cracker crumbs or dry bread crumbs.

Bake for 20 minutes in a moderate oven at 350°F, until sauce bubbles up and the top browns.  Makes 6 servings.

*see gluten-free products list at the end of the book

Note:  If you put this together earlier and refrigerated it, you will have to heat the dish a little longer until the sauce is hot and bubbly.

<u>Write your own recipes here</u>:

# PORK

## Boiled Dinner
A boiled dinner is an easy Irish dish.  I usually make this for St. Patrick's Day.

1 gluten-free smoked ham butt* or an
    assortment of smoked meats such as
    kielbasa*, frankfurters*, or corned beef*
    (See note below regarding corned beef,
    kielbasa and frankfurters).

1 bay leaf
Salt and ground black pepper
2 lbs. cabbage, cut into wedges
2 to 3 carrots per person
1 large potato, per person

Place meat in a large pot and just cover with water.  Add pepper and bay leaf and cook a half- hour.  If using pre-cooked meats, taste broth to see if it needs salt and add if needed.  Add cabbage, peeled potatoes cut into chunks, and scraped carrots.  Cook another half-hour or until all vegetables are tender.  (More time may be needed if the vegetables were cut in very large pieces.)  Remove bay leaf and discard.  Slice meats and surround with vegetables.  Moisten all with some pot liquid.  Serve with gluten-free mustard* (I prefer a spicy or a coarse mustard with this).

When my mother first made boiled dinners, she usually started with a corned beef or a smoked butt.  Now she prefers a variety of meats adding Polish or smoked sausages or even frankfurters.  Just make sure that whatever you choose that they are gluten-free.  Adjust cooking times depending on the meats you choose.  See note below.

NOTE: Some gluten-free corned beefs* are <u>not</u> precooked and require long cooking times.  Do not taste the water if the meat is raw.  Check the package for the cooking times and adjust the recipe accordingly, adding the vegetables in the last half-hour of cooking time.  If using frankfurters, add them during the last 10 minutes of cooking.  Also, use caution purchasing smoked meats.  As of this writing, Hillshire® Kielbasa* and Hatfield® are gluten-free.  Some other smoked sausages may not be, so check.

## Chinese Barbecued Spareribs and Chinese Roast Pork
When we were children, we would lick our fingers while eating these to get the taste of the sauce because we liked it so much.  Just be sure to buy gluten-free ribs.  Some are packaged in those sealed heavy plastic bags (cry-o-vac) and may contain gluten because of added solutions.  See variation below for Chinese Roast Pork.

3 pounds pork spareribs
1 ½ cups gluten-free soy sauce*
2 cloves garlic, crushed

1 ½ teaspoons salt
2 Tablespoons sugar or honey
1 Tablespoon sherry wine

Wash and remove the gristle as much as possible from the ribs.  Dry with a paper towel.  Place the rest of the ingredients in a large deep bowl and mix thoroughly.  Place the ribs in the bowl and mix well, let soak in the sauce for 10 minutes, moving the ribs occasionally so the sauce soaks in evenly.  Place the ribs on a broiler and broil until both sides are brown and they are cooked through.

*Variation:* You can use this same recipe to make Chinese Roast Pork. Instead of the ribs, cut 3 pounds of pork into strips approximately 2 inches by ½ inch thick. Soak for 10 minutes. Broil until done. Use leftovers in other Chinese dishes. It is nice for a change in the Stir Fry with Beef recipe in this book.

## Ham and Pineapple Casserole

This is a good party dish. It can be done ahead of time and reheated. Serve with rice, peas, and a green salad. The flavor of the ham gets into the sauce and the meat tastes like un-smoked pork after it is finished cooking.

1 cut up onion
1 cut up green pepper
2 cups gluten-free ham*, cut into chunks
1 lb. can pineapple chunks, reserving the juice
8 oz. can of gluten-free tomato sauce*
1 ½ Tablespoons cornstarch

2 or more Tablespoons gluten-free soy sauce*
½ teaspoon ground ginger
1 Tablespoon sugar
Oil

Heat 2 Tablespoons oil in a pan and sauté cut up onion and green pepper a few minutes. Mix the cornstarch into reserved pineapple juice and add soy sauce, ginger and sugar. Blend all together. Add ham and tomato sauce to pan and cook 5 minutes or until vegetables are tender and ham heated through. Add pineapple and sauce. Bring to a boil stirring all the while until sauce is smooth and thickened.

## Ham – Glazed

This is an easy recipe from a good friend of mine. This uses a Reynolds® brown n bag. Use caution when other people prepare foods for you in these bags! Make sure that they didn't put a Tablespoon of wheat flour in the bag as instructed on the box.

1 gluten-free ham*
¼ brown sugar*
2 cups ginger ale* (I use less and use one can or 1 ½ cups)

Reynolds® Brown 'n Bag
1 Tablespoon fine white rice flour (or other gluten-free flours may be used)

Place Brown 'n Bag in a large casserole dish that will fit the ham. Place 1 Tablespoon rice flour in the bag and shake. (This prevents the bag from bursting while cooking.) Insert the ham in the bag. Mix the brown sugar and ginger ale and pour it over the ham. Seal the bag with the provided tie. Slit as directed. Bake it according to the package directions on the ham, or if you prefer, bake it at a lower temperature for a longer amount of time. It will be delicious, juicy, and with a nice glaze.

## Ham Loaf
This is a good use of leftover ham, and a nice change from regular meatloaf.  See variation below to triple the recipe to make several at once.  They freeze and reheat well.

½ cup gluten-free fresh bread crumbs made from Gluten-Free Naturals™ Bread (put a few slices of gluten-free bread in a food processor, and pulse until crumbs)
½ pound of gluten-free ham*
1 pound of lean ground turkey or pork

2 Tablespoons milk
1 egg
Glaze:
   6 Tablespoons brown sugar
   2 Tablespoons cider vinegar
   2 Tablespoons water
   ¾ teaspoon gluten-free mustard*

Finely chop the bread in a food processor and measure out a ½ cup.  Finely chop the ham in the food processor.  Put bread crumbs, ham, ground meat, milk and egg into a bowl. (No salt is needed since ham contains salt.)  Mix together with your hands and put in a loaf pan.

Put glaze ingredients in a small pot.  Stir together using a whisk.  Heat and simmer 5 minutes.  Allow to cool a few minutes.  Preheat oven to 350°F.  Pour glaze over ham loaf.  Bake loaf for 1 hour.  (I often double the recipe and make 2 large or 3 regular size loaves and freeze the extra for another time.  If you double the recipe and put it all in one pan, bake it 1 ½ hours.)

Note: I pour the entire glaze mixture on the loaf in the beginning of baking.  The original recipe said to baste the loaf throughout the baking with the glaze.  Both methods work.  I also put some potatoes in the oven at the same time and serve the ham loaf with baked potatoes and a vegetable.

*Variation*:  We don't like things too sweet.  You may want to make half the amount of glaze, if desired.

*Variation 2*:  I sometimes triple the recipe and make 3 loaves.  I use either 2 pounds of ground turkey* and 1 pound of ham*.  Or I use 1 pound ground pork, 1 pound ground turkey and 1 pound ground ham.  I use 1 ½ cups fresh gluten-free bread crumbs, 6 Tablespoons milk and 3 eggs.  I follow directions as written above and make 3 large loaves.  I usually don't triple the glaze recipe and put a little glaze on each loaf.  (I often use honey baked ham which adds sweetness, so less glaze is needed.)  After they are baked and cooled, I freeze them.  This ham loaf recipe freezes well and reheats well in the microwave oven.

## Hot Dog/Mexican Roll-ups
A Burrito and hot dog combination that is good for weekend lunches.

10 gluten-free corn tortillas* (Use a fresh package of corn tortillas since older ones will fall apart.)
1 can gluten-free refried beans* (or see index for recipe)

Gluten-free grated cheddar cheese* or American cheese slices*
1 package gluten-free hot dogs*
Gluten-free salsa*

*see gluten-free products list at the end of the book*

Place corn tortillas on a microwave safe dish. Cover with a damp paper towel and microwave for one minute. This will make the tortillas pliable.

Open can of refried beans. Spread each tortilla with some bean mixture, cover with some cheese and a hot dog. Roll up and place in a 9 x 13 inch baking pan that is lined with aluminum foil. Put seam side down. Cover pan with foil.

Bake at 350°F for 20 minutes. Remove foil. Cover each tortilla with salsa and a little more cheese. (Some brands of tortillas may split when they bake, but the salsa and cheese covers this.) Bake uncovered until cheese melts. Eat with a fork and knife. A salad completes the meal.

*Variation*: Some canned gluten-free chopped green chilies may be added to the refried beans for a spicier dish. Or, 1 teaspoon chili powder may be added to refried beans to make it spicier.

## Kielbasa and Kraut
This can be made either on the stove top or in the oven. The stove top version is a family favorite. The oven version makes a nicer presentation for company.

1 can (1 lb. 11 oz.) sauerkraut or 2 (1 lb. each) bags of sauerkraut
1 large onion, sliced
2 stalks celery, sliced (optional)
2 Tablespoons butter or oil
1 large apple, peeled, cored and chopped (if using a Golden Delicious apple, I leave it un-peeled)

2 Tablespoons brown sugar
½ teaspoon caraway seeds (optional)
½ teaspoon leaf marjoram, crumbled
½ cup dry white wine or water
¼ cup water (if needed)
1 gluten-free kielbasa* or gluten-free smoked sausage*, about 1 pound

For stove top version: Drain the sauerkraut and rinse under cold running water in a sieve. This will give it a milder flavor. Drain water. In a large skillet with a lid, lightly sauté the onion and celery in oil (or butter) for a few minutes. Stir in sauerkraut, apple, sugar, seeds, marjoram and wine. Bring to a boil. Make deep cuts, 1 inch apart in the kielbasa, or cut into 1 inch chunks. Lay kielbasa on top of the sauerkraut mixture and cover. Simmer about 20 minutes until vegetables are done. (Kielbasa is already fully cooked.) Check after 10 minutes to make sure there is enough liquid. If not, add ¼ cup water so it doesn't burn. When finished cooking if there is too much juice in your pan, add a sprinkling of rice flour to thicken or boil a little liquid off (uncover pan) if needed. I find that a little bit of rice flour works well, and makes the juices more of a sauce. Serve with freshly boiled potatoes and prepared mustard*.

For oven version: Drain the sauerkraut and rinse under cold running water in a sieve. This will give it a milder flavor. Drain water. Sauté onion and celery in oil (or butter) in an 8 cup flameproof casserole. (If you have an electric stove, use a pot with lid that can go in the oven.) Stir in sauerkraut, apple, sugar, seeds, marjoram and wine. Bring to a boil. Make deep cuts, 1 inch apart in the kielbasa, or cut into 1 inch chunks. Lay on top of sauerkraut

*see gluten-free products list at the end of the book

mixture and cover. Bake in a 325°F oven for 1 hour 30 minutes. Stir several times and add more wine or water if necessary until sauerkraut is soft and delicately brown. Serve with freshly boiled potatoes and prepared mustard*.

*Variation 2*: For crock-pot version, put all ingredients in crock-pot <u>except</u> kielbasa. If desired, put some diced potatoes on the bottom and cover with the other ingredients. Cook on low for 8 hours. Turn to high and add kielbasa to heat it through. Serve using a slotted spoon to drain off any extra liquid. (Note: my experience is don't add the sausage until the end or it will burn.)

*Variation 3*: Hillshire Farms® Li'l Smokies® smoked sausages from Sara Lee® are gluten-free as of this writing, and can be used instead of kielbasa. I prefer the pork ones, and I think in this dish they are better than the beef ones.

## Pork Chops A L'Orange or with Peaches
This is a favorite dish of ours. I often make it for company and everyone enjoys it. I like the sauce on mashed potatoes or rice. A good friend gave me this recipe. One time I didn't have a can of mandarin oranges, so I changed it to peaches and now we enjoy both versions (see variation below).

6 1-inch thick pork chops
1 Tablespoon oil
1 (11-ounce) can mandarin oranges (or canned peaches)
¼ cup firmly packed brown sugar

½ teaspoon ground cinnamon
1 teaspoon salt
1 teaspoon gluten-free prepared mustard*
¼ cup tomato ketchup*
1 Tablespoon cider vinegar

Brown chops on both sides in oil. Drain mandarin oranges, reserving ½ cup juice in a measuring cup. Set fruit aside. Combine juice with remaining ingredients and pour over pork chops. Cover and simmer gently for 40 minutes or until chops are tender. (Shorten time if they are thinner chops.) Remove cover and boil for 5 minutes uncovered so sauce will thicken. Add oranges and cook 5 minutes more.

*Variation 1*: I often use thinner chops and it cooks in about 20 minutes.

*Variation 2*: <u>*Pork chops with Peaches*</u>: Substitute canned peaches for oranges. Use ½ cup of the peach syrup as above. If peaches are juice packed instead of syrup, mix a ½ cup juice with 1 teaspoon fine white rice flour or sweet rice flour. Follow directions as above.

## Pork Chop-Chop

This is a delicious one-pot dish with an Oriental flare.  One day I didn't have any pork but had leftover ham, so I created the second variation listed below.

4 pork chops
½ teaspoon sugar
1 large sliced Spanish onion
½ cup sliced celery
2 cups sliced, white cabbage
1 ½ cups hot gluten-free bouillon* (I use 1 cube or one teaspoon gluten-free chicken base*)

½ pound green beans, cut into 2 inch pieces
2 Tablespoons cornstarch
3 Tablespoons cold water
3 Tablespoons gluten-free soy sauce*

Heat a large skillet one minute.  Sprinkle sugar over bottom of pan and brown lightly.  Wipe chops with paper towels and add to skillet.  Reduce heat and brown nicely on both sides.  Add vegetables and hot water mixed with the bouillon cube.  Cover and simmer 15 to 20 minutes or until the celery and green beans are tender.  Mix cornstarch in cold water and add soy sauce.  Remove chops to a deep serving dish.  Now add cornstarch mixture to pan.  Cook and stir until mixture comes to a boil and thickens.  Pour over pork chops.  Can be served with rice or fried rice threads.

*Variation*:  I have also substituted frozen green beans for the fresh with excellent results.  Just add them 10 to 15 minutes after the celery.  You can also add 2 large carrots peeled and sliced at the same time as the cabbage for a variation.

*Variation 2*:  To make *Ham Chop-Chop*, substitute 1 lb. gluten-free sliced ham for the 4 pork chops.  Use 2 Tablespoons of gluten-free soy sauce, instead of 3.  Skip the step of browning the meat, since ham is precooked.

## Pork with Sauerkraut

This is a favorite of my husband's.  It is good with or without the caraway seeds.  Use a large skillet with deep sides and a cover for easy preparation.  This is a good way to use up celery tops (leaves), instead of throwing them away.

6 pork chops
Oil
1 chopped onion
Chopped tops of whole stalk of celery including all leaves (wash and then chop)
1 Tablespoon fine white rice flour or sweet rice flour

1 cup water
1 Tablespoon cider vinegar
1 pound sauerkraut (I use the canned) (I rinse the sauerkraut using a sieve for a milder flavor)
1 ½ Tablespoons brown sugar
Sprinkling of salt
1 teaspoon caraway seeds (optional)

Heat a skillet and then add some oil.  Heat until the oil shimmers, and then add the chops.  (Be careful that hot oil doesn't spatter on you.)  Brown the chops on both sides and remove from heat.  Blend the rice flour with the water and add to the pan.  (To do this, make a paste using a small amount of water and then add the rest of the water and blend.)  Add all the

*see gluten-free products list at the end of the book

remaining ingredients to the pan with the chops. Return to the heat. Now bring it to a boil, lower the heat, cover and simmer 30 minutes or until chops are tender. Serve with mashed potatoes. (I like to top the sauce from this dish on the potatoes.)

## Roast Loin of Pork
This is my mother's recipe and delicious.

| | |
|---|---|
| 1 (5 to 6 pound) pork loin | 2 teaspoons gluten-free vanilla*, or |
| ⅔ cup of currant jelly |    vanillin* |
| 3 Tablespoons Port wine | 1 teaspoon gluten-free dry mustard* |

Roast pork for 15 minutes per pound in a 350°F oven. Sprinkle salt and pepper over top. (I then insert a meat thermometer ½ way through the meat.) Place remaining ingredients in a saucepan and cook 10 minutes. Pour sauce over completely cooked roast and return to oven a few minutes to glaze.

I use a meat thermometer to be sure that the roast is cooked perfectly.

## Roast Pork Tenderloin
I frequently make this for company. I have written a lot here, but it is very easy. You are basically putting the meat in the oven and baking it.

| | |
|---|---|
| 1 (3 to 5 pound) pork tenderloin roast | 1 Tablespoon fine white rice flour or |
| Salt, ground black pepper and garlic |    sweet rice flour |
|    powder | |

Choose a pan with high sides for the roast, one that is not too much larger than the piece of meat. I use a Corningware® oval size pan. Put the roast in the pan and sprinkle generously with salt, pepper and garlic powder. Put a meat thermometer in the roast, pushing about ½ way through. Roast in a 325°F oven for 30 minutes per pound. When the thermometer shows it's done for pork, remove it from the oven. Put the meat on a cutting board.

Meanwhile, to make gravy, take some hot water (about ¾ cup) and put it in the roasting pan. Even if your pan is rather dry and doesn't have much juice from the meat, you can usually make gravy by using this method. Rub the sides and bottom with a large spoon or spatula to deglaze the pan and get all of the brown juices on the pan to dissolve in the water. (If you have a gas stove, you can take the Corningware® pan and place it on the burner and begin to heat it slowly.) Continue to mix until the brown particles on the sides and bottom dissolve in the water. Now mix a Tablespoon of the rice flour with a ¼ cup of cold water. Stir until blended. Now blend this in with the pan juices. Stir with a whisk until it boils and thickens. If it is too thin, add additional rice flour to a little bit of water. Add to the gravy and bring it to a boil again. If it's too thick add some water. Taste and adjust seasonings. Add more salt and pepper if needed. I sometimes add another sprinkling of garlic powder. If it tastes too strong, add additional water and rice flour to make a larger quantity of gravy. If it doesn't have much taste, add a little gluten-free bouillon* or gluten-free soup base* but use it sparingly.

*see gluten-free products list at the end of the book

If this method was unsuccessful in giving you enough gravy, you can make mushroom gravy. To do this take a can of mushrooms un-drained, add some additional water. Add water and rice flour blended as above, and some bouillon or soup base to taste. (I use Better than Bouillon® mushroom flavor, which is gluten-free as of this writing.) Do not add too much bouillon or it will be salty. Or instead of canned mushrooms, use fresh mushrooms. Wash and slice the mushrooms. Cook them in a covered saucepan so you retain the water. Use the same method by adding some rice flour. For a different flavor, you can add a little wine such as Madera or Marsala instead of adding extra water.

Slice meat and serve with gravy.

## Sausage, Peppers and Onions – Oven Style

I used to make this dish on the stove, but this oven method from my mother is easier, especially since there is no stove spatter to clean up. Use a large oblong pan that is non-stick for easier clean-up. Or line your pan with Reynolds® Ready Release non-stick aluminum foil.

| | |
|---|---|
| 1 lb. (or more) Italian Sausage*, sweet or hot | 2 Tablespoons olive oil |
| 1 large pepper, sliced | Salt and ground black pepper to taste |
| 1 large onion, sliced | Garlic powder to taste (I use granulated garlic) |

Cut sausage into 2 inch pieces using a poultry scissors. Cut up peppers and onions. Put in a baking pan (preferably one with 2 inch sides). Dribble oil over top. Sprinkle some salt, pepper, and garlic powder over the top. Bake uncovered at 450°F for 30 minutes (or longer if sausage pieces are large), turning every 10 minutes. (Alternatively, bake at 350°F for 1 hour.)

*Variation:* My mother puts the sausage under the broiler a few minutes first to brown it. Remove from oven, and reduce oven temperature. Add the onions, peppers and rest of the ingredients and bake as above. It cooks faster and the sausage is browner. The peppers and onions turn out a little crisper because they don't have to be baked as long.

*Variation 2*: I like the 350°F method for 1 hour, but I like my peppers and onions less cooked. I use a non-stick type baking pan (or a pan covered with non-stick aluminum foil), and add the sausage and let it bake 30 minutes. Then I add the peppers and onions and bake 30 minutes more. I usually don't add the extra oil by using the non-stick type pan, and I find that after 30 minutes there is enough fat in the pan to cook the vegetables.

*see gluten-free products list at the end of the book

## Sausage or Pork Chop Zucchini Stew

This is another dish invented by my Mother. It's an easy one-pot meal; it can be made in about 35 minutes.

4 gluten-free Italian sausages* (about 1 ¼ lbs.) or 4 large boneless pork chops very lean

¼ cup water (if using sausages)

2 Tablespoons oil

2 medium potatoes, peeled, washed and cut into 1 ¼ inch cubes

1 onion peeled and diced (or equivalent frozen chopped onions)

1 (15 ounce) can gluten-free tomato sauce*

Few dashes of ground black pepper

¼ teaspoon salt

¼ teaspoon dried basil

1 ½ pounds zucchini, ends trimmed off, washed and cut into ¾ inch chunks

½ large green pepper (or 1 small), washed, seeded and cut into 1 inch squares (or equivalent chopped frozen green peppers)

Place sausages in ¼ cup water in a 12 inch Teflon® coated fry pan with a cover. Cover and steam 10 minutes. (Meanwhile, prepare potatoes and onions.) Pour off the liquid in the fry pan after cooking 10 minutes. Add oil and brown sausages lightly. If using pork chops, place oil in the pan and brown them. When nicely browned, remove to a plate.

Add potatoes and onions to the pan and sauté briefly. Then add the can of tomato sauce, dash of black pepper, ¼ teaspoon salt and the 1 teaspoon dried basil. Bring to a boil, cover and reduce heat to a simmer and cook 8-10 minutes, until potatoes are almost tender when tested with a cake tester.

While potatoes cook, prepare zucchini and green pepper. After the potatoes cooked 10 minutes, add the zucchini and the green pepper carefully so as not to spatter the sauce. Push vegetables into the sauce and lay the sausages or pork chops on top. Cover and cook 12-15 minutes or until potatoes and zucchini are tender and the pork chops are done. Do not overcook the zucchini as it will fall apart and become unappetizing.

*Variations*: After dish is completely cooked, you can add some gluten-free grated mozzarella cheese* on top. Cover to melt and serve immediately. You can also eliminate the meat and have a delicious vegetable dish. Don't eliminate the green pepper as it adds just the right flavor to the bland zucchini.

## Sausage – Savory flavored Bulk Sausage made with Ground Pork

If you need a small amount of bulk sausage, but can't find a gluten-free brand, here is a way to make your own. I think this is very flavorful, but more herbs may be added if you like even bolder flavors.

1 pound ground pork or boneless pork chops or pork tenderloin

¼ to ½ teaspoon ground sage or rubbed dried sage may be used

¼ teaspoon marjoram

¼ teaspoon oregano or thyme

⅛ teaspoon summer savory

⅛ teaspoon ground black pepper

½ to ¾ teaspoon salt (I use ½ teaspoon)

¼ teaspoon garlic

½ teaspoon onion powder

*see gluten-free products list at the end of the book

If using boneless pork chops or pork tenderloin, put it in the food processor in pieces so the food processor is balanced when you turn it on. (Do not put it in the food processor all in one chunk or it will be off balance. Put some on each side of the cutting blade.) Add spices and process until cut up and the consistency of ground sausage.

If using commercially ground pork, mix the spices with the meat. Or if you are cooking it as bulk sausage you can heat your skillet a minute, put the meat in your skillet, and begin to cook and break it up with your spatula. Then add herbs and spices and cook until meat is done. Drain excess fat. (This method saves you from having to dirty a mixing bowl to blend the meat and spices.)

For patties, mix herbs and spices with pork. Form into patties and pan fry until browned and cooked through.

If cooking the sausage you made in your food processor, heat a skillet, add oil or cooking spray and cook until it is no longer pink. I prefer it made from pork tenderloin because you sausage will be lean, tender and not fatty. Since it is so lean, you will need oil or cooking spray to prevent sticking while cooking it.

This sausage can be used in Turkey Stuffing, Sheppard's Pie and Stuffed Acorn Squash.

## Shake-n-Bake® Type Pork Chops

Use the recipe for "Cornflake Crumb Baked Chicken" (see index). I usually make a ½ recipe of the mayonnaise mixture, since a dipping sauce is not needed. Pork Chops turn out moist and juicy. Baking times may vary depending on the thickness of the pork chops. Your butcher can tell you the baking time needed for the thickness you have. Check for doneness, especially near the bone. To prevent the possibility of trichinosis, pork should be cooked and not very pink. Do not overcook or the pork chops will be dry.

## Shepherd's Pie made with Sausage

This is a good use of leftover mashed potatoes. Heat them in the microwave while you are cooking the meat mixture. Or you can use instant prepared according to package directions. Vegetables such as drained canned mushrooms or green beans may be added to make it a more complete meal. The original recipe called for ground lamb, but we think the sausage is much more flavorful. If you would rather use ground beef (it's called Cottage Pie if using beef) or lamb, add some salt, pepper and garlic powder to the meat mixture. Sometimes ground lamb can be fatty, so be sure to drain any excess fat.

| | |
|---|---|
| 1 pound bulk pork sausage* (or see index for sausage recipe in this book) | Hot cooked mashed potatoes |
| 1 large onion, diced | Gluten-free cooking spray |

In a skillet, break up sausage with your spatula and cook until no longer pink. Drain excess fat. Add diced onion and cook until onion is translucent. Transfer to a casserole dish. Top with mashed potatoes. Spray top with cooking spray to help it brown. Bake at 400°F for about 15 minutes until the top is a little browned. Serve.

*see gluten-free products list at the end of the book

*Variation*: Ground turkey may be used instead of sausage. Add gluten-free dried onion soup mix to the meat, following the directions on the package of soup mix. (Or see index for Onion Dip/Soup mix recipe). Follow directions as above. Onion may be eliminated since it is in the soup mix.

*Variation 2*: Frozen mixed vegetables (green beans, carrots, peas, corn) may be added with the onion. Frozen diced onion may also be used.

## Smoked Sausage Casserole
My favorite sausage for this is Hillshire® beef or Polish kielbasa, which are gluten-free as of this writing. (Check packages as some of their other smoked sausages are not gluten-free.) The original recipe called for a can of mushroom soup, but this is just as easy and not as salty as with the soup.

1 large gluten-free smoked sausage* or kielbasa*
1 cup raw rice
1 medium onion
½ large green pepper chopped
2 stalks celery, chopped
1 can sliced mushrooms, un-drained

1 ½ cups milk
1 ½ cups water
3 Tablespoons fine white rice flour or sweet rice flour
2 Tablespoons gluten-free Worcestershire sauce*
Salt and ground black pepper to taste

Cut sausage into 1 inch pieces and place in the bottom of a heavily greased casserole. (It will stick very badly if you don't grease it.) Pour rice over sausage and top with chopped vegetables. Pour the milk over sausage mixture. Blend rice flour, water and Worcestershire together and pour into casserole. Cover and bake at 350°F for 55-60 minutes. Taste and adjust seasonings and serve. After serving, I suggest that you soak the casserole dish in soapy water for easier clean-up.

## Sweet and Tangy Pork Chops
This recipe comes from Hatfield Quality Meats®.

4 pork chops, less than a ½ inch thick
2 teaspoons vegetable oil
¼ cup preserves (try a flavor like peach, orange marmalade, or apricot)

1 Tablespoon gluten-free mustard*
¼ cup cider vinegar

Brown chops in oil in a large skillet over medium high heat. Turn over to brown the other side. Lower the heat. Meanwhile, combine preserves, mustard and vinegar in a bowl. Pour over chops. Cover and cook for about 10 minutes until chops are about done. Uncover and cook a few more minutes to thicken sauce. Test meat for doneness. Do not overcook the meat. (If sauce is still not thick enough, remove chops and boil sauce a minute or two to thicken.)

## Sweet and Sour Chinese Pork

There is also a crock-pot version of this dish in this book, using chicken or pork.

1 pound pork tenderloin
1 egg white, slightly beaten (or egg white powder equivalent)
1 teaspoon cornstarch
1 teaspoon gluten-free soy sauce*
1 teaspoon oil
1 onion, diced
1 green pepper, diced or cut into 1-inch pieces
⅓ cup sugar (I prefer brown sugar)

1 can (20 ounces) pineapple chunks in juice, 1 cup juice reserved
2 Tablespoons wine vinegar
2 Tablespoons gluten-free soy sauce* (I add a little more)
1 clove garlic, finely chopped or ⅛ teaspoon garlic powder
1 heaping Tablespoon cornstarch
2 plum tomatoes, cut into eighths (optional)

Cut the pork into ¾ inch pieces and trim the fat. Mix the egg white, 1 teaspoon cornstarch, 1 teaspoon soy sauce in a glass bowl and stir in the pork. Let stand 10 minutes. Meanwhile, dice vegetables. Blend sugar, juice, vinegar, soy sauce, garlic and cornstarch.

Heat a wok, put a little oil in it and add the pork. Stir-fry until no longer pink. Remove from wok and add onion and pepper. Stir-fry until crisp tender. Add sauce ingredients and bring to a boil. Cook until thick. Add the pork, pineapple and tomatoes to the wok. Cook and stir until heated through. Serve over rice or Chinese rice noodles or bean threads.

*Variation*: Use a diced red pepper instead of tomatoes. Stir fry with the onion and green pepper. Diced celery may also be added at that time.

## Tourtiere – Pork Pie

This is a Canadian specialty traditionally served on Christmas Eve. Originally this pie was made from tourtes which were carrier pigeons. Since their disappearance, fresh pork or other meats are used for tourtier pie.

Pie Filling:
1 ½ pounds pork tenderloin, ground in a food processor or ground, lean pork
1 small onion, minced in a food processor or 3 Tablespoons dried minced onion
½ cup boiling water
1 clove garlic or ¼ teaspoon garlic powder
¼ teaspoon sage (I use ground sage)
¼ teaspoon celery salt

¼ teaspoon black pepper
Pinch of ground cloves (optional)
3 medium potatoes
Double crust:
2 cups Gluten-Free Naturals™ All Purpose Flour or Sandwich Bread Flour
Sprinkling of salt
⅔ cups butter
4 Tablespoons water

Using the cutting blade of a food processor, grind the pork. Put the pork and the rest of the pie filling ingredients in a pan, except the potatoes. Cook over medium heat until the pork is no longer pink and half of the cooking liquid is evaporated. Cover and cook 30 to 45 minutes longer. (If using pork tenderloin, cook it less.)

Meanwhile, boil the potatoes. Drain and mash them. Add them to the meat mixture. Allow the meat mixture to cool.

For the pie crust, put the flour and sprinkling of salt in the food processor. (Or you can use the traditional method of making pie crust by cutting the butter into the flour, and then blending in the cold water.) Add the cold butter and cut it in with the cutting blade in the processor. Pulse and do not over-mix. After the butter is in small pieces, add the water through the feed tube with the motor on. The dough should ball up. If too dry, add a slight amount more water. If too wet, add more flour. Do not over process or the butter will start to melt. Turn off the processor and divide the dough into 2 balls.

Roll out on a piece of waxed paper. You only need to put a piece of waxed paper on the bottom, not the top. Put into a 9 inch or 9 ½ inch pie pan. If the crust tears as you are removing the waxed paper, just piece the dough together and press it. Since there is no gluten it is fine to handle the dough. It is also fine to re-roll it if needed. (If you find it difficult to roll out because you over processed the dough, refrigerate it and then roll it. Or roll it out immediately between 2 pieces of waxed paper and then refrigerate it on a flat board until it is easier to handle.) Line the pie plate with the bottom crust.

Fill the pie crust with the meat filling. Roll out top crust. Cover pie with top crust. Flute pie edges. Use a fork to poke some vent holes into the top crust. Bake at 450°F for 10 minutes. Then turn the temperature down to 350°F and bake it 30 to 40 minutes more. Makes 6 or 7 servings. In Canada they serve this pie with dill pickles. I like it served with a salad. Leftovers reheat well in the microwave oven. Store any leftovers in the refrigerator.

Write your own recipes here:

# LAMB

## Curried Lamb

This is a good way to use the last bits of a leg of lamb. My mother boils the bone with a little salted water to get the broth needed for this recipe. You can also substitute gluten-free chicken broth*, if necessary.

2 to 3 cups cubed cooked lamb
3 Tablespoons oil
1 cup thinly sliced celery
2 tart apples, peeled, cored and diced
1 medium onion, diced
2 cups lamp broth, or leftover gravy and
    water.

1 teaspoon gluten-free curry powder* (or
    see index for curry powder recipe)
2 Tablespoons cold water
2 Tablespoons fine white rice flour or
    sweet rice flour

Heat oil in a covered skillet then add celery, onions, and apples. Sauté 5 minutes. Mix curry powder into oil. Add lamb, 2 cups broth and cover. Simmer 10 minutes or until celery is tender. Taste broth to see if salt is needed. Mix the rice flour into the water and whisk together. Add to skillet and stir continuously until broth is thickened and smooth. If too thin, cook uncovered a few minutes more. Serve over rice.

## Herbed Lamb Chops

I like these prepared under the broiler, but you can also make these on a clean grill. Remember that if any bread or gluten-containing sauce is left on the grill it will contaminate your food.

16 oz. loin or rib lamb chops (3 or 4
    depending on thickness)
1 teaspoon dried marjoram

Ground black pepper, salt and garlic
    powder

Heat broiler. Line pan with foil. Rinse, dry, and trim fat from chops. Rub in spices on both sides. Broil 4 to 5 minutes per side for ¾ inch thick and 6 minutes for 1 ½ inch thick chops. Serve with Viennese Rice (see index).

## Shepherd's Pie (see recipe under Pork)

# CROCK-POT DISHES

The crock-pot® is perfect for the gluten-free diet. Use quick-cooking tapioca for the thickening. Sprinkle the granules of tapioca over the vegetables in the recipe. Also, when using chicken in a crock-pot recipe I think it is best if it is added frozen so it won't get overcooked. For easy clean-up, you can try the new Crock-pot liners from Reynolds®. If you like brown rice in dishes, add your rice and the water required to cook rice at the bottom of the crock-pot, then follow the rest of the recipe. This saves time and also saves washing another pot. The rice and meat and sauce will be all together in the crock-pot.

## Baked Beans – Crock-pot

My mother makes these for family cookouts. This recipe was a family favorite that was always gluten-free.

1 ½ pounds dried pea beans (other dried
   beans can be used but we prefer these)
6 Tablespoons light brown sugar
½ pound gluten-free salt pork* lean
   bacon*
1 large onion, chopped

½ teaspoon salt
½ teaspoon ground black pepper
½ teaspoon gluten-free dry mustard*
¼ cup molasses*
Hot water

Early the day before cooking the pea beans, soak them in a large pot with enough cold water to cover them by a couple of inches. The next day, drain the beans and cover with clean water and bring them to a boil. Boil about ½ hour and test to see if the beans are tender by blowing over a spoonful of beans. If the skins pop open, they are ready to bake.

Take out your crock-pot. Drain beans and place in the crock. Add all the other ingredients except the salt pork and mix well. Then cut the salt pork into ⅓ inch slices and place on top of the beans. Now pour hot water over the top to completely cover the salt pork by ½ inch. Place heat on high, cover and forget for 5 hours. Then remove the cover and let the water evaporate until the liquor thickens and top browns. This takes at least 1 hour more. This is a wonderful dish for a buffet or cookout.

## Barbecue Chicken – Crock-pot Style

This is tasty but not as good as on the grill. Chicken parts must be frozen when you put them in the crock, otherwise they will be overcooked and tough.

½ cup gluten-free ketchup*
2 Tablespoons brown sugar, packed
1 ½ Tablespoons quick cooking tapioca
1 teaspoon gluten-free Worcestershire
   sauce*
1 Tablespoon wine vinegar
½ teaspoon ground cinnamon

¼ teaspoon crushed red pepper (optional)
2 ½ pounds chicken pieces with bone,
   skinned and frozen (I like backless
   thighs; i.e. chicken thighs without backs
   attached)

Put sauce ingredients in the crock-pot and blend. Place chicken in the crock-pot and blend into the sauce. Cover and cook on low 10 to 12 hours or on high 5 to 6 hours. Good served over mashed potatoes.

*see gluten-free products list at the end of the book

## Chicken Cacciatore – Crock-pot Style

Use frozen, skinned chicken thighs to make this dish. (Chicken with the skin on can be used, but I find that it makes the dish greasy and I don't like the texture of the skin cooked in the crock-pot.)

1 cup brown rice (do not use white rice)
2 cups water
½ cup dry wine (I use dry Vermouth) or water
1 large Spanish onion, diced, (optional) or 2 Tablespoons dried onion flakes (optional)
1 large package of frozen chicken thighs with bone, skin removed (Note: chicken must be frozen or it will get overcooked and ruined)

Salt and ground black pepper
Garlic powder
Sliced black olives (optional)
1 can mushrooms drained (optional)
1 jar gluten-free tomato sauce (I use Classico® four cheese tomato sauce or Francesco Rinaldi® three cheese tomato sauce, which are both gluten-free as of this writing)

Put brown rice, water, and wine in the bottom of the Crock-Pot. Top with onion and then the frozen chicken. Sprinkle chicken with salt, pepper and garlic powder. Top with drained sliced olives and drained sliced mushrooms (if using). Top with the jar of sauce and make the sauce completely cover the chicken. Cook covered on low for 8 to 10 hours or on high for 4 to 6 hours.

*Variation*: Frozen chopped onion may be used instead of the fresh onion or onion flakes. Frozen green pepper may be added with the onion.

## Chili – Crock-pot Style

I frequently make this. I purchase ground meat in large quantities and brown it all at once. Allow it to cool. Then I store it in the freezer in 1 lb. or 1 ¼ lb. size bags. (I use smaller freezer bags so that the food will have a shape that will fit in the crock-pot.) To make this chili, remove the meat from the bag, put the meat in frozen, use frozen chopped green pepper and frozen chopped onion. You can quickly put it all together in the morning so it's ready when you get home from work.

2 Tablespoons oil
1 ¼ pound lean chopped meat (either ground beef, turkey, or pork)
½ cup chopped onion (fresh or frozen)
¼ to ½ cup chopped green pepper (fresh or frozen)
¾ teaspoon salt
2 teaspoons gluten-free chili powder*

1 teaspoon cumin, ground (optional some brands of chili powder contain cumin)
¼ teaspoon oregano
¼ teaspoon granulated garlic or garlic powder
1 (16 oz.) can pinto beans or red kidney beans
2 cups or 1 (15 oz.) can or 2 (8 oz.) cans gluten-free tomato sauce*

Heat a pan a minute, add oil, and allow oil to heat a minute then add meat. Cook meat until it loses its red color. Drain off any fat. (This can be done ahead of time and frozen.) When ready to make, put the meat in crock-pot. (It can be either just browned or frozen.) Add the rest of ingredients. Cover and cook on low for 8-10 hours. This makes almost 2 quarts.

*see gluten-free products list at the end of the book*

Serve over polenta (see index), rice, or baked potatoes. If desired, top with a little grated cheddar cheese.

*Variation*: A can of hominy corn can be added when you put this together. This makes it a complete meal and eliminates the need to serve it with rice, potatoes or polenta.

## Country Captain Chicken – Crock-pot Style

I often don't add the raisins and nuts when I make this crock-pot version. Note: This recipe will not work if the chicken is not frozen. Fresh chicken becomes overcooked and tough in a crock-pot. I prefer backless thighs (chicken thighs without backs attached) because they are easy to skin, and make a nice presentation. Do not use boneless chicken or it will be overcooked, and this dish will be ruined.

8 pieces of chicken, skinned and frozen (I think backless thighs are best)
1 chopped onion (fresh or frozen)
1 chopped green pepper (fresh or frozen)
1 minced clove of garlic or ¼ teaspoon granulated garlic powder
1 Tablespoon quick cooking tapioca
½ teaspoon salt

¼ teaspoon ground black pepper
1 teaspoon gluten-free curry powder*
Tiny pinch of oregano (optional)
1 (15-oz.) can tomato sauce* or use 2 (8-oz.) cans
¼ cup raisins (optional)
¼ cup slivered almonds (optional)

Ahead of time, skin chicken and freeze. I put the parts in inexpensive sandwich bags, and put those in a large freezer bag. You want to be able to get the chicken apart to fit in the crock. Chop onions and peppers and freeze, or use ones purchased chopped and frozen.

The day you want to make this dish, put the vegetables and garlic in the bottom of the crock-pot. Sprinkle with the tapioca. Remove the bags from the frozen meat, and discard bags. Place meat on top of the vegetables. Now open the can of sauce. Mix the rest of the ingredients in the can and then pour over the top. (If the can is too full, pour some sauce in the crock-pot, then mix in the ingredients and then pour the rest in.) Cook on low 10-12 hours. Serve over rice. (You can make rice ahead of time, freeze it, and reheat it in your microwave.)

*Variation*: Add 1 cup of brown rice and 2 ½ cups water on the bottom of the crock-pot. Top with vegetables and follow directions as above. This makes a one-pot dish with rice. Since brown rice takes a long time to cook, this works well. Do not substitute white rice or the rice will be too overcooked.

## Mexican Rice Casserole – Crock-pot Style
Not as pretty looking as the Mexican Skillet recipe, but just as tasty.

1 cup brown rice (do not use white rice)
2 ½ cups water (not hot)
1 pound ground meat, browned (I precook ground beef and freeze it in 1 pound packages. I add it to the crock-pot frozen)
1 green pepper, chopped (I use ½ cup frozen)
1 onion, chopped (I use ½ cup frozen)

1 (14 to 16 ounce) can gluten-free diced tomatoes*, un-drained
1 (8 ounce) can gluten-free tomato sauce*
½ teaspoon salt
¼ teaspoon garlic powder
2 teaspoons chili powder
½ to 1 cup grated gluten-free mild or sharp cheddar cheese*

Put rice and water in crock-pot. Top with rest of ingredients, except for the cheese. Cook 8 to 10 hours on low, or 4 to 6 hours on high. Top with cheese and stir in until it melts.

## Pork Stew with Cornmeal Dumplings – Crock-pot Style
You will need to use the cheese in the dumplings or they will fall apart.

1 pound boneless pork, cut in chunks
¼ teaspoon garlic powder
1 Tablespoon oil
4 medium carrots, cut into ¼ inch pieces
2 medium potatoes, peeled and diced
¼ cup quick cooking tapioca
1 (28 ounce) can tomatoes, cut up and un-drained
1 cup water
½ cup dry white wine or ½ cup of Redbridge® Gluten-Free Beer

1 Tablespoon sugar
1 Tablespoon gluten-free Worcestershire sauce*
2 bay leaves
1 teaspoon dried oregano
½ teaspoon salt
¼ teaspoon ground nutmeg (optional)
¼ teaspoon ground black pepper
Dumpling batter (recipe follows)

Sprinkle meat with garlic powder and brown it in oil. (This can be done ahead of time and frozen. Put it in the crock frozen if done this way.)

Place vegetables in crock and top with tapioca. Top with meat. Open the can of tomatoes and put the tomatoes in the crock. (I use scissors to cut the tomatoes into smaller pieces, when they're in the crock.) Use the tomato can and mix together the sauce ingredients and pour over the top. Cook on low 10 to 12 hours or on high 5 to 6 hours.

After cooking the stew, turn the crock to high temperature. Remove the bay leaves. Mix together the following dumpling batter and drop on top of the stew. Cook 50 minutes more. Do not try to make the dumpling part of this recipe without the cheese or it will not work.

Dumplings for Pork Stew:
- ⅓ cup white rice flour
- ¼ cup tapioca flour
- ½ cup shredded cheese (do not eliminate)
- ⅓ cup cornmeal
- 1 teaspoon xanthan gum

- 1 teaspoon gluten-free baking powder*
- Sprinkling of ground black pepper
- 1 beaten egg
- 2 Tablespoons milk
- 2 Tablespoons cooking oil

*Variation*: 2 cans (14 ounces each) of diced tomatoes may be used instead of canned whole tomatoes. This saves you from having to cut up the tomatoes.

*Variation 2*: To save time, I often wash and cut up the potatoes without peeling them. Or, drained canned potatoes may be used. Frozen sliced carrots may also be used. Do not defrost them, add them frozen.

## Soups (see recipes under Soup Heading)

## Soy Glazed Pork – Crock-pot Style
I prefer pork baked in the oven, but if you want to use the crock-pot this has nice flavor. The meat tends to fall apart and doesn't cut well.

- 4 to 5 pounds of pork
- ½ cup pineapple juice
- 2 Teaspoons wine vinegar
- ½ teaspoon garlic powder or granulated garlic
- ¼ cup dry white wine (I use vermouth)
- 2 Tablespoons gluten-free soy sauce*

- 2 Tablespoons honey
- ½ cup gluten-free chicken broth* (or ½ teaspoon gluten-free bouillon* plus ½ cup water)
- 2 Tablespoons cornstarch
- 3 Tablespoons cold water

Put all ingredients into the crock-pot, except cornstarch and cold water. Cook 7 to 9 hours on low. Turn on high. Mix cornstarch with cold water and add. Cook 10 to 15 minutes more until it thickens.

We like this dish served with rice.

## Spicy Lamb Shanks – Crock-pot Style
An unusual gourmet dish that uses dried apricots and prunes. Some gluten-free dishes are low in fiber; adding prunes adds fiber to your diet.

- 4 lamb shanks
- 1 teaspoon salt
- ¼ teaspoon ground black pepper
- 1 cup gluten-free dried apricots (Beware: Some brands may be dusted with oat flour)
- 1 cup pitted prunes (or dried plums)

- 1 cup water
- 2 Tablespoons wine vinegar
- ½ cup sugar
- ½ teaspoon ground allspice
- ½ teaspoon ground cinnamon
- ¼ teaspoon ground cloves

*see gluten-free products list at the end of the book

If you have a standard crock-pot, choose shanks with not too long a bone so that the lid will fit securely. A larger crock-pot works better with larger shanks. Sprinkle shanks with salt and pepper. Place in crock-pot. Add dried fruits. Combine the rest of the ingredients and pour over lamb shanks. Cook on low 7 to 9 hours. Good served with baked yams and green vegetables.

*Variation*: Remove the meat. Remove the fat from the meat juices. (I use a ladle.) Keep the crock-pot on high. Sprinkle in some fine white rice flour and stir it in. Allow juices to bubble, thicken and become gravy. Remove the bones and return the meat to the gravy. Serve over rice. I find that the slow cooking makes the prunes disintegrate into the meat juices and gives the gravy a nice dark color.

*Variation 2*: Dried cherries may be used instead of dried apricots.

## Sweet and Sour Chicken or Pork – Crock-pot Style

This can be an easy recipe to put together using frozen vegetables (see variation below). For the pork I either use frozen chops or a fresh 3-pound roast. For the chicken I skin the chicken thighs ahead of time and freeze in a freezer bag the size of the crock-pot. Or, I purchase skinless thighs and freeze them. The day you want to make it, just remove the plastic and drop it in the crock-pot frozen over the vegetables.

Another method is to freeze the chicken by putting each piece in an individual sandwich bag and put all of them in a larger freezer bag. The day you are making it, remove each from the bags. This is more time consuming but allows you to use the chicken for other dishes because they are not frozen in one big block.

3 large carrots cut into ¼ inch slices
1 large green pepper, chopped
1 medium onion, chopped
2 Tablespoons quick-cooking tapioca
2 ½ to 3 pounds chicken pieces with bone, skinned and frozen (I prefer chicken thighs without backs) or frozen pork chops

1 (8 ounce) can pineapple chunks packed in pineapple juice
⅓ cup brown sugar, packed
⅓ cup red wine vinegar
1 Tablespoon gluten-free soy sauce*
½ teaspoon gluten-free chicken base or bouillon*
½ teaspoon garlic powder
¼ teaspoon ground ginger (optional)

Put carrots, green pepper and onion in the crock-pot. Sprinkle the tapioca over the vegetables. Top with meat. Remove some of the pineapple from the can and put over meat. Now blend the rest of the ingredients together in the pineapple can and pour over meat. Cover and cook on low for 10 to 12 hours. (Or cook on high for 5 to 6 hours.)

*Variation*: You can substitute frozen carrots, pepper and onion for the fresh. It makes it easy to just grab handfuls of the vegetables and add them to the crock.

*Variation 2*: To make a one-pot dish over rice, put 1 cup of brown rice and 2 ½ cups of water in the bottom of the crock-pot. Proceed with the rest of the recipe as written above. Do not substitute white rice or the rice will be overcooked.

*see gluten-free products list at the end of the book*

# Main Dishes – Egg, Cheese, Beans, Rice, and Pasta

## Baked Ziti
I have served this to guests who had no idea this dish was gluten-free.

1 pound gluten-free ziti macaroni (we like Tinkyada® for this recipe)
½ pound cubed gluten-free mozzarella cheese*

Gluten-free tomato sauce*
Grated cheese (Parmesan or Pecorino Romano)

Cook the ziti al dente, according to package directions. Drain and return to pot. Toss in cheese cubes and a cup or two of sauce and mix. Pour a little sauce in the bottom of a deep baking dish. Pour ziti into the baking dish and cover with foil.

Bake in a 350°F oven for 30 minutes or until the cheese melts. Serve with additional sauce and grated cheese.

*Variation*: You can also vary this dish by making a layer of ziti mixture, then a layer of Ricotta mixture as made for Lasagna (see index) then top with another layer of ziti. Bake 40 minutes covered.

*Variation 2*: Sam Mills® penne or ziti pastas tend to break apart if baked in this recipe. If you want to use that brand, boil and drain the pasta as directed. In the same pot you boiled the pasta, heat the tomato sauce. Add the drained pasta and grated mozzarella cheese in the hot sauce. Mix it together. Don't bake it; serve it immediately.

## Black Beans and Rice
A good vegetarian dish. I don't use the vinegar or lemon juice, as I prefer this dish without it. It is more authentic with the "zing", so I've included it in the ingredients list.

1 Tablespoon olive oil
¾ cup onion, chopped fine
½ cup green pepper, chopped fine
1 cup tomatoes, diced (fresh or canned diced tomatoes)
1 (15 ounce) can of Black Beans, and reserve juice

½ teaspoon oregano
1 teaspoon garlic salt
1 Tablespoon cider vinegar or lemon juice (or more or less if desired)
½ teaspoon gluten-free hot pepper sauce* (or to taste)
2 cups cooked rice

Heat a skillet and add oil. Add onion and pepper and cook until crisp tender. Add tomatoes, beans, oregano and garlic salt.

Cook 3 minutes. Add the vinegar, pepper sauce and reserved juice. Continue to cook 5 more minutes. Serve over rice.

This dish reheats well in the microwave.

*see gluten-free products list at the end of the book*

## Black Beans and Rice, Cuban Style (Arroz Congri)
I prefer this recipe to the previous one.  My husband likes this dish for lunch.  Leftovers reheat well in the microwave.

½ lb. dried black beans (also called black turtle beans)
5 cups water
1 green pepper, chopped
½ lb. gluten-free kielbasa* (smoked sausage), cut in small chunks
4 Tablespoons oil
½ lb. onions (or 1 large), chopped
4 gloves garlic, minced or ½ teaspoon garlic powder
1 bay leaf

3 teaspoons salt (this amount is correct, since the dried beans and rice are unsalted)
¼ cup dry white wine or 2 Tablespoons dry red wine plus 2 Tablespoons water
¼ teaspoon cumin
½ teaspoon oregano
1 ½ cups rice
Additional onion chopped fine for garnish (optional)

Wash beans by rinsing them in a sieve.  Pick through the beans to make sure there are no small stones, as beans are dried on pebbles and you wouldn't want one to end up in your food.  Soak the beans in a large pot in the 5 cups water overnight.  Either drain and add 5 cups fresh water, or just cook in the same water until soft.  (I use the same water, since this will make the dish blacker in color.)  Put the lid on the pot, and simmer the beans about 1 hour.  When cooked, drain the water from the beans into a large measuring cup and save only 3 ½ cups of the water.  If you didn't get 3 ½ cups water, add additional water to make this amount.

Chop the kielbasa into small cubes.  (I use a poultry scissors to make it easy.)  Sauté the onion, garlic and green pepper and kielbasa in 4 Tablespoons fat (I use olive oil.)  Add the beans, reserved water, bay leaf, salt, dry wine, cumin, oregano.  When it starts to boil, add the rice and simmer covered until rice is cooked, about 20 minutes.

Remove bay leaf.  Taste to see if more salt is needed.  Garnish with chopped onions (optional).

*Variation*:  Substitute ½ lb. pork, cut in chunks and 2 slices (2 ounces) of bacon, fried and crumbled for the ½ lb. gluten-free kielbasa or smoked sausage.

Fry the bacon, crumble and set aside.  Fry the cubed pork in 4 Tablespoons of bacon fat or oil and set aside.  Sauté the onion, garlic and green pepper in the same bacon fat.  Add the cooked pork in with the beans, water, bay leaf, salt, dry wine, cumin and oregano and proceed with the rest of the recipe above.

Add the bacon back in at the end when it's finished cooking as a garnish.  This version is actually more authentic.  Or, two ounces of gluten-free salt pork may be used instead of bacon.

*Variation 2*:  To make this a quicker dish to make, use 2 (15 or 15.5 ounce) cans black beans, un-drained.  Skip the soaking/cooking dried beans step and go right to the kielbasa step.

*see gluten-free products list at the end of the book*

Use only 1 teaspoon of salt, instead of 3, since canned beans contain salt. I prefer this dish using the dried beans, but this method is a time-saver.

*Variation 3*: Substitute ½ lb. cubed ham for the kielbasa. I suggest using less salt, as sometimes ham may be saltier than kielbasa.

## Breakfast Burritos
**We enjoy these for breakfast on the weekends.**

Eggs (1 or 2 per person)
Milk
Salt and pepper
Grated mozzarella or cheddar cheese

Cooked meat (such as gluten-free ham or sausage)
Corn tortillas (about 2 per person)
Gluten-free mild salsa* (optional)

Make scrambled eggs by blending eggs with a whisk. Add some milk and salt and pepper. Heat a skillet a minute or two. Add some butter or oil to the skillet. Add the eggs. Add meat, if using. Stir until eggs are cooked. Top with the grated cheese.

Heat the corn tortillas. You can either fry them in a little oil, or heat them in the microwave. If heating in the microwave, cover with a damp paper towel and heat for about 1 minute. If using salsa and it is refrigerated, put some in a dish and warm it in the microwave.

To serve, put some eggs on corn tortillas. Top with salsa if desired. Sprinkle with a little extra cheese if desired. If you like spicy food, you can top the burritos with green chilies or use medium or hot salsa. Fold tortillas in half, pick up and eat.

## Broccoli and Spaghetti
**This is a traditional Italian recipe from my mother.**

1 bunch of broccoli (or substitute 1 large bag of frozen broccoli)
½ pound of gluten-free spaghetti*, broken into 1 ½ inch pieces
4 Tablespoons oil (I prefer olive oil)
1 clove garlic minced or ⅛ teaspoon garlic powder

1 cup water
1 teaspoon salt
Generous sprinkling of ground black pepper
Grated cheese (optional)

Cook spaghetti according to package directions. Drain in a colander.

Meanwhile, prepare broccoli by washing, cutting off tough stems and breaking into small flowerets. Peel tough stems and coarsely chop. Skip this step if using frozen.

In a pan (or the pan you just used to cook the spaghetti), put the oil, garlic, broccoli, water, salt and pepper. Bring to a boil and cook until tender. Do not overcook. Do not eliminate the oil, since the oil keeps the pasta lightly coated so it won't be waterlogged in the final dish.

Return the spaghetti to the pot and mix with broccoli. Sprinkle with additional pepper if desired, and some grated cheese.

*Variation*: Cauliflower can be substituted, but I prefer the broccoli.

## Deviled Egg Casserole
This is a good way to use up any deviled eggs leftover after a party or start from scratch.

6 hard boiled eggs
1 Tablespoon chopped parsley
1 teaspoon minced onion
1 teaspoon prepared gluten-free mustard*
⅓ cup gluten-free mayonnaise*
1 package of gluten-free noodles* or
  leftover cooked rice (or use Sam Mills® ½ pkg.
  Lasagna Corte; boil it 2 minutes longer
  than directed on the package)

Sauce:
  5 Tablespoons butter
  5 Tablespoons fine white rice flour or
    sweet rice flour
  2 cups milk
  Salt and ground black pepper to taste
  ½ pound gluten-free American cheese*,
    cut up (cubed or grated)

For eggs that are easy to peel, purchase them a week before boiling them. Prepare hard boil eggs (see index for recipe), shell and cut in half lengthwise. Remove yolks and mix with parsley, onion, mustard and mayonnaise. Fill whites.

Boil noodles according to package directions. (Or prepare 1 cup raw rice according to package directions.) Drain noodles. Make cheese sauce by adding rice flour to milk. (Add rice flour to pot, add a little milk and make a paste. Add the rest of the milk and blend.) Cook until the sauce is thick and comes to a boil. Melt in cheese. Pour half of sauce over noodles or rice and place in a buttered baking dish. Place filled eggs evenly over noodles and cover with remaining sauce. Bake at 350°F for 20 minutes or until just heated through.

## Eggs in Tomatoes
A good way to use leftover, dry (not moldy!) gluten-free bread*

1 cup flavorful gluten-free Italian tomato
  sauce* (see index). Alternatively, I take
  a can of plain gluten-free tomato sauce
  and add some garlic powder, onion
  powder, dried oregano, dried basil,
  grated Pecorino Romano or Parmesan
  cheese, and a dash of Vermouth wine.
1 to 2 eggs per person
Pinch of oregano
Grated cheese
Gluten-free toasted bread*

Heat sauce to very hot. Toast the gluten-free bread and have it ready on a plate. Beat eggs with a little grated cheese and pour slowly while stirring into sauce. Add a pinch of oregano and mix in. Pour over toast.

*see gluten-free products list at the end of the book

## Egg Foo Young

This is a Chinese style omelet. I adapted this recipe to make it easier to prepare. I would be very cautious about ordering this in a restaurant. Some deep fry it in oil used for gluten containing foods. The soy sauce used it most restaurants contains gluten.

1 cup leftover chopped cooked gluten-free ham* or gluten-free roasted pork

½ cup finely chopped onion (or 1 Tablespoon dried minced onion moistened in a little hot water)

1 cup fresh or canned bean sprouts, rinsed and drained (if you don't want to use bean sprouts, use some sliced sautéed celery)

3 Tablespoons chopped scallions (or 1 teaspoon dried chopped chives)

1 Tablespoon gluten-free soy sauce* (I use a little less if using ham)

Sprinkling of salt (optional - This varies depending on how salty the ham is; if meat has no salt use about ½ teaspoon.)

3 eggs

oil to pan fry

Sauce:

1 teaspoon cornstarch mixed

2 Tablespoons cold water

1 teaspoon molasses

1 teaspoon gluten-free soy sauce*

1 ½ cups chicken broth* (or gluten-free bouillon* and water)

Place all omelet ingredients in a bowl (except oil) and blend to incorporate eggs. Heat a large skillet and add oil. (I prefer to use an iron skillet.) Using a deep ladle, ladle the egg mixture in the pan to make 4 separate omelets. Pan-fry until browned on both sides.

If desired, serve with sauce. Mix cornstarch with 2 Tablespoons water in a pot. Then blend all sauce ingredients into the pot and cook until bubbling and thickened. If you don't wish to serve it with the sauce, serve it with a dash of gluten-free soy sauce. Makes 4 servings.

*Variation*: Substitute other meat for the ham or roasted pork, such as cooked chopped chicken, drained canned crab meat or drained canned shrimp.

*Variation 2*: For Subgum Egg Foo Young use the above recipe. In addition, add 1 cup cooked diced mushrooms, ½ cup cooked diced string beans, ½ cup diced canned bamboo shoots rinsed and drained. Mix and cook as directed above. Add a little extra salt if adding the vegetables.

*Variation 3*: Omelets can be deep fried and drained on paper towels. Carefully ladle into hot oil. Turn to cook both sides.

## Fried Spaghetti – Gluten-Free Style

I like the way this turns out with the Tinkyada® pasta. Adults and children like this.

Leftover gluten-free spaghetti that has some gluten-free tomato sauce mixed in it

1 egg per portion

1 Tablespoon grated Pecorino Romano cheese per egg

Salt and ground black pepper

2 to 4 Tablespoons oil as needed

*see gluten-free products list at the end of the book

Heat a Teflon pan and place oil and spaghetti into it. Fry until the spaghetti gets a little brown and crispy on the bottom. Stir and toss once in a while until all spaghetti is heated through and there are crispy pieces here and there. Beat eggs with cheese, salt and pepper. Pour over spaghetti mixing in the egg mixture. When eggs are set, serve.

## Frittata – Oven Baked Style
A frittata is an Italian omelet.

2 small zucchini
1 large green pepper, chopped
½ cup chopped onion
4 eggs
2 Tablespoons oil
½ lb. gluten-free ricotta* cheese

2 oz. shredded gluten-free mozzarella* cheese
2 Tablespoons grated Parmesan or Pecorino Romano cheese
½ teaspoon salt
Sprinkling of ground black pepper

Wash and remove ends of zucchini. Dry, cut in half lengthwise and cut into ½ inch chunks. Dice green pepper and onion. Heat skillet, add oil and heat a few seconds. Add vegetables to skillet and sauté on low heat a few minutes. Cover and continue to cook stirring occasionally until vegetables are tender. Beat 4 eggs in a bowl and add remaining ingredients. Blend well then add cooked vegetables. Butter an 8 inch spring-form pan and pour egg mixture in. Bake in a 350°F oven 45-50 minutes or until a knife inserted in the center comes out clean. Serves 2 to 3.

## Frittata – Skillet Style
A frittata is an Italian omelet.

Use 1 to 2 eggs per person, ½ tablespoon gluten-free grated cheese per egg (optional) and a little salt and pepper.

Choose one or the following vegetables or combinations listed below. (I frequently use leftover cooked vegetables and heat them in the microwave before making the omelet.)

- Green peppers – wash, seed, slice or dice. Sauté in oil until tender.
- Onions – chop and sauté until tender.
- Potatoes – boil, skin and dice. Fry to brown a little.
- Potatoes, onions and green peppers; prepare as above. (This is my Mother's favorite frittata.)
- Zucchini – wash; remove ends, slice or cube and sauté until tender.
- Asparagus – wash, remove woody ends, cut into 1 ½ inch pieces and cook in boiling water with some salt added until tender.
- Mushrooms – wash, slice and sauté.
- Artichokes – frozen ones cooked according to package directions. Drain and slice then sauté briefly in oil.

Now you are ready to make your frittata. Heat a Teflon skillet with straight sides. Add a little sweet butter to coat the bottom and sides of pan when melted. (Or use oil if lactose

*see gluten-free products list at the end of the book

intolerant.) Beat eggs, cheese (if using) and pepper and a little salt. Pour into the pan. Combine the cooked vegetables and add to pan. Cook over medium heat until bottom is cooked and top is a little dry.

Now carefully place a large plate over skillet and invert frittata onto plate. Place skillet back on stove and carefully push the omelet back into it uncooked side down. Cook until eggs are set but not dry. Turn onto a clean plate using the procedure as before, and serve. Using this method you can cut your frittata like a pie, for a nicer presentation.

My mother uses a small skillet and makes more than one frittata, as it is much easier to handle.

I often use grated Pecorino Romano cheese instead of grated Parmesan cheese because it is more flavorful and you can use less cheese.

## Juevos Rancheros
We enjoy this for a light meal served with the microwave polenta (see index). This is my mother's recipe.

1 Tablespoon oil
¼ cup chopped onion
1 can (14.5 ounce) gluten-free tomatoes*
   or gluten-free diced tomatoes*

Sprinkling of Cayenne red pepper to taste
   (or a few dashes of hot pepper sauce*)
4 eggs
Shredded cheddar cheese

Heat a skillet a minute and add the oil. Sauté the onion. Add the tomatoes and cayenne red pepper. Cook 15 minutes. Make 4 holes in the tomato mixture. Crack an egg and drop one into each hole. Cover and cook 2-3 minutes. Uncover and top with shredded cheddar cheese. Cover and heat 1 minute. Serve with polenta (see index).

## Juevos Rancheros – Easier Version
This is faster to make than the previous version. I make microwave polenta, and while it is cooking I make this dish to go with it. My husband likes it for brunch.

2 Tablespoons dried minced onion
1 can (14.5 ounce) gluten-free diced
   tomatoes*

2 Tablespoons (about half the can) diced
   green chilies, drained (I use mild)
4 eggs
Shredded cheddar cheese

Put onion, tomatoes and green chilies in a skillet with a lid. Cook 5 minutes uncovered. Make 4 holes in the tomato mixture. Crack an egg and drop one into each hole. Cover and cook 2-3 minutes. Uncover and top with shredded cheddar cheese. Cover and heat 1 minute. Remove from heat and serve with polenta (see index).

*see gluten-free products list at the end of the book

## Lasagna

My mother is Italian, and this is our favorite version. Most Ricotta and mozzarella cheeses are gluten-free, but check the ingredients. If it lists modified food starch, you should verify the source. When it lists vinegar in the U.S., it is usually corn vinegar. Distilled vinegar is also safe.

1 package gluten-free lasagna pasta* (I use Tinkyada®)
3 pounds gluten-free ricotta*
6 eggs
⅓ cup grated Pecorino Romano cheese

Salt and ground black pepper
Grated or sliced gluten-free Mozzarella cheese*, about 1 pound
Gluten-free tomato sauce (I use the meat sauce recipe, see index).

Boil the lasagna according to package directions. Drain into a colander and rinse with cold water for easier handling. (So that my lasagna has a better presentation, I like to lay the individual lasagna pasta on the counter after it is drained. I also piece together any that fell apart and use them in my 2ⁿᵈ layer of pasta and leave the best ones for the top layer.)

Mix Ricotta with grated Pecorino Romano cheese, eggs, and a few dashes of pepper. (I do this in the same pot I used to boil the pasta.)

Coat the bottom of a large baking pan with sauce. Place enough strips (⅓ of them – but keep the best ⅓ for the top) to cover the bottom over the sauce. Top with half of the Ricotta mixture, half of the Mozzarella and a little sauce.

Place the next strips over the layer. Top with remaining ricotta and a little sauce. Now take remaining pasta and top with it. Top with more sauce and the rest of the mozzarella cheese. Bake at 350°F for 1 hour and 15 minutes. Remove from oven and let sit 10 minutes before cutting. Serve with additional sauce and grated cheese. Serves 12.

*Variation*: If you can't find gluten-free lasagna noodles*, you can substitute gluten-free ziti pasta and layer it the same way. It won't be as pretty, but it's easier to put together and just as tasty.

*Variation 2*: You can use the crepes listed in the manicotti recipe (see index) and layer them for lasagna instead of rolling them for manicotti. For 3 pounds of ricotta cheese, I make 2 batches of crepes instead of the 3 noted in that recipe, so it is less work to make. You can also make the crepes a day ahead of time and refrigerate them. (You will be able to layer them for lasagna, but you will not be able to roll them for manicotti if they are made ahead of time.)

*Variation 3*: Use Sam Mills® Lasagna Corte Pasta prepared and drained as directed on the package. This pasta is shaped like mini lasagna pieces. Mix it in with the ricotta cheese mixture and mozzarella cheese instead of layering it. This makes it very fast to put together. Since this pasta tends to absorb a little more water than the Tinkyada® brand, I add ½ cup water to the cheese mixture. Put sauce on the bottom of the pan, pour in filling mixture, top with sauce and cheese. Bake as directed above. Top with more hot extra tomato sauce when you serve it.

*see gluten-free products list at the end of the book

## Lasagna Northern Style

I enjoy this lasagna. Instead of the ricotta filling, it has this wonderful flavored cream sauce. I often make it in the summer because you don't have to bake it. After assembling the lasagna, allow it to cool and refrigerate. Then slice it and put the servings into microwave containers. Reheat and enjoy. This is also a good recipe for those that cannot eat dairy, because you can easily convert it using a gluten-free milk substitute*.

Cream Sauce: (Note: I usually double the cream sauce recipe if using the whole box of Tinkyada® Lasagna)
3 cups milk
1 small onion, sliced, or 1 Tablespoon dehydrated onion flakes, or ½ to 1 teaspoon onion powder (I use granulated onion powder)
2 bay leaves
Salt to taste
Ground black pepper to taste or ½ teaspoon peppercorns

Sprinkling nutmeg
3 to 4 whole cloves
5 Tablespoons fine rice flour or sweet white rice flour
4 to 5 Tablespoons grated Pecorino Romano cheese
Gluten-Free Lasagna noodles*, prepared according to package directions
Gluten-free mozzarella cheese*
Gluten-free grated cheese*
Gluten-free tomato sauce* (see index)

Put milk, onion, bay leaves, cloves, sprinkling of salt and nutmeg, and peppercorns in a pot. Bring to a boil and simmer together for 10 minutes. Strain the mixture using a sieve, retaining all the liquid. Throw away the bulk left in your sieve. Put the rice flour in the pot and blend in the milk mixture using a whisk. Bring to a boil and stir. It will be thick. Turn off the heat. Add the Pecorino Romano cheese and stir in until it melts. This thick cream sauce will be used in place of the ricotta in your lasagna. Taste and add more salt if needed.

Prepare lasagna noodles* according to package directions. Once cooked and rinsed, I lay them out on the counter and choose the perfect strips for the top of the lasagna.

Put some tomato sauce in your lasagna pan first and cover the bottom with a thin layer of it. This will prevent sticking after it is baked. (See index for tomato sauce recipe or use a jar of gluten-free sauce*.) Next, add a layer of gluten-free lasagna noodles. Then add some of the cream sauce (a ½ or ⅓ depending on how many layers of lasagna noodles you have). Then add some mozzarella cheese and grated cheese. Repeat until you get to the top layer, then finish with a layer of lasagna noodles and top with sauce and cheese.

Bake at 350°F about a half hour until heated through and cheese has melted.

*Variation*: If you want a delicious lasagna without tomato sauce, use the pesto sauce (see index) instead. It is a gourmet tasting dish that we enjoy. I have made this for people allergic to tomatoes, as well as for cancer patients (chemotherapy can make tomato sauce taste like metal), and they have enjoyed this dish.

*Variation 2*: If you do not have gluten-free lasagna noodles, make the crepes as in the manicotti recipe and layer using those.

*see gluten-free products list at the end of the book

## Lentil Stew

This is a good vegetarian dish. It's flavorful with a lot of spice. My husband normally doesn't like lentils, but he likes this dish.

1 lb. lentils
5 cups water
2 medium onions, diced
1 Tablespoon gluten-free soup base*
2 cups gluten-free tomato sauce*
1 small bay leaf
½ teaspoon each of garlic powder, gluten-free dry mustard*, ground cinnamon, ground ginger, ground nutmeg, dried

savory, dried oregano and ground cloves (cloves are optional, I don't use)
2 teaspoons liquid smoke
2 cups tomato juice
3 Tablespoons molasses
2 Tablespoons barbecue sauce (see index for recipe) or ketchup

Wash and pick through lentils. Discard any pebbles. In a pot combine water, lentils and seasonings. Bring to a boil. Reduce heat and cook 30 minutes. Add remaining ingredients and simmer covered 15 minutes more. Remove bay leaf. Serves 8. This freezes well. I like it served over rice. This reheats well in the microwave.

## Macaroni and Cheese

I prefer the Tinkyada® or Sam Mills® elbow macaroni for this dish because it holds its shape better for leftovers. Mrs. Leeper's® is also good but if you use the Mrs. Leeper's, decrease the milk to 3 ½ cups and use ½ Tablespoon less fine white rice flour, and a little less salt, since the package of macaroni is 12 ounces instead of 16 ounces.

1 lb. Tinkyada® or Sam Mills® elbow macaroni or 12 oz. package Mrs. Leeper's® corn elbow macaroni
4 cups milk
4 to 6 ounces grated or cubed baby Gouda cheese or gluten-free American cheese*, or other gluten-free cheese of your choice. (I think American and Gouda melt better than cheddar cheese.

Some cheddar cheeses give cream sauces a grainy texture. See note below.)
1 teaspoon salt
⅛ teaspoon ground black pepper
4 Tablespoons fine white rice flour or sweet rice flour

Cook macaroni according to package directions and drain. If I am going to bake it, I use the least amount of cooking time recommended. Place the macaroni in a butter casserole dish. In the same pot I used to cook the macaroni, add the salt, pepper, and sweet rice flour. Add a little bit of the milk to blend. Then add the rest of the milk. Turn on the heat, and add the cheese. Cook until the sauce bubbles and cheese has melted. Pour over macaroni and bake in a 350°F oven for 20 minutes. You can eliminate the baking step and it is still good. I just boil the pasta to the longest suggested cooking time on the package.

*Variation*: You can use this cheese sauce for vegetables, over rice, or even thin it down with milk as a base for a cream soup. What is so wonderful about using rice flour is you don't need the butter (extra calories) and you can freeze this sauce without it separating.

*see gluten-free products list at the end of the book

*Variation 2*: For a more "sophisticated" version, add 1 (14 ounce) can of diced tomatoes and 8 chopped fresh basil leaves to the milk/rice flour mixture. Cook until it thickens. Add the cheese and stir until it is melted in. Follow the rest of the directions.

Note: If using a cheese such as cheddar, cook the milk/rice flour mixture until it thickens. Remove from heat and then stir in the cheddar cheese until it melts. This will help prevent the grainy texture. Boiling cheddar cheese makes it grainy.

*Variation 3*: I prefer to make my own cheese sauce using milk and real cheese. If you don't want to, you can melt some Velveeta® from Kraft (which is gluten-free as of this writing) and use it instead of the cheese sauce.

## Manicotti

This is my mother's recipe for manicotti with the crepes adjusted to be gluten-free. (This crepe recipe comes from an Argo® cornstarch recipe pamphlet. The filling comes from my mother.) If you want a special meal for company, this is it! No one would ever guess that it's gluten-free. For company, I have small porcelain baking dishes. I put two to three manicotti in each, bake and serve. It makes a nice presentation.

Crepes:
 2 eggs
 ¾ cup milk
 1 Tablespoon oil
 ¼ teaspoon salt

½ cup cornstarch or ½ cup Gluten-Free Naturals™ All Purpose Flour (The crepes made with the Gluten-Free Naturals™ All Purpose Flour are more substantial and a little easier to cook.)

Mix all ingredients except the butter in a blender. (I use my hand blender and the cup it comes with.) Heat a 6 inch Teflon® skillet, add a little butter and swirl it around to coat the pan. Heat the pan a few minutes then lift it off the heat. Pour about 2 Tablespoons or so of batter into the center of the pan and tip pan from side to side until the bottom is covered with the batter. Return to heat. When batter looks dry (about 30 seconds), take a dull table knife and lift one edge of crepe until you can take hold of it with your fingers. Now carefully pull the crepe up and flip it over. Cook a few seconds, lift pan and toss crepe out onto a linen towel or on a plate to cool. Be careful that your pan doesn't overheat. Lower heat and raise heat as needed. Add more butter after every 2 to 3 crepes if needed. (I use a new Teflon pan, so it doesn't need much butter.) This recipe makes about 10-12 crepes (8-10 crepes using the Gluten-Free Naturals™ All Purpose Flour), which is enough for this amount of filling. Triple the recipe for a crowd.

Manicotti filling for 10-12 crepes:
 1 lb. gluten-free Ricotta cheese*
 Salt and ground black pepper to taste
 2 eggs

2 Tablespoons good grated Pecorino Romano cheese
Gluten-free Mozzarella*, cut into strips
Gluten-free flavorful tomato sauce* (jar or homemade)

Mix Ricotta, salt, pepper, eggs and grated cheese together. Place 2 to 3 tablespoons filling down the center of each crepe. Top the filling with a strip of Mozzarella and roll. Place seam side down in a tomato sauce covered baking pan. Continue until all are filled and placed in neat rows in the pan. Spread a little more sauced over top and cover with foil.

*see gluten-free products list at the end of the book

Bake in a 350°F oven 45 minutes to 1 hour. Let it sit 5 minutes before serving. Top with additional sauce and grated cheese.

(If I don't have any homemade sauce, I use the small cans of sauce and add some Pecorino Romano cheese, garlic powder, dried basil and some oregano.)

*Variation*: For a lower carbohydrate gluten-free crepe, use ¼ cup defatted soy flour, 1 tablespoon oil, ¼ teaspoon salt, 2 eggs and water to get the batter the right consistency. I prefer the cornstarch crepe above, but some people watching their intake of carbohydrates, or those that must be dairy-free, prefer soy crepes.

## New Zealand Spaghetti

You can make this dish with rice instead of gluten-free spaghetti, but we prefer the pasta. It makes a lot of food and is great for a party. This also works well with gluten-free linguini. This is one of those recipes that surprise non-celiacs when they learn it's gluten-free. This recipe is a good dish to bring to church suppers.

3 onions, chopped

3 stalks of celery, chopped (I prefer it finely chopped)

Oil, about 1 Tablespoon

1 ½ pounds of lean ground beef (I use ground round or a mixture of ground beef, turkey or pork)

3 small cans (6 ounces each) of tomato paste

3 small cans of water (use tomato paste can)

1 teaspoon salt (or less if cheese is salty)

3 Tablespoons chili powder (I use less, especially if I am making this for children)

1 lb. of gluten-free spaghetti* (I like Tinkyada® or Sam Mills® in this recipe)

½ lb. grated gluten-free sharp cheddar cheese*

¾ cup canned evaporated milk (regular milk can be substituted but evaporated is better)

Boil the spaghetti according to package directions, and drain. Meanwhile, chop the onions and celery. Sauté the onions and the celery a few minutes in a little oil (I use olive oil.) Add the ground meat, break it apart and brown it. If meat is fatty, drain excess fat. Add the tomato paste, water, salt, and chili powder and cook for 10 minutes. Remove from heat. Mix in drained spaghetti and half the cheese. Pour mixture into a very large oblong pan and top with remaining cheese. Pour the milk over the top and bake it for a half hour at 350°F. Serves 10.

## Noodle Kugel

If you miss the taste of this Jewish dish, here is a way to enjoy it again.

1 (12 ounce) package gluten-free noodles* or 8 ounces (½ package) of Sam Mills® Lasagna Corte Noodles

1 Tablespoon butter

1 cup gluten-free sour cream*

1 cup milk

3 beaten eggs

3 Tablespoons sugar

½ teaspoon salt

⅛ teaspoon ground cinnamon

¼ cup raisins

*see gluten-free products list at the end of the book

Cook noodles according to package directions. (If using Sam Mills®, I cook 2 minutes longer than suggested on the package.) Drain and leave in a colander. In the same pot, melt butter. Remove from heat and add sour cream, milk, eggs, sugar, salt, and cinnamon. Mix well and toss in raisins and noodles. Pour into a buttered baking dish and bake in a preheated 400°F oven for 45 minutes.

If you would like to have a topping, mix ½ cup of gluten-free crushed cornflakes, 1 Tablespoon brown sugar and 1 Tablespoon melted butter. Sprinkle this over the kugel before baking.

## Pad Thai Noodles

This recipe originally comes from A Taste of Thai®'s website. See variation if you prefer Lo Mein or don't want to purchase the expensive packet of sauce.

6 ounces of gluten-free Pad Thai noodles*
    (A Taste of Thai® or Tinkyada®)
4 Tablespoons oil, divided
1 egg, beaten
½ pound of either: raw shrimp, deveined
    and peeled or ground pork or ground
    chicken or ground turkey or a
    combination

4 scallions or green onions, chopped
½ cup chopped peanuts (or less)
1 Packet of A Taste of Thai® Pad Thai
    sauce* (labeled gluten-free) or see
    variation below
2 cups of bean sprouts (I used canned
    bean sprouts and drain them)
Cilantro and lime wedges for garnish

Soak noodles according to package directions and drain well. (Or cook Tinkyada® according to directions.) Heat 2 Tablespoons of oil in a wok. Scramble the egg in the oil. Add the shrimp or meat and stir-fry until cooked through. Add the remaining oil and well drained noodles. Stir fry about 4 to 7 minutes until tender. Add the scallions, peanuts, and Pad Thai sauce. Stir fry a minute. Add the bean sprouts and blend in. Serve and garnish with cilantro and lime wedges.

*Variation*: When I didn't have the Thai Sauce, I substituted the sauce used in the Stir Fry with Beef recipe (see index). My husband liked it better. It is not traditional Thai, but is similar to Lo Mein. Eliminate the garnish. Substitute cashews for peanuts, if desired.

## Pasta and Chickpeas or Beans (Pasta Ceci)

A good vegetarian dish. This was one of my sister's favorite meals when she was a child.

2 Tablespoons oil
2 cloves garlic or ¼ teaspoon garlic
    powder
1 onion, minced
1 Tablespoon dried basil
½ teaspoon dried oregano
1 teaspoon salt
½ teaspoon sugar

⅛ teaspoon ground black pepper
1 (29 oz.) can tomato puree*
1 (19 oz.) can chickpeas (ceci) or
    cannelloni beans
½ pound gluten-free elbow macaroni* (I
    use either Sam Mills® or Tinkyada®)
Grated cheese (optional)

*see gluten-free products list at the end of the book*

Place oil in a saucepan and heat. Add garlic and onion and sauté until onion is translucent. Add spices and blend together. Add puree and cook about 15 minutes. Add the chickpeas or beans and continue cooking 5 minutes more to blend. Meanwhile, cook the pasta according to package directions. Drain cooked pasta and combine with sauce. Serve immediately for a soupy dish or let sit a few minutes for a thicker one, as the pasta will absorb much of the sauce. Top with grated cheese if desired.

## Pasta and Peas

You can serve this over gluten-free pasta or rice. My mother's original version did not have the bacon, but I like the bacon flavor with the peas. Or some gluten-free diced ham may be used instead of the bacon.

6 slices bacon
Oil (I prefer olive oil)
1 large onion, diced
1 can peas, un-drained

½ pound gluten-free spaghetti*, broken into 1 ½ inch pieces (I use either Sam Mills® or Tinkyada®)

Boil the water for spaghetti and cook according to package directions.

Meanwhile, in another pan cook the bacon until crisp. Remove from pan and add enough oil to make 4 tablespoons of fat. (For lower cholesterol diets, discard the bacon fat and replace it with 4 Tablespoons olive oil.) Add onions and sauté slowly until soft but not brown. Turn off heat and add peas and liquid. Return to heat; add salt to taste and some pepper. Heat until very hot. When spaghetti is cooked, drain lightly and return to pot. Crumble the bacon. Add the bacon to the spaghetti, and pour the peas and onion sauce over the top and mix together. Adjust seasonings and serve in soup bowls.

*Variation*: If you would rather have tomato sauce, drain most of the pea liquid and add an 8 ounce can of gluten-free tomato sauce*. You can eliminate the bacon.

*Variation 2*: Diced ham may be used instead of bacon.

## Quiche – Crustless Version

You can make the quiche of your choice using this recipe. This is a good use of small amounts of leftovers. For an easy spinach quiche, see the spinach pie recipe in this book.

Filling of your choice (see suggestions below)
1 Tablespoon dried minced onion flakes (optional)
⅓ cup fine white rice flour
⅛ teaspoon salt
¾ teaspoon baking powder
2 Tablespoons oil (optional, I don't use)

3 Tablespoons gluten-free cream cheese*
2 cups milk
4 eggs
1 to 1 ½ cups grated cheese, depending on your preference. (I use 1 cup of grated cheddar cheese. Swiss cheese is also good.)

Grease a 10" or 9 ½"deep dish pie plate. Put your choice of filling on the bottom of the pie plate. Cover the bottom of the plate, but do not stack the filling too high or you won't have

*see gluten-free products list at the end of the book

room for the egg mixture. Sprinkle onion flakes on top, if desired. In a large 4 cup measuring cup, put in the rest of the ingredients, except the grated cheese. Mix with a hand blender until well mixed. (Or, use a regular blender until well mixed.) Pour over the filling in your pie plate. Top with grated cheese. Carefully put in the oven (do not spill), and bake at 400°F for 35 to 45 minutes. Test by inserting a knife and checking that it comes out clean. Baking times can vary depending up the amount of vegetables added.

Some suggested filling choices:
- One (14.75 ounce) can salmon with bones and skin removed, and some diced scallions or some dried sliced chives
- Diced ham, cooked diced green pepper and cooked diced onion or dried onion flakes.
- Cooked, drained sausage with 1 small onion and ½ green pepper, diced and cooked.
- Cooked, drained sausage or ham with 1 small can mushrooms, well drained
- Frozen diced broccoli cooked and drained
- Cooked asparagus or canned asparagus well drained, cut into bite sized pieces. If desired add a ½ of a roasted red pepper, diced and drained.

*Variation*: If you don't like the grated cheese too browned on top, add it immediately as the quiche comes out of the oven. It will melt in about 5 minutes and make a nice topping.

*Variation 2*: Instead of rice flour use ½ cup Gluten-Free Naturals™ All Purpose Flour. Grease the pan well since the pie tends to stick to the pan a little more using this flour. The texture will be more like a soufflé than a pie.

## Quiche – made with Broccoli and Rice Crust
This rice "crust" is easier to make than a rolled out pie crust, and has less fat.

1 ½ cups cooked rice (I use a little less – just enough to cover the pie plate)
3 medium eggs
8 oz. grated, sharp cheddar cheese
Salt to taste
¾ cup drained, canned sliced mushrooms

1 ½ cups (10 oz. package) frozen chopped broccoli (thawed)
Sprinkling of ground black pepper
¼ cup milk

Combine rice, 1 egg (slightly beaten), half the cheese, and salt. Mix well. Press firmly in an even layer on the bottom of a well-greased 9 inch pie pan. Beat remaining eggs (I use the same bowl). Stir in mushrooms, broccoli, and milk. Season with salt and pepper. Spoon the filling mixture over the rice mixture in the pie pan. Bake at 375°F for 20 minutes. Sprinkle remaining cheese over top and bake 10 minutes longer. Cool for 10 minutes. Slice and serve. Note: this recipe will not work without the cheese in the crust.

## Quiche Lorraine – made with Shredded Potato Crust
**This is easy and delicious. I serve this quiche for brunch or dinner.**

2 cups frozen gluten-free shredded
   potatoes*
1 can of mushrooms, drained
4 slices of gluten-free cooked bacon*,
   crumbled or some cubed leftover
   gluten-free ham*
1 Tablespoon dehydrated onion (optional)

1 cup grated Swiss cheese (or grated
   cheddar cheese)
3 eggs
Salt and ground black pepper to taste
2 Tablespoons fine white rice flour or
   sweet rice flour
1 cup milk

Grease a large pie plate with oil. Spread frozen potatoes in pie plate, as for a crust. Add more potatoes if needed to cover. Microwave it on high power for 5 minutes. Be careful, they will be hot. Take ½ cup of cheese and sprinkle over the potatoes. Drain mushrooms and sprinkle over cheese. If using bacon or dehydrated onion, sprinkle over mushrooms. Beat together eggs, salt, pepper, rice flour and milk and add. Top with the rest of the cheese. Bake at 350°F for 30 to 45 minutes or until set. (Test with a fork and it comes out clean.)

*Variation*: If you can't find gluten-free frozen potatoes, take 2 fresh potatoes. Wash and grate. (There is no need to peel them. I use a food processor or Salad Shooter® to grate potatoes.) Brown them in a fry pan with some oil, and sprinkle with salt and pepper. Press the potatoes down in the pan with your spatula and do not mix. When the bottom is browned, transfer it to your pie plate. (Slide it out of the pan and into the pie plate, keeping the brown side on the bottom). Push into the pie plate with the spatula and then continue with the rest of the recipe. Using the fresh potatoes is much cheaper than the frozen, and you will know for sure that they are gluten-free.

*Variation 2*: You can use "Our Favorite Pie Crust" or the "Crepe Pie Crust" instead of the potatoes. For breakfast we liked the potatoes because it seemed more like a breakfast food with potatoes, bacon, and eggs in the pie. The choice is up to you.

*Variation 3*: If you want a browner potato crust made in the oven, follow these directions. Defrost potatoes and squeeze the moisture out of potatoes using a paper towel. Mix potatoes with 2 to 3 Tablespoons melted butter or oil. Press into pie plate using a spoon to form the crust. Bake for about 20 minutes at 450°F until golden brown. Be careful not to burn it. Remove from oven and add the rest of ingredients as directed above. Reduce oven temperature to 350°F. Bake quiche for about 30 minutes or until set. (I prefer the first method because it is easier to make, uses less baking time, and doesn't use the extra fat.)

*see gluten-free products list at the end of the book

## Quesadillas
Think of these as Mexican grilled cheese sandwiches.  You can also cut them up into small pieces for appetizers.  Quesadillas turn out the best if you cook them in an iron skillet.

1 onion, chopped
¼ teaspoon garlic powder
Sprinkling of salt
Oil or gluten-free cooking spray

1 can of mushrooms, drained or 1 (8 oz.) package fresh mushrooms cleaned and sliced
Gluten-free corn tortillas*
Monterey jack cheese

Chop onion.  Cook in a skillet and sprinkle garlic powder and a little salt on top.  Cook until onions are just about done.  Drain mushrooms and add.  Heat through.

Heat another skillet a moment (preferably an iron pan) and add some oil.  (Or spray the pan with gluten-free cooking spray.)  Add a corn tortilla and heat on one side. Flip over.  Now add a small amount of the mushroom mixture and a piece of cheese on one half. With your spatula, fold over the other half.  Cook on one side of the half, then flip and cook on the other until the cheese melts. You will have a delicious Mexican grilled cheese sandwich.

Sometimes I use a whole piece of cheese, top one-half with the mushroom mixture and fold.  It's easier to flip since the cheese sticks it together and it's more flavorful.

*Variation*:  They are also good without the vegetables.  You can use grated cheese mixed with a little sour cream.  Follow directions as above.  Serve with gluten-free salsa* (see index) for dipping.  You can also use cheese and leftover crumbled bacon.  Be creative!

*Variation 2*:  Children like the tortillas prepared as above with gluten-free American cheese and no vegetables.  We like these sandwiches served with tomato soup (see index) for a nice lunch.

## Southwestern Black Bean Pie
I like this for a very easy light meal.

1 (15 ounce) can of corn, drained
1 medium onion chopped or minced, or 1 Tablespoon dehydrated onion flakes
1 (15 ounce) can of black beans, rinsed and drained
½ cup Gluten-Free Naturals™ All Purpose Flour
⅛ teaspoon salt
¾ teaspoon baking powder

½ cup milk
½ cup gluten-free salsa* (or see index) or flavorful tomato sauce made with onions, peppers or mushrooms
2 eggs
Extra salsa or warmed tomato sauce as a garnish
½ cup shredded cheddar cheese

Heat the oven to 400°F.  Grease a 10" or 9 ½" deep dish pie plate.  Layer the corn, onions and beans in pie plate.  Sprinkle with cheese.  Blend flour, salt, baking powder with a whisk.  Blend in milk, eggs and salsa and pour over top.

*see gluten-free products list at the end of the book

Bake 45 minutes at 350ºF or until the bread part on top tests done with a cake tester. Cool 5 minutes. Serve with additional salsa or hot tomato sauce as a garnish if desired.

Note: My husband likes it best made with the tomato sauce and topped with warm sauce when served. He thinks it's slightly dry without it. I like mine without and don't think it's too dry.

## Spaghetti with Clam Sauce
Easy to make and very authentic tasting.

1 pound gluten-free spaghetti (I prefer Sam Mills® for this, but Tinkyada® is also good)
¼ cup oil
¼ teaspoon garlic powder, or 1 to 2 cloves of garlic (see variation if using garlic cloves, which is more authentic)
2 cans of clams with their juice

⅓ cup chopped Italian parsley or 3 Tablespoons dried parsley or more (I use a whole bunch of parsley)
1 bottle of clam juice (optional, I use if using Sam Mills® spaghetti)
Salt and ground black pepper
Parmesan cheese (optional)

Boil the gluten-free pasta according to package directions. (I cook it 2 minute longer than directed on the package.) Drain in a colander.

Put the oil, garlic, clams, juice and parsley in a pan and heat through. Do not overcook. Drain pasta and mix with sauce. Add salt and pepper to taste. (If using clam juice, let sit a few minutes before serving so some of the juice is absorbed in the pasta. I prefer this because I find it makes the dish more flavorful. It also makes the pasta a little bit softer with better texture for leftovers.) If desired, sprinkle with Parmesan cheese.

*Variation*: If you would rather use fresh garlic, use 1 or 2 whole cloves. Put the oil in the pot. Brown the garlic in the oil on all sides. Carefully press the garlic with a fork to release more of its flavor. (Be careful that the oil is not too hot or it can spatter.) Remove the large pieces. Let oil cool down so you can add the rest of the sauce ingredients without it spattering.

## Spaghetti with Creamy Shrimp Sauce
You can use gluten-free spaghetti or gluten-free spinach linguini for this recipe.

½ lb. of gluten-free Spaghetti*
2 cups milk
3 Tablespoons sweet rice flour or fine white rice flour
½ teaspoon salt (or to taste, if olives are salty I use less)
Ground black pepper to taste
1 (3-ounce) can mushrooms

½ cup pitted black olives*, sliced
1 Tablespoon lemon juice
½ teaspoon dill
1 ½ lb. cooked shrimp (I use the frozen cooked shrimp, defrost it and peel off the remaining shell on the tails)
Parmesan cheese

*see gluten-free products list at the end of the book*

Boil water and prepare pasta.  Cook according to package directions.  Drain in a colander in the sink.

Now use that same pot you cooked the pasta in and put the rice flour in it.  Pour in some of the milk and blend.  Add remaining milk, salt, and pepper to taste.  Bring to a boil.  Add mushrooms, olives, lemon juice, dill and shrimp.  Heat through.

Return pasta to the pot and blend with sauce.  Serve.  Sprinkle with Parmesan cheese, if desired.

## Spaghetti Pie
Some Italians occasionally like their spaghetti baked and very crunchy on the top.  When we were children we used to fight over who would get the hard top corners of the lasagna.  If you don't like crunchy spaghetti on the top, see variation below.

½ pound cooked or leftover gluten-free spaghetti*
1 pound gluten-free Ricotta cheese*
2 eggs
2 Tablespoons grated cheese*
Salt and ground black pepper to taste

A little gluten-free ham*, chopped (optional)
Sweet butter or gluten-free oil spray
Gluten-free Tomato Sauce for serving

Mix all together except the butter.  Grease a pie pan generously.  (For a double-recipe, grease a 9x13 pan.)  Pour in the mixture.  Dot the pie generously with bits of butter over the top, or spray with gluten-free cooking spray*.

Bake 30 minutes at 350°F or until the pie sets and is delicately browned.  Cut into servings and top with tomato sauce that you have heated.  This re-heats well in the microwave and freezes well.

*Variation*: Use leftover spaghetti with tomato sauce.  Eliminate ham, butter or oil.  Cook until set.  By using the tomato sauce and eliminating the butter, the top with not be so crunchy.

## Spaghetti with Walnuts, Tomatoes and Green Olives
This is an unusual combination that we had in a restaurant that served gluten-free entrees in Milan, Italy.  We make this to our liking and vary the proportions of ingredients.  The saltiness of the olives, the crunch of the walnuts and the tomato/garlic flavor all worked together in this simple dish.

1 pound gluten-free spaghetti*, cooked and drained according to package directions
Olive oil
Garlic cloves, peeled and whole (at least 2)
1 can of diced tomatoes (about 14 ounce) or fresh diced tomatoes

Walnut halves
Drained whole Green olives* stuffed with pimientos
Salt and ground black pepper to taste (not much salt is needed, since olives add salt)
Grated cheese (optional)

Cook spaghetti according to package directions.  Drain in a colander in your sink.

*see gluten-free products list at the end of the book
-303-

Heat a skillet about a minute and add the olive oil. I use about 6 Tablespoons because this is the basis of your sauce. Add the garlic (I use 2 to 3 cloves). Brown the outside of all of the sides of the garlic. Carefully press it down to release flavor (be careful it can splatter) and remove. Be careful not to burn the garlic or you will transfer a bad taste to the oil and ruin this dish.

Remove oil from heat. Add the tomatoes (be careful, if oil is too hot it will splatter). Blend into the oil. Add the walnuts (I use at least a ½ cup or more) and drained green olives (I use most of the jar) and stir in.

Return to heat and cook a few minutes until hot. This helps toast the nuts a little and incorporate the flavors. If using raw tomatoes it also cooks the tomatoes. Now mix in your drained spaghetti. If you didn't make too much sauce, add less spaghetti. Mix together. Top with grated cheese if desired.

*Variation*: For a spicier dish, some hot pepper flakes can be added to the oil with the tomatoes, after the garlic is browned and removed. Be careful not to burn them.

*Variation 2*: We also had a similar dish in Milan without the walnuts and olives. Instead they used diced tomatoes and calamari (squid). Follow the same procedure with the oil and garlic. Add the tomatoes and cleaned defrosted calamari rings. (Be careful when adding calamari, since the oil can splatter.) I use about a pound of calamari but less may be used. Cook until squid is done but not overcooked. Mix in the spaghetti. Serve with grated cheese if desired. Some parsley, fresh basil, or peas can be added to vary this dish.

## Spinach Pie
This is an easy to make crust-less pie, that is good for brunch, a light lunch or as a side dish. I have also served this as an appetizer. I enjoy the leftovers for breakfast.

1 (10 to 14 ounce) can of spinach, well drained
3 Tablespoons fine white rice flour
3 eggs
1 (8 ounce) carton gluten-free cottage cheese* (I use small curd, about 1 cup)
¼ to ½ teaspoon salt (use ¼ teaspoon if adding sausage)
⅛ teaspoon ground black pepper

4 links of gluten-free brown and serve sausage*, defrosted and sliced (optional; I use Jones Dairy Farm® which is gluten-free as of this writing.)
½ cup grated gluten-free mozzarella*, Swiss*, or cheddar cheese* (I use a little less)

Grease a 9" pie plate or quiche dish. Mix the rice flour, eggs, cottage cheese, salt and pepper together in a bowl. Open the can of spinach and drain it well over the sink. (I use a sieve and push the spinach to drain it and remove as much water as possible.)

Mix the spinach into the egg mixture. If using sausage, defrost links in the microwave according to package directions and slice; mix them in. (The cottage cheese will look lumpy in the blended mixture, but it melts in once it is baked.) Spread mixture into pie plate. Top

*see gluten-free products list at the end of the book

with grated cheese. Bake at 350°F for 30 to 35 minutes until done. The cheese on top will brown and give it a nice flavor.

*Variation*: Use 1 (10 ounce) package of frozen spinach. Defrost in the microwave and add 1 to 2 Tablespoons butter, if desired. Stir to melt in the butter. Allow it to cool. Follow the rest of the recipe. Use ½ teaspoon salt instead of ¼ teaspoon because frozen spinach contains no salt. Mix all ingredients together and bake as directed. Other cooked or canned vegetables may be used instead of spinach. See recipe for quiche for other vegetable combinations.

*Variation 2*: Mix the grated mozzarella cheese in with the other ingredients. I think using the grated cheese as a topping yields a prettier presentation, but this also works.

## Vodka Rigatoni – our favorite!

This recipe is my mother's and we prefer it because not only is it delicious but it's lower in fat and calories. Also, those with some lactose intolerance may find evaporated milk easier to digest than cream.

1 pound gluten-free rigatoni or penne (we like Tinkyada® brand or Sam Mills®)
1 Tablespoon butter
1 Tablespoon olive oil
2 pinches of dried red pepper flakes (or more if desired)
1 large (28 ounce) can of Italian whole or crushed tomatoes*

⅔ cup gluten-free vodka* (we prefer potato vodka)
2 teaspoons fine rice flour (eliminate if using heavy cream)
¾ cups evaporated milk or heavy cream
½ teaspoon salt
¾ cups grated Pecorino Romano or Parmesan cheese

Boil water and prepare pasta according to package directions. I like it cooked "al dente". Drain the pasta. (The energy saving method on the package also works well to cook the pasta.)

Meanwhile, in a large skillet, melt butter. Add olive oil and red pepper flakes and cook 2 minutes on low heat. This will release the red pepper flakes flavor, but be careful as they can burn easily. Remove from heat after 2 minutes. Now add your can of tomatoes and the vodka and blend in. Return to heat and simmer 5 minutes. This will cook off the alcohol of the vodka and make your tomatoes a little thicker.

Add the rice flour to the evaporated milk. Blend and add to the sauce. Add the salt to the sauce and stir in. Cook until thickened. If using the cream, add the cream and salt and heat through. Do <u>not</u> boil if using cream because it will curdle and ruin the texture. Add the cooked, drained pasta and the grated cheese. Mix all together and serve.

Note: Using a large skillet instead of a saucepan makes more of the liquid evaporate so that the sauce will be a good consistency. I use my 12" fryer which has deep sides.

*see gluten-free products list at the end of the book

*Variation*: I have made this without the rice flour when using evaporated milk. The sauce is a little thinner but it's still very good. (Also, leftover pasta absorbs some of the liquid.) If you choose to use rice flour, you can also add it with the tomatoes instead of with the milk.

*Variation 2*: If making this dish ahead of time, I eliminate the rice flour since the pasta tends to absorb more liquid if it sits a while. This helps to thicken the sauce.

## Vodka Rigatoni or Penne – Version 2

This recipe is from an Italian friend, and she says it's very authentic. It's richer than the previous version because it uses heavy cream and ham.

¼ cup (½ stick) butter or gluten-free margarine*

½ teaspoon crushed red pepper (more or less depending on your taste)

¼ pound chopped gluten-free ham* or bacon* or chopped gluten-free Prosciutto Italian ham

1 can (28 ounce) gluten-free crushed tomatoes*

½ cup gluten-free vodka*

¾ cup gluten-free heavy cream*

1 cup Parmesan cheese

1 package (16 ounce) gluten-free Pasta*

Boil water and prepare pasta according to package directions, and drain. If using bacon, prepare it in the microwave per package directions and blot the fat with paper towels. Crumble bacon and set aside.

In a large pot, melt the butter and add the crushed red pepper and ham (if using). Cook on low for 3 minutes and be careful not to burn the crushed red pepper.

Add vodka and cook on high for 2 minutes and then low for 2 minutes more. Add the crushed tomatoes (and bacon if using) and turn up heat for 5 minutes. Add cream, stir, then simmer on low for 12 minutes. Add cheese to pasta and mix well. Spoon some of the sauce on pasta and mix. I add extra sauce over the pasta right onto each plate right before serving.

## Write your own recipes here:

# Vegetables and Side Dishes

My mother always tried to have "all the colors" of vegetables at every meal. That is, she'd have a yellow or orange, a green, and a starch. Thanks to her, I have a variety listed here. Most of these are her recipes that we have enjoyed for years.

## Acorn Squash

This method is much easier than baking them. Instead of struggling to cut the squash when it's hard, you cut it when it's fully cooked.

Wash the outside of the squash and dry. With a cake tester or skewer, poke holes on all sides. Put on a microwave safe dish and microwave on high for 6 minutes. Using pot holders, turn them over and microwave 7 to 9 minutes more. (I use the stem to help turn them over.)

Remove from microwave with potholders. Cut in half lengthwise (be careful there will be steam) and remove seeds with a spoon. Discard seeds. The squash may be cut in half again to make 4 servings. Add a pat of butter and salt and pepper to the squash. Let butter melt. Eat out of the skin.

## Acorn Squash – Stuffed

A gourmet restaurant style dish that is nice during the Fall season.

2 acorn squash (I choose larger ones that are about 1 ½ lbs. each)
1 lb. gluten-free bulk sausage* (or see index for recipe to add spices to pork to make bulk sausage)
1 medium to large onion, peeled and diced
¼ teaspoon marjoram or thyme
2 golden delicious apples, rinsed, cored and diced (If using golden delicious there is no need to peel them. Peel if using other varieties.)
4 to 6 Tablespoons dried cranberries*
4 to 6 Tablespoons dried raisins
1 Tablespoon rice flour or Gluten-Free Naturals™ All Purpose Flour (optional)
½ cup chopped pecans (optional)
2 to 4 Tablespoons maple syrup (preferably real maple syrup)

See above recipe to prepare the acorn squash in the microwave. When cooked set aside to cool, and then cut in half lengthwise and remove seeds. Or for the traditional oven method, cut the squash in half and remove seeds. Place them cut side down and cover with aluminum foil. Bake at 350°F for 45 to 50 minutes until the squash are tender.

Cook sausage in a large skillet until it is no longer pink. (I use a 12 inch skillet so that extra moisture evaporates easily and you don't need added rice flour to thicken stuffing.) Drain any excess fat. Since I usually make my own bulk sausage (see recipe) I don't have any fat to drain.

Add the onions, marjoram, apples, raisins and cranberries. Cook until onions and applies are tender. Stir to ensure it doesn't stick while you are cooking the mixture. If your moisture is too wet, sprinkle in some rice flour and simmer to thicken. Remove from heat and add the pecans and stir them in.

Place the squash cut side up in a baking pan. I prefer to use 2 loaf pans since they have high sides and hold the squash upright. Fill the cavities with the stuffing. Drizzle some of the maple syrup on top of each. Bake at 350°F for 15 minutes.

*Variation*: I have eliminated the maple syrup and the baking, and it is also good.

## Asparagus Parmesan
This is an Italian way to make Asparagus. This is my mother's recipe.

1 pound asparagus
2 Tablespoons white wine
3 Tablespoons melted butter

Parmesan cheese
Ground Black pepper

Try to buy asparagus that is green all the way to the bottom of the spear. If not, remove the woody stems by holding asparagus with both hands. Place right hand at the white woody section and left hand next to it and try to snap the white part off. If you are not able, move left hand slowly to the left while you keep trying to break the unwanted part away. This way you won't discard any of the edible part.

Wash asparagus. Heat a little water and salt in a skillet and add a single layer of asparagus. Cook 5 minutes and spear each asparagus at its toughest part. If the fork goes in easily, it is cooked. Remove each spear of asparagus, as it is tender and place in a baking dish. Melt butter, add wine and pour over asparagus. Now sprinkle with a little black pepper and generously with Parmesan cheese. Bake in the upper third of the oven for 10 minutes at 400°F. Cheese should melt.

*Variation*: We also like asparagus cooked the same way as green beans (see index).

## Baked Beans – Western Style
This is great for a cook out as it serves 12 generously. You usually don't have any leftovers, but if you do you can use them in the baked bean soup recipe (see index). This is my mother's recipe.

8 slices of bacon, fried, drained and
  crumbled
4 large onions, sliced in rings
½ cup brown sugar
1 teaspoon gluten-free dry mustard*
½ teaspoon garlic powder
1 teaspoon salt

½ cup cider vinegar
1 (1 lb. 11 oz.) can of gluten-free Boston
  baked beans* (check labels)
1 (1 lb.) can red kidney beans, drained
1 (1 lb.) can baby lima beans, drained
2 (15 oz.) cans dried lima beans or butter
  beans, drained

Place onions, sugar, vinegar, salt, mustard and garlic powder in a large pot and cook covered for 20 minutes. Add crumbled bacon and beans and mix together. Place in a 3 quart casserole. Bake 30 minutes in a 350°F oven with cover on. Remove cover and bake 30 minutes longer. Makes 12 servings.

*see gluten-free products list at the end of the book*

## Beets and Beet Greens – Fresh
**We like beet greens as well as fresh beets.  This is an easy way to prepare them.**

Purchase beets that have fresh greens.  Prepare greens within a day or so of purchasing the beets.  Remove greens and stems.  Wash.  Use your hands to pull the greens off the stems and discard the stems.  Put greens in a pot with a little salted water and cook until tender.  Drain and add butter, salt and pepper to taste.  The greens from one bunch of beets usually serve 2 people.

For the beets, wash the outside.  Do not remove the root or the beets will "bleed" when they cook.  Put the beets whole in a microwave container.  I use something that won't stain, such as glass or Corningware®.  Choose one that isn't too large, with the beets in a single layer.  Add water about half-way up and cover (vented).  Microwave it for about 15 minutes on high.   Test for doneness with a fork.  Allow to cool.  Once cooled the outer skin and root comes off easily.  I remove it using my hands.  Since beet juice can stain, wash your hands immediately or wear rubber gloves.  I also wear an apron to protect my clothes.  Discard the skin and root.  Slice beets.  I discard the water and add butter, salt and pepper to taste.  They can be reheated in the microwave.  (If you want to make Pickled Beets [see recipe under Salads] or Harvard Beets, don't discard the water.)

## Beets – Harvard Style
**I enjoy this for a change from pickled beets (see index under salads for that recipe).**

| | |
|---|---|
| 1 can of sliced beets | 1 Tablespoon cornstarch |
| 2 Tablespoons cider vinegar | 1 ½ teaspoons sugar |
| ¼ teaspoon salt | |

Put cornstarch, sugar and salt in a pot.  Slowly pour beet liquid into a pot and stir.  Add vinegar.  Cook until it boils.  Add beets and mix in.

## Broccoli and Wine
**I like this Italian version for a change of pace.**

| | |
|---|---|
| 1 large head of broccoli | 2 Tablespoons Vermouth |
| 4 Tablespoons oil (I prefer olive oil) | Grated Parmesan cheese |
| 1 clove garlic | |

Wash and cut the broccoli about 4 to 5 inches in length, cutting away the tough stem.  Peel stems and cut in half.  Place a large pot of water on the stove, and add a little salt.  When the water comes to a boil, add all of the broccoli and cook it about 10 minutes or until just tender.  Test a stem with a fork because if it is tender the flower part will surely be so.  Turn off the heat quickly and add a cup of cold water to stop the cooking and retain the broccoli's color.  Drain and place in a deep serving dish.  Dry the pot well and add oil and heat.  Peel clove of garlic, cut it in half and sauté in hot oil until golden.  Turn off heat and mash the garlic to release its juices and flavor and then discard.  Pour oil carefully over broccoli and sprinkle on the vermouth, top with grated cheese and serve.

*Variation*: This can be made without the vermouth for a different flavor.

## Brussels Sprouts

Sometimes at our farmer's market we are able to get Brussels sprouts on the stem. They are very fresh (not strong tasting). They grow on a stem that looks a little like a mini Christmas tree with the sprouts growing around it from larger to smaller on the top.

| | |
|---|---|
| 1 box fresh or frozen Brussels sprouts | Salt and ground black pepper to taste |
| 1 small onion, chopped | Water |
| 2 slices bacon, chopped | |

If using fresh Brussels sprouts, be sure they are very fresh as they turn bitter as they age. Discard one or two outer leaves and trim a little off the stem. Then cut a cross into the stem part to help that tough part cook evenly with the leafy part of the vegetable. Sauté bacon slowly until crisp. Remove from pot and drain. Remove all but 1 Tablespoon of bacon fat and sauté chopped onion in it.

When onions are golden in color, place sprouts on top of them and add ½ cup water, sprinkling of salt, dash or two of pepper and the bacon. Cover and simmer 15 to 20 minutes until sprouts are tender. Add a little extra water if needed to prevent sticking.

## Butternut Squash

Frozen squash may be substituted to make it easier to make. I think fresh squash is more delicious, and this method allows you to peel the squash after it is partially cooked so that it is not so difficult to do.

| | |
|---|---|
| 1 butternut squash, washed | Salt and ground black pepper |
| 1 or 2 Tablespoons brown sugar | 2 Tablespoons butter |

Place the washed squash in a large pot and cover with water. Cook ½ hour or until a fork can pierce the skin. Drain and cool enough to handle. Cut open the squash and remove the seeds. Discard them, and then peel the squash and discard the peel. Cut squash into chunks and return to the pot along with some salted water. Cook until tender. Mash with a potato masher and add 2 Tablespoons butter, 1 or 2 Tablespoons brown sugar, salt and pepper to taste.

## Cabbage Sauté Side Dish

This is a good side dish vegetable. My mother cuts the cabbage in half, removes the core and slices in ½ inch slices. For guests, she leaves the core intact and cuts the cabbage in wedges. You must be more careful when cooking the wedges to retain the shape, but it looks prettier when served.

| | |
|---|---|
| 1 large Spanish onion | 2 Tablespoons water |
| 2 Tablespoons oil | 2 Tablespoons melted butter or gluten-free margarine* |
| ½ head cabbage | |
| ½ teaspoon salt | ½ teaspoon sugar |

*see gluten-free products list at the end of the book

Heat skillet and add oil and heat a minute.  Add onions and cabbage and sauté on low heat until the vegetables are a delicate golden brown.  Sprinkle the salt and sugar over vegetables as you turn the cabbage to brown both sides.  Add water, cover and cook 5 minutes.  Turn cabbage over and cook another 5 minutes until tender.  Put vegetables in a serving dish.  Melt the butter in the same pan.  Sprinkle over dish.  Serves 4.

## Cauliflower with Easy Cheese Sauce
As children (and now as adults) we always liked this recipe, and this is so easy to make.

1 head cauliflower
2 Tablespoons butter
Salt and ground black pepper

3 to 4 slices gluten-free American cheese*
    (most real cheese is gluten-free.)

Wash and trim cauliflower.  Bring a large pot of water to a boil.  Then add cauliflower and cook until tender.  Drain.  Add butter, salt and pepper and blend.  Place cheese on top of the hot cauliflower in the pot and cover.  In a few minutes, the cheese will melt into a nice light cheese sauce.

## Cauliflower – Whole
I like to make this for company because it's something different.  You leave the cauliflower whole and serve it in a large bowl topped with cheese sauce.

1 whole cauliflower
3 Tablespoons sweet rice flour or fine
    white rice flour
1 ½ cups milk

¼ cup cheese of your choice (I like Gouda
    or gluten-free American* or Cheddar)
Salt and ground black pepper

Remove some core and green leaves from the cauliflower.  Rinse it.  Put some water in a pot and bring it to a boil.  Add cauliflower.  The water will be about 2-3 inches high in the pot.  Cook in water 10 minutes on one side.  (Do not add salt to the water.)  Turn (cook 15-20 minutes total).  Drain.

Now make your cream sauce.  Put the rice flour in a pot, and pour in a small amount of the milk.  Blend.  Now add the rest of the milk and blend.  Add the cheese and bring to a boil.  Add salt and pepper to taste.

Now put the whole cauliflower in a deep casserole dish.  Pour the sauce over top.  You can make this ahead and reheat it in the oven.

## Carrots – Fried Skillet Version
These are delicious because the carrot flavor is very concentrated.

1 lb. carrots
2 to 3 Tablespoons butter

½ teaspoon sugar
Salt

Scrape and wash carrots.  Cut the carrots into ½ inch slices on the diagonal making them about 3 inches long.  The large pieces make this dish quicker to make.  Heat skillet, melt

*see gluten-free products list at the end of the book

butter and place in only enough carrot slices to cover the bottom of the pan. Sauté until carrots are golden, turn them over, reduce heat and continue until carrots are golden on the second side. Remove to a place and continue until all carrots are fried. Now place all carrots back into the skillet. Sprinkle with salt and ½ teaspoon sugar. Add a few Tablespoons of water and cover. When steam stops and you hear the carrots frying again, toss to distribute the sugar and salt and serve.

## Carrots – Hawaiian Style
**This goes well with ham.**

| | |
|---|---|
| 6 scraped and sliced carrots | ½ cup drained crushed pineapple |
| ½ cup water | 1 Tablespoon butter |
| ½ teaspoon salt | 2 Tablespoons cornstarch |
| 2 Tablespoons brown sugar | A little cold water |

Cook carrots until tender in ½ cup water and ½ teaspoon salt. Add drained pineapple, brown sugar and butter. Mix cornstarch with a little cold water and stir in and cook to thicken.

## Carrot Soufflé
**This is my mother's recipe and makes a nice company dish. People always ask for this recipe.**

| | |
|---|---|
| 2 cups cooked mashed carrots, about 1 ½ pounds | 3 Tablespoons cornstarch |
| | 1 teaspoon salt |
| 1 ½ cups rich milk (4%) | ¼ cup honey |
| 3 well-beaten eggs | 4 Tablespoons melted butter |

Boil carrots until cooked or "fork tender". Drain. Mash with a potato masher. Cool. Mix in cold milk. Then add 3 well-beaten eggs, cornstarch and salt. Mix in honey with melted butter and add in. Now butter a casserole dish. Pour mixture into casserole. Bake at 400°F for 45 minutes or until firm.

*Variation*: This is best using fresh cooked carrots. When I did not have fresh carrots on hand, I have substituted 4 cans drained canned carrots and mashed them. This saved the cooking/cooling step. Use less salt, since canned carrots are salty. Not as good, but it works if you're short on time.

## Cornbread Stuffing
**This reminds me of Stovetop® brand stuffing without the gluten.**

| | |
|---|---|
| 1 package Gluten-Free Naturals Cornbread/Corn muffin mix, prepared in an 11" x 17" pan | 1 ½ cups water with 1 teaspoon gluten-free chicken bouillon* or chicken base* |
| 2 stalks celery, washed and sliced | ¼ to ½ teaspoon garlic powder |
| 1 onion, chopped | ½ teaspoon ground sage (optional) |
| A small amount of oil | Salt and pepper |

*see gluten-free products list at the end of the book

Prepare cornbread mix according to package directions. Bake in a greased 11" x 17" non-stick pan for about 20 minutes until the top is browned. Remove from pan and allow it to cool. Cut into cubes. You can also use a poultry scissors to cut it into pieces.

In a pot, cook the onion and celery in a little oil for a few minutes. Add the water, bouillon, garlic powder and sage. Bring to a boil. Remove from heat. Add the cubed cornbread and mix in. If too dry, add a little more hot water. Taste to see if salt and pepper are needed. Some bouillon* is saltier than others.

*Variation*: Instead of chopped onion, substitute 1 Tablespoon dried minced onion. Add it when you add the water and bouillon.

*Variation 2*: Substitute the cornbread cubes in the other stuffing recipe in this book. Or use it in your own favorite recipe.

## Corn Pudding – My Mother's Version
This is nice for Thanksgiving.

| | |
|---|---|
| 1 can gluten-free cream style corn* | ⅛ teaspoon ground black pepper |
| 2 eggs | 2 Tablespoons fine white rice flour |
| ¼ cup sugar | 2 Tablespoons melted butter |
| 1 teaspoon salt | ½ cup milk |

Mix together all the dry ingredients. Beat eggs in the ½ cup milk and beat into dry ingredients. Add corn and melted butter. Grease a casserole dish and pour in the mixture over it. Place casserole in a pan of hot water and bake 1 hour 15 minutes in a 350°F oven.

## Corn Pudding – Version 2
This recipe comes from one of my mother's friends.

| | |
|---|---|
| 1 can gluten-free cream style corn* | 1 ¾ cup milk |
| 3 eggs | 1 teaspoon butter (to grease casserole) |
| 1 teaspoon grated onion | 2 teaspoons green pepper, chopped |
| 1 ½ Tablespoons sugar | 1 teaspoon salt |

Beat eggs and add milk, sugar and salt. Add corn and green pepper and fold in. Grease casserole and pour mixture in. Set it in a larger pan filled with hot water. Bake in a 1 ½ quart casserole at 325°F for 1 hour.

## Corn Pudding – Homestead Style
This is very nice on a holiday buffet table with turkey or ham.

4 cups milk, scalded
½ cup plus 2 Tablespoons cornmeal
¼ cup sugar
½ teaspoon salt
½ cup melted butter

8 oz. canned yellow corn or 3 fresh ears
1 teaspoon gluten-free vanilla*
1 teaspoon gluten-free baking powder*
4 eggs

Scald milk, remove from heat and stir in cornmeal, sugar and salt. Place on low heat and simmer 5 minutes. Remove from heat and add corn, butter, vanilla and baking powder. Stir well. Gradually add 4 eggs. Pour into a greased casserole and bake at 350°F for 45-50 minutes.

## Eggplant Parmigiana or Eggplant Parmesan
I think my mother always made the best eggplant parmigiana, and she never used bread crumbs. This version is so close to hers, that you'd never think it was gluten-free. My mother used to buy a whole bushel at the Farmer's Market, fry them up and freeze them. We'd have this tasty dish all winter. Using rice flour makes this freeze well.

1 eggplant
Fine white rice flour
Egg
1 Tablespoon water
Salt and ground black pepper
Oil to fry in (I like olive or corn oil)

Mozzarella cheese* (sliced or grated, make
  sure it's gluten-free)
Oregano
Grated Italian cheese (I like Pecorino
  Romano but Parmesan is good too)
Gluten-free tomato sauce* (see index)

Peel and slice eggplant into ¼ inch slices. Place the rice flour on a piece of waxed paper. Beat eggs, water, salt and pepper in a pie pan type dish and place next to rice flour. Set out a flat pan and cover it with a couple of layers of paper towels and place it next to your range. Now dip both sides of each slice of eggplant into flour and completely cover. Shake off excess and dip into beaten egg mixture, turning eggplant over to moisten both sides. Place eggplant slices to one side of the pie pan and continue in the same manner with each slice stacking them one on top of the other. This allows the excess egg to run off and gives enough egg to finish the job. If, however, you run out of egg, just add another one to the pie pan along with the water, salt and pepper as you did before. When all slices have been dipped in egg and stacked, let set a while so egg excess drains off. This makes the frying step easier and cleaner as egg doesn't drip all over the stove.

Heat a skillet and add just enough oil to cover the bottom, and heat a minute. Place a few slices of eggplant in skillet and fry both sides to a delicate golden brown. Drain on paper towels and continue until all slices are cooked. Add more towels and continue until all slices are cooked. Add more oil if needed. Sometimes a foam forms on top of the frying eggplant. When this happens, it is best to discard that oil, wipe the skillet with a paper towel and add fresh oil before continuing.

Take a suitable baking dish and layer eggplant, sauce and mozzarella and continue until all ingredients are used up ending with mozzarella. Sprinkle top with oregano and grated cheese. Bake at 350°F for 30 minutes or until bubbly and cheese melts.

You can make ahead of time and freeze the eggplant, with or without the sauce. Do not substitute cornstarch for the rice flour, because the cornstarch will not freeze well.

*Variation*: For a company dish, instead of layering the eggplant you can make eggplant rolls. Sprinkle the fried eggplant with mozzarella cheese. Roll. Put in a small baking dish, so each person gets one. Or line them up in a larger dish. Top with tomato sauce and a little oregano. I give each guest two rolls as a side-dish.

*Variation 2*: See recipe for grilled zucchini and follow same procedure to grill eggplant. Grilled eggplant can be used instead of frying it.

## Eggplant Manicotti
If you like eggplant parmesan and manicotti, you have both flavors in one dish.

Prepare the eggplant by frying as in eggplant parmesan recipe. Drain well on paper towels to remove the excess oil. Prepare the cheese filling as in the recipe for manicotti (see index). Take a large baking dish and put a little tomato sauce in the bottom and spread around until covered. This will keep your eggplant from sticking. Now, take a slice of eggplant and put some cheese mixture in the middle. Roll and put in the pan with the "seam" side down. Continue until all of the eggplant slices are used up. Top with tomato sauce and sprinkle with grated mozzarella cheese. (Or use slices of mozzarella cheese cut in long strips and top each manicotti roll.) Cover with foil. Bake at 350°F for 45 minutes to 1 hour until cheese is set. Remove foil after ½ hour of baking.

## Escalloped Tomatoes
This is a quick and easy winter-time vegetable dish that uses stale gluten-free bread.

3 slices day-old gluten-free bread (do not use moldy bread)
4 slices gluten-free American cheese*

1 pound can gluten-free stewed tomatoes*
Butter or gluten-free margarine*

Butter a loaf pan or small casserole generously. Spread some butter on the day old bread and then cut them into tiny cubes. Place half of the bread on the bottom of the pan. Top with 2 slices of cheese. Open can of stewed tomatoes and pour on top. Cover with 2 more slices of cheese. Last, put the rest of the buttered gluten-free bread cubes on top. Bake at 350°F for 20 minutes.

*see gluten-free products list at the end of the book

## Escarole

My mother used to make escarole pie (see next recipe for crust). Even before I started cooking gluten-free foods, I used to just make the filling and enjoy it as a side-dish with a piece of bread. (Now I enjoy it with gluten-free bread!)

3 pounds escarole
½ cup water
2 to 3 Tablespoons oil (I use olive oil)
1 large clove garlic
¾ cup black pitted olives, sliced

3 Tablespoons pine nuts
2 Tablespoons capers* (optional). Use less salt if using capers.
½ to 1 teaspoon salt
Ground black pepper to taste

Cut away ¼ to ½ inch of the bottom of the escarole heads. If you wish, you can remove the tender yellow leaves, which are delicious in salads. Cut the rest of the leaves into 2 inch pieces and wash well in cold water. Now put escarole in a pot, sprinkle on a little salt and add ½ cup water. Cover and cook 20 minutes or until escarole is tender. (Test the escarole with a fork to make sure it is fork tender.) Drain well in a colander. Dry the pot and add oil and heat. Peel and cut garlic in half and sauté in hot oil until golden brown. Turn off heat to cool slightly. Now mash garlic with a fork to release its juice and flavor. Remove any large pieces and discard. Add escarole to pot along with olives, pine nuts, capers (if using), salt and pepper. Mix together and heat a few minutes. Serve.

## Escarole Pie

My mother invented this pastry, and I converted it to gluten-free. It has yeast it in and is more bread-like. You can use "our favorite pie crust" if you prefer. I enjoy this pie for lunch.

Pastry:
2 cups Gluten-Free Naturals™ Sandwich Bread Flour or Gluten-Free Naturals™ All Purpose Flour (do not substitute any other flour blends or this will not work.)
6 Tablespoons butter

4 to 6 Tablespoons hot milk
2 ¼ teaspoons yeast (1 yeast packet)
Escarole Filling: See previous recipe. Escarole filling should be freshly made and still warm in the pot

Put the gluten-free flour in a food processor. Cut in the butter with the cutting blade. Do not over process. Heat ¼ cup (4 Tablespoons) of the milk to warm (not hot) and add the yeast to it. Let it sit a few minutes. Turn the processor back on, and while it is running pour the milk down the feed tube. The dough should ball up to one side. If too dry, add a little more milk a Tablespoon at a time. If too wet, add a little more flour.

Make 2 balls of dough. Put a piece of waxed paper on your counter. Roll out the bottom crust. Place it in a buttered 9 inch pie plate. Roll out the top crust. Now place the warm escarole in the lined pie plate and cover it with the top pastry. (When you remove the escarole from the pot use a slotted spoon so that you don't put too much of the liquid in the pie or it can make your pie boil oven when it bakes.) Seal the edges by fluting and then prick the top of the crust with a fork.

Let pie crust rise for 45 minutes. The warm escarole will help the dough rise. Bake in a 375°F oven for 1 hour until golden brown. Cool 10 minutes before cutting and serving.

*see gluten-free products list at the end of the book

## Escarole – Baked
My friend from church gave me this recipe. I adjusted it to gluten-free. This is one of those Italian recipes without exact measurements.

1 head escarole
Olive oil
Garlic powder

Day-old gluten-free bread (not moldy!) I use 2 to 3 slices, depending how thick the bread is.
Ground black pepper

Cut away ¼ to ½ inch of the bottom of the escarole head. Wash in cold water and remove any dirt. Spin in a salad spinner to remove all of the moisture. Break leaves into 2 inch pieces and put ⅓ of the escarole in a casserole dish. You will be making 3 layers of escarole. Drizzle a little olive oil over the top of the escarole in the casserole. Sprinkle on a little garlic powder and black pepper. Take a slice of your gluten-free bread and crumble it with your hands over the top. I find that with most gluten-free breads that rubbing my hands together with the gluten-free bread in-between makes it turn into crumbs. (Or pulverize bread in a food processor to make fresh breadcrumbs.) Repeat for the remaining layers. Bake at 350°F for 30 minutes or until the escarole tests done with a fork.

Note: It is important to have the escarole really dry after you wash it. Otherwise it will be too watery, and the gluten-free bread crumbs will become waterlogged.

## Fruit Casserole with Cream Sherry
This is nice on a Christmas buffet table.

1 can sliced pineapple
1 can (large) peach halves
1 can (large) pear halves
1 can apricot halves
1 jar apple rings
½ cup brown sugar

½ cup butter
2 Tablespoons sweet rice or fine white rice flour
1 cup gluten-free cream sherry (I use Gallo®, which is gluten-free as of this writing)

Drain fruit. Cut pineapple slices and peach halves in half. Mix all fruit together in a casserole dish. In a saucepan, melt butter and add flour and blend. Then add sugar and stir in sherry. Cook and stir over low heat until smooth and thick. Pour over fruit and chill overnight. About ½ hour to 45 minutes before serving, place in an oven and set to 350°F. Do not preheat oven. Heat the fruit about 30-45 minutes until hot and bubbly. Serves 12.

## Fruit Casserole with Curry
This is nice served with poultry or ham.

1 can pineapple slices
1 can peach halves
1 can pears
1 can apricots
1 (16 oz) jar gluten-free maraschino
  cherries*

1 cup brown sugar
¼ cup butter
2 to 4 teaspoons gluten-free curry
  powder* (or see index for recipe)
Slivered almonds

Drain fruit well and mix all together and place in a buttered refrigerator to oven baking dish. Cook sugar, butter and curry in a saucepan until sugar and butter melt. Pour over fruit and refrigerate covered overnight. Bake in a preheated 350°F oven for 45 minutes uncovered. Sprinkle with nuts.

## Green Beans

Make green beans as you would make broccoli or Brussels sprouts. Wash green beans and remove the stems. (Some people remove a little on both ends, but I only remove the stem side since this is what restaurants do so you know they are fresh green beans.) Place the green beans in a pot of boiling salted water. Watch and test the beans often as you only want to cook them to the crisp tender stage. Overcooking makes the green beans turn a sick grayish green and they lose their sweet taste. As soon as the beans are cooked, quickly remove from heat and immediately pour some cold water into the pot to stop the cooking process. Now your green vegetables will remain a bright green. Drain promptly and keep only about ¼ cup of water in the pot. Place a lump of butter or gluten-free margarine*, salt and pepper to taste, return the beans to coat with butter sauce, heat a minute and serve. If you prefer a thick sauce, melt 1 teaspoon cornstarch in a little cold water then add to boiling liquid in the pot while stirring. Cook until liquid thickens, then continue to heat beans and serve. For a restaurant style presentation, top with some slivered almonds before serving.

## Green Beans and Potatoes
This is an Italian side-dish. The potato thickens the sauce.

2 Tablespoons oil
1 clove garlic
1 pound green beans
1 (8 ounce) can gluten-free tomato sauce*
1 large potato, peeled and cut into large
  dice

½ cup water (I pour the water in the
  tomato can to get any remaining sauce).
Salt and ground black pepper
Oregano

Heat oil and add peeled clove of garlic. Sauté garlic until lightly browned. Remove pot from heat and cool a minute. Mash garlic with fork to release its entire flavor and remove any large pieces. Add potatoes and tomato sauce and ½ can of water (½ cup). Place pan back on heat and cook until potatoes are half cooked. Wash, remove stems and slice green beans and add to pot along with salt and pepper. Cook until all vegetables are tender and add a pinch of oregano. Taste to correct seasonings. If there is a slight bitter taste given off by oregano, add a pinch of sugar. Toss and serve.

## Grits and Cheese (easy)

Grits* are good for breakfast or as a main meal side dish. They are granulated white corn, and when cooked have a similar texture as farina. I think their flavor is a lot nicer because of the mild sweet corn taste, whereas farina doesn't have much taste. Just be sure to purchase brands that are gluten-free without contamination. Some companies say their regular and instant grits are contaminated because they are processed on the same lines with wheat.

To prepare, follow the package directions. Once cooked, add one slice of gluten-free American cheese* per serving. You can also use grated cheddar cheese*. Stir and melt it in.

Children like grits and cheese as a side dish with hot dogs, and they are easier to make than macaroni and cheese. They are also good for breakfast alone, or with eggs and bacon.

## Grits Casserole, Southern Style

This is nice for a side-dish or brunch entrée. This is easy to make in the microwave.

4 cups water, hot  
½ teaspoon salt  
1 to 1 ¼ quick cooking gluten-free grits*  
    (use amount on package directions for 4  
    cups water)  
8 ounces grated cheddar cheese  

¼ cup butter or gluten-free margarine  
¼ teaspoon garlic salt  
Dash of ground red pepper (optional)  
3 eggs  
⅓ cup milk  

*Microwave directions (these instructions were developed using an 800 watt microwave oven)*: In a large glass or Corningware® casserole, add hot water and salt. Microwave it on high about 5 to 7 minutes until boiling. Stir in grits and cover with waxed paper. Microwave for 5 minutes or until thickened. Carefully stir grits, and then stir in cheese, butter, garlic salt, and red pepper (if using), until cheese melts. Microwave on high, with waxed paper cover, for 5 more minutes. Beat eggs and blend in milk in a bowl. Blend the egg mixture into grits (see note below). Microwave it 5 minutes more. Let stand for 10 minutes, covered, before serving. (Note: Microwave temperatures and times may vary depending on the wattage of your oven.)

*Oven directions*: Heat oven to 325°F. Prepare grits according to package directions by boiling the water and salt in a pot, adding the grits and cooking for 10 minutes in a large saucepan. Remove from heat and stir in the cheese, butter, garlic salt, and red pepper (if using). Continue stirring until cheese melts. Beat eggs and milk in a bowl. Stir it into grits mixture (see note below). Grease a 1 ½ casserole and add grits. Bake for 1 hour. Let stand 10 minutes before serving.

Note: Whenever you want to mix eggs into a hot mixture, it is a good idea to first carefully stir some of that hot mixture into the eggs (as you would for puddings.) After doing so, then blend the egg mixture into the hot mixture. If you just dump the eggs on top of the hot mixture they could cook on top or turn into "egg drop". By incorporating some hot mixture into the eggs first and mixing it well, then the eggs will blend in instead of cooking at the wrong time.

*Variation*: American cheese can be used instead of cheddar, for a milder flavor that children like.

## Halushkie Russian Noodles and Cabbage
**This is nice for a side-dish.**

8 ounces (½ package) of Sam Mills®
   Lasagna Corte Noodles or ½ recipe of
   Spaetzle (see index) or a full recipe of
   Spaetzle you like a lot of noodles
1 small head of cabbage
1 medium onion

1 stick of butter or gluten-free margarine*
   (separated, use ¼ cup at a time); I use a
   little less
½ teaspoon salt
¼ teaspoon pepper

Cook the noodles according to package directions. (I cook the noodles 2 to 3 minutes longer or they will be too hard and dry for this dish.) Drain noodles in a colander and then put them back into the pot you boiled them in. Add ¼ cup of butter and stir in. (If using Spaetzle, add ¼ cup butter and not what is listed in that recipe.)

Finely grate the cabbage and onion in a food processor. (Do not over process and turn it into puree. It should be grated not totally pulverized.) Melt ¼ cup of butter in a skillet. When skillet is hot, add the cabbage, onion, salt and pepper. Cook the vegetable mixture until they are soft and lightly browned. This adds flavor. Add to the noodles and blend.

You can place the mixture into a buttered casserole and reheat it in the oven. This dish improves in flavor the second day. It can also be reheated in the microwave oven.

## Mushroom Casserole
**This is a recipe from my mother and grandmother. We always have this at Thanksgiving. It works well with the dry gluten-free bread crumbs (see index).**

1 pound cleaned and sliced mushrooms
¼ cup oil (I use olive oil)
1 large clove garlic
Salt and pepper

½ cup dry gluten-free bread crumbs made
   from Gluten-Free Naturals™ Bread,
   with Italian seasonings added (see index
   for recipe)

Wash and slice the mushrooms. Steam in a pot with a little salted water in it, until the mushrooms are limp. Drain and put mushrooms in casserole dish or glass baking dish. (I use a shallow Corningware® casserole.)

Let pot cool a few minutes and dry it. Heat the oil in the same pot. (Be sure pot is dry or oil will splatter.) Add the garlic and sauté it over low heat until lightly browned. Remove from heat and let it cool a minute. Then mash the garlic with a fork and discard any large pieces. Remove 2 Tablespoons of oil and toss with mushrooms in the casserole dish. Add some salt and pepper and blend in.

*see gluten-free products list at the end of the book

To the remaining oil in the pot, mix in the gluten-free bread crumbs. If the mixture is too dry, add a little more oil until all crumbs are moistened. Sprinkle the crumbs over the top of the casserole and bake it at 350°F for 20 minutes, or until the crumbs are lightly browned.

*Variation*: Make artichoke casserole exactly the same way, but only use 2 boxes of frozen artichoke hearts (check ingredients to be sure they are gluten-free). Cook according to package directions and then proceed.

## Mushroom Newburg

Freeze the leftover egg whites in a container for another use. (When I get enough I make an angel food cake.)

1 pound cleaned and halved mushrooms
1 to 2 Tablespoons fine white rice flour or
  sweet rice flour
¼ cup melted butter
1 ¼ cups half and half (half milk/half
  cream)

⅛ to ¼ cup dry sherry
¼ teaspoon salt
⅛ teaspoon ground nutmeg
Dash ground black pepper
3 egg yolks

Dredge mushrooms in rice flour and sauté in butter. Add half and half, sherry, salt, pepper and nutmeg. Stir until slightly thickened. Beat 3 yolks in a metal or Pyrex® measuring cup. Add a little hot liquid to them while beating constantly with a whisk. Now pour egg yolk mixture back into pot. Cook and stir until mixture just comes to a boil, approximately 2 minutes. Serve over rice or toasted gluten-free bread cut into quarters. My favorite is to serve it over a combination of brown and wild rice.

## Onion and Cheddar Cheese Casserole

I prefer the creamed onions recipe below, but this one is also good and a lot easier to make.

2 lbs. onions
Water
½ teaspoon salt
3 Tablespoons butter or gluten-free
  margarine*

½ teaspoon gluten-free Worcestershire
  sauce*
1 cup sharp grated cheddar cheese

Skin and slice onions into ¼ inch thick rings. Place in a pot and just cover with water. Add salt and cook just until the water comes to a boil and drain. Mix the butter and the Worcestershire sauce into the onions. Turn onions into a shallow baking pan and top with grated cheese.

*see gluten-free products list at the end of the book

## Onions, Creamed

My mother considers these a must for Thanksgiving dinner.  She makes them early in the day and re-heats them in the oven.

1 ½ to 2 pounds small white boiling onions

3 Tablespoons fine white rice flour or sweet rice flour

1 ½ cups milk

¼ cup gluten-free grated cheddar*, Gouda, or American cheese*

Salt and ground black pepper to taste

Rinse onions and pierce each one with a cake tester.  This helps the onions retain their shape.  Place into boiling water a few minutes and drain.  When cool enough to handle, cut off root section and the onion should peel easily and quickly.  Now boil some salted water and return onions to the pot.  Cook until tender, testing with a cake tester.  When tender, drain and place in a casserole or serving dish.  Now make the white sauce by pouring 1 cup milk in pot and begin to heat.  Meanwhile, mix the rice flour with the remaining milk.  Add and stir in.  Add the cheese and cook over low heat stirring all the while until it thickens and bubbles.  Add the salt and pepper and pour over the well-drained onions.

## Polenta – Firm, Easy Microwave Version

This is much easier than standing before a hot stove stirring.  I usually make this as a quick side-dish for dinner, and then put the leftovers in a greased loaf pan.  Allow to cool, cover with plastic wrap and refrigerate.  The next day slice the polenta and fry the slices in a pan with a little oil.  Note:  these directions were developed using an 800 watt microwave oven.  Reduce cooking times for higher wattage ovens, or use medium instead of high.

4 cups water

1 ¼ cups cornmeal*

1 teaspoon salt

2 Tablespoons butter

⅛ teaspoon ground black pepper

2 Tablespoons grated Pecorino Romano or Parmesan cheese (optional)

Combine water, cornmeal and salt in a 2 quart dish.  (I use a deep Corningware® casserole dish.)  If using fine cornmeal, I prefer to slowly mix it in.  Cook on high uncovered for 12 minutes, stirring after 6 minutes with a whisk.  (To stir, begin gently and then stir more vigorously as the polenta and water blend.  Do not mix too vigorously at first as it is possible to splash hot water on you.)  Remove from microwave and add butter and salt.  Stir.  Let stand 3 minutes.

Grease a loaf pan.  Pour polenta into the pan and allow it to cool.  Cover and refrigerate until firm.  To fry, slice into ½ inch slices.  For easier frying, I am told you can dry the polenta slices on a rack for 20 minutes.  I do not do this and just fry it in olive oil until crusty.  It is also delicious deep fried.

This makes a wonderful side dish.  I like polenta served with Country Captain Chicken (see index), or entrees with sauces.  I also like it with the Peppers and Onions Oven Style (see index).

*Variation*: For quicker preparation directions, boil the 4 cups of water. Add all the ingredients into the casserole and stir with a whisk. If using fine cornmeal, add it in gradually and stir. Microwave the polenta on High Power for 6 minutes. It will be thicker on the bottom, but gently stir it with your whisk. (Stir gently so that the water on top does not splash and burn you.) It will blend and become free of lumps. You can stir more vigorously once the water on the top is blended in. Once blended, put into the greased loaf pan as above.

## Polenta – Soft Microwave Version

I like this version when I am serving polenta immediately. It is nice for breakfast or as a side dish. I also like this version with Juevos Rancheros (see index for recipe). Note: These directions were developed using an 800 watt microwave oven. Reduce cooking times for higher wattage ovens, or use medium instead of high.

| | |
|---|---|
| 4 cups water | ⅛ teaspoon ground black pepper |
| ¾ cups cornmeal* | 3 to 4 Tablespoons grated Pecorino |
| 1 teaspoon salt |    Romano or Parmesan cheese |
| 2 Tablespoons butter | |

Combine water, cornmeal and salt in a 2 quart soufflé dish. Cook on high uncovered for 6 minutes. Stir well, starting gently so that the hot water does not splash you. Cover loosely with a paper towel and cook 6 minutes more. (If your dish is deep enough, the paper towel may not be necessary. I use a deep Corningware® casserole dish and I do not use the paper towel.) Remove, uncover and stir in butter and cheese. Let stand 3 minutes. Serve hot. Delicious topped with tomato sauce.

*Variation*: For cornmeal mush for breakfast, do not add the black pepper or the grated cheese. I like it plain for breakfast, but you can also serve it with sugar and milk if desired.

## Polenta – Traditional Stovetop Version

I normally do not make this recipe, because it takes long and I have burned myself when the polenta bubbles. I am including this recipe here for those that like the traditional method.

| | |
|---|---|
| 1 ½ quarts of water | 1 ½ cups cornmeal* |
| 2 teaspoons salt | |

In a 4 quart saucepan, bring water and salt to a boil. Pour in cornmeal while stirring so it remains lump free. Continue to stir and cook 30 minutes.

## Polenta with Mushrooms – side dish

This is a fancier way to serve polenta. It's nice for company because you can make it ahead of time. Slice and reheat it in the microwave.

| | |
|---|---|
| Firm Microwave Polenta or Traditional | 2 Tablespoons dehydrated onion flakes |
|    Polenta (see index for recipe) |    (or use about 2 medium onions, diced) |
| 1 can mushrooms (or use 1 package fresh) | Pecorino Romano, Parmesan or |
| |    mozzarella cheese |

*see gluten-free products list at the end of the book

Prepare the microwave or traditional polenta. Grease a loaf pan. Meanwhile, re-hydrate the onions in the mushroom water. Drain. Sauté both the mushrooms and the onions in a pan.

When the polenta is done, pour ½ of the polenta in the pan. Top with the mushroom and onion mixture. Top with cheese. Pour the rest of the polenta on top. Top with more cheese. Allow to cool and set. Slice and arrange on a plate. Microwave it to heat it through.

## Potato Casserole Using Instant Potato Flakes

I admit that I prefer homemade potatoes, but this recipe is easy if you're in a hurry. The cream cheese and herbs cover the instant potato flake taste.

Instant Potato Flakes* or Potato Buds*
    for 6 servings (see package directions)
1 (8 ounce) package of gluten-free cream
    cheese*

2 Tablespoons chopped green onion or 1
    Tablespoon dried chives
2 Tablespoons minced fresh parsley or 1
    Tablespoon dried parsley flakes
1 Tablespoon butter (optional)

Prepare potatoes for 6 servings as directed on the package, but use the 8 ounces of cream cheese in place of the 4 Tablespoons butter. (Cream cheese is half the calories of butter, so the calories will remain the same.) Stir in the onions and parsley. Grease casserole that holds 1 quart or a baking dish. Spread potatoes in casserole and dot with butter if desired. Bake at 400°F for 30 minutes.

## Potatoes – Del Monico Style

If you like scalloped potatoes, you will like this.

3 Tablespoons sweet rice or fine white
    rice flour
1 ½ cups milk
1 clove garlic, pressed in a garlic press
Paprika

½ cup grated gluten-free Swiss or gluten-
    free Fontina cheese
4 cups cold cooked potatoes, sliced ¼
    inch thick
Salt and ground black pepper

Wash and boil potatoes. Drain and allow them to cool. Pour 1 cup milk into a saucepan and begin to heat. Mix ½ cup milk with the rice flour and add and blend with a whisk. Add garlic, salt and pepper and cook while stirring until thick and smooth. Now peel (if desired) and slice the potatoes to ¼ inch thick slices and place in a greased baking dish. Sprinkle cheese over potatoes; pour hot cream sauce over top and top with a little paprika. Bake in a 400°F oven for 20 minutes.

*see gluten-free products list at the end of the book

## Potato Filling

I make this when I have leftover mashed potatoes and day-old gluten-free bread.  If you use leftover potatoes, don't add the extra milk or too much salt and pepper.

1 medium onion, chopped
½ cup chopped celery
3 Tablespoons butter or gluten-free margarine
2 cups cubed Gluten-Free Naturals™ bread
1 egg
¼ cup milk

2 cups (about 1 ½ lbs.) hot mashed potatoes
1 teaspoon salt (use less if using leftover potatoes)
1 Tablespoon minced parsley
3 dashes black pepper
Paprika

Sauté the onion and the celery in 3 Tablespoons of butter.  Cook until tender.  Meanwhile, add the egg to the hot mashed potatoes along with milk, parsley, salt and pepper.  Add the onion and celery mixture to the potato mixture.

Brown bread cubes in a little butter and fold into the potato mixture.  Butter a 1 quart casserole and place the potatoes in it.  Sprinkle the top with paprika and bake at 350°F for 35 minutes.  This serves 4.

## Potato Fingers

This recipe was created by my Grandmother, who was a wonderful cook.  This tastes like a restaurant dish.  Do not use leftover mashed potatoes with milk and butter in them, or this dish won't work.  The potatoes must be boiled with the skin on, then peeled and mashed.  If there is too much moisture in the potatoes, they will fall apart.

4 medium potatoes
Chopped parsley
¼ cup gluten-free grated Italian Cheese (I use less if I use Pecorino Romano Cheese)
2 eggs
Salt and pepper to taste

Gluten-Free Mozzarella cheese, cut into strips about 2 inches long by ½ inch thick
Plain gluten-free dry bread crumbs made with Gluten-Free Naturals™ Bread (see index for recipe)
Oil for frying

Wash potatoes.  Do not peel.  Boil the potatoes "in their jackets" until they are tender.  Peel when they are cool enough to handle, and then mash.  Add a little chopped parsley, grated cheese, eggs, salt and pepper.  Mix well and cool.

Take some of the cooled potato mixture in your hands, and make a flat cake out of it.  Place a strip of Mozzarella cheese in the center.  Mold potato around the cheese to completely cover it and seal in the cheese.  Your potato finger should be about 3 inches long and 1 ¼ inches in diameter.

Roll the potato fingers in dry bread crumbs.  When all "fingers" are molded, heat a skillet.  Add oil to skillet and heat until the top looks like it has a little shimmer to it.  (Or drop a little of the gluten-free bread crumbs in the oil and see if they sizzle.)  Add the potato fingers, lower heat and brown on all sides. Drain on paper towels. Serve hot so that the cheese will be melted and ooze out when cut into. Leftovers are best when reheated in a toaster oven so that the crumbs stay crispy.

*Variation*: If you make these potato fingers smaller, cracker crumbs or cornflake crumbs may be used. These crumbs brown faster than the dry gluten-free bread crumbs. By making them a smaller size they cook faster and do not burn.

## Potato Litchfield
This is a nice dish for company.

6 large potatoes
½ of a stick (¼ cup) butter or gluten-free margarine*
Salt and pepper

Generous sprinklings of garlic and onion powder
½ cup milk
1 cup grated cheddar cheese*

Boil potatoes in their skins. Allow to cool. I boil them ahead of time and put them in the refrigerator when cool enough. Then I prepare this the next day.

Butter a soufflé or Pyrex® dish. Peel and shred potatoes and put them in the buttered dish. (Or peel and put potatoes through a ricer into the dish.)

Mix the potatoes with the spices. I taste to see if it is to my liking. I lightly salt if the cheese is salty. Pour milk over them and dot with butter. Cover with cheese. Bake at 350°F, uncovered, for 45 minutes.

## Potatoes Pan Fried
Instead of loading up potatoes with butter, try this version. It has lower cholesterol and tastes like French Fries without all the fat of deep frying. I also use this method with leftover baked potatoes.

Baked potatoes (in the microwave or the oven)
Oil

Adobo® seasoning* or salt, pepper and garlic powder

Wash potatoes and bake them in either the oven or microwave. Do not remove skins. Cut cooked potatoes in 4 pieces the long way. (It looks like you have 4 large French fries.)

Sprinkle potatoes with Adobo® or seasonings. Heat a 12 inch non-stick fryer skillet. Add some oil and swirl around. (I use just a few Tablespoons.) Do not allow Teflon® pan to get too hot and overheat. Add potatoes. Brown the potatoes on the sides that don't have the skin on them. Serve hot.

*see gluten-free products list at the end of the book

## Potato Pancakes
**We enjoy this as a side dish, or even for breakfast.**

2 eggs
½ cup yogurt
A little milk or water if batter is too thick
¼ teaspoon granulated onion powder or
    ⅛ teaspoon fresh onion juice (optional)
¼ cup Gluten-Free Naturals™ All
    Purpose Flour (or other gluten-free
    flour may be used)

2 teaspoons baking powder
1 teaspoon salt
3 cups grated raw potatoes (about 4 large
    potatoes. I grate these in my food
    processor or use a Salad Shooter®)
Oil for pan frying

Blend eggs, yogurt, onion powder and flour together in a bowl. Set aside. Grate the potatoes and blend all ingredients together. Or, if you have a salad shooter, wash potatoes, and use the Salad Shooter® to grate them into the batter. Quickly blend in so that the potatoes do not discolor. (They turn a gray color when exposed to air.) Otherwise, grate the potatoes in a food processor and add them in. If using a food processor, you may find water on the bottom so drain it off and do not add this extra liquid to the batter.

Heat 1 Tablespoon of oil in a pan. Use a ⅓ cup or a ½ cup measure to dip out the mixture and put it in the pan. Fry over medium heat until brown and crusty. Turn and finish cooking. Serve immediately. Makes 8, 8-inch pancakes. I enjoy these with applesauce on the side. My husband likes them with gluten-free ketchup*.

*Variation*: Milk may be used in place of yogurt, but add a ¼ to ½ teaspoon xanthan gum to make the batter thick enough.

## Potato Pancakes – Food Processor Version
**These are easy and nice served with applesauce. No xanthan gum is needed for this recipe.**

1 ½ cups raw potatoes, washed. (I leave
    the skin on.) This is about 2 medium
    potatoes or 3 small potatoes.
¼ cup milk
2 eggs
¼ teaspoon granulated onion powder or 1
    Tablespoon diced fresh onion

¼ cup fine white rice flour
¼ teaspoon baking powder
1 teaspoon salt
A little butter or oil for the skillet

Wash potatoes. Cut potatoes into quarters and add to the food processor. Pulse them with the chopping blade until chopped fine. (Note: you want them chopped, not whipped). Immediately add the milk, eggs and rice flour and pulse again. This will keep the potatoes from discoloring. Add the rest of the ingredients and pulse again until blended.

Drop by Tablespoons onto a hot greased griddle. Brown them on both sides. Makes thirty 2" pancakes.

## Potatoes – Hash Brown Style
I think this is easy to make, and is tastier than frozen hash browns.  It is also less expensive.

4 large Potatoes (I prefer russets)
Oil

Adobo® seasoning* or salt, pepper and garlic powder

Wash potatoes.  I prefer to clean them using a soft nail brush.  (I think they work better than a kitchen brush.)  Dry the potatoes.  Heat a 12 inch non-stick fryer skillet.  Add a little oil and swirl around.  Do not allow Teflon® pan to get too hot.

To grate potatoes, I use a salad shooter® and the grating disk to "shoot" the potatoes into the fry pan.  Once potatoes are in the pan, press them with your spatula into an even layer.  Sprinkle with Adobo® or seasonings.  Cook until browned on that side.  Take your spatula and cut the large round fried potatoes into 4 pieces.  Flip over each quarter section and brown other side.

## Potatoes O'Brien (Potatoes with Peppers and Onions)
I enjoy peppers and onions, so this is a favorite of mine.

4 large potatoes (I use Russets, Red Potatoes, New Potatoes, or Gold Potatoes)
Oil

1 large green pepper, diced
1 large onion, diced
Salt, pepper, garlic powder or Adobo® seasoning may be used.

Wash potatoes.  I do not peel.  Dice and put into a microwave container.  Cover and vent.  Microwave them on high for 5 minutes.  While potatoes are cooking, dice green pepper and onion.  Be careful opening the lid of the potatoes as there will be a lot of steam that could possibly burn you.

Heat a large 12 inch skillet.  Add some oil.  Put in hot potatoes and the peppers and onions.  Sprinkle generously with salt, pepper and garlic powder.  Cook and stir until potatoes are browned and peppers and onions are cooked.

This method of precooking the potatoes in the microwave saves time, as well as insures that the peppers and onions aren't overcooked while waiting for the potatoes to be done.

*Variation*:  Leftovers are good in a frittata (see index for recipe).

## Potatoes – Roasted
**A nice side-dish for company.**

6 potatoes, small enough to fit into a large
  metal serving spoon; (I have an old
  spoon that I use for this purpose).

3 Tablespoons melted butter or gluten-
  free margarine*
1 teaspoon salt
2 Tablespoons Parmesan cheese

Peel potatoes and place in the spoon. Cut slits in potatoes every ⅛ inch. The sides of the spoon will stop your knife from cutting too deeply into the potatoes. Place in a bowl of cold water to prevent discoloration until all potatoes are prepared. Dry potatoes with paper towels and place potatoes in a generously buttered baking dish with the slit side up. Baste with melted butter. Sprinkle salt on top and bake in a 475°F oven for 30 minutes. Baste again with butter. Bake 10 minutes more and then sprinkle on the Parmesan cheese. Bake an additional 5 minutes. Potatoes should be tender and a golden brown.

## Potatoes – Roasted – Easy Stovetop Style
**A good side dish using canned potatoes.**

Canned whole potatoes
Fine white rice flour
Salt
Garlic powder

Sage (crumbled dry sage or powdered can
  be used)
2 Tablespoons butter or oil or gluten-free
  cooking spray

Drain canned potatoes. Place a little rice flour on a piece of waxed paper, add a few dashes of sage, garlic powder, salt and roll the potatoes in this mixture. Melt 2 Tablespoons butter or oil in an iron skillet and fry or place in the oven and roast 20 minutes. (If making them in the oven, I spray them with cooking spray.) Shake pan to roll potatoes over and roast another 20 minutes.

## Potatoes – Stuffed
**These are delicious and make a nice presentation for company.**

Potatoes (I use 2 medium potatoes per
  person or 1 very large)
Gluten-free sour cream*
Butter*
Milk

Salt and pepper
Gluten-free bacon*, cooked and crumbled
  for garnish or gluten-free bacon bits*
Parsley for garnish (optional)
Paprika for garnish (optional)

Wash potatoes and prick with the tines of a fork. Either bake in the oven for 1 hour at 350°F, or bake in the microwave for 5 to 7 minutes or until done. Test with a fork or cake tester to be sure they are not hard in the middle.

When done, remove from oven and place on a heat resistant plate. Allow to cool until you are able to handle them. Slice in half lengthwise. Scoop out the inside, but leave about a ¼ inch or so of potato in the skin. Keep the potato pulp. Either put the potato pulp through a

*see gluten-free products list at the end of the book

ricer (I prefer this) or mash in a bowl. Add some butter, milk, sour cream, salt and pepper to taste. They should be creamy and smooth. Taste and adjust seasonings.

Fill the potato skins and make the filling go high (heaping) above the skins and round off the top. You will have extra skins leftover. (You can use these for another use. You can top with bacon bits and cheese for an appetizer. I also use the leftover skins filled with chili for a lunch.) Garnish your stuffed potatoes with the bacon bits and/or the parsley and paprika. For variation, you can also top with grated cheese. I make these ahead and reheat in the microwave or oven. This makes a nice presentation for company. Serve either one half of a large potato or two halves of the medium potatoes per person.

*Variation*: Instead of going through the effort of scooping out the potatoes and making mashed potatoes; just top potato halves with cooked leftover vegetables such as broccoli, mushrooms, onions or green peppers. Top with cheese. Cover and microwave until it is heated through and the cheese melts. (I take leftover baked potatoes; place in a microwave container, top the potatoes with frozen vegetables and cheese. Microwave it at lunchtime for an easy light lunch.)

## Ratatouille
This makes a lot of food. I enjoy it as a light lunch topped with mozzarella or provolone cheese.

1 Tablespoon olive oil
1 clove garlic, minced
1 chopped onion
½ to 1 cup chopped green pepper
2 to 3 zucchini sliced
1 large eggplant, peeled and cubed
1 teaspoon sugar
1 teaspoon salt
¼ teaspoon chili powder

¼ teaspoon ground nutmeg
1 lb. 9 oz. can of crushed tomatoes
1 lb. 9 oz. can of whole tomatoes, cut up
1 cup dry white wine (I use vermouth)
2 large pinches oregano
2 large pinches basil, or add fresh
I Tablespoon Pecorino Romano cheese
   (optional)

Heat the oil in a large pot. Add garlic and lightly brown. (Do not burn the garlic or you will ruin the dish.) Add all other ingredients and cook. This tastes better the next day. Serve hot in a bowl topped with melted provolone cheese or mozzarella cheese.

## Red Cabbage
This dish must be made the day before for best results. It is wonderful served with Sauerbraten (see index). My mother recently made this and my 14-month old niece loved it! This is my mother's recipe.

3 lbs. red cabbage
3 Tablespoons butter or gluten-free
   margarine*
¼ cup sugar
½ cup wine or cider vinegar

1 teaspoon salt
½ cup water
¼ cup currant jelly

*see gluten-free products list at the end of the book

Cut cabbage in quarters, remove core and slice in half inch slices. Place cabbage in a large pot with butter, salt, vinegar and sugar and ½ cup water. Bring to a boil, cover, lower heat and simmer 1 hour 15 minutes. Every once in a while, stir the cabbage and check to see if a little more water is needed so that you don't burn the vegetables. By the end of the cooking time, the cabbage should be tender and all but ¼ cup liquid should be evaporated. If too much liquid is left just uncover and boil a few minutes until ¼ cup is remaining. Now add the jelly and stir in. The jelly gives the cabbage good color and a shiny appearance as well as good flavor. The cabbage may not be as tasty as you would like but do not fear. Cool and refrigerate and the next day reheat the cabbage slowly and it will be delicious.

## Refried Black Beans

When I noticed that many of the refried beans contained unknown ingredients, it just seemed easier to make my own. What I discovered was that I not only liked these better, but that they are one-fourth the price of canned refried beans. These also don't contain lard or other fats. You will need a hand blender to make these. We prefer the black beans but pinto beans are good too.

1 can of black beans un-drained (I like Goya® brand which is gluten-free as of this writing. Many store brands are gluten-free. Check ingredients).

Sprinkling of granulated garlic powder
Sprinkling of granulated onion powder

Put the beans in a pot, including the juice in the can. Don't add any salt, because the liquid is providing enough salt. Sprinkle with the spices. Take the hand blender and pulverize the beans. Heat beans through, stirring so they don't burn. Continue cooking (about 5 minutes) until desired thickness is achieved.

We like this served on corn tortillas*. (Heat the tortillas in the microwave according to package directions.) Top tortillas with refried beans, lettuce and tomato, salsa*, and shredded cheese. Hot sauce* and sour cream* may also be added according to your preferences.

## Rice Balls – "Arancini"

This is an Italian dish and a family recipe. They look like little oranges. Some people put a pinch of saffron into the water while cooking the rice to give the proper color. Do not use converted rice to make this dish, or it will not work.

1 lb. white rice (I use Carolina® Brand since it has the right starch content)
1 stick (½ cup) butter or gluten-free margarine*
1 ½ Tablespoons salt
3 eggs
3 Tablespoons parsley flakes
4 Tablespoons grated gluten-free Italian cheese* (I use Pecorino Romano cheese)

½ teaspoon pepper
Pinch of salt
Mozzarella Cheese (I like Polly-O®, which is gluten-free as of this writing)
Unseasoned dry gluten-free bread crumbs made from Gluten-Free Naturals™ bread (see index for recipe)
Additional eggs for coating (about 2)
Pinch of salt for beaten eggs
Oil for frying

Place rice in a 5-quart pot. Fill pot halfway with water, and add the butter and 1 ½ Tablespoons of salt. Cook over medium heat for about 20 minutes. Rice should be soft and the water evaporated. If water evaporates before rice is fully cooked, add more water. While rice is cooking, beat 3 eggs, parsley, cheese, pepper and a pinch of salt together with a fork. Remove cooked rice from heat when done. Stir in the egg mixture. Pour rice into a platter and cool.

While rice is cooling, cut up the mozzarella into cubes. I start with cutting up half of the package, and cut more if needed. Beat 2 eggs, pinch of salt and a dash of pepper in a pie plate. Place some bread crumbs on a piece of waxed paper.

When rice is cool enough to handle, cup some in your hand, add a Mozzarella cube and cover with a little more rice to form a ball. Don't make them too big. Roll rice ball into egg mixture and roll in bread crumbs. Fry in oil until golden brown, spooning hot oil of them while they are frying so that all sides get cooked. Drain and serve hot. This recipe makes about 28 rice balls.

## Rice – Chinese Fried Rice

I often make fried rice with leftover meat and rice. This stretches a ½ cup meat to serve 4 people. I always keep frozen diced green pepper and onion in my freezer. (They are the easiest vegetables to freeze since no blanching is needed. Just dice, put in a freezer bag and freeze.) I also keep diced ham in the freezer. If you don't have leftover rice, while the rice is cooking start to stir-fry the other ingredients. You will have the meal completed in less than 30 minutes.

About 6 cups cooked rice (I cook 2 ½ cups raw rice in 6 cups water. I don't add salt since I will add soy sauce to this dish. Or you can add some soy sauce to the rice water now and add less later.)
3 eggs, beaten
1 cup diced mushrooms (fresh or canned, drained)
½ cup diced, green pepper

4 Tablespoons oil
½ cup diced cooked chicken, pork, shrimp, beef or gluten-free ham*
2 cups diced onions
½ cup diced, Chinese water chestnuts, drained (optional)
4 finely chopped scallions
About 4 Tablespoons gluten-free soy sauce*

Heat a wok, and place a little oil in the pan. Pour in the eggs and cook like for scrambled eggs. Remove and cut into pieces. Add more oil, and add the green pepper and onions. Stir-fry for about 4 minutes. Add the rice, the cooked meat, water chestnuts (if using) and mix well, stirring constantly for 4 minutes. Add the scallions and the soy sauce. Mix thoroughly and heat through.

*Variation*: Make your rice the day ahead of time and refrigerate. Your fried rice will turn out less gummy if you do.

*Variation 2*: Fried rice can be an excellent dish to use leftovers. Sometimes I start with some diced onions and celery. Stir fry in a little oil. Sprinkle them with a little garlic powder. Add a bag of frozen stir fry vegetables, some frozen peas, some drained canned mushrooms. Choose vegetables you like. Once your vegetables are stir fried, add your cooked rice and

*see gluten-free products list at the end of the book

some gluten-free soy sauce. Add the meat. Leftover chicken, turkey, or ham cut into small pieces are good choices. Or leftover cooked ground beef or gluten-free sausage may be used. I have even used gluten-free pepperoni cut up into small pieces. You can use some drained canned shrimp or frozen shrimp. Cook as above.

## Rice – Boiled

I often buy rice in 25 pound bags, and put it into smaller ones to store in my pantry. These large bags sometimes don't have cooking directions on them, so here is the recipe. See variation below for Brown Rice.

| | |
|---|---|
| 1 cup white rice | ½ teaspoon salt |
| 2 ½ cups water | |

Bring water to a boil. Add the rice and the salt. Cover and cook 20 minutes on low heat. Uncover and fluff with a fork.

You can also prepare the rice in the microwave. Cook uncovered in a microwave safe bowl for 20 minutes. Do not cover the bowl or it will boil-over. Cooking it using this method keeps your stove and microwave clean.

*Variation*: Add 2 ½ teaspoons gluten-free chicken base to the water, eliminate the salt, add a Tablespoon of dehydrated onion, drained canned mushrooms and a handful of frozen peas for an easy rice pilaf. Cook as noted above.

*Variation 2*: If you want to use brown rice instead of white rice, cook it about 50 minutes instead of 20 minutes. Some packages suggest an hour, but I find cooking it that long makes it gummy. To speed up the cooking time of brown rice you can soak it overnight and the next day cook it for about 30 minutes. See recipe "Mushroom Sauce Bianca" under Sauces, for the health benefits of pre-soaking rice. Note: If you are going to keep a package of uncooked brown rice for a long time, store it in the refrigerator so that it won't go rancid. Or vacuum package it.

## Rice – Mexican Style

A nice side dish with Mexican food.

| | |
|---|---|
| 2 Tablespoons oil | 1 Tablespoon chopped parsley |
| 1 cup uncooked rice | 1 cup chicken broth* |
| ½ cup chopped onions | 1 cup (8 oz.) tomato sauce* (I use canned sauce) |
| 1 clove garlic, minced | |
| 1 teaspoon salt | ½ cup water |
| 2 tomatoes, chopped | |

Heat the oil in a skillet over medium heat. Add rice, and sauté until lightly browned. Add onion and garlic. Sauté until rice is golden brown. Add the rest of ingredients, and bring to a boil. Cover and cook 20 minutes.

## Rice – Risotto – Microwave Version

Risotto normally is made by cooking it on the stove uncovered, and stirring it for 20 minutes or so. You also have to heat your chicken broth in separate pot and constantly add it in. Made in the microwave it is much easier and eliminates these steps, but it must be covered or you won't get that creamy texture. Conversely, regular rice (also called long grain rice) is made cooking on the stove covered for 20 minutes. However, in the microwave it must be cooked uncovered or it boils over and doesn't cook properly. So, in both cases stovetop versions are opposite the microwave versions.

2 cloves garlic, chopped
1 small onion, chopped
1 Tablespoon oil
2 ¾ cups gluten-free chicken broth* (or
    water plus gluten-free bouillon* or
    gluten-free chicken base*)

1 cup Arborio rice
6 to 8 ounces sliced fresh mushrooms
2 Tablespoons Pecorino Romano or
    Parmesan Cheese
Salt and Pepper to taste

In a large microwave dish (I use a Corningware® casserole with a lid) combine the oil, garlic and the onion. Cover and microwave on high 5 minutes.

Add oil and rice and stir so that the oil coats the rice. Add broth, stir together, cover and microwave on high for 15 minutes. (If using chicken base and water, stop it after 7 minutes and stir to mix in the bouillon.) Meanwhile, clean and slice mushrooms.

Stir in mushrooms. Cover and microwave on high for 8 minutes more. Use pot holders to remove from microwave oven. Stir in cheese. Add salt and pepper to taste. Some chicken soup/bouillon is saltier than others.

Note: Microwave oven wattage may vary. I have an older microwave that may have less power than the model you have. The first time you make this, check it to be sure it doesn't boil over halfway through the 15 minute cooking time. Also, the onions should be steamed and not browned. You may want to check them a minute or two early the first time you make this.

*Variation*: Peas may be added to make "Risotto e Piselli".

## Rice – Risotto

Risotto is delicious and creamy, but it takes more work than regular rice because you have to stir it throughout the time it's cooking. I included this recipe here, but admit that I enjoy my mother's Viennese Rice recipe just as much and it's easier to make. You can make this without the cheese and butter if you're lactose intolerant.

4 Tablespoons olive oil
1 clove minced garlic (optional)
1 ½ cups raw Arborio rice
1 medium onion, minced
4 to 5 cups chicken broth (I use chicken
    base* and water, and I use a little less
    base as it can be salty)

2-4 Tablespoons white wine or sherry
    (optional)
8 ounces sliced mushrooms
2 Tablespoons parsley
½ cup Parmesan cheese, grated (optional)
2 Tablespoons butter (optional)
Salt and pepper to taste

*see gluten-free products list at the end of the book*

Check your package of rice. They may suggest different amounts of rice and water depending on the size of the rice. If so, adjust recipe accordingly.

Heat your chicken broth. (I use boiling water and gluten-free chicken base*.)

In another pot, heat the oil and add the onion and garlic and cook a few minutes. Add the rice and stir in to coat the rice with oil. Begin to add the chicken broth about a ½ cup at a time to the rice and cook until absorbed. Be careful that your first addition doesn't spatter on you because of the oil. Lower heat if needed. Add the wine if using. Continue to keep adding broth, and cook and stir until absorbed. This takes a while. You don't have to stir constantly but stir every 1-2 minutes. Keep adding broth so it doesn't stick. After about 10 minutes of this process, add the mushrooms and parsley. Continue until rice is cooked and creamy. (Total cooking time is usually about 20 minutes.) Top with cheese and butter if desired. Add salt and pepper if needed.

## Rice – "Stuffing" with Mushrooms for poultry
I like this in Cornish game hens. See index for Turkey Stuffing if you want a traditional bread cube stuffing.

Prepare the recipe of Mushroom Sauce Bianca (see index), following the recipe using brown rice. I usually make half of the recipe and use only a ½ of pound of mushrooms instead of 1 ¼ pounds. Allow to cool and stuff Cornish game hens, chicken, or turkey with it. It also is a good side dish. You may also add some cubes of ham or crumbled bacon to this for a variation.

## Rice – "Stuffing" made with Wild Rice and Mushrooms
This is an easy gourmet stuffing. For a traditional bread stuffing, see index for Turkey Stuffing. For a wild rice stuffing without sausage and cheese, see recipe for Chicken with Wild Rice Stuffing.

¾ cup brown rice

¼ cup wild rice, rinsed

½ teaspoon salt or 1 teaspoon gluten-free chicken base or bouillon* (use less bouillon if your brand is salty)

1 onion, diced or 1 Tablespoon dehydrated onion flakes

½ pound sausage* cooked (optional)

1 small can of sliced mushrooms

1 stalk of celery, diced

¼ cup grated Pecorino Romano or Parmesan or ½ cup grated Mozzarella cheese

Rinse the wild rice. Prepare the rice by boiling 3 cups water. Add the salt and the rice. Cook covered on low heat for 40 minutes. Drain. Meanwhile, sauté the onion, sausage (if using), and celery in a little oil. Drain if too much fat from the sausage. Cook until sausage is cooked through and vegetables are tender. Add the drained mushrooms. Add the cooked rice. If your brand of sausage is very salty, use less cheese first and taste it. Mix in the cheese. Add more if needed. (I like adding cheese because it helps to keep the stuffing together.) I enjoy this with turkey and Cornish game hens.

## Rice – Spanish Style
We like this side-dish served with chicken or enchiladas.

½ cup onion, diced
½ cup diced celery
1 Tablespoon oil
1 cup uncooked rice
½ cup diced tomato
1 bay leaf
¼ teaspoon paprika

¼ teaspoon chili powder
½ teaspoon salt
¼ teaspoon garlic powder
Dash of ground black pepper
1 cup water
1 ½ cups tomato juice
1 teaspoon chicken base*

Cook onion, celery and rice in oil for a few minutes.  Add the rest of ingredients in the pot.  Bring to a boil.  Cover and simmer 20 to 25 minutes.  Remove bay leaf and serve.

## Rice – Viennese Style Rice
A family favorite!  We like this dish for company.  I especially like it served with Chicken Marsala.  For family members that don't like to see large onion pieces, I sometimes chop the onion fine with the mincing blade in my food processor.  This is my mother's recipe.

4 Tablespoons butter, gluten-free
    margarine* or oil (I use ½ the amount)
1 cup rice
1 medium onion, chopped

2 ½ cups hot water
2 teaspoons gluten-free chicken base* or
    gluten-free bouillon*

Melt the butter or margarine in a skillet.  (Or add oil to heated skillet.)  Add the rice and cook, stirring constantly until rice is golden.  Add onion and continue cooking until onion and rice are golden brown.  Turn off heat and cool a minute then add hot water into which the chicken base or bouillon cube has been dissolved.  (Be careful; if your pot is too hot it can splatter when the water is added.)  Put on a low flame, cover pot and simmer 18-20 minutes.

## Sauerkraut Casserole
This is very good served with ham and baked beans or any pork dish.

2 (16 ounce) cans sauerkraut
2 Macintosh apples
2 to 4 Tablespoons brown sugar

4 Tablespoons butter or gluten-free
    margarine*

Drain sauerkraut and place in a sieve.  Rinse with tap water and press out all the water.  Put kraut in a bowl and add the brown sugar, use 2 Tablespoons and mix in.  If you think it should be sweeter, add 2 more Tablespoons.  Peel, core and coarsely grate the apples (I use a food processor) and add to the sauerkraut.  (I prefer grated apples but they can be chopped.)  Toss and place in a buttered casserole dish.  Dot top with butter, cover and bake in a 350°F oven for 20 minutes to heat through, then remove cover and bake 10 more minutes to dry it out a little.

*see gluten-free products list at the end of the book

## Spaetzle

These are little German dumplings. This is delicious served with sauerbraten (see index) and red cabbage (see index) for an authentic German dinner. You can also use Spaetzle in place of pasta or as a noodle in soup or with Gulyash (Goulash) or in the Halushski Noodles recipe. This version is a little lighter than the second version, but both are very good. You need a colander with large holes or a Spaetzle maker to make these.

| | |
|---|---|
| 4 eggs | 1 teaspoon salt |
| 1 cup water | Few pinches of nutmeg |
| 3 cups Gluten-Free Naturals™ All Purpose Flour or Gluten-Free Naturals™ Sandwich Bread Flour (do not substitute other flour blends) | 2 Tablespoons butter |
| | Pot of boiling water with about 2 quarts water and 1 teaspoon salt added |

Beat eggs and water together. Add flour, salt and nutmeg. Blend together. Check consistency; I find I sometimes need to add an additional Tablespoon of water. They need to hold together but also be thin enough to be pushed through or drip through the holes into boiling water.

Either use a plastic colander with large holes (about ¼ inch or so, I found mine at a dollar store), or a spaetzle maker. For the colander method, I suggest using a pot with high sides that the colander will fit over, but the bottom will not be in the boiling water. You want the dough to fall from the colander or spaetzle maker through the holes and drop down into the water. Push the dough through the colander with a spoon. For spaetzle maker, place over boiling water. Fill with dough and move sides back and forth.

Stir water from time to time to release any spaetzle that may stick to the bottom. Let boil a few minutes and remove spaetzle that rise to the top of the water with a slotted spoon. Put in a bowl with 2 Tablespoons of butter. When all are in the bowl, mix to blend butter. Leftovers may be reheated in the microwave.

## Spaetzle – Version 2

This version uses rice flour. This version is also very good and the noodles freeze well.

| | |
|---|---|
| 3 eggs | 1 teaspoon salt |
| ½ cup water | Additional 2 Tablespoons water |
| ¾ cup fine white rice flour | 1 Tablespoon butter |
| ¾ cup brown rice flour | Pot of boiling water with about 2 quarts water and 1 teaspoon salt added |
| ½ teaspoon xanthan gum | |

Beat eggs and ½ cup water together. Add flour and salt. Blend together. Check consistency; I find I sometimes need to add an additional 2 Tablespoons water. They need to hold together but also be thin enough to be pushed through or drip through the holes into boiling water.

Either use a plastic colander with large holes (about ¼ inch or so, I found mine at a dollar store), or a spaetzle maker. For the colander method, I suggest using a pot with high sides that the colander will fit over, but the bottom will not be in the boiling water. You want the dough to fall from the colander or spaetzle maker through the holes and drop down into the water. Push the dough through the colander with a spoon. For spaetzle maker, place over boiling water. Fill with dough and move sides back and forth.

Stir water from time to time to release any spaetzle that may stick to the bottom. Let boil a few minutes and remove spaetzle that rise to the top of the water with a slotted spoon. Put in a bowl with a Tablespoon of butter. When all are in the bowl, mix to blend butter. Leftovers may be reheated in the microwave.

Note: I have the best success using this recipe as written without substitution.

## Spinach Casserole with Rice
This is a good use for leftover plain cooked rice.

½ cup melted butter (or use less)
½ cup chopped onion (fresh or frozen)
1 package frozen spinach, cooked and
   drained
1 ½ cups sharp cheese, grated

2 eggs
2 cups milk
Sprinkling of salt to taste
½ teaspoon gluten-free dry mustard*
2 ½ cups cooked rice

Melt the butter in the microwave on defrost in a large casserole. Carefully swirl around to grease the bottom and sides of casserole. Set aside. Cook spinach in the microwave according to package directions. If using frozen onion, cook it with the frozen spinach. Mix in the onion, spinach, cheese with the melted butter in the casserole. Mix in the 2 eggs and 2 cups milk. Sprinkle with salt if desired. Add ½ teaspoon dry mustard and the 2 ½ cups cooked rice. Blend in. Bake in the large casserole at 325°F for 1 hour.

## Spinach Pie
See recipe under Main Dishes, Egg and Cheese. This is a good main dish for brunch or a light lunch, or a nice side-dish that is very easy to make. I make this for company because I can put it in the oven with a roast or chicken. It also can be made ahead of time and reheated in the microwave oven.

## Spinach Ring
This is my mother's recipe. It looks nice on a dinner party buffet.

3 (10 ounce) packages frozen leaf spinach
3 Tablespoons fine white rice flour or
   sweet rice flour
1 cup milk
3 eggs
¾ teaspoon salt

⅛ teaspoon ground black pepper
⅛ teaspoon ground nutmeg
½ cup grated Pecorino Romano cheese
Sweet butter
A few cooked carrots for color (optional)

Cook frozen spinach according to package directions and drain. Make a white sauce by heating ¾ cup milk in a pan. Blend the rice flour with the remaining milk and add to the pan. Cook until mixture is smooth and thick, stirring with a whisk.

When spinach cools, squeeze out the water and place in a food processor to puree. Combine the spinach and white sauce. Then add the eggs, grated cheese and seasonings. Mix well. Butter one large tube mold (ring mold) or individual molds. You will have enough spinach to fill 8 to 10 individual molds or custard cups. For a more colorful dish, place a few cooked carrots in each mold. Then fill with the spinach filling. Place molds in a larger pan and pour hot water into it to come up half way on the molds. Place in a preheated 350°F oven and bake 30 minutes or until a knife inserted in one mold comes out clean. Remove molds from water and invert onto a serving dish.

This can be made earlier in the day and reheated in the oven. Keep spinach in the molds. Bring to room temperature and place in the oven in freshly boiled water in a larger pan for 10 minutes.

## Spinach Soufflé with Cream Cheese
This recipe comes from Philadelphia® Cream Cheese.

½ cup chopped onion
1 clove garlic, minced
1 Tablespoon butter or gluten-free margarine*, melted
1 (8 ounce) package gluten-free cream cheese*
8 ounces gluten-free farmer cheese*
⅛ teaspoon salt

⅛ teaspoon ground black pepper
3 eggs
2 (10 ounce) packages frozen spinach, thawed, well drained and chopped
¼ teaspoon paprika
⅛ teaspoon ground nutmeg

Cook the onion and garlic in butter. Beat the cream cheese, farmer cheese, salt and pepper with an electric mixer. Beat in the onion mixture. Add the eggs, 1 at a time, mixing well after each addition. Blend in the spinach.

Pour the cheese mixture into a greased 9 inch square baking pan. Sprinkle with paprika and nutmeg. Cover and bake at 325°F for 30 minutes. Uncover and bake an additional 15 minutes.

## Spinach Soufflé with Swiss Cheese
This is my mother's recipe and it's delicious. I've served it at Thanksgiving.

2 packages frozen chopped spinach
5 Tablespoons fine white rice flour or sweet rice flour
1 ¼ cups half and half cream (or substitute evaporated milk)

⅛ teaspoon ground nutmeg
Salt and ground black pepper
4 eggs, separated
1 ¼ cups grated Swiss cheese

Cook frozen spinach according to package directions and drain. Cool and then squeeze dry and set aside. Make a white sauce by warming 1 cup cream in a pan. Blending the rice flour with the remaining cream and add to the pan. Gradually add the cheese. Add seasonings and cook until mixture is smooth and thick, stirring with a whisk. Add spinach to the sauce and blend. Cool. Add 4 yolks to spinach and mix well. Beat egg whites until stiff and fold

*see gluten-free products list at the end of the book

into spinach mixture.  Place in a buttered 2 quart baking dish and bake 45 to 50 minutes in a 325°F oven.

### Turkey Stuffing – Traditional Style

I developed this recipe for GFN foods™/Gluten-Free Naturals™, using their pizza crust mix.  This is the traditional stuffing you remember!  The bread cubes have excellent flavor and texture.  My non-celiac guests love it.  They are surprised to learn it is gluten-free.  Or, if you prefer using leftover Gluten-free Naturals™ Bread or Cornbread, see variations.

For the bread cubes: (This can be done
  ahead of time)
1 package Gluten-Free Naturals™ Pizza
  Crust Mix prepared according to
  package directions (or Gluten-Free
  Naturals™ Bread or Cornbread
  prepared; see variations)

½ teaspoon garlic powder
¼ teaspoon ground black pepper
¼ teaspoon salt
1 teaspoon dried marjoram
½ teaspoon ground sage or rubbed dried
  sage crumbled

Prepare pizza crust mix according to package directions, but in addition to the water, eggs, and oil specified, add the garlic powder, black pepper, salt, marjoram and sage.  Blend it in.  Spread in prepared pan (a pizza pan or oblong pan may be used.)  Bake the full amount of time for the pizza as listed on the package.  Allow to cool so that it is not too hot to handle.  Cut the pizza crust into cubes using a pizza cutter, knife or poultry scissors.

Place the cubes on a larger baking pan, and spread them apart so that they will dry evenly.  Bake at 200°F for about an hour until they are dry, hard and not bendable.  This can be done ahead of time.  After the cubes are dried and cool, store in a plastic bag until ready to use.

For the stuffing:
½ pound gluten-free bulk sausage* or
  sausage with casing removed* (Or see
  index for recipe to make bulk sausage
  using pork.)
2 large stalks celery, diced (if desired, also
  chop and add the leafy tops)

1 large onion, diced
1 ½ cups gluten-free chicken broth* or
  use 1 ½ cups water plus 1 teaspoon
  gluten-free chicken bouillon*
2 eggs

Put the gluten-free bread cubes into a large bowl.  Put sausage in a fry pan and break up with your spatula into small pieces.  Cook until brown.  Remove the sausage using a slotted spoon, and put it in the bowl with your bread cubes.

Drain all fat except for 1 Tablespoon.  Add the vegetables to the pan.  Cook on medium heat until the vegetables are tender.  Add the vegetables to the bowl with the gluten-free bread cubes.

Heat the chicken broth in the same pan until hot.  Add the liquid to the bread cube mixture and blend using a large spoon.  Let the mixture cool down.  (This is so that the raw eggs don't become scrambled eggs when you add them.)  Add the 2 eggs and blend in.

*see gluten-free products list at the end of the book*

Grease a casserole or oblong pan and spread the stuffing evenly in the pan. Bake at 350°F for 30 to 40 minutes.

You may also use this to stuff your turkey. The stuffing should be completely cooled. Never stuff a turkey ahead of time. It should be stuffed right before you put it into the oven. Follow the directions on your turkey regarding adding stuffing and baking times. We found this makes enough stuffing to stuff a 25 pound turkey.

Note: I have made the bread cubes a month or so ahead of time. If they are thoroughly dry, they will keep a long time. Another make-ahead tip is you can cook the vegetables and the sausage a day or two ahead of time and refrigerate them. The day you are ready to make the stuffing, add the cooked vegetables and cooked sausage to the gluten-free bread cubes and continue with the directions from that point.

*Variation*: For a bolder flavored stuffing, use 1 teaspoon ground sage instead of ½ teaspoon. If you like rosemary, a ½ teaspoon or a little more may be added to the bread cube batter.

*Variation 2*: Gluten-Free Naturals™ bread can be used instead of the pizza crust mix. Make cubes using day-old bread. I do this ahead of time, and dry the cubes in a 200°F for about an hour. I store them in an airtight container. I add the seasonings when I make the stuffing. For a large turkey, I use the entire loaf and double the recipe.

*Variation 3*: Prepare Gluten-Free Naturals™ cornbread mix can be used instead of the pizza crust mix. Prepare according to package directions except bake in a greased 11" x 17" non-stick pan for about 20 minutes until the top is browned. Remove from the pan and allow it to cool. Cut into cubes and follow recipe above. (Or see index for Cornbread stuffing recipe.)

*Variation 4*: For a bolder flavored stuffing, use the whole pound of sausage.

## Tomatoes – Stuffed
These are best when you can get vine-ripened beefsteak tomatoes. If you use blue cheese be sure it is a safe brand because some brands grow the blue mold on wheat bread. If you can't find a safe brand, substitute gluten-free goat cheese (fromage de chèvre) or Pecorino Romano cheese. My husband prefers this dish without the blue cheese.

3 large tomatoes at room temperature
3 Tablespoons gluten-free blue cheese* or
   Pecorino Romano cheese or gluten-free
   goat cheese
3 Tablespoons cream cheese, softened

1 teaspoon gluten-free Worcestershire
   sauce*
½ teaspoon onion powder
Paprika

Plunge the whole tomatoes into boiling water a minute then plunge them into cold water, to allow the skins to slip off easily. Cut out stem part and cut in half. Mix the 2 cheeses, onion powder and Worcestershire sauce together and spread equally on all 6 halves. Sprinkle with a dash of paprika. Broil about 5 minutes or just until cheese melts.

*see gluten-free products list at the end of the book

## Yams and Sweet Potatoes
These are easy to make in the microwave.

Wash yams or sweet potatoes and dry. Prick with a fork. Take some oil and coat each yam and place on a microwave safe dish. This helps to seal in the moisture and keep them from drying out. Microwave on high for 7 to 9 minutes or until done. To serve, cut in half. Top with butter, salt and pepper and eat out of the skin. If you prefer, you can remove the skin before serving, but be careful as they will be very hot.

*Variation*: You can use this oil method if you want to bake yams in an oven. You can then wrap them in foil and bake with the meat you are baking. They will be moister inside by using the oil.

## Zucchini, Baked Italian Style
Since bread crumbs made with Gluten-Free Naturals™ Bread are so close to regular bread crumbs, we can enjoy this easy dish again. Sometimes the zucchini and yellow squash come in a package together, which is why I use both kinds of squash. Growing up we only used zucchini for this dish.

Zucchini, washed and sliced in ¼" to ½" slices, the long way
Yellow squash (like zucchini, only yellow), washed and sliced and sliced in ¼" to ½" slices, the long way

Bread crumbs made from Gluten-Free Naturals™ bread, flavored with seasonings and grated cheese if desired (see index for recipe)

Wash and dry the zucchini and yellow squash. Cut into slices. They can also be cut into rings if you prefer. Dip in oil, then the bread crumbs, covering both sides. Place on a foil-lined pan. (I use Reynolds® Release Foil). Bake 20 to 30 minutes at 350ºF. If you cut the zucchini into rings instead of lengthwise, bake it a little less. Test for doneness with a fork.

*Variation*: Sometimes my mother only breads it on the top, instead of both the top and bottom.

## Zucchini Fritters
I like to make these during the summer when I get zucchini fresh from the Farmer's Market.

1 cup Gluten-Free Naturals™ All Purpose Flour
1 teaspoon gluten-free baking powder*
1 teaspoon salt
1 teaspoon oil

2 eggs
½ cup milk
1 ½ cups grated zucchini

Whisk together all dry ingredients. Beat eggs, milk and oil together and add to dry ingredients and beat well. Wash and dry tender zucchini and grate on the coarse side of a grater or in a food processor. Holding a handful of grated zucchini over the sink, squeeze as much water out of the zucchini as possible. Now add to the fritter batter and drop by spoonfuls into hot oil to fry until golden. I use a wok or fryer or a 12" fry pan for this purpose. Drain and serve.

*see gluten-free products list at the end of the book

## Zucchini – Grilled

We like this served with grilled steak. Always be sure your barbeque grill is clean, because gluten from previously grilled foods can transfer to your food.

Zucchini, washed and sliced the long way, about ¼ inch thick
Olive oil

Garlic powder or granulated garlic
Salt
Pepper

Choose zucchini that are not too large, so that they won't be seedy inside. Wash, dry and cut off stems. Slice them the long way. I usually get about 3 slices per zucchini. Place zucchini on a dish and drizzle them with some olive oil. Season them with garlic powder, salt and pepper. Place on a hot barbeque grill and grill on each side, until tender. Do not over-cook or they will get mushy. (If you don't have an outdoor grill, one of those indoor grill pans with the lines can be used to cook it on the stove.)

*Variation:* For a "kick" sprinkle them with some hot pepper flakes, in addition to the other spices.

*Variation 2*: Eggplant and other vegetables can be grilled the same way. Eggplant and zucchini grilled using this method can be used in the Parmigiana recipes in this book. I prefer the traditional method, but grilling the vegetables saves time as well as the extra calories from frying.

## Zucchini Parmigiana or Zucchini Parmesan

One day I bought a bushel of zucchini from the farmer's market, and didn't know what to make with so many. I came up with this recipe.

6 zucchini (choose ones that are not too large because they will be seedy)
Fine white rice flour
Egg
1 Tablespoon water
Salt and ground black pepper

Oil to fry in (I like olive or corn oil)
Mozzarella cheese* (sliced or grated, make sure it's gluten-free)
Oregano
Grated Italian cheese (I like Pecorino Romano but Parmesan is good too)

Peel and slice zucchini into ¼ inch slices, lengthwise. Place the rice flour on a piece of waxed paper. Beat eggs, water, salt and pepper in a pie pan type dish and place next to rice flour. Set out a flat pan and cover it with a couple of layers of paper towels and place it next to your range. Now dip both sides of each slice of zucchini into flour and completely cover. Shake off excess and dip into beaten egg mixture, turning zucchini over to moisten both sides. Place zucchini slices to one side of the pie pan and continue in the same manner with each slice stacking them one on top of the other. This allows the excess egg to run off and gives enough egg to finish the job. If, however, you run out of egg, just add another one to the pie pan along with the water, salt and pepper as you did before. When all slices have been dipped in egg and stacked, let them set awhile so egg excess drains off. This makes the frying step easier and cleaner as egg doesn't drip all over the stove.

*see gluten-free products list at the end of the book

Heat a skillet, and then add just enough oil to cover the bottom and heat a minute. Place a few slices of zucchini in skillet and fry both sides until it is tender when you insert a fork, but not overcooked. Drain on paper towels and continue until all slices are cooked. Add more oil if needed.

Take a suitable baking dish and layer zucchini, sauce and mozzarella and continue until all ingredients are used up ending with mozzarella. Sprinkle top with oregano and grated cheese. Bake at 350°F for 30 minutes or until bubbly and cheese melts.

## Zucchini Side-dish
**An Italian side-dish.**

1 whole Spanish onion, diced
1 Tablespoon oil
1 can (1 lb. size) gluten-free stewed
   tomatoes*

2-3 small tender zucchini
Pinch or 2 of oregano and basil
Salt and ground black pepper to taste

Heat a medium saucepan. Add oil and heat. Add onions to hot oil and sauté on medium heat for 5 minutes. Add the can of stewed tomatoes and cook gently 10 minutes. While this is cooking, wash and remove stems from zucchini. Cut each zucchini in half lengthwise, then cut each half lengthwise again having 4 long strips. Now cut each strip into 1 inch chunks. Add to pot along with spices. Cook 5 to 7 minutes. Remove from heat and let rest with cover 5 or more minutes and serve.

## Zucchini Stew
**We enjoy this dish in the summer when zucchini is plentiful. The potatoes help to thicken the sauce.**

2 onions
3 small potatoes
2 Tablespoons oil
1 (15 oz.) can gluten-free tomato sauce*

4 (7 inch) long thick zucchini
3 basil leaves or 1 teaspoon dry basil
1 or 2 pinches oregano
Salt and ground black pepper to taste

Peel potatoes and cut into 6 pieces each. Peel and slice onions. Heat a large pot a minute, add the oil and heat. Dry potatoes with a paper towel to be sure they will not stick to the pan or spatter. Place the potatoes in hot oil. When potatoes are lightly cooked on one side turn them over. Now add onions and continue to sauté vegetables until potatoes are lightly browned. Remove from heat and then add the can of tomato sauce, basil, oregano, salt and pepper. Return to heat and cook gently for about 10 minutes until potatoes are almost tender. While this is cooking, clean zucchini, remove stem end, cut in half lengthwise and then into 1 inch chunks. Add to sauce and cook 15-20 minutes more, just until the zucchini is cooked and the potatoes help to thicken the sauce. Remove from heat. Do not overcook as zucchini will fall apart and be mushy and totally unappetizing.

## Breads, Rolls, Pancakes and Muffins

# BAKING POWDER BREADS, PANCAKES, MUFFINS, AND DONUTS

Baking powder breads are easier to make than their wheat counterparts, because you don't have to worry about over-mixing! You don't have to mix them with a fork until just blended. You can beat them with an electric mixer. Since there is no gluten that will make them tough, they remain tender.

## Applesauce Muffins

These muffins are moist and light in texture.

1 cup Gluten-Free Naturals™ All Purpose
    Flour
¾ cup sugar
¼ teaspoon gluten-free baking powder*
1 teaspoon baking soda
¾ teaspoon salt
1 ½ teaspoons ground cinnamon
¼ teaspoon ground nutmeg (or less)

1 egg
¼ cup oil
⅓ cup plain gluten-free yogurt* or gluten-
    free buttermilk*
¾ cup unsweetened applesauce (I use
    canned)
½ cup chopped nuts

Blend all ingredients until thoroughly mixed. Pour into greased muffin tins or line with cupcake papers. Bake them for 20-25 minutes or until done at 400°F. Makes 12 large muffins.

*Variation*: Add ¼ cup raisins

## Banana Bread

This bread is a favorite of ours for breakfast or snacking. By using the smaller pans you save baking time, as well as ensure that the center of the bread is cooked. The size provides easier cutting and the slices hold together better. My baking pans are by Ecco® and measure a little over 3" x 5 ½". This bread freezes very well.

Another tip – if you have a lot of leftover ripe bananas; peel and freeze them. I put one banana per sandwich bag and put them all into a larger freezer bag, so I can grab the exact number of bananas I need. When you defrost them they will look watery and dark, but they work perfectly in baking your recipe. (You can also defrost them in the microwave.) The freezing also saves you the "mashing" step.

1 cup mashed ripe bananas
¾ cup sugar
1 teaspoon gluten-free vanilla*
2 eggs
¼ cup oil

1 ½ cups Gluten-Free Naturals™ All
    Purpose Flour
¼ cup chopped nuts
¾ teaspoon baking powder
½ teaspoon baking soda
¼ teaspoon salt

Combine mashed bananas, sugar, vanilla, eggs, and oil. (I mash the bananas with the sugar, and then blend in the rest. I beat the egg and oil in with a whisk.) Add the rest of

*see gluten-free products list at the end of the book

ingredients and blend in using a spoon. (It will get too thick to use a whisk.) Put in 3 small greased loaf pans. Bake at 350°F for 30-35 minutes. Or put it in one large greased loaf pan and bake 45 to 50 minutes. Test with a cake tester to be sure it's done.

*Variation*: You can make muffins out of this batter and bake for about 25 minutes. I prefer the bread but if you want a faster baking muffin that freezes well, this works.

*Variation 2*: You can substitute ¾ cup fine white rice flour and ¾ cup defatted soy flour and 1 ½ teaspoons xanthan gum for the Flour. The bread will turn out a little denser if you make this substitution, but it will work.

## Banana Pecan Muffins

These are easier to make than wheat muffins, because you can use an electric mixer. Wheat muffins must be mixed with a fork until just moistened. Mixing wheat muffins a lot makes the gluten come out of the flour and then makes them tough. Since these contain no gluten, you can mix them well.

This is a good recipe to use leftover bananas. If you have a lot of leftover ripe bananas, peel and freeze them. When you defrost them they will look watery and dark, but they work perfectly in baking your recipe. (You can also defrost them in the microwave.) The freezing also saves you the "mashing" step. These muffins also freeze well.

1 cup mashed ripe bananas (2 bananas)
¾ cup sugar (or use a little less if bananas
　are very ripe)
1 teaspoon gluten-free vanilla*
2 eggs
¼ cup oil
1 ½ cups Gluten-Free Naturals™ All
　Purpose Flour

¼ cup chopped pecans (or other nuts may
　be used)
¾ teaspoon baking powder
½ teaspoon baking soda
¼ teaspoon salt
¼ cup milk or gluten-free milk substitute

In an electric mixer, blend bananas and sugar until bananas are mashed. Add eggs and oil and blend in. Add the dry ingredients and the milk and blend in with the mixer until mixed.

Line muffin tins with cupcake papers, and fill. Makes 12 muffins. Bake at 350°F for 20 to 25 minutes until they test done with a cake tester. If you didn't measure your bananas, and 2 large ones were used, bake them about 25 to 30 minutes.

Note: When mixing using a heavy duty mixer, I sometimes add a good sized handful of whole pecans instead of chopped nuts. Since pecans are a softer nut, the mixing paddle of my machine breaks them up into chunks, and I can avoid the chopping step.

*see gluten-free products list at the end of the book

## Banana Fritters

3 firm bananas
Cornstarch or Gluten-Free Naturals™ All
    Purpose Flour
1 cup Gluten-Free Naturals™ All Purpose
    Flour
2 teaspoons gluten-free baking powder*

1 ¼ teaspoons salt
¼ cup sugar
1 well beaten egg
⅓ cup milk
2 teaspoons melted butter

Use only firm bananas or this won't work.  Cut bananas cross-wise into 4 pieces each, making 12 pieces.  Roll in cornstarch.  Blend together the Flour with the baking powder, salt and sugar.  Beat eggs and mix with milk and melted butter.  This will be a thick batter.  Heat about 1 ½ to 2 inches of oil in a fry pan and allow the oil to heat to 375°F.  Spear a piece of banana with a fork and completely cover it with batter.  Fry until golden brown and drain on paper towels.  Serve with a main course or sprinkle with sugar and serve as dessert.

## Banana Peanut Butter Bread
This bread is light and delicious.  Children (and adults) like this.

¼ cup sugar
¼ cup brown sugar*
1 large ripe banana, mashed
3 Tablespoons gluten-free chunky peanut
    butter*
½ cup milk or gluten-free milk substitute*
1 Tablespoon oil
½ teaspoon gluten-free vanilla*
1 egg

1 cup Gluten-Free Naturals™ All Purpose
    Flour
1 ½ teaspoons gluten-free baking
    powder*
¼ teaspoon salt
⅛ to ¼ teaspoon ground cinnamon
½ cup gluten-free semi-sweet chocolate
    chips*

Mash the bananas with the sugar.  Blend in the peanut butter.  Add the milk, oil, vanilla and eggs and blend in.  Add the dry ingredients.  Blend with the banana mixture.  Blend in the chocolate chips.  Bake at 350°F in a greased 8 x 4 inch loaf pan for 50-55 minutes, or use 3 greased smaller loaf pans and bake about 30-35 minutes.  If using the large pan, allow it to sit for 10 minutes on a wire rack before removing it from pan.  If using the smaller pan you can remove them immediately onto a wire rack.  Cool and serve.  If you are not going to eat it all in the next couple of days, freeze it.

*Variation*:  You can also use this batter to make muffins or mini-muffins.

## Bread Sticks with Garlic

My husband invented these crispy corn bread sticks.  These are quite a bit of work, but look like those store-bought ones from Italy.

1 cup Masa Harina (corn flour treated with lime, it's used to make tortillas)
½ cup cornstarch
1 ½ teaspoons baking powder
2 Tablespoons olive oil
½ teaspoon garlic

⅛ teaspoon onion powder
½ teaspoon xanthan gum
½ teaspoon salt
1 ¼ to 1 ½ cups water

Blend all ingredients.  If too thick, add additional water and blend.  Put into a heavy plastic bag (freezer type).  Make a small cut in one corner, and squeeze the dough onto a greased baking sheet.  You will have long sticks about ¼" in diameter.  Or, use a pastry bag for this purpose.  Bake at 400°F for 25 minutes until done.  (Time may vary depending on the thickness of the breadsticks).

## Biscuits – Roll Out Version

1 cup Gluten-Free Naturals™ Sandwich Bread Flour or Gluten-Free Naturals™ All Purpose Flour
⅓ cup butter*, cold from refrigerator (I use less)
Sprinkling of salt
1 teaspoon baking powder

¼ teaspoon baking soda
6 Tablespoons to ½ Cup Gluten-Free Plain Yogurt (add slowly as needed so dough won't be too wet to roll out)
Water

Prepare biscuits by putting cold butter, Sandwich Bread flour, sprinkling of salt, and baking powder and soda in a food processor.  Process until butter is cut in.  If you don't have a processor, cut in butter with a pastry blender.  Add the yogurt and process until the dough balls up.  If dough is too wet, add 1 to 2 Tablespoons more of the gluten-free flour and blend in.  You can knead dough to improve blending it.  Roll out on waxed paper to about ½ inch thick.  You shouldn't need to have to put extra flour on the waxed paper.  It should roll out without it.  Cut using a biscuit cutter or a juice glass.  Place on a foil lined pan, or foil lined toaster oven pan.  (I like using Reynolds® Release foil so they don't stick.)  Since there is no gluten, it is fine to re-roll the leftover pieces and cut them into biscuits.  Continue until dough is gone.  Or, if you prefer not to roll out the dough, divide it into 12 balls.  Flatten and put onto the foil lined pan.

Brush with some cold water so that the dough will absorb it and rise better.  If you are not baking them immediately, cover them with plastic wrap so that they don't dry out. If they look a little dry, brush with water again before baking.  (Note:  If they get too dry they won't rise properly.)

Bake for 10 to 15 minutes at 450°F until cooked and lightly browned.  They can be cooked in a toaster oven set to 450°F.

*see gluten-free products list at the end of the book

*Variation*: Milk can be used instead of yogurt. Use 1 ¼ teaspoons baking powder instead of baking powder and soda. For drop biscuits increase milk by ¼ cup and drop the dough into a greased muffin pan. Bake as directed above.

*Variation 2*: For Scones, add 2 Tablespoons sugar. Use ⅓ cup milk and add 1 egg instead of yogurt. Follow directions listed above if dough is too wet or dry. Roll out and cut into triangle or diamond shapes. Or roll out into balls and flatten them. Brush with milk and sprinkle with sugar. Bake as directed above. Or use ½ cup milk and make dropped biscuits by putting the dough in a greased muffin pan.

## Bisquick® Substitute

You can make this ahead of time and keep it on hand in your refrigerator. You can use it in Bisquick® Recipes.

| | |
|---|---|
| 1 cup Gluten-Free Naturals™ All Purpose Flour | 1 ½ teaspoons gluten-free baking powder* |
| ½ teaspoon salt | 6 Tablespoons butter (or 4 Tablespoons can be used and it will work) |

Mix all together in a food processor. Or blend the flour and cut the butter in by hand using a pastry blender. To make biscuits add about ½ cup milk. Sprinkle flour on waxed paper and roll out the dough, or make drop biscuits. Bake at 450°F for 8 to 10 minutes.

## Carrot Muffins

These are moist and light muffins that are easy to make. You don't have to peel any carrots. My husband thought these were just spice muffins and didn't realize they contained carrots.

| | |
|---|---|
| 1 can (14.5 ounces) of cooked carrots, drained | 1 ½ teaspoons ground cinnamon |
| 1 cup Gluten-Free Naturals™ All Purpose Flour | ¼ teaspoon ground nutmeg (or less) |
| ¾ cup sugar | 1 egg |
| ¼ teaspoon gluten-free baking powder* | ¼ cup oil |
| 1 teaspoon baking soda | ½ cup plain gluten-free yogurt* or gluten-free buttermilk* |
| ½ teaspoon salt (use ¾ teaspoon salt if carrots are unsalted) | ¼ cup chopped nuts |
| | ¼ cup raisins |

Drain the carrots. I use a hand blender to pulverize them. (I put the hand blender right inside the opened can.) You could also mash the carrots with a masher until fine, but I prefer them pulverized with the blender. Or you can use a food processor.

Blend all ingredients until thoroughly mixed. Pour into greased muffin tins or line with cupcake papers. Bake them at 400°F for 20-25 minutes or until done. Makes 12 large muffins.

*see gluten-free products list at the end of the book*

## Corn Bread/Corn Pudding Style – Bundt Pan Version

This bread is crispy on the outside yet creamy inside like a corn pudding. Serve directly onto your dinner plate and top with a pat of butter or gluten-free margarine*. It is nice for Thanksgiving or whenever serving poultry or pork. Half the recipe and bake in a loaf pan for smaller groups.

1 cup yellow cornmeal
1 cup Gluten-Free Naturals™ All Purpose
   Flour
1 ½ teaspoons salt
4 teaspoons gluten-free baking powder*
4 Tablespoons sugar

2 eggs
½ cup oil
2 (16 ounce) cans gluten-free creamed
   corn*
Sweet butter

Mix cornmeal, flour, salt, baking powder and sugar together. Add oil and eggs and beat well. Add creamed corn and stir until blended. Butter a Bundt pan generously with sweet butter. Pour batter into prepared pan and bake in a preheated 350°F oven for 45-50 minutes. Top should be golden and dry. Shake pan to see if batter moves, and if it does not, it is done. Serves 16.

## Cornbread with Sage and Cheddar Cheese

One summer I grew a lot of sage and came up with this cornbread for a change. I like to reheat leftovers in the microwave for about 10 to 20 seconds to re-melt the cheese.

Gluten-Free Naturals® Cornbread Mix
   prepared according to package
   directions

5 to 6 fresh sage leaves, washed and cut
   up
¼ to ⅓ cup grated cheddar cheese*

Prepare mix according to package directions, and add the sage and cheese. Bake according to package directions. Serve warm.

## Corn Bread – Square Pan Version

This cornbread is good the day you make it, but will be very stale and fall apart the next day. I use the leftovers the next day by crumbling them in a bowl and topping them with chili (see index). We prefer Gluten-Free Naturals™ Cornbread mix because it stays fresher longer, and it is light and moist without being gritty.

1 ½ cups yellow cornmeal
½ cup fine white rice flour
2 Tablespoons sugar
1 ½ teaspoons gluten-free baking
   powder*
1 teaspoon salt

2 eggs
⅔ cup milk
¼ cup oil
1 can (8.5 ounces) of gluten-free creamed
   corn*

Combine the cornmeal, rice flour, sugar, baking powder and salt. In a large Pyrex® measuring cup, measure the milk. Beat in the eggs, oil and creamed corn in the same cup. Pour into the cornmeal mixture and blend until moistened. Put into a greased 8 x 8 inch baking pan. Bake at 400°F for 20 to 25 minutes. It will become lightly browned.

*see gluten-free products list at the end of the book

*Variation*: Add some gluten-free grated cheese and/or some leftover cooked peppers to the batter for a more Mexican flare.

## Crepes

Crepes have a lot of uses. They are delicious rolled with jam on them. They can be cut up and used as noodles in soup. They can be used in place of pasta in Manicotti or Lasagna. These taste like the real thing.

2 eggs
¾ cup milk
1 Tablespoon oil
¼ teaspoon salt

½ cup Gluten-Free Naturals™ All
    Purpose Flour
Butter for the pan (not much is needed if
    using a Teflon® Pan

Mix all ingredients except the butter in a blender. (I use my hand blender and the cup it comes with.)

Heat a 6 inch Teflon® skillet, add a little butter and swirl it around to coat the pan. Heat the pan a few minutes then lift it off the heat. Pour about 2 Tablespoons or so of batter into the center of the pan and tip pan from side to side until the bottom is covered with the batter. Return to heat. When batter looks dry (about 30 seconds), take a dull table knife or a plastic spatula and lift one edge of crepe until you can take hold of it with your fingers. Now carefully pull the crepe up and flip it over. (If you have a thin plastic spatula sometimes you can flip it using that, so you don't have to use your fingers.)

Cook a few seconds, lift pan and turn crepe out onto a plate to cool. Be careful that your pan doesn't overheat. Lower heat and raise heat as needed. Add more butter after every 2 to 3 crepes if needed. (I use a new Teflon pan, so it doesn't need much butter.) This recipe makes about 8 crepes.

*Variation*: You can substitute ½ cup cornstarch for the Gluten-Free Naturals™ All Purpose Flour. The crepes will be very thin and a little more difficult to work with. They are blander in flavor. I think that they are too thin to serve with jam, but they work in recipes such as Manicotti.

## Cornbread – Cornmeal Only Version

This is only good the day you make it. It's a good recipe if you don't have any special gluten-free ingredients like xanthan gum on hand. Just be careful in purchasing cornmeal. Some brands may have contamination. We prefer Gluten-Free Naturals™ Cornbread mix because it stays fresher longer, and it is light and moist without being gritty.

2 cups gluten-free cornmeal, course grind*
2 teaspoons sugar
2 teaspoons gluten-free baking powder*
½ teaspoon salt
¼ cup oil, gluten-free shortening* or
    gluten-free butter or margarine*

½ cup boiling water
½ cup gluten-free buttermilk* or gluten-
    free plain yogurt*
2 eggs
2 Tablespoons butter*

*see gluten-free products list at the end of the book

Mix dry ingredients together with a whisk. Add the ¼ cup fat and boiling water and mix well. Add buttermilk. If too dry, add 1 to 2 Tablespoons more buttermilk or water. (If using a very fine cornmeal, a little more liquid may be needed.)

Heat the oven to 350°F. Take an 8 x 8 x 2 inch baking pan and put the 2 Tablespoons of butter in it. Heat in the oven until the butter is melted. Take a spatula and spread butter around. (If lactose intolerant; use gluten-free cooking spray*, shortening or lactose-free gluten-free margarine*.)

Spread the batter in the pan. Bake for 10 minutes at 350°F. Increase the oven temperature to 375°F and bake for 20 to 25 minutes more. It is done when it's lightly golden brown and tests done with a cake tester.

Cut into squares and serve with additional butter or gluten-free jam.

## Cranberry Nut Bread

If you like cranberries, this is a tasty bread that is full of fruit. It is also milk and dairy-free. This was adapted from the recipe on the Ocean Spray® cranberries package.

2 cups Gluten-Free Naturals™ All
  Purpose Flour
1 cup sugar
1 ½ teaspoons gluten-free baking
  powder*
½ teaspoon baking soda
1 teaspoon salt

1 egg
1 cup orange juice
2 Tablespoons oil
1 ½ cups fresh cranberries, chopped
  course
½ cup walnuts, chopped

Blend flour with sugar, baking powder, baking soda, and salt. Beat egg with juice and oil and add all at once to dry ingredients. Since there is no gluten in these, you may mix them well. Add the fruit and nuts and mix in. Put in a greased 9 x 5 inch loaf pan. Bake at 350°F for 55 to 60 minutes. Cool 15 minutes in the pan on a rack, then remove from the pan and cool completely. Slice and enjoy. It has a delicate cake-like texture with nice flavor from the nuts and cranberries.

## Date or Raisin Nut Bread

This is a soft, springy bread. Enjoy it at breakfast topped with gluten-free cream cheese. Also nice served at a brunch or afternoon tea. My non-celiac taste testers said this is "phenomenal."

½ pound (2 cups) Gluten-Free Naturals™
  Bread Flour (Multi-Grain or Sandwich)
  or Gluten-Free Naturals™ All Purpose
  Flour
½ cup sugar
½ teaspoon salt
2 teaspoons gluten-free baking powder*
1 teaspoon ground cinnamon (optional)
1 egg

1 to 2 Tablespoons oil
1 ¼ cups milk
½ cup gluten-free chopped dates or raisins
  (check ingredients, some brands of
  chopped dates contain oats and are not
  gluten-free.)
½ cup chopped walnuts

*see gluten-free products list at the end of the book*

Whisk flour, sugar, salt, baking powder, and cinnamon together in a mixer bowl. Add egg, oil, and milk and blend in. Stir in dates and nuts by hand. Pour into a greased 8 ½" non-stick loaf pan. Bake at 350°F for 1 hour, until it tests done. Remove from pan and cool on a cooling rack. Slice when cool.

*Variation*: You can substitute raisins, dried cranberries, dried cherries or other dried fruits for the dates.

## Doughnut Holes

If you miss having donuts, these are very delicious and easy. We like them best when still a little warm. They look like "real" donut holes and taste like them too. These are my mother's recipe.

1 cup Gluten-Free Naturals™ All Purpose
　　Flour
2 teaspoons gluten-free baking powder*
½ teaspoon salt
2 Tablespoons sugar
1 cup gluten-free Ricotta Cheese*

2 eggs
¼ teaspoon gluten-free vanilla*
Oil for frying
Powdered sugar or granulated sugar or
　　cinnamon sugar mixture

Whisk flour, salt and baking powder together. In a large bowl, combine Ricotta cheese, sugar, eggs and vanilla and blend well. Add dry ingredients and mix thoroughly. Heat the oil in a deep fryer to 375°F. Measure 1 level Tablespoon of dough for each doughnut and push into hot oil. They will become nicely shaped round balls about the size of a walnut. Be careful not to make them too big or they won't cook through properly. Drain and dust with sugar or shake in a bag of granulated sugar or cinnamon sugar.

## Focaccia Bread (Easy)

We enjoy this served with an Italian dinner. Or heat up some gluten-free tomato sauce for dipping and enjoy this as an appetizer. This recipe comes from my brother.

2 packages Gluten-Free Naturals™
　　Pizzeria Style Pizza Crust Mix
2 eggs
2 cups warm water
4 Tablespoons oil (I prefer olive oil, but
　　corn oil can be used)
½ teaspoon garlic powder

½ teaspoon oregano
¼ teaspoon sea salt
Extra virgin olive oil (for drizzling)
2 ounces shredded gluten-free mozzarella
　　cheese

Empty the two bags of Pizza Crust mix into a large mixing bowl. Add 2 eggs, 4 Tablespoons oil and 2 cups of water. Mix thoroughly into a batter with a rubber spatula. (Or a heavy duty mixer may be used.) Grease an 11 ¼" by 17 ¼" non-stick jelly roll pan. (Or a cookie sheet with a lip around the edge.) Baker's Secret® makes this exact size.

Scoop the batter from the bowl into the pan. Wet the rubber spatula with water repeatedly as you spread the batter evenly around the cookie sheet into a layer of uniform thickness.

*see gluten-free products list at the end of the book

Bake at 400°F for 18 minutes.  Remove from the oven and drizzle with extra virgin olive oil. Sprinkle with about 2 ounces of mozzarella cheese, oregano, garlic powder, and sea salt. (Other herbs or spices maybe used, such as rosemary, roasted garlic pieces, sundried tomatoes, parmesan cheese, or pepper may be added to make the focaccia your own special creation.)

Return the pan to the oven for 4 to 6 minutes to melt the cheese.  Remove from the oven and enjoy while hot, or let cool.  Cut into slices or bite-size pieces for an appetizer.

## Funnel Cakes
This is the traditional funnel cakes you remember from Carnivals.

3 large eggs
3 Tablespoons sugar
1 cup milk
1 ¾ cups Gluten-Free Naturals™ All Purpose Flour or Gluten-Free Naturals™ Sandwich Bread Flour
2 teaspoons baking powder
½ teaspoon salt

¼ teaspoon gluten-free vanilla*
6 Tablespoons water (or a little more if batter is too thick)
Oil for frying
Confectioner's sugar to sprinkle on the funnel cakes after they are fried

Beat together all ingredients but the oil and confectioner's sugar.  I find it easier to blend together using a wire whisk.  Pour batter into a food-safe plastic bag.  Cut off a small hole on one corner.  It should be smaller than ¼ inch.  Do not make the hole too large or your funnel cakes will be too big and they won't be crispy.  (Although you can use a funnel the dough gets thicker as you work with it and I found squeezing it through the plastic bag to be easier.)

Fry in a large skillet in hot oil.  I prefer using an iron pan because the heat radiates better. Swirl the batter in a spiral and fry until golden brown.  Turn over with a pancake turner and fry until done.  Drain on paper towels and sprinkle with confectioner's sugar.

## Ginger Bread
This is light colored bread has a cake-like texture and a mild, not too sweet ginger ale flavor.  Try it for breakfast topped with cream cheese.  Or try it as an accompaniment to pork, chicken or ham at dinner.

1 ¾ cups Gluten-Free Naturals™ Sandwich Bread Flour or Gluten-Free Naturals™ All Purpose Flour
½ cup sugar
1 teaspoon baking soda
1 to 1 ½ teaspoons ground ginger (I use 1 teaspoon only)

1 teaspoon ground cinnamon (optional)
¼ teaspoon salt
¼ cup oil
1 egg
1 cup gluten-free plain yogurt*

*see gluten-free products list at the end of the book

Put all ingredients in a heavy-duty mixer and blend. Or, to prepare by hand, whisk all dry ingredients together and then add oil, egg and plain yogurt all at once, stirring with a sturdy spoon. Put in a well greased loaf pan. Bake in a preheated 375°F oven for 35-40 minutes.

## Ginger Bread – Version 2
This version uses soy flour and milk instead of yogurt. It's a little more dense, but still good.

½ cup cornstarch
½ cup defatted soy flour
¾ cup white rice flour
1 teaspoon xanthan gum
½ cup sugar
1 teaspoon baking powder

1 to 1 ½ teaspoons ground ginger (I use 1)
1 teaspoon ground cinnamon (optional)
¼ teaspoon salt
¼ cup oil
1 egg
1 cup milk

Put all ingredients in a heavy-duty mixer and blend. Or, to prepare by hand, whisk all dry ingredients together and then add oil, egg and milk all at once, stirring with a sturdy spoon. Put in a well greased loaf pan. Bake in a preheated 375°F oven for 35-40 minutes.

## Great-Grandma's Italian Spoon Bread
We always enjoyed this recipe even before we knew about the gluten-free diet. When we started the gluten-free diet, we purchased a new iron fry pan for this recipe, because we didn't know if the old one harbored any gluten in the black coating.

1 quart boiling water
1 teaspoon salt
1 cup cornmeal*
4 Tablespoons butter

¼ cup grated gluten-free Italian cheese (I use Pecorino Romano or Parmesan)
Ground black pepper
3 eggs
Additional butter

Add salt to water and bring to a boil. Using a long wooden spoon slowly add cornmeal to water and stir until mixture becomes thick and bubbly. Remove from heat and add butter, grated cheese and a good sprinkling of black pepper. Mix well, then add eggs and beat them into the batter. Grease a 10 inch iron fry pan heavily with sweet butter and pour the batter into it. Dot the top with more butter and bake in a 375°F oven for 35 minutes or until bread is golden brown and nicely crusted.

## Irish Soda Bread
A delicious bread that is nice to serve on St. Patrick's Day, or anytime. I usually double the recipe and make 2 loaves; one to enjoy and one to share. This bread freezes well.

1 ¾ cups Gluten-Free Naturals™ Sandwich Bread Flour or Gluten-Free Naturals™ All Purpose Flour
½ cup sugar
1 teaspoon baking soda
¼ teaspoon salt (use a little less if using salted butter)

¼ cup oil or butter (butter makes it taste more like Irish Soda bread)
1 egg
1 cup gluten-free plain yogurt* or buttermilk*
¼ cup raisins

Blend dry ingredients together. Add softened butter or oil. (You can use a heavy-duty mixer.) Add egg and yogurt or buttermilk and blend in. Put in a well greased loaf pan, preferably glass or a metal non-stick pan. Bake in a preheated 375°F oven for 35-40 minutes. All to cool completely on a wire rack before cutting. This bread freezes well.

## Lemon Poppy seed Bread
This bread has a cake-like texture with a nice lemon flavor. It's nice served with a cup of tea. I like it as part of a Sunday brunch.

1 ¾ cups Gluten-Free Naturals™ Sandwich Bread Flour or Gluten-Free Naturals™ All Purpose Flour
½ cup sugar
1 teaspoon baking soda
¼ teaspoon salt
¼ cup oil

1 egg
1 cup gluten-free plain yogurt* or ½ cup yogurt and a ½ cup milk
½ teaspoon lemon extract
1 teaspoon poppy seeds

Put all ingredients in a heavy-duty mixer and blend. Or, to prepare by hand, whisk all dry ingredients together and then add oil, egg and milk all at once, stirring with a sturdy spoon. Put in a well greased loaf pan. Bake in a preheated 375°F oven for 35-40 minutes. Cool before slicing.

## Muffins: Basic Muffins, "Donut" Muffins, Apple Muffins, & Blueberry Muffins
If you miss the flavor of donuts, donut muffins (see variation below) will help fill that craving without eating all the fat in fried donuts. This is my mother's recipe that I converted to make it gluten-free.

1 ½ cups Gluten-Free Naturals™ Sandwich Bread Flour or Gluten-Free Naturals™ All Purpose Flour
1 teaspoon baking powder
1 teaspoon baking soda
½ teaspoon salt
½ cup sugar

1 egg
⅓ cup oil
½ cup milk
Cinnamon sugar mixture (see below; this is optional)

*see gluten-free products list at the end of the book

Blend dry ingredients in a large bowl. Beat egg with oil and yogurt. Add all liquid at once to dry ingredients and combine. If batter is too thick, add a few Tablespoons additional water or milk. (Some yogurts are thicker than others and additional liquid may be needed.) Grease muffin tins well with sweet butter or oil. Place batter into tins about ⅔rds full. If desired, top each muffin with a good sprinkling of cinnamon sugar. Bake in a preheated 400°F oven for 20 minutes. Makes 10 to 12 muffins. If making 12 instead of 10, test for doneness a few minutes sooner.

Cinnamon sugar mixture – 1 Tablespoon sugar and 1 teaspoon cinnamon

*Variation*: For a Donut muffins, add ½ teaspoon ground nutmeg. Top with cinnamon/sugar mixture.

*Variation 2*: For apple muffins, add ½ teaspoon cinnamon to the batter. Add 1 peeled and grated or finely chopped apple. If desired, top with a mixture of ⅓ cup brown sugar, ½ cup nuts and ½ teaspoon cinnamon. (I like them plain.) Bake for 25 to 30 minutes. Makes 12 to 14 muffins.

*Variation 3*: For blueberry muffins, eliminate cinnamon/sugar topping. Add 1 teaspoon vanilla and 1 cup of blueberries to the batter.

## Muffins: Basic, "Donut", Apple, & Blueberry Muffins – Version 2
By using yogurt instead of milk, these muffins are a little more moist in texture.

½ cup cornstarch
½ cup defatted soy flour
½ cup white rice flour
1 ½ teaspoons xanthan gum
1 teaspoon baking powder
1 teaspoon baking soda
½ teaspoon salt
½ cup sugar

1 egg
⅓ cup oil
¾ cup gluten-free plain yogurt*
2 to 4 Tablespoons additional yogurt or
    milk (may or may not be needed)
Cinnamon sugar mixture (see below; this
    is optional)

Blend dry ingredients in a large bowl. Beat egg with oil and yogurt. Add all liquid at once to dry ingredients and combine. If batter is too thick, add a few Tablespoons additional water or milk. (Some yogurts are thicker than others and additional liquid may be needed.) Grease muffin tins well with sweet butter or oil. Place batter into tins. If desired, top each muffin with a good sprinkling of cinnamon sugar. Bake in a preheated 400°F oven for 20 minutes. Makes 8 to 9 muffins.

Cinnamon sugar mixture – 1 Tablespoon sugar and 1 teaspoon cinnamon

*Variation*: For a Donut muffins, add ½ teaspoon ground nutmeg. Top with cinnamon/sugar mixture.

*Variation 2*: For apple muffins, add ½ teaspoon cinnamon to the batter. Add 1 peeled and grated or finely chopped apple. If desired, top with a mixture of ⅓ cup brown sugar, ½ cup

*see gluten-free products list at the end of the book*

nuts and ½ teaspoon ground cinnamon. (I like them plain.) Bake for 25 to 30 minutes. Makes 12 muffins.

*Variation 3*: For blueberry muffins, eliminate cinnamon/sugar topping. Add 1 teaspoon vanilla and 1 cup of blueberries to the batter.

## Pancakes – Apple Pancake Bake
This can be made ahead of time and reheated in the microwave. Makes 2 round 9" pancakes that you slice and serve. These are also good as a snack. My husband sometimes takes a couple of leftover slices for an on-the-go breakfast, and eats them cold.

1 packet Gluten-Free Naturals™ Pancake
  Mix, prepared according to package
  directions

2 large or 3 to 4 small apples, peeled,
  cored and thinly sliced
Sugar and Cinnamon
Maple Syrup (optional)

Prepare pancake mix as directed on the package using the additional water for a slightly thinner batter. (The directions are: add 1 cup milk, ½ cup water, 1 Tablespoon oil and 1 egg.) Blend well with a whisk.

Grease two 9" round non-stick baking pans. Slice the apples very thinly, and put half in each pan. Spread apples to evenly distribute them on the pan. Sprinkle apples with cinnamon and sugar. I use approximately 1 teaspoon sugar and ¼ teaspoon cinnamon in each pan. Cover each pan with half of the pancake batter. Smooth to cover apples. Sprinkle with a little more cinnamon sugar.

Bake at 350°F for 20 minutes. Turn out onto 2 round plates. Slice into wedges. Serve with maple syrup* if desired. We enjoy them plain. Or, sprinkle with a little confectioner's sugar if desired. Store any leftovers in the refrigerator. They reheat well in the microwave the next day.

## Pancakes – Version 1
We prefer the Gluten-Free Naturals™ pancake mix, because they are the traditional pancakes you remember. These pancakes are good but with a different flavor and texture. I prefer the Gluten-Free Naturals™ All Purpose Flour in this recipe, but the Cookie Blend is also good. My mother came up with this recipe and I converted it to gluten-free. They are not the prettiest pancakes because they are not uniformly round, but they taste good. We use real maple syrup because it's gluten-free. See list in the back of this book for other pancake syrups.

1 cup Gluten-Free Naturals™ All Purpose
  Flour or Gluten-Free Naturals™
  Cookie Blend
¼ to ½ teaspoon salt
2 teaspoons baking powder
½ teaspoon baking soda

2 teaspoons sugar
1 egg
1 cup buttermilk* or plain yogurt*
¼ cup milk or water
1 Tablespoon oil

*see gluten-free products list at the end of the book

Mix together dry ingredients with a whisk. Add all wet ingredients and blend with the whisk. If too thick, a little more milk or water may be added. Sometimes gluten-free pancake batter becomes thicker as it sits, so you may have to add a little more water as needed while you are cooking them.

Cook on a lightly greased griddle, at a moderate (not high) temperature. I use a ladle to pour the batter on the griddle then use the back of the ladle to spread batter out to a 5 inch circle. Flip after bubbles form and it's lightly browned. Serve with butter* and maple syrup*.

## Pancakes – Buckwheat Pancakes

If you like the flavor of buckwheat then you will like these pancakes. Buckwheat has a very strong distinct flavor, and can be an acquired taste for most people. These are very hearty and thick pancakes. Make sure you purchase a brand of buckwheat flour that is not contaminated. See some suggested brands at the back of this book.

½ cup Gluten-Free Naturals™ All
   Purpose Flour
1 cup buckwheat flour*
2 ½ teaspoons gluten-free baking
   powder*
½ teaspoon salt
1 egg

1 Tablespoon oil
1 Tablespoon molasses*
½ cup milk
1 ½ to 2 cups water, or a little more if
   needed

Mix together the dry ingredients with a whisk. Add egg, oil, molasses, milk and water. Start with the 1 ½ cups water and add more to get the desired consistency. Blend with the whisk.

Cook on a lightly greased griddle, at a moderate temperature. A Teflon® coated type griddle works best. I use a ladle to pour the batter on the griddle then use the back of the ladle to spread batter out to a 5 inch circle. Flip after bubbles form and it's lightly browned. (If batter is way too thick you will not get many bubbles, so you may need a little more water.) These will rise and be thick, so be sure they are cooked through. Add additional butter or gluten-free cooking spray to the griddle as needed to prevent sticking.

Serve with butter and maple syrup. These pancakes keep well in a covered container in the refrigerator and any leftovers can be reheated in the microwave the next day.

## Pizza Crust – Version 1

We prefer the Gluten-Free Naturals™ Pizzeria Style Pizza mix. If you don't have it or you are allergic to soy, you can use this method. The herbs add flavor, but they can be eliminated. I use a plain small can of tomato sauce*, since the herbs are in the crust. By using baking powder, you can bake it right away but it will have a biscuit-like flavor and texture.

4 cups (1 lb.) Gluten-Free Naturals™ Bread Flour (Sandwich or Multi-Grain) or Gluten-Free Naturals™ All Purpose Flour
1 ½ teaspoons salt
2 Tablespoons sugar
1 Tablespoon gluten-free baking powder*

2 eggs
¼ cup olive oil
½ teaspoon garlic powder (optional)
½ teaspoon dried basil (optional)
¼ teaspoon oregano (optional)
1 ¾ cups water

Blend all ingredients in a bowl, by mixing dry ingredients first and then wet ingredients. Spread dough in two greased 12" pizza pans. If it is difficult to spread, wet your rubber spatula with water.

Bake at 350°F for 20 minutes or until done. Or it can be baked at 400°F for about 15 minutes. Top with gluten-free sauce* and cheese*. Bake until the cheese melts (about 4 to 5 minutes).

*Variation*: For a yeast pizza, increase the sugar to 3 Tablespoons instead of 2. Use 1 yeast packet and eliminate baking powder. Prepare crusts and let rise in a warm, draft-free place for one hour. Then bake as directed above.

## Pizza – Version 2

We prefer the Gluten-Free Naturals™ Pizza Crust Mix. This recipe is good for those with allergies, but be aware that it is very crumbly. It doesn't hold together as well and doesn't brown well on the outside like the Gluten-Free Naturals™ product does.

½ cup cornstarch or tapioca starch or tapioca flour
1 cup fine white rice flour
¼ teaspoon salt
1 teaspoon baking powder
¾ cup milk
¼ cup oil

1 egg
Sprinkling of garlic, dried basil and oregano
¼ cup (4 oz.) gluten-free tomato sauce*
8 ounce package of gluten-free grated mozzarella cheese*

Preheat oven to 425°F. Blend together the dry ingredients with a whisk. Add the milk, egg, and oil and stir to blend. Grease a 9 ½ x 13 ½ oblong dark non-stick type pan. Spread the dough into the pan with a spatula. Sprinkle generously with the garlic, basil and oregano. Bake for 13 minutes. Remove from oven and take a spatula and make sure that the crust is not stuck anywhere on the bottom. This will make for easy removal after you have the toppings on. Pour tomato sauce on top and spread around. Sprinkle with the mozzarella cheese. You can add any toppings if you choose. Bake another 6 minutes or until the cheese is melted. Remove from pan and cut with a pizza cutter. For a crispier pizza, cool it

*see gluten-free products list at the end of the book

slightly on a cooling rack.  Reheat leftovers in microwave for a softer crust.  Leftovers may also be frozen.

*Variation*: Omit the baking powder for a crunchier, flatter pizza.  You will have to push down the puffed up parts with the back of a spoon before you add the sauce.

## Pizza Bread Sticks

Use Gluten-Free Naturals™ Pizzeria Style Pizza crust mix or follow one of the recipes above for pizza crust.  Put dough in pan as directed.  Sprinkle it with garlic powder, Parmesan cheese, and oregano.  Bake according to directions.  Remove from oven.  Using a pizza cutter, slice the pizza crust in half lengthwise, then cut into 1" strips and then in serving pieces.  Serve with gluten-free pasta dishes, salads and soups.  Or serve at an Italian dinner with a dish of olive oil with garlic powder mixed in for dipping.  Or serve with hot tomato sauce for dipping as an appetizer.

## Pizza Turnover or Stromboli
My husband came up with this recipe and it is delicious!  You need Reynolds® Release Foil to make this.  The dough will stick to regular foil, but doesn't stick to the Release Foil.

Gluten-Free Naturals™ Pizzeria Style Pizza Mix prepared according to package directions
Gluten-Free Pepperoni*

Gluten-Free Provolone Cheese* and/or Mozzarella Cheese*
Gluten-free Tomato Sauce from a jar*
Reynolds® Release Foil

Blend the Pizza crust dough as directed (I use a heavy-duty mixer).  Grease half of a large pizza pan.  Lay the Reynolds® Release Foil over the other half of the pan that you didn't grease.  Be sure the foil hangs over the edge and the non-stick side is up.  This will help you flip that half over.

Spread dough on the entire pizza pan using a rubber spatula.  Top the half of the pizza that doesn't have the foil with pepperoni and cheeses, placing them 1 inch from the rounded edges of the pan.  This will allow an edge so you can press and seal the Stromboli together.

Using the foil, lift and flip the other half to cover the pepperoni and cheese, being careful not to rip it in the fold area.  Gently remove the foil.  With wet hands, smooth edges and press seams.  Bake for 35 to 40 minutes at 350°F.  Slice into 4 large slices.  Serve with warmed tomato sauce.

## Popovers

When we first started the gluten-free diet, I never thought my husband would be able to have popovers. They are a golden brown muffin/roll that are hollow inside, that "pop over" while baking. My mother used to make these for us when we were children.

1 cup Gluten-Free Naturals™ All Purpose Flour or Gluten-Free Naturals™ Sandwich Bread (do not substitute other flours)

½ teaspoon salt
1 cup milk
2 eggs

Blend all ingredients together. Pour into well greased muffin cups or glass baking cups. Fill to ⅔ full. Bake at 425°F for 35 to 40 minutes, until golden brown. Serve immediately with butter. Makes 6 to 9 popovers, depending on the size of your pan.

## Pumpkin Muffins

Moist and delicious muffins. You wouldn't think that chocolate and pumpkin goes well together, but in this case they certainly do. These are nice at a brunch or for dessert.

1 ⅓ cups Gluten-Free Naturals™ All Purpose Flour
⅓ cup white rice flour
1 cup sugar
2 teaspoon ground cinnamon
½ teaspoon ground ginger
¼ teaspoon ground allspice
¼ teaspoon ground nutmeg or ground cloves
1 teaspoon baking soda

¼ teaspoon baking powder
¼ teaspoon salt
2 large eggs
1 cup canned pumpkin
½ cup oil
¼ cup water (Note: some pumpkin is drier than others. If batter is too thick, add a little more water).
1 cup gluten-free chocolate chips*

Blend all the dry ingredients together in a large bowl. Mix oil with the pumpkin and then the eggs. Stir in chocolate chips and combine with the dry ingredients. Blend only until all flour mixture is moistened. Use a fork so you won't be tempted to beat the batter. Place into greased muffin tins. Bake 20-25 minutes in a 350°F oven. Makes 8 large muffins or 36 miniature muffins. If making miniature muffins only cook about 15 minutes. For the mini muffins you can use either regular size chocolate chips or the mini chips.

*see gluten-free products list at the end of the book*

## Pumpkin and Spice Bread

**Moist and flavorful.**

¼ cup oil
¾ cup sugar (it will turn out using ½ cup sugar but it will not be sweet)
4 eggs
¼ cup molasses
1 cup canned plain pumpkin
½ cup plain yogurt
1 teaspoon gluten-free vanilla* or 2 Tablespoons dark rum* (optional)
1 teaspoon baking powder

1 teaspoon baking soda
2 ⅓ cups Gluten-Free Naturals™ All Purpose Flour
½ teaspoon ground cinnamon
½ teaspoon ground nutmeg
½ teaspoon ground allspice
¼ teaspoon ground ginger
½ teaspoon ground cloves (optional)

Blend oil, sugar, eggs, yogurt, molasses, rum and pumpkin together. Add the flour, baking soda, baking powder and spices. Blend well with a sturdy spoon or use a heavy duty mixer. Bake at 350°F in a greased 8 inch loaf pan or 3 greased mini loaf pans. Bake 1 hour 10 minutes for the large pan or 40 minutes for the small pans.

## Rolls

These are easy to make because they don't use yeast. They have a nice biscuit-like flavor, and bake in about 20 minutes. They stay fresh for several days. If you have a "top of the muffin" pan, you can make 6 hamburger rolls.

1 ½ cups Gluten-Free Naturals™ Sandwich Bread Flour or Gluten-Free Naturals™ All Purpose Flour
¼ teaspoon salt

1 teaspoon baking powder
¾ cup milk
¼ cup oil
1 egg

Preheat oven to 425°F. Blend together the dry ingredients with a whisk. Add the milk, egg, and melted butter and stir to blend. I use a heavy duty mixer. The dough will get thicker as it mixes.

Grease a jumbo muffin pan. (A regular muffin pan may also be used for smaller rolls.) Drop the dough into your pan. Wet your rubber spatula and smooth the tops of the rolls. Bake at 425°F for 20 to 25 minutes using the jumbo muffin pan. Bake for 18 to 20 minutes for smaller rolls. Test them to be sure they are done with a cake tester. They should be lightly browned on the top. You will be able to slice them better if you wait for them to cool.

*see gluten-free products list at the end of the book

## Rolls – Version 2

These are quick and easy to make, with a nice biscuit-like flavor. They are only soft and springy the day you make them. I like to make these before leaving on an outing. Allow them to cool (or they can be sliced warm) and then pile on gluten-free deli meat*, cheese* and condiments* for an "on-the-go" lunch. Use Gluten-Free Naturals™ Pizza crust or Gluten-Free Naturals™ Bread Flour to make more authentic Italian style rolls, by following the directions on the packaging and using the same baking time and temperature below.

| | |
|---|---|
| ½ cup cornstarch | 1 teaspoon baking powder |
| ½ cup defatted soy flour | ¾ cup milk |
| ½ cup white rice flour | ¼ cup oil |
| 1 ½ teaspoons xanthan gum | 1 egg |
| ¼ teaspoon salt | |

Preheat oven to 425°F. Blend together the dry ingredients with a whisk. Add the milk, egg, and melted butter and stir to blend. Grease a jumbo muffin pan. (A regular muffin pan may also be used for smaller rolls.) Drop the dough into your pan. Wet your rubber spatula and smooth the tops of the rolls. Bake at 425°F for 15 to 18 minutes using the jumbo muffin pan. (Or bake 13 to 15 minutes for smaller rolls.) Test to see if they are done with a cake tester. They should be lightly browned on the top. They're good hot out of the oven to make a cheese sandwich.

Note: These are good the day you make them and are soft and springy. Since they have no preservatives, they do start to become stale the next day. I suggest once they cool that you freeze what you're not going to eat that day. They freeze well and microwave on the defrost cycle. Another way to enjoy them the next day if you forgot to freeze them is to cut in half, butter each side and put them on a hot griddle butter side down. This toasts and steams them at the same time.

## Rolls – Cottage Cheese and Chive

These are easy to make and are nice for a ham and cheese sandwich or a hamburger roll. They bake in about 20 minutes. They stay fresh for several days. If you have a "top of the muffin" pan or English Muffin Rings, you can make 6 hamburger rolls.

| | |
|---|---|
| 1 cup Gluten-Free Naturals™ Sandwich Bread Flour or Gluten-Free Naturals™ All Purpose Flour | 1 ½ teaspoons baking powder |
| ¼ teaspoon salt | ½ cup milk |
| 1 Tablespoon sugar | ¼ cup gluten-free cottage cheese* |
| 2 teaspoons dried chives | 2 Tablespoons oil |
| | 1 egg |

Preheat oven to 425°F. Blend together all ingredients in a heavy duty mixer for several minutes so that the cottage cheese breaks up and becomes incorporated.

Grease a non-stick pan top of the Muffin Pan to make 6 large rolls or use a jumbo muffin pan. (Wet your rubber spatula and smooth the tops of the rolls. Bake at 425°F for 15 to 20 minutes. They should be lightly browned on the top. You will be able to slice them better if you wait for them to cool.

## Rolls – Crescent Rolls
Biscuit-like rolls that are nice to serve during the Holidays.

1 cup Gluten-Free Naturals™ Sandwich
   Bread Flour or Gluten-Free Naturals™
   All Purpose Flour
Sprinkling of salt
1 teaspoon baking powder
¼ teaspoon baking soda
⅓ cup butter*, cold from refrigerator

6 Tablespoons to ½ Cup Gluten-Free
   Plain Yogurt (add slowly as needed so
   dough won't be too wet to roll out)
1 Tablespoon Butter, softened
Herbs or Parmesan cheese (optional)
 Water

Blend the gluten-free flour, salt, baking powder, and baking soda in a bowl. Either cut in the butter using a pastry blender, or put it in a food processor and cut it in with the cutting blade. Add the yogurt to make a soft dough that you are able to roll out. Don't make it too stiff or your crescent rolls will be dry.

Put a little flour on some waxed paper and roll the dough out. Spread the 1 Tablespoon butter on the dough. If using herbs or Parmesan cheese, sprinkle some on now. Cut into 6 pie shaped wedges. Roll each wedge from the wide end to the triangle point. Put on a greased baking pan or place on a pan lined with Reynolds® Release Foil. Curve the rolls at the ends a little to have a crescent moon shape. Brush with a little water to put some moisture in the flour used to roll them out. Bake at 450°F for 10 to 12 minutes. They can be baked in a toaster oven, if desired.

*Variation*: Milk or water can be used instead of yogurt, but the texture will be a little drier. Use 1 ½ teaspoons baking powder instead of the baking powder and baking soda. They brown better if made with milk or yogurt rather than with water.

## Scones
I like the flavor that the sour cream gives these scones. See recipe under variation for Biscuits for another version of scones.

2 cups Gluten-Free Naturals™ Cookie
   Blend
1 teaspoon xanthan gum
2 Tablespoons sugar (I use 3 Tablespoons
   if using raisins)
½ teaspoon salt
2 teaspoons baking powder

½ cup gluten-free sour cream
½ cup milk
1 egg
1 Tablespoon oil
½ teaspoon cider vinegar
Raisins (optional)

Blend together dry ingredients with a whisk. Add in wet ingredients and blend. If the dough is too dry, you can add a little more milk. Drop into 12 cup greased muffin tins. Bake for 35 to 40 minutes at 350°F.

*Variation:*  Gluten-Free Naturals™ All Purpose Flour can be used in place of the Cookie Blend and xanthan gum.

## Tortillas

I like fresh tortillas made with Masa Flour.  This recipe comes from Maseca® Brand and I adapted it to use my mixer that has a dough hook.  They also suggested using plastic wrap on the tortilla press but I found using circles cut out of heavy duty freezer bags to work better.  Not only were they reusable, but they also didn't put depressions from the folding plastic wrap onto my tortillas.

Maseca® brand of corn Masa flour is gluten-free as of this writing.  I usually make half of the recipe, since this makes a lot of tortillas.  You will need a tortilla press to make these quickly.  Otherwise you can roll them out with a rolling pin.  To get that authentic texture, cook them in an iron skillet.  I do not recommend using a Teflon® pan because you need high heat to cook tortillas.

4 cups gluten-free Masa corn flour*          ½ teaspoon salt
2 ½ cups water

In a KitchenAid® mixer put all the ingredients.  Blend using the dough hook.  Continue to knead with the dough hook until you have a smooth, soft dough.  If your dough is too dry, you can add some additional water a Tablespoon at a time.  If too wet, add some more corn Masa flour a tablespoon at a time.

Divide the dough into 32 equal balls.  Flatten with a tortilla press lined on the top and bottom with 2 circles that you cut out of a heavy duty freezer bag.  (I find it easier to press and cook as I go, instead of pressing all of them at once.  If you are going to use that method, put all of the dough balls back in your bowl and cover it with a damp paper towel until you press them so that they don't dry out.)

Heat an iron skillet or tortilla griddle.  I put a little oil in the griddle when I cook the tortillas because I prefer them that way, although this isn't necessary if your skillet is well seasoned.

Put cooked tortillas on a plate and cover with a cloth napkin until ready to serve to keep them soft and warm.  Store any leftover tortillas in the refrigerator.

## Waffles – Our favorite

These are our favorite waffles, using the Gluten-Free Naturals™ Pancake Mix.

1 package Gluten-Free Naturals™          Additional 2 to 3 Tablespoons oil per
Pancake Mix, prepared as directed on          batch (Instead of 1 Tablespoon as
the package          directed for pancakes, I use ¼ cup oil
          for waffles)

Use one package of pancake mix, and follow the directions.  Add the additional oil and blend in.  Bake on a clean waffle iron.  (Gluten can be transferred if you used it for wheat and did not thoroughly clean it.  Once the waffle iron is cleaned, I suggest you discard the first gluten-free waffles you make or give them to a person who can eat gluten.  Do this just in case some gluten gets transferred to them.)

*see gluten-free products list at the end of the book

Grease waffle iron with oil (I use gluten-free cooking spray*) or use butter. (Place a pat of butter on the iron and let it melt. Spread with a clean natural bristle type pastry brush.) Bake the waffles for about 3 to 5 minutes according to your waffle iron.

## Waffles – Version 2

These are our favorite waffles from scratch, and my husband likes to make extra and microwaves them the next day for breakfast. We store leftovers covered in the refrigerator. Eliminate the sugar and vanilla if you want to use them as part of a main course under Chicken a la King (see index).

| | |
|---|---|
| 1 ¾ cups Gluten-Free Naturals™ Cookie Blend | 2 eggs |
| 4 teaspoons baking powder | ¼ cup corn oil |
| 1 teaspoon xanthan gum | 1 ¾ cups milk |
| 2 Tablespoons sugar | 1 teaspoon gluten-free vanilla* |
| ¼ teaspoon salt | |

Blend flour, baking powder, xanthan gum, sugar and salt together with a whisk. Add eggs, oil, milk and vanilla and whisk together. Bake on a clean waffle iron. (Gluten can be transferred if you used it for wheat and did not thoroughly clean it. Once the waffle iron is cleaned, I suggest you discard the first gluten-free waffles you make or give them to a person who can eat gluten. Do this just in case some gluten gets transferred to them.)

Grease waffle iron with oil (I use gluten-free cooking spray*) or use butter. (Place a pat of butter on the iron and let it melt. Spread with a clean natural bristle type pastry brush.) Bake the waffles for about 3 to 5 minutes according to your waffle iron.

## Waffles – Version 3

These have a different flavor/texture than version 1 or 2, but are also good. Eliminate the vanilla and reduce the sugar to 1 Tablespoon if you want to use these waffles as part of a main course under Chicken a la King.

| | |
|---|---|
| 1 ¾ cup Gluten-Free Naturals™ All Purpose Flour | 2 eggs |
| 2 Tablespoons sugar | ½ cup oil |
| 5 teaspoons gluten-free baking powder* | 1 teaspoon gluten-free vanilla* |
| ½ teaspoon salt | 1 ¾ cup milk |

Mix together the dry ingredients with a whisk. Add all wet ingredients and blend with the whisk. If too thick, add a little more milk. Cook on clean (gluten-free) waffle iron. (Gluten can be transferred if you used it for wheat and did not thoroughly clean it.) Either spray with gluten-free cooking spray* or put some butter to help prevent sticking. These are incredibly light with some crunch. They almost melt in your mouth. Bake 5 minutes.

## Waffles with Ricotta Cheese

You don't notice the cheese in these. We like these because the added protein seems to "stick with you better" and you won't get hungry as quickly afterwards.

| | |
|---|---|
| 1 cup Gluten-Free Naturals™ All Purpose Flour | 3 eggs |
| 1 Tablespoon sugar | ½ to ¾ cup gluten-free Ricotta cheese* |
| 2 teaspoons baking powder | 3 Tablespoons oil |
| ½ teaspoon salt | 1 ¼ cups milk |

Blend flour, sugar, baking powder and salt with a whisk. Add eggs, ricotta, oil and milk. Blend well. Cook on a hot, gluten-free waffle iron. (Gluten can transfer to your waffles if you did not clean your waffle iron well after making regular waffles.) Makes 6 waffles about 7" in size.

## Wraps

These are like a crepe but are a little thicker and more flexible so they can be used as a sandwich wrap. This recipe makes 4 wraps.

| | |
|---|---|
| 4 heaping Tablespoons Gluten-Free Naturals™ All Purpose Flour or Gluten-Free Naturals™ Sandwich Bread Flour | 2 eggs |
| Pinch of salt | 2 Tablespoons oil |
| | 4 Tablespoons milk |
| | 4 Tablespoons water |

Blend in a blender. (I use a hand blender.) The batter will be somewhat thick. Cook on a buttered gluten-free griddle or non-stick pan. (Gluten can transfer to your food if you grilled wheat on it; clean it well before using.) When you pour the batter, use the back of the ladle to spread the batter to make a circular wrap. If too thick you can add a little more water. Don't add too much water or they will be too wet. Cook immediately after mixing batter, because if the batter sits it will get thicker and be difficult to cook.

Cook one side and then turn over and cook the other side. Remove from pan and put on a plate. Fill with gluten-free cold cuts, cheese, etc. and then roll to eat.

*see gluten-free products list at the end of the book

## Zucchini Bread

This is a sweet cake-like bread. Sometimes children don't like seeing green zucchini in their bread. If so, use a carrot peeler and scrape away the green outside before shredding it. When the bread is baked, you can't tell it contains the zucchini. I tried this trick and my husband didn't know he was eating zucchini bread. He thought it was moist spice bread. This recipe makes 2 loaves.

3 eggs
1 cup oil
2 ½ cups sugar
3 cups zucchini grated finely (wash well,
    remove stems and grate)
3 teaspoons gluten-free vanilla*
1 teaspoon baking soda

¼ teaspoon baking powder
1 teaspoon salt
2 teaspoons ground cinnamon
3 cups Gluten-Free Naturals™ All
    Purpose Flour
1 cup chopped walnuts (optional)

Grease 2 loaf pans. Beat eggs, oil, and sugar with a whisk. Grate zucchini (I use a food processor.) Add zucchini and the rest of the ingredients and blend using a sturdy spoon. The batter will get thick. Bake for 1 hour at 325°F or until done. Depending on the loaf pans you use, you may have to bake it 10 to 15 minutes longer. Use a cake tester to see if it is done. Cool completely, or it will crumble when you try to slice it.

## Write your own recipes here:

# BREAD CRUMBS

Gluten-free breads are made differently, so you have to make bread crumbs differently. When you are first learning the gluten-free diet, you may sometimes create breads that don't turn out as well as they should have. Perhaps they didn't rise high or they crashed because you took them out of the oven too soon. Instead of throwing them away, turn them into bread crumbs!

## Bread Crumbs – using leftover gluten-free bread
Instead of wasting leftover gluten-free bread, here is how to make bread crumbs.

For bread crumbs using Gluten-Free Naturals™ bread, put the bread in a food processor and pulverize until they are in very small pieces. They can be used immediately in recipes calling for fresh bread crumbs. For traditional dried bread crumbs, dry them in the oven so they will keep a long time. Spread pulverized bread evenly in a layer on a baking sheet. Bake in the oven at 200°F. It usually takes about 1 hour for them to completely dry. I stir them after 30 minutes of baking to ensure all of the crumbs dry evenly. Once cooled, add gluten-free spices if desired. (See the next recipe for some suggestions.) Store unused dried bread crumbs in a jar or tightly sealed container.

Alternatively, you can air dry bread crumbs. Spread the crumbs in a very thin single layer on a plate or baking sheet. Whenever I make bread, I usually take the ends and pulverize them and use this method. In winter months the bread crumbs usually dry within one day, because the humidity is less in the house than in the summer. Be sure they are thoroughly dry before you put them in a container. If they are still moist, mold could grow on them.

For gluten-free rice breads, they fall apart easily so you can crumble them in your hands, or break them up using a food processor. Get the pieces as small as possible. (Rice breads make very, very hard bread crumbs, so you want the crumbs to be very small.) Spread evenly in a layer on a baking sheet. Bake in the oven at 200°F for about 1 hour. When completely dry and cooled, put in a jar. Add gluten-free spices if desired.

You will notice in my recipes, that I do not use bread crumbs made from rice breads. I find the crumbs are hard and the texture can be grainy in meatloaf or meatballs. Rice bread crumbs that are toasted sometimes stick in your teeth when you eat them, because they are so hard.

## Bread Crumbs – Flavored Italian Style

I like the texture of bread crumbs made with Gluten-Free Naturals™ breads, but sometimes I don't have the time to make them. I find the texture of bread crumbs made with gluten-free crackers better than those made with rice breads. Sometimes crackers are hard to find, and coating meat with Gluten-Free Naturals™ All Purpose Flour is another good alternative. There are many choices that work for bread crumbs, and you can add the spices listed to give your coating that traditional flavor.

8 Tablespoons Gluten-Free bread crumbs made in the previous recipe OR 4 Ener-G® low protein crackers, pulverized in a food processor to make 8 Tablespoons OR 8 Tablespoons Gluten-Free Naturals™ All Purpose Flour
Dash of dried oregano
Dash of dried basil

¼ teaspoon garlic powder
¼ teaspoon salt
¼ teaspoon parsley flakes
⅛ teaspoon sugar
⅛ teaspoon onion powder

See previous recipe if you want traditional dried bread crumbs from bread. Or, pulverize crackers in a food processor. Add spices and blend well.

If you used crackers, they may be stored in an airtight container. If you made "fresh" bread crumbs (see previous recipe), use them immediately. If you dry the bread in the oven as explained in the recipe above, you may store these crumbs in an airtight container. Use as you would use regular bread crumbs.

If using the Gluten-Free Naturals™ All Purpose Flour, mix with spices and then coat your meat. Spray your meat with cooking spray before baking. (Spray pan, place coated meat in pan and spray meat.) If frying, coat with the flour mixture and fry. For example, for oven baked chicken parts, dip in coating mixture, spray with gluten-free cooking spray and then bake. The oil from the cooking spray makes it crispy instead of dry. Or, dip chicken in gluten-free buttermilk* and then the coating and deep fry for southern fried chicken.

*Variation*: Add 1 Tablespoon Pecorino Romano or Parmesan cheese. (If cheese is salty, eliminate the salt.) Store any extra crumbs in the refrigerator if using cheese.

*Variation 2*: Pulverize gluten-free cornflakes* or gluten-free Rice Chex® or tortilla chips* or Asian rice crackers* in a food processor. Add the spices above if desired. These pulverized crumbs are best used on meats you are baking instead of frying.

*Variation 3*: Gluten-Free Naturals™ Cookie Blend may be used instead of the Gluten-Free Naturals™ All Purpose Flour. Spray meat with cooking spray before putting it in the oven to bake, as noted above.

## Breading Cornmeal Crumbs – Southern Style

This is a traditional Southern recipe, for breading fish, chicken, chops, oysters or vegetables for frying.

1 cup gluten-free yellow Cornmeal* (I prefer finely ground cornmeal)
½ cup grated Parmesan* cheese
½ cup sesame seeds (see note below)
2 Tablespoons dried chives
2 Tablespoons dried parsley flakes

2 Tablespoons dried marjoram or oregano (or thyme may be used)
2 teaspoons garlic powder
2 teaspoons ground sage
½ teaspoon ground red pepper

Blend all ingredients.  Store this mixture in a tightly sealed jar in the refrigerator until ready to use.

To use, dip the fish, meat or whatever you are breading in beaten egg.  Then dip in this crumb mixture to coat.  Fry in oil until done.  (I use a 12 inch frying skillet with about a ¼ inch of oil.  Or, a deep fryer may also be used.)  Drain the food on paper towels to remove any excess oil.  (Although printed paper towels do not contain gluten, I prefer to use un-printed ones for draining the oil of fried foods.)

I fry the foods until the sesame seeds begin to get golden brown in color.  This brings out their nutty flavor.

*Note*:  We like this coating on whiting fish, since it is a mild fish and this coating adds a lot of flavor.  Since fish cooks quickly, you may want to toast the sesame seeds before preparing the crumb mixture.  This will ensure that nutty flavor without overcooking the fish.  You can toast the seeds in a toaster oven at 300°F for about 3 to 5 minutes.  Watch carefully as they can burn easily.

*Variation*:  Gluten-Free Corn Flour may be used instead of the cornmeal in this recipe.

## YEAST BREADS

Yeast breads are by far the hardest thing to duplicate. I spent over 8 years developing bread flour that would create a bread that was soft, light, held together well for a sandwich, and wouldn't crumble. I think breads using Gluten-Free Naturals™ Bread Flour are the closest in flavor and texture to wheat breads. Unlike other flour blends, you can use it to convert wheat recipes for the bread machine. You can make sandwiches, grilled cheese, French toast, croutons, bread crumbs, and turkey stuffing. It holds together and has excellent flavor. Most other breads are crumbly, grainy or have a "beany" taste. Even non-celiacs tell me that the Gluten-Free Naturals™ products tastes like homemade bread.

I don't have very many rice bread recipes, but if you have allergies and prefer breads made with brown rice there are many free recipes on the Red Star Yeast® web page, www.redstaryeast.com.

As with wheat breads, all yeast breads may require some practice. I remember when I got a bread machine for a wedding gift. It took some trial and error to learn my machine in order to make the best breads.

As with wheat breads, fresh ingredients and fresh yeast yields better breads. (Store yeast in the freezer to keep it fresh. If you purchase yeast in bulk or in a jar, store it in the freezer. If using bread machine yeast, use 2 ¼ teaspoons. If using regular yeast I use 1 Tablespoon. Once exposed to air, sometimes the regular yeast can lose some of its strength, which is why I use more.)

Also, the water can't be too hot or you will kill the yeast. It will take time for you to learn how the consistency of the batter should be. Too much water can create breads that fall, but too little yields dry breads that don't rise as high. I suggest that in the beginning when you make breads, hold back a little water while blending and check consistency. Add the extra water if needed. The time of year and type of day can also make a difference. Summer breads usually rise higher than those made in the winter. A wet or dry day can affect the moisture content. With a bread machine, baking breads is the most fool-proof, but even so on hot summer days the breads rise a little higher than in the winter.

### Bagels
These taste like bagels!

2 eggs
1 ½ cups warm (not hot) water
2 Tablespoons oil
4 cups (16 ounces) Gluten-Free
   Naturals™ Sandwich Bread Flour (not
   Multi-Grain) or Gluten-Free Naturals™
   All Purpose Flour
1 ½ teaspoons salt
3 Tablespoons sugar
1 Tablespoon ground flax seed, also called
   flax meal. (If your dough is very wet,

you can add a little more of the flax but
don't add more than 2 Tablespoons.)
1 packet of gluten-free yeast* (2 ¼
   teaspoons) or 2 ¼ teaspoons gluten-free
   bread machine yeast* or 1 Tablespoon
   regular yeast* from jar (I use Red Star®
   brand)
6 cups of boiling water in a pot
½ teaspoon baking soda

Prepare dough. You can blend it in a heavy duty mixer with a paddle or dough hook. Or, mix by hand with a sturdy spoon. The dough should be thick.

*see gluten-free products list at the end of the book*

Take a baking pan, cover it with foil and spray it with cooking spray. With hands wet with water, grab large amounts of dough. (Or use a very large wet spoon.) Using wet hands, smooth the dough into a round ball and form a hole in the middle. Flatten it a little so it looks like a bagel.

Place bagels on the baking sheet. Let rise 15 minutes. I cover them with saran wrap and a warm wet towel and leave then on the counter. Meanwhile, get your water boiling and add the baking soda to it. Preheat your oven temperature to 350°F.

Boil the bagels in the water for about 3 minutes or so. (You will find it easier to remove from the pan if you wet the spatula with water first.) They will float to the top and start to expand somewhat. Remove from the boiling water and put them back on the baking sheet. If you want seeds on your bagels, sparingly brush the top with egg white and sprinkle with seeds. (Too much egg white can burn on the bottom.) Bake in a 350° oven for 35 minutes, until bagels are done.

Note: Just like regular bagels get stale the next day, these will also get stale. I suggest you freeze leftovers. I wait until they are completely cooled and then slice them. I put them in individual sandwich bags, and then in a large freezer bag. Or toast leftovers. Makes 8 to 10 bagels.

*Variation*: For Cinnamon Raisin bagels, add 1 Tablespoon cinnamon, use 4 to 6 Tablespoons brown sugar instead of granulated sugar, and add ¼ to ⅓ cup raisins.

*Note*: Using the ground flax helps to make the dough thick enough so that it can withstand the boiling. If your dough seems a little thin initially, wait a few minutes to see if the flax thickens it. If not thick enough, add a little more but don't add more than 2 Tablespoons. Be sure that your flax is fresh. It can go rancid quickly, and rancid flax will impart a terrible flavor. It is also not good for you to eat rancid foods. When flax is fresh, it is mild and nutty tasting. Smell it before using it. If the smell is unpleasant, it is probably rancid. I store flax in the refrigerator or vacuum package it so that it stays fresh a long time.

## Banana Yeast Bread
**Delicious served with peanut butter or cream cheese. My husband likes this for breakfast.**

1 ripe banana
2 eggs
1 cup warm (not hot) water
½ cup plain gluten-free yogurt*
2 Tablespoons oil
1 ½ teaspoons salt
4 Tablespoons sugar
½ teaspoon baking soda
1 package (4 cups / 16 ounces) Gluten-Free Naturals™ Bread Flour (Sandwich or Multi-Grain) or Gluten-Free Naturals™ All Purpose Flour
1 packet of gluten-free yeast* (2 ¼ teaspoons) or 2 ¼ teaspoons gluten-free bread machine yeast* or rapid rise yeast, or 1 Tablespoon regular yeast* from jar (I use Red Star® brand or 1 packet of Rapid Rise.)
2 to 3 Tablespoons chopped pecans

Follow directions for basic bread, using these ingredients.

*see gluten-free products list at the end of the book

## Basic Bread – our favorite (Bread Machine, Oven and Crock-pot® Methods)

I make this bread the most out of all the yeast breads listed. This bread is soft, springy, and even is soft for several days!! You can slice it in thinner slices than other gluten-free breads. You can eat it warm, but it slices best when fully cooled. It "domes" on the top. It's not gritty like rice breads. It makes a great sandwich and holds together very well. Even our non-celiac taste testers loved it. You can use this bread to make just about anything you'd make with regular bread.

For higher rising breads in the summer, consider putting your bread machine in your garage! This may sound unusual but in summer months when your air conditioner is running your home may be actually too cool to make high rising breads. As long as the temperature is not above 100°F (as hot as 90°F to 95°F is ok), your garage can be a great place to rise and bake your bread and not add additional heat to your kitchen. Check on it periodically. Set a timer so you know when to remove the bread from the machine. (I don't recommend putting the machine outside where breezes/drafts can cause bread to fall, or where animals can come and try to get it!)

**Note: The directions look long but I've tried to be very detailed. It is not difficult to make gluten-free bread, especially if you have a programmable bread machine. You basically put in the wet ingredients, top with the dry ingredients and turn on the machine! For best results, weigh the gluten-free flour instead of measuring it in a measuring cup.**

2 eggs

1 ¾ cups warm (not hot) water (Note: Check dough consistency and add 1 to 2 Tablespoons if too thick. Do not add more than 2 cups water or your bread may "fall". You may also use a combination of 1 cup milk and ¾ cup water. The addition of milk adds protein and makes the crust brown nicely. Or use all milk.)

2 Tablespoons oil

1 ½ teaspoons salt

3 Tablespoons sugar or ¼ cup honey

1 package (16 ounces/4 cups) Gluten-Free Naturals™ Bread Flour (Sandwich or Multi-Grain) or Gluten-Free Naturals™ All Purpose Flour

1 packet of gluten-free yeast* (2 ¼ teaspoons) or 2 ¼ teaspoons gluten-free bread machine yeast* or rapid rise yeast, or 1 Tablespoon regular yeast* from jar (I use Red Star® brand or 1 packet of Rapid Rise.)

For a bread machine method:

- Set program as follows:
- To program the Zojirushi® programmable bread machine, set the homemade cycle to knead 10 minutes, rise 50 to 60 minutes, second rise and punch-down off, and bake 1 hour 10 minutes. (If you have a Zojirushi® machine that has 3 rises, choose your rise time in the 3rd rise since that is a warmer temperature than rise 1.) Choose dark crust. (This sets the baking temperature and doesn't mean your bread will be dark. However, some bread machine temperatures may vary. You may want to try medium, but if your bread is losing height when it cools, that means it is under-baking and you need to select dark crust to get a higher baking temperature.)
- For the Regal KitchenPro® use the dark crust setting and the quick bread cycle. This cycle mixes, rises and bakes. It doesn't have a punch-down. Test for doneness. You will most likely have to press bake again, because it has a short baking cycle. Be sure to be there when it beeps because if it is not baked enough it can crash very

*see gluten-free products list at the end of the book

quickly and the bread will be ruined. If not done, press bake and test again in 10 more minutes. It usually requires the extra baking time. Our experience was at least another 10 to 20 minutes additional time. Temperatures of the bread machines can vary, so if you use a non-programmable machine make sure it is one that allows you to bake it longer.

- For other bread machines, follow your machine directions. Most will tell you to use the dough cycle. Smooth the top of the bread. Let rise 1 hour. If the machine won't allow you to bake it longer than one hour, you may want to consider baking it in the oven.

Add ingredients:
Remove the pan from the machine and put the 2 eggs, water and oil in the pan. Add salt and sugar to the liquid. Top with the Bread Flour and then the yeast. Turn the machine on. Let the machine mix it for a few minutes. Then open the lid and with a rubber spatula finish blending the wet and dry ingredients. Pay special attention to the corner areas and around the paddles. Smooth batter evenly in pan. Close the lid and let the machine finish mixing the bread dough. The machine starts with a slow mix and then does a faster blending. After the machine does the faster mixing, the dough should have a smooth texture similar to a wheat bread and not look crumbly. If too dry, add up to 2 Tablespoons more water and see how it looks. Once it stops mixing, you may want to smooth the top with a spatula that is wet with water so it looks nicer.

When finished baking, remove pan from machine, remove bread and cool on a wire rack. The bread slices best when completely cooled.

*This bread remains soft for several days. However, as with any homemade bread without preservatives, this bread doesn't last longer than 3 to 4 days in a plastic bag on your counter or in a breadbox, because it contains no preservatives. I usually leave a good part of the loaf in a plastic bag on the counter because we enjoy it fresh. But I also put some in the freezer for later. I use sandwich bags and put two slices in each. I then put them in a large freezer bag and put them in the freezer. The frozen bread is delicious defrosted, and it is also good toasted. If you didn't freeze the bread, day old bread is good for French toast, grilled cheese, or toast. This is a bread that holds together well for a sandwich and is soft and springy.*

*Note: The reason for putting the wet ingredients in the bread machine first is that if you put the dry in first you often end up with flour under the paddles. This flour will bake and make it difficult for your bread to be removed from the pan. If you put the wet in first, it blends better. The bread is easier to remove from the pan. This is true of any bread made in a bread machine.*

*What do you do if you made the bread at night and it is too hot to put away, and you don't want to stay up waiting for it to cool down? Wrap the bread in a couple of clean kitchen towels. Put it in a large plastic bag. In the morning, remove the bag and remove the towels. They will be wet. Put the bread in a dry plastic bag. This method yields a softer crust, and your bread will be fresh and moist in the morning. If you left it out all night to cool on a cooling rack, it would be dried out and stale. Don't let your bread sit in the moist towels/wet plastic bag longer than overnight or it will get moldy more quickly.*

*\*see gluten-free products list at the end of the book*

For the oven method: Grease a large 10 inch by 5 to 5 ½ inch (2 pound size) non-stick metal loaf pan. Or grease two 8 inch by 4 ½ inch (1 pound size) loaf pans. Non-stick metal works best, but glass pans may also be used. For best results, use a heavy duty mixer to blend the wet and dry ingredients; using the paddle or dough hook. It can also be mixed by hand if you don't have a mixer. If doing it by hand, first mix the dry ingredients together and then add the wet ingredients.

Put batter in your prepared loaf pan(s). Let rise in a warm, draft-free place for 50 to 60 minutes, until double in size. (I often set it in the oven with the light on. If it is in the winter, I turn the oven on and let it get to 100°F, but no hotter than that. Turn the oven off, put the loaf in the oven with the light on, close the door and let it rise.)

To get additional rise after the 60 minutes, you can leave the bread in the oven and preheat the oven with the bread in the oven. My oven has a 10 minute preheat, and I set the timer as soon as I turn the oven on. Bake at 350°F for approximately 1 hour and 15 minutes (including the 10 minute preheat). For 2 pans, bake for 1 hour (including the 10 minute preheat). Test for doneness with a cake tester. Do not under-bake or your bread may fall after it is removed from the oven. It should be nicely browned on the outside. Cool on a wire rack.

*Note*: If your bread is falling in the middle as it cools, it may be under-baked. Next time bake 5 to 10 minutes longer. Oven temperatures can vary.

*Variation*: If you wish to have your bread topped with sesame or poppy seeds, mix 1 teaspoon egg white powder with 1 Tablespoon water and 1 Tablespoon of seeds. Once the bread has completely finished mixing and is just starting the rise cycle, top the bread with this mixture.

For Crock-Pot®/oven method: If you are having trouble getting your bread to rise because you home is too cold or drafty in the winter, a crock-pot can be a way to resolve this. Unfortunately, temperatures vary dramatically from model to model. So the first time you try this, you will have to determine if the "low" or "high" setting works better for your bread. For the models that I have, I found that the high setting worked better.

You can use a large oval 7-quart crock-pot and choose a 1 pound loaf pan that fits inside. A non-stick metal pan works best. Prepare half the bread recipe. Mix and put dough into the greased loaf pan. Set loaf pan in crock-pot, cover, and set to either high or low and secure the lid. After 45 minutes, it should be doubled in size. Remove it and immediately put it in the preheated oven to bake. Don't allow it to get to the point that it starts to bake in the crock-pot, or when you lift the lid it will deflate and not regain height. Once gluten-free bread starts to bake, you need to maintain baking temperature or it will fall in the middle and be ruined.

On high, my bread rose to the top of the pan within 45 minutes. At this point I removed the bread and put it in a 350°F oven and baked it (see oven method.) Don't leave the bread in the crock for an hour on high, or it will crash when you remove it to put it in the oven.

*see gluten-free products list at the end of the book*

Some of the GFN Foods® testers baked good bread in their Crock-pots®. They loved how easy it was to prepare bread. One tester used a round Hamilton Beach® model 33401, which is a 4 quart model. This crock-pot worked well because it has temperature core all around the sides and is a taller crock-pot. The taller height eliminated the problem I had of water condensation dripping on the bread.

She greased the crock with cooking spray or oil. She mixed the dough and put it right into the crock-pot. She turned it on high temperature and placed the lid securely on top. The bread rose and then baked in the crock-pot. It took between 2 hours 20 minutes to 2 hours 40 minutes for the rising and baking. She used the handle of a wooden spoon to loosen the sides. Then she carefully tilted it and used pot holders to place the bread on a cooling rack. Slice the bread when completely cooled. The sides of the bread will be very hot until it cools, so be careful removing it. Since the bread is touching the sides of the crock where the heat is, do not attempt to touch the sides of the bread with your bare hands until it is cooled.

I didn't have consistent success with the crock-pot models I have. Using the loaf pan method it didn't maintain a high enough temperature to bake it as well as my oven. That is why I suggest only using the large oval crock-pot with a baking pan inside it for rising.

My best success was using an old round Rival® Crock-Pot® that did not have a removable crock. (It measures 7 inches in diameter/6 inches deep.) I also had success with a very old no-name model that did not have a removable crock. For this method, I greased the sides, put the dough directly in the crock-pot, set it to high and slightly vented the lid. It rose to the top and made bread in about 2 ¼ hours. I found that the old models with the interior coils all around the sides have much more consistent heat. The temperature was also better for baking bread than the newer models. (Perhaps this is because the older crock-pot models by Rival® could be used for baking and this was a selling feature. They used to have a metal baking pan insert. It had a lid with a knob for easy removal. The lid had vents. The temperature was probably designed to be more consistent in order to use this baking pan.) It seems that the new models are not manufactured for this use.

I tested a lot of models, but some of the newer ones I tested were too hot, and water dripped all over the bread from condensation so it didn't bake properly. Others were too cool and took hours, and then the sides burned and the center wasn't cooked enough so it was too doughy. Some models with removable crocks had less uniform heat. They seemed to have most of the heat on one side (maybe because the removable crocks do not fit securely?) so that one side rose higher and burned while the other side was too cool.

So keep this in mind, if you want to try this method. It is easy but results can vary, depending on the model of crock-pot that you have.

## Beer Bread

Now that Redbridge® Gluten-Free Beer is available, here is a way to make beer bread. I like adding both poppy seeds and sesame seeds, but it is also good without them.

2 eggs
1 cup Redbridge® Gluten-Free Beer
  (room temperature, not cold)
½ to ¾ cup warm water
2 Tablespoons oil
1 ½ teaspoons salt
4 Tablespoons brown sugar
1 package (4 cups / 16 ounces) Gluten-
  Free Naturals™ Bread Flour (Sandwich

or Multi-Grain) or Gluten-Free
  Naturals™ All Purpose Flour
1 packet of gluten-free yeast* (2 ¼
  teaspoons) or 2 ¼ teaspoons gluten-free
  bread machine yeast* or rapid rise yeast,
  or 1 Tablespoon regular yeast* from jar
  (I use Red Star® brand or1 packet of
  Rapid Rise.)
1 Tablespoon sesame seeds (optional)
1 Tablespoon poppy seeds (optional)

Follow directions for basic bread, using these ingredients.

## Brown Rice Bread

For a rice bread, this one is soft. It is good warm out of the oven and not as gritty as other rice breads I have made. You can slice it in thinner slices and eat it warm, unlike other rice breads.

1 ½ cups warm water
4 tablespoons oil
1 teaspoon cider vinegar
3 eggs or 2 Tablespoons egg white
  powder and 6 Tablespoons water
2 cups fine brown rice flour
½ cup gluten-free yellow corn flour or
  sorghum flour
½ cup tapioca starch or tapioca flour

⅓ cup defatted soy flour or other bean
  flour
1 Tablespoon xanthan gum
1 ½ teaspoons salt
3 Tablespoons sugar
1 Tablespoon active dry yeast or 1 packet
  of yeast (I use Red Star® brand)

Follow directions for Basic Bread, using these ingredients. The water may have to be adjusted if substituting bean flour for soy flour.

*Variation:* One day making this bread I made a mistake and used ½ cup soy flour instead of ⅓. I added a little additional water to get the right consistency and the bread turned out fine.

*Variation 2:* If you wish to have your bread topped with sesame or poppy seeds, mix 1 teaspoon egg white powder with 1 Tablespoon water and 1 Tablespoon of seeds. Once the bread has completely finished mixing and is in the rise cycle, top the bread with this mixture.

*Variation 3:* For a soy free bread, you can substitute cornstarch for the soy. The bread will be a little more crumbly but it will work. It will also be lower in protein.

## Brown and White Rice Bread

Thanks to my brother-in-law for this recipe he created for the programmable bread machine. It's good, especially if you like very moist rice bread.

| | |
|---|---|
| 3 large eggs | ⅓ cup cornstarch |
| 1 Tablespoon cider or wine vinegar or wine or gluten-free vanilla* | ½ cup tapioca flour or tapioca starch |
| | 1 cup white rice flour |
| ¼ cup corn oil | 1 cup brown rice flour |
| ¼ cup plain yogurt* | ¼ cup sugar |
| 1 ½ cups water | 1 teaspoon salt |
| ¼ cup gluten-free corn flour or sorghum flour | 1 Tablespoon gluten-free yeast* |
| | 1 Tablespoon xanthan gum |
| ¼ cup defatted or full fat soy flour | |

Mix dry items in a 2 quart Tupperware® and shake them to mix. Mix wet items in Bread machine, then add dry ingredients.

The bread program is as follows on the Zojirushi machine: Homemade Mode is Crust: Medium, Preheat for 10 minutes, Knead for 11 minutes, Rise 1 is 40 minutes, Rise 2 is off, Rise 3 is off, Bake is 1:00 hour, Keep Warm is 1:00 hour.

Leave overnight in machine for bread to cool and set. (It will stay moist for several days.) For ready to eat Bread, Bake 1:10 min, Crust: Dark. (This bread dries out faster.)

## Buttermilk Bread

Some brands of buttermilk are very thick because of added gums, so you may have to add a little more water. If your dough is too thick it may not rise properly.

| | |
|---|---|
| 2 large eggs | or Gluten-Free Naturals™ All Purpose Flour |
| 2 Tablespoons oil | |
| 1 cup gluten-free buttermilk* or gluten-free plain yogurt* | ¼ cup sugar |
| | 1 ½ teaspoons salt |
| ¾ cup warm water | 2 ¼ teaspoons gluten-free yeast* |
| 4 cups (1 lb.) Gluten-Free Naturals™ Bread Flour (Sandwich or Multi-Grain) | |

Follow directions for Basic Bread, using these ingredients.

If using the bread machine, add wet ingredients first and then dry ingredients.
If using oven method, follow as directed using these ingredients.

## Buttermilk Powder Bread

As of this writing, Saco® buttermilk powder is gluten-free. Check the status to be sure it still is. I think fresh buttermilk is better, but the powdered is very convenient to use.

2 large eggs

2 Tablespoons butter*

1 ¾ cups warm water (Add 2 Tablespoons more if dough looks too thick or dry. Do not add more than 2 cups of water total.)

4 cups (16 ounces) Gluten-Free Naturals™ Bread Flour (Sandwich or Multi-Grain) or Gluten-Free Naturals™ All Purpose Flour

3 Tablespoons sugar (white or brown)

1 ½ teaspoons salt

½ cup gluten-free powdered buttermilk*

2 ¼ teaspoons gluten-free yeast*

Follow directions for Basic Bread, using these ingredients. Check for doneness. Breads made with buttermilk powder tend to brown more on the outside, so you need to test that the inside is fully baked.

## Cheese Bread

A little bit denser than the regular bread, but it has a nice cheese flavor. We like it for ham sandwiches.

2 large eggs

2 Tablespoons oil

1 ¾ cups water (Add more water if dough looks too thick or dry. Do not add more than 2 cups water total.)

4 cups (1 lb.) Gluten-Free Naturals™ Bread Flour (Sandwich or Multi-Grain) or Gluten-Free Naturals™ All Purpose Flour

2 ¼ teaspoons gluten-free yeast*

1 Tablespoon instant minced onion or 1 teaspoon onion powder (optional)

¼ cup non-fat dry milk powder (optional, I don't use since cheese already adds milk)

1 Tablespoon poppy seeds (optional)

1 ½ teaspoons dill weed (optional)

¾ cups or 3 ounces grated sharp cheddar cheese (or other flavorful cheese)

Follow directions for Basic Bread, using these ingredients.

## Cinnamon Raisin Bread
Nice for breakfast served with cream cheese.  I use leftover bread in bread pudding.

2 large eggs
1 ¾ cups warm water (Add 2 Tablespoons more if dough looks too thick or dry. Do not add more than 2 cups of water total.) Or use ¾ cup water and 1 cup milk.  (I heat milk 1 minute in the microwave so it is not cold.)
2 Tablespoons oil
4 cups (16 ounces) Gluten-Free Naturals™ Bread Flour (Sandwich or Multi-Grain) or Gluten-Free Naturals™ All Purpose Flour
1 ½ teaspoons salt
4 ½ to 6 Tablespoons brown sugar
1 Tablespoon ground cinnamon
½ cup raisins (regular or sultanas)
1 packet of gluten-free yeast* (2 ¼ teaspoons) or 2 ¼ teaspoons gluten-free bread machine yeast* or rapid rise yeast or 1 Tablespoon regular yeast* from jar (I use Red Star® brand)

Follow the directions under Basic Bread.

## Cinnamon Rolls
My husband invented these using Gluten-Free Naturals™ Sandwich Bread.  These look and taste like the real thing.

1 package (16 ounces) Gluten-Free Naturals™ Sandwich Bread or Gluten-Free Naturals™ All Purpose Flour
1 ½ teaspoons salt
3 Tablespoons sugar
1 ¾ cup warm milk
2 eggs
2 Tablespoons cooking oil
1 yeast packet
2 Tablespoons very soft butter
½ cup sugar
2 teaspoons of ground cinnamon
Drizzle:
  ½ to ¾ cup sugar
  ¼ to ½ teaspoon gluten-free vanilla*
  Milk to make it the right consistency, about a Tablespoon or so

Blend the Sandwich Bread Flour, salt, sugar, milk, eggs, oil and yeast together using a heavy duty mixer using the dough hook.  Or use the mixing paddle on medium speed.  Mix it for 5 to 10 minutes until it is completely smooth.  Then let it sit for 10 minutes.  Grease a non-stick 9 inch square pan.  Or you can use a 9 x 13 inch pan.

Grease a large piece of aluminum foil with butter to roll out your dough to a size of about 9 x 13 inches.  If you use Ready Release® foil, grease it with butter.  Spread the dough on the foil in a rectangle to ½ to ¾ inch thick.  We prefer ¾ of an inch thick for cinnamon rolls made in a 9 x 9 inch square pan.  The thicker dough produces softer rolls.

Dust the top of the dough with some gluten-free flour to keep the top from sticking.  Sprinkle gluten-free flour on the counter top and flip the dough onto the counter and peel away the foil.

*see gluten-free products list at the end of the book

Spread the 2 Tablespoons butter on the dough. If you are having trouble spreading it, melt the butter and brush it on. Mix cinnamon and sugar together. Pour sugar mixture over butter. Put leftover sugar mixture in the pan.

Roll up the dough as you would for a jelly roll, rolling at the short end. Have a cutting board at the end of your dough and roll it onto the cutting board. Cut the cinnamon rolls into 1 inch thick slices and place them in your prepared pan. There should be a ½ inch gap between them but they can touch if need be to fit in the pan.

Let rise in a warm place, covered with plastic wrap, for 45 minutes or until doubled in size. (I put them in the oven with the oven light on, so they are away from drafts.) After rising, remove plastic wrap and turn on the oven to 375°F. Leave the rolls in the oven during the preheat time so that they will rise some more. Bake for 35 minutes (including the 10 minute oven preheat) or until they appear done.

Remove from oven and immediately take them out of the pan. Be careful because the sugar will be hot. If you don't remove them from the pan right away, the sugar will harden and you will not be able to get them out. Put on a dish. Make a drizzle using some confectioner's sugar, vanilla, and milk. The cinnamon rolls can be eaten warm, but not hot because the cinnamon/sugar could burn you. I prefer them cooled.

*Variation*: If you greased the foil well, you will be able to roll it from the foil and skip the step of putting the dough on the counter. I find that the rolls rise higher if you don't have to add much additional flour. Brush the top of your rolled dough with melted butter and sprinkle with cinnamon. Roll by peeling the dough away from the foil and rolling the dough onto itself. Then roll the dough onto the cutting board and cut. Follow the rest of the recipe.

## Egg Free Bread

Flax is gluten-free and adds fiber, healthful omega 3 trans-fatty acids, and works as an egg replacement. When using as an egg replacement, your bread will be a little heavier, denser and chewier. (Note: For some people the addition of fiber can have a laxative effect so you may want to try the bread in small amounts at first to see how your body will react.)

Basic bread recipe (see index) eliminating eggs

2 Tablespoons ground flax seed or flax meal
¼ cup hot water

Follow the basic bread recipe, eliminating the 2 eggs and adding the flax and ¼ water in addition to the other water and ingredients in the recipe. Soak the water and flax together about 15 minutes for best results. It should be goopy and not too hot.

If using whole flax seeds, grind it in a food processor immediately before using. If using flax meal, it should be stored in the refrigerator to keep it from going rancid.

*Variation*: Use the cinnamon raisin bread recipe. The cinnamon helps to cover the flax flavor, if you don't like flax.

*see gluten-free products list at the end of the book*

## French Loaf #1
You don't need a bread machine for this one, but you do need a heavy duty mixer and a pan.  This makes 2 loaves.

Follow directions for our favorite basic bread.  Mix in a heavy duty mixer using either the paddle or the bread hook.  Or mix the dough by hand.

Put a piece of aluminum foil on your baking pan.  Spray with cooking spray.  Using hands wet with water make 2 large loaves and put them on the pan.  If you want a darker brown color crust, brush dough with egg white.  Sprinkle on seeds if desired.  Let rise for 1 hour in a warm, draft free place.  (I put it in my oven and leave the light on.)

Put loaves in oven.  Set temperature to 375°F.  Let loaves continue to rise while oven gets to the right temperature.  Bake for about 35 minutes until it tests done.

*Variation*:  Sprinkle loaves with garlic powder before baking for a different flavor.

*Variation 2*:  For a yeast-free loaf that you can bake right away, substitute 2 ¼ teaspoons baking powder for the yeast.  The loaves will have a biscuit-like flavor.

*Variation 3*:  Instead of using the egg white on the outside, spray the loaves with gluten-free cooking spray.  The bread won't brown as much.  Don't use seeds because they won't stick.

## French Loaf #2
You don't need a bread machine for this one, but you do need a food processor and a baguette mold or double French bread pan.  This makes 2 loaves.

4 teaspoons potato starch
1 cup water
1 cup brown rice flour
⅓ cup cornmeal
½ cup tapioca starch
1 cup Gluten-Free Naturals™ Cookie
  Blend
1 Tablespoon xanthan gum
½ teaspoon salt

1 ½ teaspoons sugar
2 packages gluten-free yeast or 2
  Tablespoons yeast (or 2 Tablespoons
  baking powder if you want to bake it
  right away)
1 teaspoon cider vinegar
1 large egg
1 cup warm water (or more if needed)

Boil the 1 cup water and potato starch until thick.  Set aside to cool so that it's warm but not hot.

In your food processor, add the dry ingredients and blend with the cutting blade.  After blended, start the machine and slowly pour in the warm (not hot) potato starch mixture.  Keep blade going and slowly add the cider vinegar, egg and water.  It should be a thick, pasty, goopy dough.

*see gluten-free products list at the end of the book

Grease two sheets of aluminum foil.  Lay foil on a two-loaf French bread loaf pan.  Sprinkle with additional cornmeal if desired.  Spread batter evenly in the pan.  With oiled hand you can smooth out the tops if desired.  If you used yeast, place in a warm, draft free place for 20-30 minutes until the dough is doubled.  If you used baking powder, you can bake it right away.

Bake at 400°F for 35-40 minutes until done.  Cool a little and carefully remove from foil.  My husband likes this served warm.

Use leftovers the next day to make Bruschetta or Crostini by slicing it about ¼ inch thick or so, brush with olive oil and bake in a 375°F oven for 12 minutes.  Turn the bread over, brush other side with oil for Crostini.  For Bruschetta, top the bread with chopped tomatoes and mozzarella cheese.  Bake 5 to 10 minutes more.

*Variation*:  Sprinkle loaves with garlic powder before baking for a different flavor.

*Variation 2*:  1 Tablespoon ground flax seed and 2 Tablespoons water may be substituted for the egg in this recipe for those who can't have eggs.  Flax will add fiber to the bread, but it will be dense in texture.

## Herb Bread
My husband likes the Italian Herb flavor.

Basic Bread recipe (see index)
Use olive oil instead of other oil
Add ½ teaspoon garlic powder

½ teaspoon dried basil
¼ teaspoon oregano

Follow directions for Basic Bread, adding the garlic and herbs, and using olive oil for the oil.  To bring out a stronger herb flavor, put the olive oil, garlic powder, basil and oregano in a glass measuring cup and microwave for 30 seconds to warm it.  Then add it to the wet ingredients.

## Milk and Honey Bread
This bread is slightly sweet and nice for breakfast.  Using milk adds a nice texture to the bread.  This is good using either the Gluten-Free Naturals® Multi-Grain or the White Bread flour.

2 large eggs
1 cup milk, at room temperature (I warm it in the microwave for 20 seconds)
¾ cup warm water (add 2 Tablespoons more if dough looks too thick or dry but do not add more than 2 cups of water total)
2 Tablespoons oil

4 to 6 Tablespoons honey (I prefer ¼ cup)
4 cups (1 lb.) Gluten-Free Naturals™ Bread Flour (Sandwich or Multi-Grain) or Gluten-Free Naturals™ All Purpose Flour
1 ½ teaspoons salt
2 ¼ teaspoons gluten-free yeast* (1 packet)

Follow directions for Basic Bread, using these ingredients. Sometimes it is easier to measure out the honey if you measure the oil first. The oil helps to release it from the Tablespoon.

## Naan – Indian Flatbread

This recipe was invented by Mike, and he cooks the Naan on a baking stone on his outdoor gas grill. They can also be cooked on a cast iron skillet on the stove. Don't use a Teflon™ pan because the Teflon™ breaks down at high heat and you need high heat to make this flatbread.

1 cup water
2 Tablespoons sugar
2 ¼ teaspoons gluten-free yeast* (1 packet)
2 cups (1/2 lb.) Gluten-Free Naturals™ Sandwich Bread Flour or Gluten-Free Naturals™ All Purpose Flour

1 teaspoon salt
Clarified butter or Ghee *(To make it, melt butter in a pan or microwave oven on low. Let it sit a few minutes until the solids settle. The clear part is the Ghee. Skim it off and use it. You can strain it and pour it into a container.)*

Mix the water with the yeast and sugar. Wait for the yeast to activate. Mix in the flour and salt. Let the mixture rise 1 hour.

Form into balls about the size of golf balls. Let rise 1 hour more. Roll out the balls between waxed paper or use 2 Silpat® silicon non-stick pads. Place on a hot stone on an outdoor grill, or cook on a cast iron skillet. Cook about 2-3 minutes. Brush with clarified butter. Flip and cook 2 minutes or so on the other side.

## Pecan Bread

This bread has a lot of protein and the nuts add flavor.

2 large eggs
2 Tablespoons oil or butter
1 ¾ cups warm water (Add 2 Tablespoons more if dough looks too thick or dry. Do not add more than 2 cups of water total.)
¾ cup pecan meal

2 cups Gluten-Free Naturals™ Bread Flour (Sandwich or Multi-Grain) or Gluten-Free Naturals™ All Purpose Flour
¼ cup brown sugar
1 ½ teaspoons salt
2 ¼ teaspoons gluten-free yeast* (1 yeast packet)

Follow directions for Basic Bread, using these ingredients. Add the wet ingredients and then the dry ingredients to the bread machine. Or if using the oven method, this mixes well using a mixer with a dough hook. It can also be mixed by hand.

*see gluten-free products list at the end of the book

## Pizza Crust – Version 1

We prefer the Gluten-Free Naturals™ Pizza mix. If you don't have it, you can use this method. The herbs add flavor. I use a plain small can of tomato sauce*, since the herbs are in the crust.

1 pound (4 cups) Gluten-Free Naturals™ Bread Flour (Sandwich or Multi-Grain) or Gluten-Free Naturals™ All Purpose Flour
1 ½ teaspoons salt
3 Tablespoons sugar
1 gluten-free yeast packet
2 eggs
¼ cup olive oil
½ teaspoon garlic powder (optional)

½ teaspoon dried basil (optional)
¼ teaspoon oregano (optional)
1 ¾ to 2 cups warm water (I suggest you use less water initially and check dough consistency. Add 2 Tablespoons more if dough looks too thick or dry. You should be able to spread this dough.)
Gluten-free tomato sauce*
Mozzarella cheese*

Blend all ingredients in a bowl, by mixing dry ingredients first and then wet ingredients. Spread dough in <u>two</u> greased 12" pizza pans. If it is difficult to spread, wet your rubber spatula with water. Let rise in a warm, draft free place for 1 hour. (I let it sit in the oven with the light on.)

Bake at 350°F for 20 minutes, or until done. Top with gluten-free sauce* and cheese*. Bake until the cheese melts (about 4 to 5 minutes).

*Variation*: Use 1 Tablespoon baking powder instead of yeast, to avoid the rising time and bake it right away. Your pizza crust will have a biscuit-like flavor.

## Pizza Crust – Version 2

This pizza is a crust using rice flour. It will begin to crumble after a few days in the refrigerator, so it's best eaten the day you make it. This pizza crust has yeast and baking powder so it doesn't need the rising time. See variation below for directions on how to rise the crust using only yeast. Other versions of pizza are under the baking powder bread section of this book.

2 cups white rice flour
2 cups tapioca flour
¼ cup sugar
1 Tablespoon xanthan gum
1 teaspoon salt
1 teaspoon gluten-free yeast* (optional)
1 Tablespoon gluten-free baking powder*
¼ cup oil
½ cup non-fat dry milk powder

2 cups warm water
1 teaspoon cider vinegar
1 (8 ounce) can gluten-free tomato sauce*
Oregano, garlic, basil, Pecorino Romano or Parmesan cheese
1 (16 ounce) package of grated gluten-free mozzarella cheese*
Toppings of your choice

Mix all dry ingredients together with a whisk. Add wet ingredients. Blend.

Grease two non-stick rectangular pans (mine are approximately 9 x 13 inches, with black non-stick finish). Spread dough with a rubber spatula. Bake at 350°F for 12 to 14 minutes. Loosen edges with a pancake turner and loosen under the dough. Let cool a few minutes.

*see gluten-free products list at the end of the book

Then flip the dough over and put it back in the pan. This is to prevent sauce from soaking in, because the bottom will have a crispier crust. This also makes it easy to get your pizza out of the pan once you have your toppings on it.

Top the pizza with sauce. I use one 8 ounce can of tomato sauce for 2 pizzas. Then I sprinkle it with some dried oregano, garlic powder, dried basil, Pecorino Romano cheese and gluten-free shredded mozzarella cheese. I use one 16 ounce package of mozzarella cheese for 2 pizzas. Add gluten-free toppings if desired. Bake until cheese melts.

*Variation*: If you would prefer a pizza that is risen using yeast, increase the yeast to 1 Tablespoon or 1 yeast packet. Decrease baking powder to 1 teaspoon or eliminate it. Let rise in a warm, draft free place for 1 hour. Then bake as directed.

*Variation 2*: If you cannot have yeast, eliminate it and use only the baking powder. Reduce the sugar to 2 Tablespoons. The flavor is better with the yeast, but this will work.

*Variation 3*: For a higher rising pizza using both the yeast and the baking powder, let pizza rise 15 to 30 minutes before baking.

## Potato Bread
This is a soft, very moist bread.

Basic Bread recipe (see index)
Use the water from boiled potatoes (see instructions below)

¼ cup light brown or granulated sugar instead of 3 Tablespoons

When you boil potatoes to make mashed potatoes, keep the water. Wash and cut potatoes into chunks. (I have found that the best way to wash potatoes is to use a nail brush that I designate for that purpose. Since they are designed to clean under your nails and not harm your skin, they work much better than vegetable brushes and last longer too.) We prefer our potatoes unpeeled, so cut them so that the cooked peels are about a ½ to ¾ inch square. Boil the potatoes in an uncovered pot until potatoes are tender. Remove from heat.

Save the water from the potatoes to use in your bread. Put a bowl under your sieve or colander and drain the potatoes retaining the water.

Put potatoes back in your pot and make mashed potatoes. I add butter, salt, pepper, and milk and use a masher.

Allow the potato water to cool somewhat so it is warm but not too hot. Follow directions for Basic Bread, using the potato water in place of the liquid. The potato water adds nutrients. In the old days they wasted nothing and used potato water in bread or soup.

*Note*: Since this bread has more moisture, it can get moldy much more quickly, especially in the summer months. I suggest that you freeze or refrigerate leftovers.

## "Pumpernickel" Bread
**A good bread for those who like dark breads.**

2 large eggs
3 Tablespoons molasses
1 ¾ cups warm water (Add 2 Tablespoons more if dough looks too thick or dry. Do not add more than 2 cups of water total.)
2 Tablespoons oil
4 cups (1 lb.) Gluten-Free Naturals™ Bread Flour (Sandwich or Multi-Grain)
or Gluten-Free Naturals™ All Purpose Flour
2 ¼ teaspoons gluten-free yeast* (1 packet)
1 Tablespoon caraway seeds (optional)
1 ½ teaspoons salt
⅓ cup non-fat dry milk powder (optional)
1 Tablespoon cocoa powder
3 Tablespoon sugar, brown or white
1 teaspoon grated orange peel (optional)

Follow directions for Basic Bread, using these ingredients.

*Variation*: To add a darker color as well as some protein, use 1 cup of water that you cooked black beans in (also called turtle beans) as part of the water in this recipe.

## Raisin or Dried Fruit Bread
**For bread that reminds me of Panettone, eliminate the cinnamon and use golden raisins for the fruit. You can also add a little lemon or orange zest. Use the 4 Tablespoons sugar. (My husband doesn't like the candied citron, or I would use half citron and half golden raisins).**

2 large eggs
2 Tablespoons oil
2 cups water (I suggest you use 2 Tablespoons less water initially and check dough consistency. Add remaining 2 Tablespoons if dough looks too thick or dry.)
4 cups (1 lb.) Gluten-Free Naturals™ Bread Flour (Sandwich or Multi-Grain) or Gluten-Free Naturals™ All Purpose Flour
3 to 4 Tablespoons sugar (white or brown)
1 ½ teaspoons salt
½ cup non-fat dry milk powder (optional)
⅔ cup dried fruit such as dried cranberries or raisins (If using apricots or dates, be sure they aren't dusted with wheat flour)
2 ¼ teaspoons active dry gluten-free yeast*
1 teaspoon ground cinnamon (or more if desired)

Follow directions for Basic Bread, using these ingredients. (This bread uses more water since the fruit draws in some of the water).

## Raisin Cardamom Bread
The cardamom flavor reminds me of some of the breads I had in Norway.

2 large eggs
1 ¾ cups warm water (Add 2 Tablespoons more if dough looks too thick or dry. Do not add more than 2 cups of water total.)
2 Tablespoons oil
4 cups (1 lb.) Gluten-Free Naturals™ Bread Flour (Sandwich or Multi-Grain) or Gluten-Free Naturals™ All Purpose Flour

2 ¼ teaspoons gluten-free yeast*
1 ½ teaspoons salt
¼ cup non-fat dry milk powder (optional)
1 Tablespoon cocoa powder
3 Tablespoon sugar, brown or white
2 teaspoons ground cardamom (or 1 teaspoon cardamom and 1 teaspoon ground cinnamon)
6 ounces raisins

Follow directions for Basic Bread, using these ingredients.

If your bread machine "beeps" to add raisins/nuts, add the raisins at that time.

## Rolls #1

Follow the recipe for our favorite Basic Bread or the directions on the Gluten-Free Naturals™ package.  Mix the dough in a heavy duty mixer.

Using a large spoon, drop the dough onto a non-stick baking sheet.  If dough is sticking to your spoon, wet the spoon with water.  Leave space in-between the rolls since they will double in size when they rise.  If you have a "top of the muffin" pan or mini pie pans, this will help you make perfect hamburger roll shapes.  Grease the pan(s) if they are not the non-stick type of pan.  I put about 6 mini pie pans onto a large baking sheet so it is easy to put them in the oven.

*Or you can make your own gluten-free Pepperidge Farm® style "Deli-Flats™" round breads by putting the dough in the "top of the muffin" pan or on a baking sheet with 6 English muffin rings. Flatten the dough, using a wet spatula.  Instead of doming the dough in the middle so it rises like a regular roll, evenly flatten it deliberately so it will look very flat like the Deli-Flats™ bread.*

Wet your hands with water.  Shape the dough into the shape of roll that you want (i.e. dinner rolls, hamburger rolls or hot dog rolls).  Smooth tops.  Brush with egg white and sprinkle with seeds, if desired.

Rise and (about 1 hour) and bake as directed.  You can either set your pan in the oven with the light on, or you can cover the rolls with plastic wrap and a warm wet towel.

Or if you prefer to eliminate the rising, substitute 2 ¼ teaspoons baking powder for yeast to bake immediately.  Rolls made with baking powder will have a biscuit-like flavor.

Place rolls in the oven and set temperature to 350°F.  The rolls will rise as the oven heats up. Bake for about 20 to 25 minutes for small rolls.  If you made larger rolls, they may need to bake longer.  Torpedo rolls may take 30 to 35 minutes, depending on the size.  Cool on a cooling rack.  Slice when they are completely cooled.

## Rolls #2

Follow the recipe for French Bread #1.  Roll into roll shapes (dinner rolls, hamburger rolls or hot dog rolls) using your hands wet with water. Smooth tops.  Brush with egg white and sprinkle with seeds if desired.  Rise and bake as directed in the other recipe, or substitute 2 ¼ teaspoons baking powder for yeast to bake immediately.  Rolls made with baking powder will have a biscuit-like flavor.

If using yeast, set rolls in the oven during the pre-heat so that they continue to rise.  Bake at 375°F for 20 to 25 minutes.  Torpedo rolls may take 30 to 35 minutes.

## Rolls #3

If you can find a "top of the muffin" pan or "mini pie pans", you can use this recipe to make hamburger rolls.  For smaller rolls I use an English tart pan (a rounded bottom muffin pan).  These are a plain and simple roll.  They contain no eggs for those who are allergic to them.  They also contain no soy flour.

1 cup white rice flour
1 cup tapioca flour
2 Tablespoons sugar
2 teaspoons xanthan gum
¼ cup nonfat dry milk powder

½ teaspoon salt
2 teaspoons gluten-free active dry yeast*
2 Tablespoons oil
1 cup warm water
½ teaspoon cider vinegar

Mix all dry ingredients together with a whisk.  Add wet ingredients. Blend.

Grease a 12 "top of muffin pan" or English tart pan.  Put dough in pan and let rise 1 hour in a warm place.  Bake at 350°F for 20 to 25 minutes.

## "Russian" Black Bread

A dark bread, that is nice for a change of pace.

2 large eggs
2 Tablespoons oil
2 Tablespoons molasses
1 ¾ cups warm water (Add 2 Tablespoons more if dough looks too thick or dry.  Do not add more than 2 cups of water total.)
4 cups (1 lb.) Gluten-Free Naturals™ Bread Flour (Sandwich or Multi-Grain)

or Gluten-Free Naturals™ All Purpose Flour
3 Tablespoons dark brown sugar, packed
1 ½ teaspoons salt
¼ cup instant non-fat dry milk (optional)
1 teaspoon instant coffee
4 ½ teaspoons cocoa
2 Tablespoons caraway seeds (optional)
2 ¼ teaspoons gluten-free active dry yeast*

Follow directions for basic bread using these ingredients.

*see gluten-free products list at the end of the book

*Variation*: You can use 1 cup of Redbridge® Beer in place of 1 cup of the water in this recipe.

*Variation 2*: To add a nice black color as well as some protein, use 1 cup of the water used to cook black beans in (also called turtle beans) as part of the water in this recipe. You can eliminate the non-fat dry milk.

## "Rye" Bread (mock Rye)
**Try a Ruben sandwich (corned beef, Swiss cheese, sauerkraut and Russian dressing) on this bread.**

2 large eggs
2 Tablespoons oil
1 Tablespoon molasses
1 ¾ cups warm water (Add 2 Tablespoons more if dough looks too thick or dry. Do not add more than 2 cups of water total.)
4 cups (1 lb.) Gluten-Free Naturals™ Bread Flour (Sandwich or Multi-Grain)

or Gluten-Free Naturals™ All Purpose Flour
2 ¼ teaspoons gluten-free yeast*
¼ cup brown sugar, firmly packed
1 ½ teaspoons salt
Caraway seeds and egg white for the top of the bread (optional)

Follow directions for Basic Bread, using these ingredients.

*Variation*: If you want caraway seeds on top of your bread, mix 1 teaspoon egg white powder, with 1 Tablespoon water and 1 Tablespoon caraway seeds. Blend and spoon this mixture on the top of the bread before baking it, for the oven method. For the bread machine method, wait until after the bread is mixed. Smooth top of bread with a rubber spatula when the mixing stops. Put egg/seed mixture on top before it starts the rising time.

## Seed Bread
**Seeds add texture and protein to the bread.**

2 large eggs
2 Tablespoons oil
1 ¾ cups warm water or 1 cup milk and ¾ cups water (Add 2 Tablespoons more if dough looks too thick or dry. Do not add more than 2 cups of water total.)
4 cups (1 lb.) Gluten-Free Naturals™ Bread Flour (Sandwich or Multi-Grain) or Gluten-Free Naturals™ All Purpose Flour

2 ¼ teaspoons gluten-free yeast*
3 Tablespoons sugar
1 ½ teaspoons salt
1 Tablespoon unsalted, shelled sunflower seeds
1 Tablespoon poppy seeds
1 Tablespoon sesame seeds (optional)

Follow directions for Basic Bread, using these ingredients.

*Variation*: 1 Tablespoon to 2 Tablespoons of uncooked teff grain may be used instead of the seeds.

*see gluten-free products list at the end of the book

## Soft Pretzel Bites
These taste like soft pretzels.

2 eggs
1 ½ cups warm (not hot) water
2 Tablespoons oil
4 cups (16 ounces) Gluten-Free Naturals™ Sandwich Bread Flour (not Multi-Grain) or Gluten-Free Naturals™ All Purpose Flour
1 ½ teaspoons salt
2 to 3 Tablespoons sugar

1 Tablespoon ground flax seed (flax meal)
1 packet of gluten-free yeast* (2 ¼ teaspoons) or 2 ¼ teaspoons gluten-free bread machine yeast* or rapid rise yeast, or 1 Tablespoon regular yeast* from jar (I use Red Star® brand)
6 cups of boiling water in a pot
½ teaspoon baking soda

Prepare dough. You can blend it in a heavy duty mixer with a paddle or dough hook. Or, mix by hand with a sturdy spoon. It will be a very thick dough.

Take a baking pan, cover it with foil and spray it with cooking spray. With hands wet with water, grab small amounts of dough to make pretzel bites. Dough also can be put in a heavy duty plastic bag, cut the corner and make longer pretzel logs. Smooth them with hands wet with water. Although it is possible to make pretzel shapes, it is more time-consuming and more difficult to boil them. This is why I recommend doing the bites or logs.

In a pot, boil water and add the baking soda to it. Set your oven temperature to 350°F.

Boil the pretzels in the water for about 3 minutes or so. They will float to the top and start to expand somewhat.

Remove from water and put them on a foil covered baking sheet that is sprayed with cooking spray. If you want the course salt to stick really well, brush them with egg white and sprinkle with coarse salt or seeds.

Bake in a 350° oven for 35 minutes, until pretzels are done.

Just like regular hot pretzels get stale the next day, these will also get stale. I suggest you freeze leftovers.

*Note*: If you don't boil the pretzels in the boiling water with the baking soda, they will not brown properly on the outside like a regular pretzel.

Also, your dough must be somewhat thick or it will not hold up in the boiling water. The ground flax helps to make the dough thick enough for it to be boiled in the water. If your dough seems a little thin initially, wait a few minutes to see if the flax thickens it. If not thick enough, add a little more but don't add more than 2 Tablespoons. Be sure that your flax is fresh. Flax can go rancid quickly, and rancid flax will impart a terrible flavor. It is also not good for you to eat rancid foods. When flax is fresh, it is mild and nutty tasting. Smell it before using it. If the smell is unpleasant, it is probably rancid. I store flax in the refrigerator or vacuum package it so that it stays fresh a long time.

*\*see gluten-free products list at the end of the book*

Write your own recipes here:

## Cakes, Icings, Pies and Cookies

## CAKES

### Angel Food Cake – Our Favorite Version

This cake is very light in texture.  I served it at a party with whipped cream and it was gone in no time!  Or try it with the mocha or cocoa frosting (see recipe under Angel Food Cake – Mocha).

1 ½ cups egg whites (about 12) or
    substitute egg white powder [½ cup]
    and water [1 ½ cups]
1 ½ teaspoons cream of tartar
¾ cup sugar
¼ teaspoon salt
1 teaspoon gluten-free vanilla extract*

½ teaspoon almond extract
¼ cup fine white rice flour
¾ cup Gluten-Free Naturals™ Sandwich
    Bread Flour or Gluten-Free Naturals™
    All Purpose Flour
¾ cup sugar

If using fresh egg whites, beat egg whites and cream of tartar in a large clean bowl on medium speed until foamy.  Beat in ¾ cup sugar on high speed, adding it 2 Tablespoons at a time.

If using egg white powder, mix ¼ cup sugar and cream of tartar with the egg powder.  Put the water in your mixer bowl and slowly mix in the powder.  Adding in some sugar first will help prevent the egg white powder from getting lumpy.  Beat until foamy.  Then beat in the rest of the sugar on high speed, adding it 2 Tablespoons at a time.

Add the salt, vanilla, and almond extract (if using) with the last addition of sugar.  Now gradually beat in the rice flour with the mixer.  Once blended, remove from mixer.  Mix the ¾ cup Gluten-Free All Purpose Flour or Sandwich Bread Flour and ¾ cup sugar together in another bowl.  Gently fold into the egg white mixture a ¼ cup at a time using a rubber spatula.  (Do not attempt to beat in the flour mixture using the mixer.  The xanthan gum in the gluten-free flour will deflate the egg whites if whipped in.)  Put into an ungreased tube pan, 10 x 4 inches.  Use a rubber spatula to gently cut through the batter.  This removes any large air holes.  Bake at 375°F for 30 to 35 minutes.  Invert the pan and keep it upside down until the cake is cool.  (You must cool it upside down or your cake will fall).

This is a moist light cake that keeps well for several days unrefrigerated, or about a week refrigerated.  Refrigerate it if you frost it with whipped cream.  Use a knife with a serrated edge to gently "saw" the cake when you cut it.

## Angel Food Cake – "Snow White" version
This cake is good the day you make it. The next day I find it has a grainy texture.

3 Tablespoons plus 1 teaspoon egg white powder
⅓ cup sugar (granulated)
¾ teaspoon cream of tartar
½ cup plus 2 Tablespoons water
½ cup confectioner's (powdered) sugar
¼ cup cornstarch

¼ cup potato starch
¼ teaspoon salt
1 teaspoon orange or lemon zest or ¼ teaspoon lemon extract* or ½ teaspoon gluten-free vanilla extract*

With a whisk, blend the egg white powder, granulated sugar, and cream of tartar in a large clean bowl of an electric mixer. Add the water and mix with a whisk until blended. Then beat the egg whites on medium speed until stiff peaks form. Blend the cornstarch, potato starch, salt and zest (if using) in a bowl. Gently fold in the flour mixture and flavoring. Put into an ungreased 8 x 4 inch loaf pan. Use a spatula to gently cut through the batter. This removes any large air holes. Bake at 375°F for 30 to 35 minutes. Invert the pan on a cooling rack and keep it upside down until the cake is completely cool. This recipe may be doubled for a 10 inch tube pan. This is nice served with fresh strawberries and whipped cream, or frosted with whipped cream frosting (see index for recipe).

## Angel Food Cake – Mocha
This is my mother's recipe, and it is light and delicious. This mocha whipped cream frosting is also nice on other cakes.

1 angel food cake recipe for a 10 inch tube pan (see previous recipes) or 1 package gluten-free angel food cake mix
1 Tablespoon hot water
1 Tablespoon instant coffee
1 teaspoon gluten-free vanilla*
1 ½ cups gluten-free heavy cream*

3 Tablespoons sugar
2 tablespoons dry cocoa
2 teaspoons instant coffee
2 teaspoons hot water
¾ teaspoon gluten-free vanilla*

Melt 1 Tablespoon instant coffee in the 1 Tablespoon of hot water and add to cake mix with the teaspoon of vanilla when adding the required liquid. Proceed according to recipe or package directions. Cool cake completely.

For mocha topping, melt two teaspoons of instant coffee in hot water and add to heavy cream with all the rest of the ingredients. Whip until stiff. Cover cake with cream in swirls and refrigerate until serving time. It can be made hours ahead of time.

*Variation*: If you don't like coffee flavor, you can make the whipped cream with just the cocoa.

## Apple Cake with Grated Fresh Apples

1 ¾ cups grated apples
1 cup sugar
1 ½ cups Gluten-Free Naturals™ All
   Purpose Flour
½ teaspoon salt
1 teaspoon baking soda

½ teaspoon ground allspice
½ teaspoon ground nutmeg
1 teaspoon ground cinnamon
1 egg
½ cup oil

Grease a ring mold pan generously with butter. Peel, core and grate apples with the course grater disk of your food processor. Add sugar to apples and let stand 10 minutes. Blend flour and dry ingredients with a whisk. Add egg and oil to the apple mixture. Then mix in the dry ingredients. Pour batter into prepared pan and bake 45 minutes in a preheated 375°F oven.

## Apple Cake with Sherry

1 cup butter
2 cups sugar
3 eggs
3 cups Gluten-Free Naturals™ All
   Purpose Flour
1 ½ teaspoons baking soda
1 teaspoon ground cinnamon

½ teaspoon salt
⅛ teaspoon ground nutmeg
3 cups peeled and chopped apples
2 cups chopped walnuts or pecans
2 teaspoons gluten-free vanilla*

Glaze:  1 ½ cups sugar

½ cup sherry

Whisk together flour, baking soda, salt, cinnamon and nutmeg. Cream butter and sugar with a mixer. Add eggs one at a time. Mix in dry ingredients. When blended, add apples, nuts and vanilla. Bake 1 ½ hours in a greased tube pan in a 325°F oven. When tests done, cool and remove from pan. Place on a platter and pour sherry glaze on top.

To make glaze, put sugar and sherry in a pot. Heat on low until syrupy.

## Apple Upside-down Cake
This is my mother's recipe. It's moist and delicious.  It makes its own topping so no icing is needed.

2 Tablespoons butter, melted
2 apples, peeled, cored and thinly sliced
1 teaspoon ground cinnamon

⅓ cup brown sugar, packed
1 Gluten-Free Naturals™ Yellow Cake
   Mix, batter prepared as directed

Melt butter and spread in the bottom of an 8 x 8 inch square or 9 inch round non-stick pan. (I melt butter in a Pyrex® measuring cup using the defrost cycle in the microwave.)

Peel apples, core and slice them very thin. Place over butter mixture. Sprinkle cinnamon and brown sugar over apples.

*see gluten-free products list at the end of the book

Prepare cake mix as directed. Pour over the top of apples. Bake for 40 minutes or until it tests done. Remove from pan and allow to cool.

*Variation*: Substitute drained canned sliced peaches for apples.

*Variation 2*: Add chopped walnuts or pecans with the apples.

*Variation 3*: Prepare the cake without apples. Use butter, ground cinnamon, brown sugar, and a handful of whole or chopped nuts.

## Apple Upside Down Cake Version 2
This is a delicious cake that is moist and easy to make. We like it served with brunch or as a dessert. These directions are on the mix package.

2 Tablespoons melted butter
2 medium apples, peeled and thinly sliced
½ cup brown sugar

½ teaspoon ground cinnamon
1 Gluten-Free Naturals™ Yellow Cake
   Mix, batter prepared as directed

Use pan sizes specified on the mix package. In the baking pan pour 2 Tablespoons melted butter. Peel and thinly slice two medium sized apples and place around the bottom of the pan in the butter. Take ½ cup brown sugar and ½ tsp. cinnamon and sprinkle around the bottom of cake pan over the apples and butter. Mix the Yellow Cake as directed on the package and pour the batter into the pan on top of the apple mixture. Add 5 minutes of baking time for the pan used.

## Applesauce Cake
This is a good "snacking-cake". I often make half the recipe.

2 ½ cups Gluten-Free Naturals™ All
   Purpose Flour
¼ teaspoon gluten-free baking powder*
1 ½ teaspoons baking soda
1 ½ teaspoons salt
¾ teaspoon ground cinnamon
½ teaspoon ground cloves
½ cup oil

½ cup water
1 ½ cups unsweetened applesauce (I use
   canned)
2 eggs
½ cup chopped nuts
1 cup cut up raisins (optional)
½ teaspoon ground allspice

Blend dry ingredients together. Add oil and water and mix, then add eggs and applesauce. Beat 2 minutes. Bake in a greased tube pan or 2 small loaf pans in a 350°F oven for 35 to 40 minutes.

*Variation*: 1 ½ cups rice flour and 1 cup defatted soy flour and 2 ½ teaspoons xanthan gum may be used for the Gluten-Free Naturals™ All Purpose Flour in this recipe. The cake will be heavier if you make that substitution.

*see gluten-free products list at the end of the book

## Applesauce Cake – Loaf pan
This cake is nice served with breakfast.

1 cup Gluten-Free Naturals™ All Purpose
   Flour
¾ cup sugar
¼ teaspoon gluten-free baking powder*
¾ teaspoon baking soda
½ teaspoon ground cinnamon

1 egg
¼ cup oil
½ cup plain gluten-free yogurt*
¾ cup unsweetened applesauce (I use
   canned)

Blend all ingredients until thoroughly mixed. Bake in a greased loaf pan for 35 minutes until it tests done.

## Banana Cake
I often put the less sugar amount and enjoy this cake for breakfast. Double the recipe and make a delicious layer cake. I recently made this for a coworker's child on the gluten-free diet, and everyone liked this cake better than the store-bought one that she purchased for everyone else at the party.

2 ripe bananas
½ cup to ¾ cup sugar, depending how
   ripe bananas are (If bananas are very
   ripe and syrupy, I use a ½ cup,
   otherwise use the ¾ cup)
1 egg
¼ cup oil
1 teaspoon gluten-free vanilla*

¾ cup plain yogurt* (if bananas are not
   very large, use a little more)
1 cup Gluten-Free Naturals™ All Purpose
   Flour
1 ½ teaspoons baking soda
½ teaspoon salt

Mash bananas in a bowl with the sugar and blend. Add the egg, oil, vanilla and yogurt and blend. Add the flour, baking soda and salt, and blend until the flour is mixed in. Pour into a greased 11 x 7 inch pan. Bake for 30 minutes at 350°F. It's good as a breakfast cake unfrosted, or frost it for a layer or sheet cake.

*Variation*: Double the recipe and put in a larger pan (9 ¾ x 14 ¾ inch or so. My Pyrex® glass pan says 38x25x4cm on it). Bake 40 minutes until it tests done (cake tester comes out clean). Cool completely and frost. (My husband likes cream cheese frosting. See index for recipe.) This is an easy sheet cake for birthdays.

*Variation 2*: If you have an old style crock-pot with the non-removable crock and the aluminum baking insert and rack; bake this cake on high for 2 ½ hours. Be sure to grease the inside of the baking pan before pouring in the batter and to secure the cover. Put the rack inside the bottom of the crock before putting in the baking insert. This makes a very moist cake.

*\*see gluten-free products list at the end of the book*

## Banana Chocolate Cake

It was my mother's idea to add the chocolate to the banana cake. I've never seen this type of recipe elsewhere. Our family always enjoys this cake.

| | |
|---|---|
| 1 cup Gluten-Free Naturals™ All Purpose Flour | 2 very ripe bananas |
| ¾ cup sugar | 1 egg |
| ¼ to ⅓ cup cocoa | ¼ cup oil |
| 1 ½ teaspoons baking soda | 1 teaspoon gluten-free vanilla* |
| ½ teaspoon salt | ¾ cup gluten-free buttermilk* or gluten-free plain yogurt* |

Mash the bananas. If they are syrupy and sweet use ⅓ cup cocoa. If they are not, use ¼ cup cocoa. Combine dry ingredients. In a large bowl mix the egg, oil, buttermilk and vanilla. Then add the dry ingredients all at once and beat in. Pour into a buttered loaf pan or a layer cake pan and place in a preheated 350°F oven and bake 30-35 minutes. To make a layer cake, double the recipe and use two 9" round cake pans. Slice and serve with cream and sliced bananas.

*Variation*: You can replace the Gluten-Free Naturals™ All Purpose Flour with ½ cup fine white rice flour and ½ cup defatted soy flour and 1 teaspoon xanthan gum. It will be a little denser if you make this substitution, but it will work.

*Variation 2*: Sometimes I make one 9" layer as directed above, and cut it in half making two half circles. Place one half on a nice plate, put frosting on the top of it and top with the second half. Frost the rest of the cake. Now you have half a layer cake. Put plastic wrap on the cut side if you didn't frost it. I find that ½ a layer cake is the right amount for a small dinner party. There are a few brands of gluten-free frostings you can buy, or use the recipes found in this book. This cake is good with or without frosting.

*Variation 3*: One time I didn't have buttermilk. I used ¾ cup milk instead. I used 1 ½ teaspoons baking powder instead of baking soda. I used 1 ¼ cups Gluten-Free Naturals™ All Purpose Flour instead of 1 cup. It was a slightly denser cake, but very moist. It was nice served with some whipped cream topping.

*\*see gluten-free products list at the end of the book*

## Blueberry Cake

This cake is delicious with the crunchy topping and buttery cake. The cake is not too sweet and works well with the fruit. However, if you like things very sweet, add an additional 2 to 4 Tablespoons sugar. This cake is best the day you make it. The next day the blueberries will make the topping a little wet, but it is still very tasty. This is nice as a coffee cake or for dessert.

½ cup oil
½ to ¾ cup sugar (if blueberries are sweet,
   I use ½ cup)
1 egg
3 teaspoons gluten-free baking powder*

2 cups Gluten-Free Naturals™ All
   Purpose Flour
¼ teaspoon salt
1 cup milk
¼ cup water
2 cups blueberries

Topping:
⅔ cup Gluten-Free Naturals™ Cookie
   Blend
½ cup sugar

⅓ cup butter
½ teaspoon ground cinnamon

Beat oil, sugar and egg in an electric mixer. Add in the baking powder, All Purpose Flour, salt, milk and water and blend well with the mixer. Spread into a buttered 13 x 9 inch pan (or a 9" spring-form pan may be used). Top with blueberries (use less with the spring-form pan). Blend topping ingredients and sprinkle on top. Bake at 350°F for 50 minutes.

*Variation*: Instead of the Gluten-Free Naturals™ Cookie Blend and butter for the topping, you can top with sugar, nuts, and cinnamon. We prefer it with the topping recipe above, but this is nice for a change.

## Blueberry Cake – "English" Version

6 Tablespoons oil
1 cup sugar
1 egg
2 cups Gluten-Free Naturals™ All
   Purpose Flour

4 teaspoons gluten-free baking powder*
Pinch of salt
¾ cup milk
1 cup blueberries

Preheat oven to 375°F. Grease a 9 inch square baking pan. In an electric mixer, blend together the oil, sugar and egg. Add dry ingredients and milk. If batter is too dry, add a few more Tablespoons of milk or water. Stir in blueberries. Place batter in prepared pan and smooth top with a spatula. Bake for 35 minutes or until golden brown and done.

## Buttermilk Cake

2 cups light brown sugar  
½ cup oil  
1 cup gluten-free buttermilk* or plain yogurt*  
2 eggs  
1 teaspoon gluten-free vanilla*  

2 cups Gluten-Free Naturals™ All Purpose Flour  
¼ teaspoon salt  
1 teaspoon baking soda  
Cinnamon  
Sugar  
Sliced almonds  

Blend oil and sugar together in a mixer. Add buttermilk, eggs and vanilla and blend in with the mixer. Mix flour, salt and baking soda together. Add flour mixture to wet mixture. Grease a 9 x 14 inch pan and pour in the batter. Sprinkle top with sliced almonds or other chopped nuts. Then top with a sprinkling of cinnamon and sugar. Bake at 350°F for 35 minutes.

## Carrot Cake

*This cake is a very moist cake. The reason I have a range for the flour is that some cans of crushed pineapple have more juice in them than others. If your batter is too wet you will need to add more flour. If your batter is too thin (i.e. wet) the cake will not bake properly. It will sink in the middle after it bakes. I suggest you try other cake recipes first so you know the proper batter consistency you need for this cake.*

2 ¼ to 2 ½ cups Gluten-Free Naturals™ All Purpose Flour  
2 teaspoons gluten-free baking powder*  
1 ½ teaspoons baking soda  
2 teaspoons ground cinnamon  
1 teaspoon salt  
2 cups sugar  

1 ½ cups oil (I use less)  
4 eggs  
2 cups grated carrots (6 to 7 medium carrots)  
1 (8 ½ ounce) can crushed pineapple  
½ cup chopped nuts  

Cream Cheese Frosting:  
½ cup butter or gluten-free margarine*  
8 ounce package of gluten-free cream cheese*  

1 teaspoon gluten-free vanilla*  
1 pound sifted confectioner's sugar  
Milk or gluten-free milk substitute*  

Add dry ingredients in a mixer bowl and blend together. Add oil and eggs and mix well. Add carrots, pineapple and nuts. The batter should be somewhat thick, and not come off the beaters too quickly. If the batter does, add more of the All Purpose Flour. (The amount of juice in the canned pineapple can vary, which is the reason I have a range.)

Turn into two greased 9 inch round pans. Bake at 350°F for 45-50 minutes or until done. Cool and turn onto a wire rack.

To make frosting, blend ingredients. If too thick, add a little milk until mixture is the right consistency.

*see gluten-free products list at the end of the book

## Carrot Cake – Version 2

This cake is an alternative recipe that uses less expensive flours. It is heavier than the other recipe, but the rice flour is more forgiving as far as the range of differences in the liquid from the canned pineapple. Sometimes I use homemade leftover carrot salad (shredded carrot, pineapple, mayonnaise and walnuts) to make this cake.

| | |
|---|---|
| 1 cup fine white rice flour or sweet rice flour | 2 eggs |
| ¼ cup cornstarch | 1 cup sugar |
| 1 ¼ teaspoons xanthan gum | ½ cup gluten-free mayonnaise* |
| 1 teaspoon baking soda | 1 can (8 ounces) crushed pineapple, packed in its own juice, un-drained |
| ¼ teaspoon salt | 1 ½ cups shredded carrots |
| 1 teaspoon ground cinnamon | ½ cup chopped walnuts |
| ¼ teaspoon ground ginger | |

Cream Cheese Frosting:

| | |
|---|---|
| ½ package (4 ounces) gluten-free cream cheese*, softened | ⅓ cup confectioner's sugar (I use more) |
| | 1 teaspoon orange juice |

Whisk together the flour, xanthan gum, cornstarch, soda, salt and spices. Set aside. In an electric mixer bowl, blend together the eggs, sugar, mayonnaise and pineapple at medium speed. Add the flour gradually until it is blended in. (Note: Your batter should not be too thin. When you lift the beaters it should slowly pour off the beaters. If it pours off fast and is thin, add a little more rice flour. Some cans of crushed pineapple have more liquid than others.)

Generously grease a 9-inch square baking pan. Pour in the batter and bake at 350°F for 40 minutes, or until it tests done with a cake tester. Cool on a wire rack. Once cool, make frosting by combining those ingredients. Frost and serve.

*see gluten-free products list at the end of the book

## Carrot Cake – Version 3

This version has no pineapple. This has a sweeter frosting since there is less sugar in the cake.

¾ cup sugar

½ cup oil

2 eggs

1 cup Gluten-Free Naturals™ All Purpose Flour

½ teaspoon baking soda

¼ teaspoon salt

¾ teaspoon ground cinnamon

¼ teaspoon ground nutmeg

1 ½ cups shredded carrots

½ cup chopped walnuts

Cream Cheese Frosting:

½ package (4 ounces) gluten-free cream cheese*, softened

½ teaspoon gluten-free vanilla*

1 to 2 teaspoons milk (Start with 1 and add more if necessary)

2 cups confectioner's sugar

In a heavy-duty electric mixer, blend sugar, oil, and eggs. Add the flour, soda, salt and spices. Blend well. Stir in the carrots and walnuts. Pour into a greased 8 x 8 inch pan, or a 9 inch round pan. Bake 35 to 40 minutes. Allow to cool completely.

Blend cream cheese and vanilla together in an electric mixer. Add the rest of the ingredients and blend until smooth. If too thick, add an additional teaspoon of milk. Frost the completely cooled cake. Recipe can be doubled to make a 9 x 13 inch cake. If doubling, bake 35 to 45 minutes.

## Cassata

A delicious Italian cake.

1 chiffon cake, baked in a 10 inch spring-form pan, cooled completely (see index)

3 pounds gluten-free Ricotta cheese*

2 teaspoons gluten-free vanilla*

¾ cup sugar

½ cup gluten-free chocolate bits*

¼ to ½ cup rum* or other gluten-free liquor*

2 cups gluten-free heavy cream*

Gelatin and sugar

Chopped pistachio nuts

Make the chiffon cake a day before serving and slice in 3 layers. Mix Ricotta, sugar, tiny chocolate bits (or chop larger variety) and add vanilla together. Place the bottom layer in the spring-form pan and pour on half of the rum. Top with half Ricotta mixture. Place second layer on top. Pour on the rest of the rum and the rest of the Ricotta cheese. Place top layer on cake, cover the pan and refrigerate. On the day you serve the cake, beat cream and sugar (4 teaspoons) together lightly. Take 1 Tablespoon plain gelatin and mix with 1 Tablespoon cold water in a Pyrex® cup. Place cup in a pan of hot water and melt until liquid is clear. (Or, this may also be done in the microwave oven.) Cool and add gradually to whipped cream and beat until nice and thick. Frost cake with cream and refrigerate until serving time. Garnish frosting with chopped pistachio nuts.

*see gluten-free products list at the end of the book

## Cheesecake, No-Crust Version – Our Favorite

This is our absolute favorite and it's so easy. By whipping in the food processor or blender it's lighter and creamier. (My mother's original recipe suggested using a mixer, but the food processor or blend makes it lighter.) This was our favorite recipe long before we ever knew about the gluten-free diet.

| | |
|---|---|
| 1 lb. gluten-free cream cheese* at room temperature | ½ pint (1 cup) gluten-free sour cream* |
| ⅔ cup sugar | 3 Tablespoons sugar |
| ½ teaspoon gluten-free vanilla* | 1 teaspoon gluten-free vanilla* |
| 3 eggs | Ground cinnamon (optional) |

Place cream cheese, ⅔ cup sugar, ½ teaspoon vanilla and eggs in a food processor or mixer or blender and whip until smooth. (For an extra-light cheesecake, whip it in the food processor for an extra 3 minutes after the ingredients are combined.) Pour into a buttered pie pan. I use a 9 inch Pyrex® glass pan. Bake in a preheated 350°F oven for 30 minutes. It will rise during baking if you whipped it the extra 3 minutes. Remove from oven and cool 10 minutes. The center will sink and the rim looks like a crust. Take the sour cream and mix with sugar and vanilla. Pour on top of cheese mixture leaving the rim uncovered and bake 15 minutes longer. Sprinkle top with a little cinnamon if desired. I prefer it plain, but for a change the cinnamon gives it a nice flavor.

*Variation*: You can serve it topped with some canned gluten-free cherry pie filling*. (See list in the back of this book for some gluten-free brands.)

## Cheesecake, No-Crust Version (with cottage cheese)

This is a little heavier consistency than some of the other versions, but also very good. This is the more traditional type in a spring-form pan.

| | |
|---|---|
| 1 pound gluten-free cottage cheese* | 3 Tablespoons sweet rice or fine white rice flour |
| 1 pound gluten-free cream cheese*, softened | ½ cup (1 stick) melted butter or gluten-free margarine* |
| 1 ½ cups sugar | 1 pint gluten-free sour cream* |
| 4 eggs | 1 teaspoon ground cinnamon and 1 teaspoon sugar (optional) |
| 2 Tablespoons lemon juice | |
| 2 teaspoons gluten-free vanilla* | |
| 3 Tablespoons cornstarch | |

Put cottage cheese in a food processor or blender. Add the softened cream cheese and blend. Gradually add the sugar and beat well. Add the eggs, lemon juice and vanilla and mix well. Mix the cornstarch and rice flour together and add to the cheese mixture along with the melted butter. Add the sour cream last and mix thoroughly.

Pour into a greased spring-form pan. Sprinkle with cinnamon and sugar if desired. Bake at 350°F for 1 hour. Turn heat off and leave in the oven about 1 hour with oven door open slightly.

*see gluten-free products list at the end of the book

After cake is very cool, loosen the clips on the side of the pan and place the whole pan in the refrigerator to set well overnight. Put cake out a while before serving it, as it is better at room temperature.

## Cheesecake with Macaroon Crust

If you miss cheesecake with the cookie crust, here is a way to have it. You can use leftover homemade coconut macaroons (see index) or other gluten-free cookie crumbs. Be careful with some store-bought macaroons and check for yourself. I checked with some brands made for Passover, such as Manischewitz®, and in 2002 they are not made on dedicated equipment. This may no longer be the case because I noticed in 2005 they listed some macaroons on a gluten-free list on their web page. Check for yourself to be sure.

1 ½ cups of soft gluten-free coconut macaroon cookie crumbs*
1 Tablespoon butter, melted (I do this in the microwave on defrost)
2 packages (8 oz. each) of gluten-free cream cheese*, softened
½ cup sugar
½ teaspoon gluten-free vanilla*

2 eggs
1 cup sweetened gluten-free whipped cream (1 cup gluten-free heavy cream* plus 2 teaspoons sugar, whipped)
2 Tablespoons strawberry jelly melted or raspberry syrup* (optional)

Mix the macaroon cookie crumbs with the melted butter. Press into the bottom and sides of a greased 9-inch pie plate. Beat the cream cheese, sugar and vanilla with an electric mixer or food processor. Add the eggs and blend in. Pour into the crust. Bake at 350°F for 40 minutes. Cool. Refrigerate 3 hours or overnight before serving. I find this is tastier if you make it a day ahead. Spread the whipped cream over the cheesecake. Drizzle with the jelly or syrup if desired.

## Cheesecake with Mock Oreo® crust

This is a great use for leftover Gluten-Free Naturals™ brownies. This is very easy to make and delicious! I served it to non-celiacs, and they thought it was a regular Oreo® crust. I often double the recipe to make 2 cheesecakes for a crowd. You can make the brownies and the cheesecake ahead of time.

½ batch of Gluten-Free Naturals™ Brownies, prepared as directed
2 (8 ounce) packages of gluten-free cream cheese*

½ cup sugar
½ teaspoon gluten-free vanilla*
2 eggs

Prepare brownies as directed on the package. Remove ½ of the brownies and crumble them over a 9 inch round glass pie pan. Press them along the sides and bottom to form a crust.

Preheat oven to 325°F. Put the rest of the ingredients into a food processor, and blend until smooth. (An electric mixer can also be used; however the cheesecake will be smoother in texture if you use a food processor.)

*see gluten-free products list at the end of the book

Pour cheesecake mixture into chocolate crust. Bake for 35 to 40 minutes, until the center of the pie is almost set. Allow to cool. Refrigerate 3 hours or overnight. This is best made a day ahead of time. Store any leftover cheesecake in the refrigerator or in the freezer.

*Variation*: If desired, sprinkle some chocolate chips or some of the brownie crumbs into the cheesecake mixture after pouring it into the pan, to add more chocolate flavor.

## Cheesecake with Pie Crust
Do not eliminate the sugar in the pie crust, or this recipe will not work.

½ cup butter
1 ¼ cups Gluten-Free Naturals™ Cookie Blend or Gluten-Free Naturals™ All Purpose Flour
½ cup sugar (do not eliminate)
1 yolk of a hard cooked egg

1 pound gluten-free cream cheese* (4 cups)
1 pint gluten-free sour cream*
5 eggs
1 cup sugar (I use a little less)
1 teaspoon gluten-free vanilla*
1 teaspoon lemon juice

Melt butter in a heavy saucepan. With a sturdy spoon blend in the flour, sugar, and egg yolk. Press into the side and bottom of a 9 or 10 inch spring-form pan about 3 inches high. Bake at 325°F for 20-25 minutes or until set.

Separate eggs. Beat eggs whites. Set aside. In another bowl, add yolks and beat, adding the sugar until creamy. Turn to low speed and add cream cheese, sour cream, and flavorings. Beat on high speed until thick (no more than 5 minutes). Fold the egg whites into cheese mixture.

Bake at 300°F for 1 hour. Let cake remain another 3 hours in the turned off oven. Do not open door. Remove and refrigerate.

## Cheesecake with Pineapple
If you like pineapple in your cheesecake, this recipe is for you. This recipe comes from Argo® cornstarch. They used to have a wonderful gluten-free recipe brochure that has since been discontinued. As of this writing, their cornstarch is gluten-free with no contamination.

2 (8 ounce) packages gluten-free cream cheese*
1 cup sugar
½ cup milk
3 eggs
¼ cup cornstarch

2 teaspoons gluten-free vanilla*
1 (8 ounce) can of crushed pineapple packed in its own juice. Drain and reserve juice.
Ground cinnamon (optional)

In a blender or food processor, combine the cream cheese, sugar, milk, eggs, cornstarch, vanilla and the pineapple juice. Blend until smooth. Pour into a greased 9 inch square or 10 inch or 9 ½ inch round deep dish pie pan. Spoon the pineapple evenly into the batter. It will sink to the bottom. If desired, sprinkle with cinnamon. Bake at 300°F for 50 to 60 minutes. Cook 1 hour on a wire rack and then refrigerate.

*see gluten-free products list at the end of the book

## Chiffon Cake – Our Favorite

This is my mother's favorite cake and mine too. It is light and delicious, and I like it even better than sponge cake because I think it is more flavorful. I served it at a party and the non-celiac guests were surprised to learn it was gluten-free.

I usually bake this cake in a spring-form pan. Use this cake for birthday cakes, Cassata cake, or Rum cake (see index). This cake rises high, and works best if your spring-form pan has deep sides. Otherwise, I suggest you use a deep tube pan with the tube higher than the sides. Mine rose almost to the top of the center tube (about 2 inches beyond the sides). I cooled it upside down, and it was perfect.

| | |
|---|---|
| 1 cup egg whites (7 large or 5 jumbo) | 1 teaspoon salt |
| ½ teaspoon cream of tartar | ½ cup oil |
| 2 cups of Gluten-Free Naturals™ All Purpose Flour | 7 egg yolks large size or 5 jumbo |
| 1 ½ cups sugar | ¾ cup water |
| 3 teaspoons gluten-free baking powder* | 2 teaspoons gluten-free vanilla* |

Separate the eggs placing the whites in your large mixer bowl. Add cream of tartar to whites, put the mixer on high speed and beat until very stiff. You will know the whites are stiff enough if you push them to one side and they stay as placed. While the whites are being beaten, blend the dry ingredients together into a large bowl. Add the egg yolks, water, oil and vanilla and mix well. It will get very thick because of the xanthan gum in the gluten-free flour. Pour this mixture gently over the egg whites and fold the two mixtures together. Pour into an ungreased large tube pan or a 10 inch spring-form pan.

Bake in a preheated 325°F oven for 55 minutes and test for doneness with a cake tester. If not done, raise the heat to 350°F and bake 10 minutes longer. Invert cake onto cake rack immediately and leave upside down until completely cooled. (Your cake will fall if you do not cool it upside down.) If the cake rose higher than the sides, still turn it over and cool it upside down.

For birthday cakes, we often slice it in the middle to make 2 layers after it is completely cooled. Remove the spring-form. Slice the cake into two layers with a knife or wire cake-slicer for this purpose. Remove the top layer carefully. You may need to put two large spatulas under it and set it aside. Place the bottom layer on a plate. (I leave the metal base on, but you can remove it if you choose to.) Replace the spring-form. Add the filling in the middle, put the top layer back on. Allow filling to cool if you used a pudding type filling. (You replaced the spring-form to center the cake to have a perfect shape.) Remove spring-form and frost the top and sides. Decorate if desired.

*see gluten-free products list at the end of the book

## Chocolate, Chocolate Cake

Very nice cake that is good for birthdays. I think the cake is even better the next day, which allows you to make it ahead of time. I've included the mousse filling and frosting recipe, but this cake is also excellent frosted with other frostings (see index) or gluten-free store-bought frosting. If you use whipped cream it must be refrigerated.

1 ¼ cups boiling water
¾ cups unsweetened cocoa
1 ½ cups Gluten-Free Naturals™ All
   Purpose Flour
¼ cup sorghum flour or rice flour
1 teaspoon baking soda
½ teaspoon gluten-free baking powder*
¼ teaspoon salt

¾ cup oil or ¾ cup butter or gluten-free
   margarine* (1 ½ sticks) softened
1 ½ cups sugar
3 eggs
1 teaspoon gluten-free vanilla extract*
Chocolate Mousse (recipe below)
Chocolate butter-cream frosting (recipe
   below)

Grease two 9-inch round cake pans. In a small bowl, combine the water and the cocoa. Do not boil the cocoa. Allow to cool.

Mix the flour, baking soda, baking powder and salt and set aside. Cream the oil (or butter) and sugar in a large bowl, until fluffy. I use a heavy duty electric mixer for best results. Add the eggs, one at a time, beating after each addition. Alternately add cocoa and flour mixtures. Beat in vanilla.

Pour batter into the prepared pans. Bake at 350°F for 20 to 25 minutes, or until a cake tester comes out clean. Cool in pans on wire racks for 10 minutes. Remove from pans, cool completely on the wire racks. Prepare chocolate mousse filling. Place one cake layer on a serving plate. Spread with the mousse and refrigerate 30 minutes. Then top with the second layer and refrigerate. Prepare frosting. Let the cake filling set; then frost the cake and then layers won't shift.

Chocolate mousse filling:
  2 ounces gluten-free semisweet
    chocolate*
  2 eggs, separated

2 Tablespoons sugar
½ cup gluten-free heavy/whipping cream*

Melt chocolate in a small saucepan over low heat, or melt in the microwave. Remove from heat and then rapidly stir in egg yolks until blended. Set aside. Beat egg whites until soft peaks form. Gradually beat in sugar. Beat until firm peaks form. In another bowl, whip cream until stiff. Stir about half the egg whites into the chocolate mixture. Fold chocolate mixture into remaining whites. Fold in whipped cream.

Chocolate butter-cream frosting:
  6 ounces semisweet chocolate*
  1 cup butter or gluten-free margarine*
  1 pound confectioner's sugar

1 egg yolk (you can save the egg white in
  the freezer for another use, or substitute
  egg powder for the yolk)
1 teaspoon gluten-free vanilla*
4 or 5 Tablespoons gluten-free heavy
  cream* or milk

Melt chocolate in a small saucepan over medium heat, or in the microwave. Remove from
heat then rapidly mix in egg yolk. Using a heavy duty mixer, beat the butter until smooth.
Beat in the chocolate. Add remaining ingredients. Beat until smooth and easy to spread.

## Chocolate Cupcakes
**These are easy to make. These cupcakes are not too sweet and need frosting.**

1 cup Gluten-Free Naturals™ All Purpose
  or Gluten-Free Naturals™ Sandwich
  Bread Flour
¾ cup sugar
¼ cup cocoa
½ teaspoon baking soda
¼ teaspoon baking powder

¼ teaspoon salt
¼ cup oil
¼ cup milk
¼ cup hot tap water
1 egg
½ teaspoon gluten-free vanilla*

Blend dry ingredients. Add the rest of the ingredients and blend well with an electric mixer.
Put into paper-lined cupcake tins. Bake at 350°F for 20 to 30 minutes. Makes 12 cupcakes.
Allow to cool. Frost with your favorite frosting (see index for recipes.)

## Chocolate Mousse Cake
**A very, very rich dessert.**

1 (8 ounce) package gluten-free semisweet
  chocolate chips*
½ cup (1 stick) butter or gluten-free
  margarine*
6 eggs, separated

⅓ cup sugar
2 Tablespoons cornstarch
Confectioner's sugar for decoration
  (optional)

In a microwave safe container, melt the chocolate and the butter on the defrost cycle. Once
melted, blend together and set aside. I put it in for a minute and stir, then try another 30
seconds or so until melted. Separate the eggs and put the whites into a clean mixer bowl.
Beat the eggs with the mixer on medium speed until foamy. Gradually add the sugar,
increase the mixer speed to high. Beat until you have soft peaks.

Your chocolate should be melted and cool. Add the egg yolks to the chocolate and blend in.
You don't want to cook the egg yolks, so be sure the chocolate is not too hot. Stir in the
cornstarch.

Now gently fold the chocolate mixture into the egg white mixture. Pour into a greased 9-
inch spring-form pan. Bake at 300°F for 40 minutes until set. Cool on a wire rack. Run a

*see gluten-free products list at the end of the book

knife around the edge and remove the sides of the pan. If desired, sprinkle with confectioner's sugar.

## Coffee Cake
A tasty cake that is nice served with a cup of coffee. It is a little crumbly but not gritty. It is very flavorful and easy to make.

| | |
|---|---|
| 2 cups Gluten-Free Naturals™ Cookie Blend | 1 teaspoon gluten-free vanilla* |
| 1 ½ cups sugar | ¾ cup milk or gluten-free milk substitute |
| 2 teaspoons baking powder | 2 eggs |
| ¼ teaspoon salt | 3 teaspoons xanthan gum (do not eliminate or the cake will fall apart) |
| ¾ cup butter, softened | Ground cinnamon |

In a heavy duty mixer, blend together the Cookie Blend™, sugar, baking powder, salt and butter. When butter is the size of small peas, turn off mixer. Remove ½ cup of this mixture for the crumb topping and set aside.

Add vanilla, milk, eggs and xanthan gum, and blend well. Pour into greased 11 x 7" glass pan, or a 9" x 9" square pan. Top with the crumb topping that you set aside. Sprinkle with cinnamon. Bake 35 to 45 minutes at 350°F. Allow to completely cool before serving or it won't hold together.

*Variation*: Use 2 cups of Gluten-Free Naturals™ All Purpose Flour instead of the Cookie Blend and eliminate the xanthan gum. The crumb topping will melt together and sink a lot more than with the Cookie Blend, but the flavor will be delicious. For this version, the cake looks nicer if you mix the cinnamon in the topping instead of sprinkling it on the cake. (The cake texture is better with the Gluten-Free Naturals™ All Purpose Flour.)

## Coffee Marble Pound Cake
This is my mother's recipe.

| | |
|---|---|
| 4 teaspoons instant coffee (I use decaf. Caution – some flavored coffees may contain gluten) | 1 teaspoon gluten-free vanilla* |
| | 2 cups Gluten-Free Naturals™ All Purpose Flour |
| 1 ¼ cups sugar | ½ teaspoon salt |
| ⅔ cup oil | 1 teaspoon gluten-free baking powder* |
| 3 eggs | 3 squares gluten-free semi-sweet chocolate*, grated |
| ⅔ cup cold water | |

Melt the instant coffee in 1 or 2 teaspoons of hot water and set aside and allow to cool a minute or two. Mix sugar and oil in a bowl with a whisk or an electric mixer. Add eggs one at a time and blend in. Add ⅔ cup cold water and vanilla. Add cooled coffee mixture. Add flour, salt, and baking powder. Blend in with a sturdy spoon or a mixer.

Butter the bottom of a tube pan and pour in half the batter and then half the grated chocolate. Top with the rest of the batter and the rest of the chocolate. Take a spoon and

*see gluten-free products list at the end of the book

fold the batter a little to form a marble effect. Bake in a 350°F oven for 1 hour or until the cake tester tests clean. Cool in pan ½ hour, run a knife around the edges and remove from pan. Dust with powdered sugar when completely cooled.

This may also be made in a decorative dark color silicon tube pan. (I have tested this in dark blue and black pans and had success, but for me the red color silicon pan did not work.) The outside doesn't brown much when baked in this type of pan. Cool about 10 minutes in the pan and remove to a wire rack. Cool completely and dust with powdered sugar, if desired. Note: Since silicon pans can be difficult to clean and could harbor gluten, use a pan dedicated to gluten-free baking.

## Crumb Cake

This is a favorite snacking cake of ours. Nice served at a breakfast buffet, at an afternoon tea, or for dessert.

| | |
|---|---|
| 1 Gluten-Free Naturals™ Yellow Cake Mix, prepared as directed | ⅓ cup sugar |
| Crumb Topping: | Pinch of salt |
| ¼ cup butter | Glaze: |
| ⅓ cup Gluten-Free Naturals™ Cookie Blend | Confectioner's sugar (about 1 cup) |
| | About a ½ Tablespoon butter |
| 2 teaspoons ground cinnamon | About a teaspoon of gluten-free vanilla* |
| | Water |

Prepare cake mix as directed on the package. I frequently use an 8 x 8" square disposable pan. Prepare Crumb topping by blending together the butter, Cookie Blend, cinnamon, sugar and pinch of salt. Using your hands, put the crumble topping on the cake batter. For an 8 x 8" disposable pan, bake about 40 to 45 minutes until cake is done. For other cake pan sizes, bake about 5 minutes longer than directed for the yellow cake mix. Test cake for doneness.

For the glaze, cream the butter in a bowl. Add some confectioner's sugar (I use about a cup). Blend together. Add the vanilla and blend. Add a little bit of water to make it drizzle consistency. If too wet, add more confectioner's sugar, if too dry, add more water. I drizzle it over the warm cake so it melts in a little bit. Or allow cake to thoroughly cool, and then drizzle it on top for the streusel look.

*Variation*: Gluten-Free Naturals™ All Purpose Flour can be substituted for the Cookie Blend. It will be a different topping than with the Cookie Blend but it is also good.

*see gluten-free products list at the end of the book

## Danish Cream Cake
We love this cake. It's easy to make and I make it often. It has excellent taste and texture. Do not eliminate the cream or it will not work.

1 cup gluten-free heavy cream* (minus 1 Tablespoon used in topping)
2 eggs
¼ teaspoon gluten-free almond extract*
1 cup sugar

1 ½ cups Gluten-Free Naturals™ All Purpose Flour
2 teaspoons gluten-free baking powder*
¼ teaspoon salt

Topping:
2 Tablespoons butter
⅓ cup sugar
1 Tablespoon gluten-free heavy cream* (removed from the 1 cup)

1 Tablespoon fine white rice or sweet rice flour
¼ teaspoon gluten-free almond extract*
¼ cup finely sliced or slivered almonds

Remove 1 Tablespoon cream and place in a small saucepan and set aside. Whip remaining cream until stiff. Lightly beat eggs and stir in almond extract. Gently add to whipped cream. Blend together sugar, flour, baking powder and salt with a whisk. Fold into cream mixture and pour into a greased 8 or 9 inch spring-form pan. Bake the cake in a preheated 350°F oven for 45 minutes, or until lightly browned.

Meanwhile, add butter, sugar and rice flour to the saucepan along with the Tablespoon of heavy cream. After the cake has baked 40 minutes, begin heating and stirring the topping in the saucepan. (This way you'll have the topping ready at 45 minutes). Blend and cook until it is a thickened milky glaze. Turn off heat, add almond extract and nuts. Remove cake from oven and pour over hot cake. Return cake to oven and bake about 10 minutes longer.

## Dr. Bird Cake
A very moist cake.

3 cups Gluten-Free Naturals™ All Purpose Flour
1 teaspoon baking soda
1 teaspoon ground cinnamon
2 cups sugar
1 teaspoon salt

1 ½ cups oil (or for a nice buttery flavor, use 1 cup oil and ½ cup melted butter)
1 (8 ounce) can crushed pineapple, not drained
1 ½ teaspoons gluten-free vanilla*
3 eggs
2 cups diced bananas – (2 large ones)

In a large bowl, whisk together the dry ingredients. Add everything else and mix until blended. (I use a heavy duty mixer.) The batter should be somewhat thick. If it is too thin, add a little more of the All Purpose Flour. (Some brands of crushed pineapple have more liquid than others.)

Bake in a greased round tube pan at 350°F for 1 hour 20 minutes. Cake will crack a little at the top. Cool in pan on a rack. This cake will stay moist and fresh in the refrigerator.

*see gluten-free products list at the end of the book

## German Apple Cake and Cherry Crumble

I really think the name of this should be "Easier than pie". This is my mother's recipe. For an easier version, instead of making the apple filling use a gluten-free canned pie filling. It's nice served warm with gluten-free vanilla ice cream or whipped cream. It's best the day you make it, as the topping will be crunchy. The crust will absorb moisture the next day.

For the Apple Filling:
5 cups peeled and sliced apples
2 Tablespoons minute tapioca
½ cup sugar

¾ teaspoon ground cinnamon
¼ teaspoon ground nutmeg

For the Crumb Crust:
1 ½ cups Gluten-Free Naturals™ Cookie
  Blend (do not substitute)
½ cup sugar (do not eliminate)
Dash of salt

1 stick (½ cup) butter or 6 Tablespoons
  gluten-free margarine* plus 2
  Tablespoons butter
Nuts (optional)
½ teaspoon ground cinnamon (optional)

Prepare apples, (my mother prefers Cortland variety for this cake but any good baking apple will do). Mix apples with tapioca, ½ cup sugar and spices.

For topping, mix flour with ½ cup sugar, salt and cinnamon (if using). Mix in 6 Tablespoons of butter with a form or fingers until all is mixed well and crumbs form. Remove ¾ cup of crumbs and put the rest into a greased 8 or 9 inch silver spring-form pan. (Note: do <u>not</u> use a dark non-stick spring-form pan, because the dark color will make this cake burn.)

Press the crumb mixture on the bottom and sides of the pan. (On the sides of the pan, go up about 1 inch so the filling won't stick to the sides, and also the filling won't discolor your pan.)

Pour in the apple mixture and cover pan with foil. Pour in the apple mixture and cover pan with foil. Place in a preheated 425°F oven and cook for 20 minutes. While the cake is baking, add the 2 Tablespoons of butter to the leftover crumbs and mix well. Now add the chopped nuts if desired. After 20 minutes of baking, remove the cake from the oven and remove foil. Take a handful of the crumb mixture and press tightly to form a big compressed lump. Now crumble this lump into good sized crumbs over the apples. Continue until all of the crumb mixture is used.

Return cake to oven and bake an additional 20-25 minutes until crumbs are golden and apples cooked. Test with a cake tester to see if apples are soft. A little visible juice near the outer edge is a good indicator that the apples are done. If not done, cover lightly with foil and cook a little longer. Remove from oven and cool slightly. Run a knife around the outer edge of pan and sprinkle with confectioner's sugar. Remove sides of pan. Nice served warm. Serves 6-8.

*Variation*: Sometimes my mother cooks the apples and all the filling ingredients on top of the stove. Alternatively, use the "Delicious Apples" recipe for the filling. It's very good with the apples and raisins.  Prepare the crumb mixture as above.  Put the cake together and bake 20 minutes covered with foil.  Then remove foil and bake 20 minutes more until crumbs are golden.

*Variation 2*:  Use a gluten-free pie filling of any flavor instead of the apple filling.  As of this writing, Comstock® and Wilderness® brands are gluten-free.  I particularly like cherry filling.  I often prepare the crumb crust and use all butter.  I blend it at once, set aside the amount for the top without the nuts.  I press the crumb mixture on bottom and sides, top with filling, put the topping on and bake with the foil for 20 minutes and then without the foil for 20 minutes.

## "Gingerbread" Cake – Buttermilk Version

⅔ cup brown sugar
⅓ cup oil
1 egg
½ cup molasses
¾ cup gluten-free buttermilk* or gluten-free plain yogurt*
2 cups Gluten-Free Naturals™ All Purpose Flour

1 ¼ teaspoons baking soda
½ teaspoon salt
1 teaspoon ground ginger
1 teaspoon ground cinnamon
½ teaspoon ground allspice
¼ teaspoon ground cloves

In a heavy duty mixer, blend together the sugar and the oil.  Beat in the egg, molasses and buttermilk.  Add in the rest of the ingredients and mix until blended. Pour into a buttered 9 x 9 inch pan and bake at 350°F for 35-45 minutes.  Top with whipped cream and chopped pecans if desired.

*Variation*:  You can replace the 2 cups of Gluten-Free Naturals™ All Purpose Flour in this recipe with 1 cup fine rice flour and 1 cup defatted soy flour and 2 teaspoons xanthan gum.  It will be a heavier cake if you make this substitution, but it will work.

## "Gingerbread" Cake – Hot Water Version

½ cup sugar
½ cup molasses
1 teaspoon salt
½ cup hot water
1 Tablespoon butter or gluten-free margarine*

½ teaspoon baking soda
1 cup Gluten-Free Naturals™ All Purpose Flour
1 teaspoon ground ginger or a little less
1 egg

Melt butter in hot water.  Mix the sugar and molasses together.  Whisk together the dry ingredients.  Add hot water and butter to sugar and molasses.  Add dry ingredients and mix to blend.  Pour in a buttered 8 x 8 inch pan.  Sprinkle some sugar and cinnamon on top. Bake 30 minutes at 350°F.

*see gluten-free products list at the end of the book

*Variation*: May substitute ½ cup fine white rice flour and ½ cup defatted soy flour plus 1 teaspoon xanthan gum for the Gluten-Free Naturals™ All Purpose Flour. It will be lighter if you use the All Purpose Flour.

## Ice Box Cake

Sponge cake (see index) cut into the size of lady fingers
Chocolate Angel Pie filling (see index)

Grease and line the bottom of an 8 x 4 x 3 inch loaf pan with butter and a piece of waxed paper on the bottom. Line the bottom and sides of the pan with the sponge cake to form a lady finger crust. Fill with the chocolate angel pie filling. Chill for 2 hours before serving.

## Jelly Roll Cake – Vanilla and Chocolate Versions

This is an impressive dessert, especially to celiacs since most gluten-free cakes don't have the elasticity to allow them be rolled. Until I invented Gluten-Free Naturals™ All Purpose Flour, it was impossible to make this cake. Other flour blends will fall apart and crumble; so do not substitute. See variation for Chocolate Jelly Roll. Have a kitchen towel dusted with confectioner's sugar ready when you remove the cake from the oven.

3 eggs (large size)
1 cup sugar
5 Tablespoons water
1 teaspoon gluten-free vanilla*
1 cup Gluten-Free Naturals™ All Purpose
   Flour (for chocolate version, use ¾ cup
   Gluten-Free Naturals™ All Purpose
   Flour and ¼ cup cocoa)
1 teaspoon baking powder
1/4 teaspoon salt

Gluten-Free Jam or Jelly* (I like black
   cherry or raspberry, but any flavor is
   good. Polaner® is labeled gluten-free.)
Chocolate Whipped Cream Frosting
   (optional):
1/2 cup whipping cream
1 Tablespoon sugar
2 teaspoons cocoa
1/2 teaspoon gluten-free vanilla*

Grease and line the bottom of a 15 ½ inch by 10 ½ inch jelly roll pan with parchment paper. Grease the parchment paper.

Beat the eggs in a mixer for 5 minutes until thick. Gradually beat in the sugar. Beat in the water and vanilla. Add the flour, baking powder and salt. Blend it in until smooth. Pour into prepared pan.

Bake at 375°F for 12 to 15 minutes. Do not over-bake or it will be difficult to remove from the pan and difficult to roll. Do not under-bake or it will stick to the towel. Make sure you use a cake tester to test the cake.

Loosen edges of cake and turn it upside down on a clean, old kitchen towel that has been sprinkled with confectioner's sugar. Carefully remove the parchment paper. Do this immediately or you won't be able to get it off. Spread the hot cake with the jam. Roll it up from the short end, using the towel to help you roll it. Wrap the cake in the towel and put it

*see gluten-free products list at the end of the book*

on a cooling rack. Allow it to cool completely, which will take about a half-hour. Put the cake on a pretty platter and remove the towel, once it has cooled.

Put the cream in a mixing bowl and add the sugar, cocoa and vanilla. Beat until cream is whipped. Frost it with the whipped cream. Refrigerate leftovers.

*Variation*: For a chocolate glaze instead of whipped cream frosting, you can make a chocolate glaze by melting ½ cup semisweet chocolate chips with 2 Tablespoons butter and 1 Tablespoon light corn syrup. Cook it over low heat (be careful it can burn), stirring constantly, until the chocolate is melted. Cool slightly and pour the glaze over the jelly-roll cake.

*Variation 2*: To make a mini 3-layer cake, do not roll the cake. Instead, cut the cake into thirds that measure about 5 x 10 ½ inches. Frost and layer it.

## Margherita Tart

This cake is an old Italian recipe. It is very plain, and best when served with fruit. Note: it has a slight potato flavor. Some of my other recipes are more geared to what Americans prefer, but I have included this recipe because it may be good for those with allergies to other gluten-free flours.

| | |
|---|---|
| 6 egg whites | ½ cup (1 stick) butter (melted and cooled) |
| 6 egg yolks | 1 teaspoon gluten-free vanilla* |
| 1 ¾ cups confectioner's sugar | 1 teaspoon grated lemon rind |
| 1 ⅓ cups potato flour (not potato starch) | |

Grease a 9 ½ or 10 inch spring-form pan. Preheat oven to 375°F. Beat the egg whites until they form very stiff peaks. In a separate bowl, beat the egg yolks and sugar together until foamy. Fold together the yolks and the whites gently, and add the potato flour gradually. Mix well but gently, folding in. Add the melted butter and the lemon rind, gently folding in.

Pour into the prepared pan and bake for 30 minutes. Turn over on cake rack and cool.

*Variation*: For lactose intolerant you can substitute oil for the butter but it will not be as flavorful. If you are allergic to corn, you can substitute 1 ¼ to 1 ½ cups granulated sugar for the confectioner's sugar which contains cornstarch. Whip the egg yolks and sugar until you do not feel any grit.

## Nut Cake or Nut Torte – Flourless Version

To make this cake lighter, I use less nuts. If you want a denser cake, use the full amount. This cake contains 11 Tablespoons sugar total. I kept adding all the sugar to the egg whites, instead of putting 5 Tablespoons in the whites, 5 in the yolks, and 1 for the top.

6 egg whites
5 Tablespoons sugar (or for a sweeter
  cake, use ½ cup)
6 egg yolks
5 Tablespoons sugar
1 (12 ounce) package nuts, finely ground
  in a food processor. (I use less nuts
  since 12 ounces produces a
  heavier/denser cake. I prefer using 10

ounces of nuts. I use hazelnuts, or
  almonds or almond meal)*
1 teaspoon gluten-free vanilla*, or almond
  extract* if using almonds
2 teaspoons baking powder
1 pint gluten-free heavy cream*
1 Tablespoon sugar
2 teaspoons cocoa (sifted)

In an electric mixer, whip up egg whites in a clean bowl. Gradually beat in 5 Tablespoons sugar (or ½ cup if using more), until stiff. Set aside. In another mixer bowl, whip the egg yolks beat in 5 Tablespoons sugar. Beat in vanilla or almond extract and the baking powder.

Fold the egg yolk mixture into the egg white mixture. Fold in the nuts. Pour into a 9 x 9 ½ inch greased spring-form pan. Bake in a 325°F oven for 1 hour or up to 1 hour 15 minutes until the top of the cake springs back lightly when tapped. Cool cake completely on a wire rack. When cake is cooled, split into 3 layers.

Take a small sieve, and sift the cocoa into the cream. Add the 1 Tablespoon sugar. Whip the cream until stiff. Spread between the layers of the cake and on the top and the sides.

*Variation*: If you prefer, one of the whipped cream frostings from this book may be used instead (see index). Use either the one with a little gelatin or instant pudding so that it holds up nicely.

*Variation 2*: I don't like things too sweet. You can use additional sugar in you wish. Instead of 5 Tablespoons which is about ⅓ cup, a ½ cup of sugar may be used each time.

## Nut Cake or Nut Torte

This cake is good for those who don't have a lot of gluten-free special baking supplies on hand. If you have nuts and cornstarch, you can make this cake. We were served a cake like this one in Norway. They piled on the whipped cream and it was delicious.

1 cup shelled nuts, chopped fine (6 ounces
  of nuts of your choice. You can use
  walnuts, pecans, almonds, or hazelnuts)
⅓ cup potato starch or cornstarch
3 egg whites
¼ teaspoon cream of tartar
½ cup sugar
3 egg yolks

¼ cup sugar
½ teaspoon gluten-free vanilla*
½ teaspoon gluten-free baking powder*
¼ teaspoon salt
Whipped cream frosting (see index) or see
  recipe above and use that frosting

*see gluten-free products list at the end of the book*

In a food processor, chop the nuts until fine, or use nut meal. Blend in the gluten-free flour and set aside.

Separate eggs. Be careful not to get any of the egg yolk into the egg whites or they will not whip. Whip egg whites in a clean bowl with cream of tartar. Gradually add the ½ cup sugar and continue beating until stiff. Set aside. (I always whip the egg whites first because you can use the same beaters to whip the yolks but you cannot do this the other way around.)

In another bowl, mix together the egg yolks, sugar, vanilla. I use the electric mixer. Beat in the baking powder and the salt. (The original recipe said to beat in the flour and nuts, but I found this created a mixture that was too difficult to fold into the whites.)

Gently fold the egg yolk mixture and then the nut mixture into the egg white mixture. Put in a 9 inch spring-form pan. Bake at 325°F for about 45 minutes until the cake springs back to the touch. Cool completely. Slice cake into two layers and frost with whipped cream frosting.

## Nutmeg Cake

This cake is good and most people like it as written. I use a little less sugar when I make it because it is a little sweet for my taste. You need a food processor to make this.

| | |
|---|---|
| 2 cups brown sugar | 1 egg |
| 2 cups Gluten-Free Naturals™ All Purpose Flour | 1 teaspoon ground nutmeg |
| | 1 teaspoon baking soda |
| ½ cup cold butter or cold gluten-free margarine* | 1 cup sour cream |
| | ½ cup chopped nuts |

In a food processor, combine sugar, flour and butter. Process until crumbly and butter is cut in. Press half of the "crumbs" in a well buttered 9 x 9 inch pan. Add the remaining ingredients to the leftover crumb mixture. Pour carefully over crumbs and bake at 350°F for 35-40 minutes. The crumbs form a crust at the bottom of the cake. Does not need frosting.

*Variation*: You can substitute 2 cups of Gluten-Free Naturals™ Cookie Blend and 2 teaspoons xanthan gum for the Gluten-Free Naturals™ All Purpose Flour. The cake will be a little more crumbly, but still be very delicious! I like the crumbs made with the Cookie Blend.

## Orange Rind Cake

This is a very old recipe.  It's an unusual cake made with orange and lemon rinds.

2 oranges
2 lemons
¾ cup sugar
4 eggs
1 cup Gluten-Free Naturals™ All Purpose
   Flour

3 teaspoons gluten-free baking powder*
½ teaspoon salt
⅔ cup oil
½ cup chopped toasted almonds

Wash the oranges and lemons.  Boil the oranges and lemons whole until tender.  Cool.  Discard the pulp and pulverize skins in a food processor.  Add ¾ cup sugar as pulverizing.  Taste the pulp mixture.  If it's very bitter, add more sugar.

Beat the 4 eggs until yellow with a whisk.  In a separate bowl, mix the flour, baking powder, salt and oil.  Add the orange skin mixture and the eggs alternately to the flour mixture.  Add the nuts.  If the batter is very thin, add a few Tablespoons more All Purpose Flour.

Bake in an 8 inch spring-form pan at 350°F for at least an hour until done.

## Paradise Cakes

An Australian sponge cake.

3 eggs
⅔ cup sugar
¼ teaspoon salt
3 Tablespoons oil or melted butter

1 teaspoon gluten-free vanilla*
2 Tablespoons fine white rice flour
⅓ cup potato starch

Beat eggs in an electric mixer until thick.  Add sugar and salt and continue to beat.  Blend together oil, vanilla, rice flour and potato starch.  Fold this mixture in.  Bake in 12 buttered and floured muffin tins at 350°F for 20 minutes.

## Peanut Butter Tandy Cakes Squares

TastyKake® Kandy Kakes® are a Philadelphia tradition.  Here is an easy way to make your own gluten-free version.  This makes a lot of squares and they freeze well.  We store the leftovers in sandwich bags and then put them in a larger freezer bag and freeze.  This makes it easy to grab a Tandy Cake in the morning to add to your lunch box.

2 Gluten-Free Naturals™ Yellow Cake
   mixes
½ cup oil
2 teaspoons gluten-free vanilla*
4 eggs

1 cup milk
1 cup (8 ounces) creamy peanut butter*
12 ounces (about 2 cups) milk chocolate
   chips*
½ to 1 Tablespoon oil

Put cake mixes in a large mixer bowl.  Add the oil, vanilla, eggs and milk.  Blend until smooth with an electric mixer.  Grease an 11 x 17 inch non-stick jelly roll pan.  Spread the

*see gluten-free products list at the end of the book*

batter in the prepared pan and bake at 325°F for 25 minutes. The top should be golden brown.

Immediately after the cake comes out of the oven, heat the peanut butter for 1 minute in the microwave. Pour the peanut butter on the top of the hot cake and spread it completely over the top. Allow the cake and the peanut butter to cool. Once the peanut butter is set and "tacky" to the touch you are ready to do the chocolate layer. Melt the chocolate and the oil in the microwave for 2 to 3 minutes. Stir to melt. Spread over the top of the entire cake. Allow to cool. Cut into squares. (Note: If you eliminate the oil in the chocolate, the chocolate will be hard. If you forget to add the oil, score the chocolate before it is completely set, and later cut the squares once completely cooled.)

## Pineapple Cake
**This recipe comes from Tiffany, and is on the GFN Foods™ website. (Reprinted with permission)**

⅔ to 1 cup canned crushed pineapple, well drained and juice reserved
1 Gluten-Free Naturals™ Yellow cake mix, blended according to package directions

2 to 3 ounces gluten-free cream cheese*
¾ to 1 cup confectioner's sugar
Reserved pineapple juice

Prepare yellow cake mix according to package directions. Add pineapple and blend in. Pour mix into greased pan and bake according to package directions. You may have to increase the baking time an extra 5 minutes, due to the addition of the pineapple.

While cake is baking, mix reserved pineapple juice, 2-3 ounces of softened cream cheese and confectioner's sugar. You may have to add additional sugar or liquid to get desired consistency. Cover bowl with a damp paper towel until cake is cooled and glaze is ready to be used. After cake is completely cooled, drizzle glaze over cake. It will cover about ¾ of the surface area. Make a larger batch of glaze if you want to cover the entire surface.

*Variation*: Instead of a cake, make cupcakes or mini cupcakes for a great brunch treat.

## Pineapple Upside Down Cake, Version 1
**Very easy and delicious.**

2 Tablespoons melted butter
½ cup brown sugar
Canned pineapple slices, drained

Pecan halves or gluten-free maraschino cherries*
1 Gluten-Free Naturals™ Yellow cake mix, blended according to package directions

Use the pan size specified on the yellow cake mix. In the baking pan pour 2 Tablespoons melted butter. Arrange slices of canned pineapple on the bottom of the pan in the butter. Place pecan halves (or cherries) in the center of the pineapples slices if desired. Take ½ cup brown sugar and sprinkle around the bottom of cake pan over the pineapples and butter.

*see gluten-free products list at the end of the book*

Mix the Yellow Cake as directed on the package and pour the batter into the pan on top of the pineapple mixture. Add 5 minutes of baking time for the pan used.

## Pineapple Upside Down Cake, Version 2
This is my mother's recipe. I usually use the pecans in the center of the pineapple slices, because I know they're gluten-free. Some maraschino cherries may not be safe.

2 Tablespoons butter or gluten-free margarine
½ cup brown sugar, firmly packed
3 to 4 slices of canned pineapple, drained reserving juice
2 eggs
1 cup Gluten-Free Naturals™ All Purpose Flour

1 teaspoon gluten-free baking powder*
⅛ teaspoon salt
½ cup sugar
1 Tablespoon pineapple juice (or a little more if batter is too dry)
Pecans (which I usually use) or gluten-free maraschino cherries*

Melt butter in a heavy iron 10 inch skillet. Remove from heat and add brown sugar, spreading it evenly over the bottom of the skillet. (If you do not have a skillet, use a 10 inch spring-form pan. Melt the butter in the microwave and pour in. Add the sugar and spread evenly.) Arrange pineapple and pecans attractively over sugar. Preheat oven to 350°F. Whisk together flour, sugar, salt and baking powder. Using a deep narrow bowl, beat the 2 eggs with a rotary beater or electric mixer. Add sugar gradually and continue beating. Add flour mixture and the 1 Tablespoon pineapple juice and beat until well blended. Pour carefully over arranged pineapple and bake 30 minutes. Let sit 5 minutes. Loosen sides and place a plate over skillet and invert. If you used a spring-form pan, remove the outer ring, place a plate on the bottom and invert.

## Poppy seed Cake – Version 1
Easy and delicious.

1 Gluten-Free Naturals™ Yellow Cake Mix

1 teaspoon lemon extract
1 teaspoon poppy seeds

Prepare cake mix in an electric mixer according to package directions, substituting lemon extract for vanilla. Add poppy seeds and blend in. Pour into a greased 9 inch pan and bake at 350°F for 25 minutes.

*Variation*: Frost cake with an icing made of butter, confectioner's sugar and lemon juice.

## Poppy seed Cake – Version 2

Two hours before you want to bake this cake, soak the poppy seeds.  Otherwise, soak them overnight in the refrigerator.

2 cups Gluten-Free Naturals™ All
  Purpose Flour
½ teaspoon salt
2 teaspoons gluten-free baking powder*
1 ½ cups sugar

¾ cups oil
4 egg whites, stiffly beaten
½ cup poppy seeds soaked in 1 cup milk
  for 2 hours.

Filling:
  2 cups milk
  2 Tablespoons cornstarch
  ½ cup sugar

4 egg yolks
¼ cup broken walnuts

Whisk flour with salt and baking powder.  Whisk together the oil and sugar.  Add dry ingredients alternately with milk and poppy seeds.  When well blended, fold in stiffly beaten egg whites.  Pour into 2 (9 or 10 inch) greased pans.  Bake at 350°F for 25 minutes.

To prepare filling, scald 1 ½ cups milk.  Blend sugar, cornstarch and the remaining ½ cup milk together in a very large Pyrex® measuring cup.  Add yolks to cold milk mixture and blend well.  Add the scalded milk slowly, stirring constantly until thick.  Add nuts and cool. Spread this between cooled cake layers.

## Pound Cake – Our Favorite

This is our favorite pound cake recipe.  It is not too sweet a cake.  It's nice served with some whipped cream and strawberries, or with ice cream.  You can slice it in thin slices when made in a loaf pan.

½ cup (1 stick) butter, softened; not
  melted
1 cup sugar
2 cups Gluten-Free Naturals™ All
  Purpose Flour
3 teaspoons baking powder

1 teaspoon salt
¾ cup milk
1 teaspoon gluten-free vanilla*
1 teaspoon almond extract* (optional)
2 eggs

Beat together all ingredients for about 3 minutes in an electric mixer.  Grease a 9" x 5" x 3" loaf pan.  Pour in batter and smooth top with rubber spatula.  Bake at 350°F for 60 minutes. Test with a cake tester.  Cool for 10 minutes before removing from pan.  Cool completely on a wire rack.

This batter can also be used in 2 greased 8" round pans.  Bake at 350°F for 30 to 35 minutes. Cool 10 minutes and remove from pan.  Cool completely on a wire rack.

*see gluten-free products list at the end of the book

## Pound Cake made with Rice Flour

This recipe comes from my sister-in-law, who made this as their wedding cake. The texture and taste are very good, considering it is made with rice flour. Slice in thin slices because it's very rich. This is a good recipe for people that are allergic to other grains, since it only has rice flour. I normally don't like cakes with just rice flour but this one works. Double the recipe to make it in a Bundt® pan.

Note: Ingredients should be at room temperature so that they will mix properly. If you are in a rush, put the butter in the microwave on defrost for 10 seconds at a time. Less than 30 seconds in my microwave is more than enough. Do not melt it, just soften it. Do the same with the milk and just take the chill out but do not heat it. A minute on defrost usually is more than enough for the milk.

¼ pound (1 stick) butter
¾ cups sugar
2 large eggs
¼ cup milk
¾ teaspoons gluten-free vanilla*

1 cup fine white rice flour
1 teaspoon xanthan gum (optional)
¾ teaspoons baking powder
¼ teaspoon salt

In a large mixer bowl, beat the butter until fluffy. Add the sugar and cream it in. Add the eggs and milk and vanilla and beat it on low speed to blend. Add the rest of the ingredients and beat on medium speed for a few minutes to combine. Scrape down the sides of bowl and beat for 10 minutes. Pour batter into one greased loaf pan. Bake at 350°F for 45 to 55 minutes, or until cake tester comes out clean. Cool on a wire rack. Remove from pan. Once it is thoroughly cooled, frost if desired.

For a wedding cake you can use different size pans, but you will have to adjust the baking times. Use the butter frosting so you can decorate it, as the cake may sit out a long time. A whipped cream frosting would be more difficult to decorate and could go bad sitting out on a hot day.

## Pound Cake made with Splenda® Sugar Blend

This recipe was converted from the www.splenda.com web page. My converted version has lower cholesterol because I used some oil instead of all butter as in the original recipe.

½ cup oil
¼ cup soft butter
3 ounces gluten-free cream cheese*
¾ cup Splenda® sugar blend (white or brown sugar blend; not the granulated) or ¾ cup sugar and 36 packets of Splenda® (if you like things less sweet use 24 to 30 packets)

½ teaspoon salt
1 ¾ cup Gluten-Free Naturals® All Purpose Flour
1 teaspoon baking powder
2 teaspoons gluten-free vanilla* extract
1 teaspoon almond or lemon extract (I use less)
5 large eggs

Using a heavy duty mixer, beat together the oil, butter, and cream cheese in a large mixer bowl. Beat in Splenda® sugar blend, or the sugar and contents of Splenda® packets. Add salt, flour, baking powder and continue to mix. The batter will be stiff. Add the extracts followed by one egg. Continue to add the eggs one at a time, beating at least a minute in-between each egg.

*see gluten-free products list at the end of the book*

Pour into a well greased 9" x 5" or 8.5" x 4.5" loaf pan. Bake at 350°F for 55 to 60 minutes. Test for doneness. If unsure, it is better to slightly over-bake than under-bake so it won't collapse when cooled. Place pan on wire rack to cool. Remove from pan once cooled. Put in a plastic bag so that the outer crust will not be so crispy. This cake is a high riser and can be sliced thinly if desired. Nice served with strawberries and some whipped cream.

## Pumpkin Cake

This is a cake with a lot of spice. You can use a Bundt™ pan or tube pan for this recipe. Or, make half the recipe in a loaf pan.

3 ½ cups Gluten-Free Naturals™ All Purpose Flour
1 teaspoon gluten-free baking powder*
3 teaspoons baking soda
½ teaspoon salt
1 teaspoon each ground allspice, ground cinnamon and ground nutmeg

½ teaspoon ground cloves (optional)
4 large eggs
2 cups sugar
1 cup oil
1 lb. can pumpkin
⅔ cup water

Grease a 12 cup Bundt® pan. In a bowl, whisk together the dry ingredients. In a large bowl, beat the eggs until foamy and add the sugar and oil and beat thoroughly. Add the pumpkin blend well. Add the flour mixture a half at a time alternately with the water, beating well after each addition, until smooth. Pour into the prepared pan and bake in a preheated 350°F oven until a cake tester inserted comes out clean (about an hour). Place the pan on a cake rack to cool 10 minutes. With a spatula, loosen the edges and turn out on a rack to cool completely. When cool, sprinkle with confectioner's sugar if desired.

## Rum Cake

A recipe from my sister. She thinks this cake tastes just like the Bacardi® rum cakes you can buy. You must make this a day ahead of time for the filling to firm up before you frost the cake.

2 Gluten-Free Naturals™ Yellow Cake mixes baked in two 9" pans or 1 recipe chiffon cake, baked in a 10 inch spring-form pan (see index)
½ cup gluten-free light rum* (I use Bacardi®)
½ cup sugar
2 Tablespoons cornstarch

½ teaspoon salt
2 cups cold milk
2 egg yolks, slightly beaten
2 Tablespoons butter
2 teaspoons gluten-free vanilla*
2 cups gluten-free heavy cream*
4 teaspoons sugar
1 Tablespoon plain gelatin

Make filling by mixing cornstarch, sugar and salt in a saucepan. Gradually add cold milk while stirring to make a smooth mixture. (I use a whisk.) Bring to a boil and stir until thick. Remove from heat. Beat egg yolks lightly in a metal or large Pyrex® measuring cup. Pour ½ of the milk mixture over them while stirring rapidly. Pour mixture back into pot and boil 1 minute while stirring. Add butter and vanilla and blend. Cool, stirring occasionally so as not to form a skin on the pudding.

*see gluten-free products list at the end of the book

Cool layers of cake. If using chiffon cake cut cooled cake into 2 layers. Place bottom layer back into the spring-form pan and sprinkle on 4 Tablespoons of rum evenly over cake. Spread on the filling that should now be cool. Now turn your top layer upside down and pour on the last 4 Tablespoons of rum on it. It is important to turn the layer upside down. Otherwise the rum will ruin the whipped cream frosting on top. Now place the top layer on the cake, right side up. Leaving the cake in the spring-form pan assures a cake that won't be lopsided. If using the two layers made in the 9" pan, wrap some plastic wrap around the sides to stabilize it, if needed. Cover and refrigerate the cake 24 hours. This will firm the filling so your cake will stay together well.

On the day of serving, make the cream frosting by blending the cream and 4 teaspoons sugar. Take the 1 Tablespoon plain gelatin and mix it with 1 Tablespoon cold water in a Pyrex® cup. Place cup in a pan of hot water and melt until liquid is clear. Cool and add gradually to the whipped cream and beat until nice and thick. Frost cake with cream and refrigerate until serving time. Refrigerate until serving time.

## Sour Cream Coffee Cake

This is the traditional sour cream coffee cake recipe, converted to be gluten-free.

½ cup butter or margarine*
1 cup sugar
2 eggs, beaten
1 teaspoon gluten-free vanilla*
2 cups Gluten-Free Naturals™ All
    Purpose Flour
1 teaspoon gluten-free baking powder*
1 teaspoon baking soda
¼ teaspoon salt

1 cup gluten-free sour cream*
½ cup water
½ cup chopped nuts (optional)
½ cup sugar
1 teaspoon ground cinnamon
½ cup gluten-free miniature chocolate
    chips* (optional)

Cream the butter and sugar. (I use a mixer.) Add eggs and vanilla and blend. In a separate bowl, whisk together flour, baking powders, baking soda and salt. Add dry ingredients to creamed mixture alternately with sour cream and water. In a separate bowl mix the nuts, sugar, cinnamon and chocolate chips. Pour half the batter into a greased tube pan or Bundt® pan. Top with cinnamon mixture. Pour the rest of the batter on top and smooth it. Bake 350°F for about 50-60 minutes. (A silicon pan may be used, but it must be black or dark blue in color or it won't bake properly. Baking time may need to be increased.)

## Sponge Cake – Lady Finger Substitute

This cake is easy to make, but is a little too plain and too spongy by itself. It is nice topped with strawberries and whipped cream or gluten-free vanilla ice cream. It's also very good sliced thinly to replace lady fingers in recipes like Trifle (see index) or as a lady finger crust for some desserts.

4 eggs
¾ cup sugar
1 teaspoon gluten-free baking powder*

1 cup Gluten-Free Naturals™ All Purpose
    Flour

*see gluten-free products list at the end of the book

Beat eggs for 8 minutes in an electric mixer, preferably one with a mixer stand. (I set a timer to make sure it's beaten long enough.) Then beat in the sugar, adding it gradually until dissolved. (Take a little on your finger and rub together. If you don't feel the grit, it's dissolved. This test is also the secret for wonderful meringues.) Blend together the flour and baking powder. Gently fold into the egg mixture. Put in a greased 9 x 13 inch pan. Bake at 350°F for 20-25 minutes. When completely cooled, it can be cut into pieces the size of lady fingers.

This sponge cake is good for a rum cake or just frosted with the cream as for the mocha angel food cake recipe (see index). It is also good for a Trifle (see index), using cream sherry, pudding and whipped cream. You could also use it for a base for Baked Alaska (see index) or in Zuccato (see index).

## Sponge Cake – "Grand Champion"

This cake is a family favorite. Because of the xanthan gum in the All Purpose Flour, be warned that your egg yolk mixture may seem a little thick and mixes best using a heavy duty mixer. This cake will rise quite a lot as it bakes. I took it to a family gathering and I received compliments on my homemade cake – they didn't realize it was gluten-free.

| | |
|---|---|
| 1 ¼ cups Gluten-Free Naturals™ All Purpose Flour | 1 teaspoon cream of tartar |
| 1 cup sugar | ½ cup sugar |
| ½ teaspoon gluten-free baking powder* | 6 egg yolks |
| ½ teaspoon salt | 5 Tablespoons water |
| 6 egg whites | 1 teaspoon gluten-free vanilla* |

Whisk together flour, sugar, baking powder and salt. Set aside. In a large clean bowl, beat egg whites with a mixer until frothy. Add cream of tartar. Gradually beat in ½ cup sugar, a little at a time. Beat until whites form stiff, not dry, peaks.

In a small bowl combine egg yolks, water, vanilla and blended flour mixture. Then beat at high speed for 4 minutes until mixture is smooth and satiny. It will be somewhat thick, but don't worry – it will fold into the egg white mixture. (Note: it should pour down from the beater in a thick ribbon. It should not be so thick that it stays on the beaters and doesn't pour. If it is too thick add another Tablespoon of water and blend in with the mixer.)

Add the egg yolk mixture to egg white mixture and fold in lightly and thoroughly by hand. Then put in a 10 inch un-greased tube pan. Bake at 350°F for about 45 minutes. Test for doneness. Allow pan to cool upside-down before removing cake. (Very important: your cake will fall and be ruined if you don't cool it upside down.)

*Variation*: Slice and top each piece with strawberries and whipped cream. Or, frost this cake with Pineapple Creamy Frosting (see index for recipe).

## Sponge Cake – Italian Style

I prefer the Grand Champion recipe, but this one is also good.  It's a European cake and not as sweet.

5 egg whites
½ cup sugar
5 egg yolks
1 cup sugar

1 ¼ cups Gluten-Free Naturals™ All
    Purpose Flour
1 teaspoon gluten-free vanilla*
½ teaspoon grated lemon rind

Carefully separate the egg whites from the egg yolks.  Be careful not to get any yolk in the whites or the whites will not whip.  Beat egg whites in a clean bowl with clean beaters until stiff.  Add ½ cup sugar and beat until well blended.  (Beaters must be clean or they will not whip.)  Place egg yolks and 1 cup sugar in a separate mixing bowl and beat until lemon colored.  Add flour, a little at a time, blending in well.  Add vanilla and lemon rind.  Fold the egg whites into the cake mixture.  Butter a cake pan, about 18 inches square (or two 9 inch pans).  Bake at 375°F for 40 minutes for large pan, less for two smaller pans.  Turn over cake(s) onto a wire rack to cool.

## Zuccato

This cake is an Italian specialty from the Florence area.  It's good for company as it must be made a day or two before serving.  The cake is shaped like a dome, so you must have a 1 ½ quart rounded bottom bowl for best appearance.

1 (12 ounce) gluten-free chiffon cake or
    gluten-free sponge cake (see index)
2 ounces almonds
2 ounces hazelnuts (or filberts)
3 Tablespoons Cognac* or light Rum*

3 Tablespoons Grand Marnier®*
5 ounces gluten-free semi-sweet tiny
    chocolate chips*
2 cups gluten-free heavy cream*
4 teaspoons sugar

Heat your oven to 250°F.  Skin the almonds by placing in boiling water and then drain and slip skins off.  Place on a shallow pan and toast a few minutes to a golden brown color.  Be careful not to burn.  Remove and chop.  Put oven up to 400°F.  Place hazelnuts on the baking sheet and bake 5 minutes.  Remove from oven, put in a towel and rub to remove most of the skins.  Chop coarsely.  Set nuts aside.

Now line your bowl with plastic wrap or foil, leaving some overhanging the edge for easy removal.  Cut cake into ½ inch slices lengthwise and then in half on the diagonal.  Moisten cake with the Cognac or rum and Grand Marnier® that you have mixed together.  Now place the slices around the sides of the bowl, being sure to leave no gaps for filling to fall through.  Leave enough cake to completely cover the top of the cake, when completed.

Whip cream and sugar until thick and fold in nuts and chocolate chips.  Pour cream into cake lined bowl and top with reserved cake that you also moistened with liquors.  Cover with more plastic wrap and refrigerate at least 24 hours before serving.  When ready to serve, remove top plastic wrap and invert on a serving dish.  Remove bowl and carefully remove plastic wrap covering cake.  Dust generously with confectioner's sugar or a mixture of confectioner's sugar and cocoa.

*see gluten-free products list at the end of the book

# ICINGS / FROSTINGS

## Butter Creamy Frosting

I find this type of frosting too sweet, but my sister-in-law used it on the pound cake recipe for her wedding cake and it was good. If you are lactose intolerant you can use shortening or gluten-free margarine*, and also substitute water or a gluten-free milk substitute for the milk.

⅓ cup butter, softened
4 ½ cups sifted powdered sugar
¼ cup milk (add slowly by Tablespoon since less may be needed)

1 ½ teaspoons gluten-free vanilla*
Food coloring optional

In a mixing bowl beat the butter until fluffy. Gradually add 2 cups of the powdered sugar, beating well. Slowly beat in the milk and vanilla, adding the milk one Tablespoon at a time until the right consistency is achieved. This makes enough for two 8 or 9 inch layer cakes.

*Variation:* For lemon frosting, substitute the milk with lemon juice and add ½ teaspoon finely shredded lemon peel.

## Chocolate Creamy Frosting

This is also very sweet for my taste, but children like it on chocolate cake.

3 Tablespoons sweet butter, softened or melted
½ cup cocoa
⅓ cup milk

1 ½ teaspoons gluten-free vanilla*
3 ½ cups sifted confectioner's sugar
Dash of salt

Beat all together, adding milk a little at a time to get the right consistency.

## Chocolate Whipped Cream

A very, very rich whipped cream frosting using powdered sugar.

3 cups chilled whipping cream
1 ½ cups powdered sugar
¾ cup cocoa (I use less)

¼ teaspoon salt

Sift the powdered sugar, cocoa and salt. Whip together and frost the chocolate angel food cake.

## Cream Cheese Frosting

This frosting is nice on carrot or spice cake. It can be used on Hermit cookies, if desired (see index).

½ cup butter or gluten-free margarine*
8 ounce package of gluten-free cream cheese*
1 teaspoon gluten-free vanilla*

1 pound sifted confectioner's sugar
A teaspoon or more milk or gluten-free milk substitute*, if needed

*see gluten-free products list at the end of the book

Blend ingredients. If too thick, add a little milk to make it the right consistency. Good on carrot cake.

## Mocha Whipped Cream Frosting
This is my mother's recipe on Angel Food Cake. It also holds up well because the cocoa gives the whipped cream a wonderful texture.

1 ½ cups gluten-free heavy cream*           2 teaspoons instant coffee
3 Tablespoons sugar                         2 teaspoons hot water
2 Tablespoons sifted dry cocoa              ¾ cup gluten-free vanilla*

Melt two teaspoons of instant coffee in hot water and add to heavy cream with all the rest of the ingredients. Whip until stiff. Cover cake with cream in swirls and refrigerate until serving time. Cake can be frosted and made hours ahead of time, as long as it is refrigerated.

## Ornamental Icing for Decorating
Use this icing for writing on cakes or decorating cookies.

1 ¼ cups sifted confectioner's sugar        ¼ teaspoon gluten-free vanilla*
⅛ teaspoon cream of tartar                  Food coloring
1 egg white (or use equivalent egg white
   powder and water)

Beat all together with an electric mixer and fill a pastry bag using the tiniest writing tube. Cover what icing is left with a dampened paper towel to prevent it from drying out. Decorate cooled cookies or a frosted cake.

## Pineapple Creamy Frosting
Use this frosting on the "Sponge Cake — Grand Champion" recipe.

½ cup butter                                ⅛ teaspoon salt
3 cups confectioner's sugar, sifted         ¼ teaspoon gluten-free vanilla*
1 (8.5 ounce) can drained, crushed          ½ teaspoon grated lemon rind, optional
   pineapple

Cream the butter. Gradually add sifted confectioner's sugar. Beat until light and fluffy. Blend in pineapple, salt, vanilla, and grated lemon rind (if using). Good on Sponge Cake, "Grand Champion" (see index for recipe).

*see gluten-free products list at the end of the book

## Whipped Cream Frosting
This holds up well because of the gelatin. My mother often uses this recipe. See below for an even easier version.

Be sure to check the ingredients on the cream. Some brands are now including additives that may or may not be safe, which may give you less cream because cream is the expensive ingredient. I noticed this with Land O'Lakes® "premium" cream. It contained additives and milk. They could not tell me at that time whether or not it was gluten-free. (This may change in 2006 with the new labeling law.) I called several times and they told me that they would call back but never did. I normally use Hood® brand, which is gluten-free as of this writing.

2 cups gluten-free heavy cream* (be sure
  to check ingredients.)

4 teaspoons sugar
1 Tablespoon plain gelatin

Blend cream and 4 teaspoons sugar. Take the 1 Tablespoon plain gelatin and mix with 1 Tablespoon cold water in a Pyrex® cup. Place cup in a pan of hot water and melt until liquid is clear. Cool and add gradually to whipped cream and beat until nice and thick. Frost cake with cream and refrigerate until serving time.

## Whipped Cream Frosting – Easier Version
My mother gave me this recipe. It's delicious, holds up well, and is easier to make than the recipe with the gelatin. It's my mother's idea to use the cheesecake flavor, and we prefer it over the vanilla. Be sure the instant pudding is gluten-free.

1 cup gluten-free heavy cream* (be sure to
check ingredients)
1 teaspoon sugar

1 teaspoon gluten-free instant pudding
mix*, cheesecake flavor or vanilla flavor

I usually double this recipe. Blend cream and the sugar and pudding mix. Whip immediately and beat until nice and thick. Frost cake with cream and refrigerate until serving time.

*Variation*: If you are lactose intolerant and you tolerate Cool Whip® better than real whipped cream, frost your cake with Cool Whip® immediately before serving. This works well on cupcakes.

## Waldorf Astoria Frosting
This is a very buttery frosting. It is not very sweet.

4 Tablespoons fine white rice flour or
  sweet rice flour
¾ cup milk
½ cup sweet butter at room temperature

½ cup gluten-free margarine* or
  shortening
¾ cup sugar
1 teaspoon gluten-free vanilla*

Mix flour and milk together and cook until it loses its glossy appearance and is very thick, stirring constantly. Remove from heat and cool to room temperature, stirring every now and then so that a skin doesn't form on top.

*see gluten-free products list at the end of the book

In an electric mixing bowl, place butter, shortening and sugar and beat well for 5 minutes. Add vanilla. Then add flour mixture gradually to butter mixture one spoonful at a time and beat another 5 minutes or more until creamy.

## White Peaks Frosting

You need a candy thermometer to make this. It tastes like a marshmallow frosting.

½ cup sugar                               2 egg whites
¼ cup light corn syrup*             1 teaspoon gluten-free vanilla*
2 Tablespoons water

Mix sugar, corn syrup and water in one-quart saucepan. Cook over medium heat until it boils. Continue to boil until a candy thermometer registers 242°F or when a small amount is dropped into some cold water it forms a firm ball.

Beat egg whites until stiff peaks form. Pour hot syrup in very slowly in a thin stream and keep beating. Add vanilla and beat until stiff peaks form.

## Write your own recipes here:

# PIES AND PASTRIES

I spent many years working on pie crust. That is why there are so many versions in this book. Some things I was able to develop quickly, but bread and pie crust took me years. If you're not sure which recipe to try first, try the "Our Favorite" crust. If you don't want to try a roll out a crust first, then try the mock Oreo®. I've got a lot of versions so I'm sure you'll find one that fits your needs. Whatever crust you choose, you don't have to worry about overworking it and making it tough, because there is no gluten!

## Apple Dumplings
This is my mother's recipe. She adds the apple peels to the syrup to make it a pretty red color. If it is not red enough you can add a little red food coloring.

Our Favorite Pie Crust for 2 crusts (9 inch) pie – Do not try the other crusts in this book for this recipe
6 apples, medium size, preferably the Cortland variety
½ cup sugar
1 teaspoon ground cinnamon
¼ teaspoon ground nutmeg

2 Tablespoons butter
For the Syrup:
⅓ cup sugar
2 Tablespoons lemon juice
4 ½ Tablespoons butter
¼ teaspoon ground cinnamon

Wash, peel and core applies leaving them whole. Place the peels in a saucepan with the 2 cups of water and simmer for 10 minutes. Meanwhile, make the pie crust. Sprinkle some gluten-free flour on waxed paper. Separate the dough into 6 balls. Roll them out thin, and do your best to make them into a 7 inch square shape. Loosen the crust from the waxed paper. I use a new piece of waxed paper for each piece of dough.

Mix ½ cup sugar, 1 teaspoon cinnamon and ¼ teaspoon nutmeg together. Place an apple on each piece of pie crust. Fill each center of apple with a heaping tablespoon of sugar/spice mixture and dot it with butter. Draw up the 4 corners of pastry and pinch closed. Use a little water if necessary to keep the pastry together. Chill while making syrup.

Add remaining sugar, lemon juice, cinnamon and butter to a saucepan and cook 10 minutes or until slightly syrupy. Place the dumplings in a baking dish being sure they do not touch each other. Strain the syrup and pour it around the apple dumplings. Sprinkle a little syrup over the dumplings and bake in a preheated 375°F oven for 40-45 minutes or until apples test done with a cake tester and pie crust is lightly browned.

Serve warm with some of the syrup spooned over the top.

## Apple Sour Cream and Walnut Streusel Pie
My husband likes this pie.

Our Favorite Pie crust or Crepe Pie Crust (see index) may be used
8 to 10 very large apples, peeled & cored
½ cup sugar (or can substitute light brown sugar) – (use more if tart tasting)
⅔ cup gluten-free sour cream (I use a little less)
1 teaspoon ground cinnamon

2 Tablespoons cornstarch
¾ cup finely chopped walnuts (I use less, enough to cover top)
1 Tablespoon butter
½ to 1 cup confectioner's sugar
Dash of milk
¼ teaspoon gluten-free vanilla* (optional)

Prepare a pie crust to line a 10" or 9 ½" deep dish pie pan. Blend together sour cream, sugar and cinnamon. Chop and slice the apples and blend well into the sour cream. (Blend the apples into the sour cream as you chop them to keep them from turning brown.) Taste the mixture to see if it is too tart or if more sugar is needed. Blend in the cornstarch. Pour into the pie crust. Top with chopped nuts. (The sour cream and the nuts will keep the apples moist without a top crust.) Bake for 20 minutes at 400°F. Turn heat down to 350°F and bake 20 minutes more. Remove from oven and test apples with a cake tester to be sure they are cooked. Bake longer if needed. Allow the pie to cool a little. Make a drizzle frosting by blending the butter into the confectioner's sugar and adding milk and vanilla (if using), to get the right consistency. My directions aren't too specific because I add some milk and sugar as I go. Drizzle over the top of the pie. Serve.

Even though this pie has sour cream if you use the crepe crust it seems lighter. Without the sugar topping this is good for a breakfast treat.

*Variation*: Instead of the frosting topping, prepare the following rich sugary topping before you bake the pie. Blend ½ cup sugar and ½ cup butter together. Add ½ cup Gluten-Free Naturals™ Cookie Blend and the nuts. Take large pieces of topping, form into a ball and then flatten with the palm of your hand. Lay these flat pieces on the top of the pie like sections of crust. Bake as above for 20 minutes and check the top and lower the oven temperature as above. If the top is getting too dark cover it with foil and bake 20 minutes more.

## Bisquick® Type Substitute for Impossible Pies™
I came up with this formula to covert Bisquick® Impossible Pie™ recipes. It works well and it has no saturated fat if using oil. I substitute this recipe for every ½ cup used in a pie recipe. Whip it in as part of the ingredients of the recipe you are using. You can also use the other recipe in this book.

⅓ cup fine white rice flour or ½ cup Gluten-Free Naturals™ All Purpose Flour
⅛ teaspoon salt

¾ teaspoon gluten-free baking powder*
2 Tablespoons oil (or melted butter)

Mix all together and let it sit a few minutes so the oil absorbs into the rice flour. Blend into recipes for Impossible Pies™. (Note: It is best if you put this together immediately before

*see gluten-free products list at the end of the book

you use it.)  This makes the right amount to substitute a ½ cup of Bisquick® in the pie recipe.

Shortening can be used in place of oil for a better texture, but I think oil is a healthier choice. Most shortening contain trans-fats.  If you use shortening, cut it in with a pastry blender.  A mixer may also be used.  Another choice of fat to use is butter.  It will add more flavor, but must also be put together immediately before you use it.  Use less salt if using salted butter.

## Blueberry Miniature Tarts

These are a good use for the homemade blueberry jam in this book, or use store-bought jam.  You need a non-stick mini-muffin pan that makes 24 muffins to make these.  I like to make these for a party because they are easy to serve and they give your guests a taste of pie without having to eat a large piece.

1 ½ cups Gluten-Free Naturals™ All Purpose Flour or Gluten-Free Naturals™ Sandwich Bread flour (do not substitute other flour blends)
Pinch of salt
½ cup butter

3 Tablespoons cold water
Blueberry jam*
Rice flour (use only if your homemade jam is thin or a little watery)
Cinnamon and Sugar (optional)

Preheat oven to 425°F.  In a food processor, put the flour, salt and butter.  Pulse the food processor to cut in the butter.  (If you don't have a food processor, cut the butter in using a pastry blender).  Add the water through the feed tube and process until the dough balls up on one side.

Remove the dough and make 24 balls.  Using your fingers, press one ball into each cup of a mini-muffin pan to form a crust on the bottom and sides.  Fill with blueberry jam until each one is two-thirds full.  (If you jam is thin, mix in a little rice flour into it before filling the pastry.)  Sprinkle with some cinnamon and sugar, if desired.  Bake for 15 minutes.

## Cherry Custard Pie – Crustless Version

1 ½ cups milk
¼ cup oil
1 ½ teaspoons gluten-free vanilla*
4 eggs
¾ cup sugar
⅓ cup fine white rice flour

⅛ teaspoon salt
¾ teaspoon baking powder
2 Tablespoons oil
1 (21 ounce) can cherry pie filling*
Gluten-free whipped cream* (optional)

Preheat oven to 400°F.  Grease a 10 inch or 9 ½ inch deep dish glass pie plate.  Beat all ingredients (except the cherries and whipped cream) until smooth in a blender or food processor.  Pour into pie plate.  Drain pie filling, reserving the syrup in a microwave safe dish.  Spoon the cherries evenly over the top.  Bake for 30-35 minutes until a knife inserted comes out clean.  Cool for 5 minutes.  Serve with warm syrup heated in the microwave.  If desired, serve with whipped cream.

*see gluten-free products list at the end of the book

## Chocolate Angel Pie

This is a meringue pie that is upside-down, so that the meringue is the crust.

Meringue shell
2 egg whites
⅛ teaspoon cream of tartar
⅛ teaspoon salt
½ cup sugar

½ cup nuts, chopped fine (optional)
½ teaspoon gluten-free vanilla*

Filling
1 (¼ lb.) pkg. Baking Sweet German
    Chocolate*
2 Tablespoons water

1 cup whipping or heavy cream*
1 teaspoon gluten-free vanilla*

Whip the egg whites, cream of tartar and salt with clean beaters. Add the sugar 2 Tablespoons at a time and beat after each addition until stiff peaks form. Fold in the vanilla and nuts. Grease an 8 inch pie plate generously and spoon in the filling. Spread gently to build up the sides a ½ inch above the top of the pan. Bake in a 300°F oven for 50 to 55 minutes. Cool to room temperature.

Make the filling by melting the chocolate and water in the microwave on defrost. Stir until melted. Cool until thickened. Add the vanilla. Whip the cream and fold in the chocolate. Fill the shell and chill for 2 hours before serving. This may be made 1 day ahead of time.

## Chocolate Pie – Crustless Version

2 eggs
1 cup milk
¼ cup oil
1 teaspoon gluten-free vanilla*
2 ounces melted semi-sweet chocolate* (I
    melt in the microwave on defrost)
1 cup brown sugar

⅓ cup fine white rice flour
¾ teaspoon gluten-free baking powder*
Pinch of salt
Whipped cream or Cool Whip® for
    garnish

Preheat oven to 350°F. Put everything in a blender. Whip about 1 minute. Put in a greased pie plate. Bake for 30 minutes until it tests done with a knife. Cool. Top with whipped cream or Cool Whip®.

## Chocolate Pecan Pie

1 recipe gluten-free pie crust (see index), to fit a 9" pie pan (Our Favorite Pie Crust works best)
3 eggs
6 Tablespoons butter or gluten-free margarine, melted
¾ cup light corn syrup*
½ cup sugar
¼ cup firmly packed brown sugar

2 Tablespoons rum (optional) or gluten-free bourbon (optional)
1 Tablespoon fine white rice flour or sweet rice flour
1 teaspoon gluten-free vanilla* or vanillin*
1 cup chopped pecans
1 cup gluten-free semi-sweet chocolate morsels*

Beat eggs well. Add cooled melted butter and blend. (I melt the butter in the microwave on the defrost cycle.) Add sugars, syrup, rum, rice flour and vanilla and mix well. Add pecans and stir in. Sprinkle chocolate morsels on the bottom of an <u>un</u>baked 9 inch gluten-free pie shell or use my pie crust recipe. Carefully pour the pecan mixture over the chocolate. Bake in a preheated 350°F oven for 1 hour. Cool.

## Coconut Cream Pie – Crustless Version

My husband doesn't like coconut, but if you like it this is a delicious pie that it easy to make. Don't use a smaller pan or it will spill over in the oven as it bakes and make a mess.

2 cups milk
¼ cup oil
1 ½ teaspoons gluten-free vanilla*
4 eggs
1 cup coconut, flaked or shredded

¾ cup sugar
⅓ cup fine white rice flour
⅛ teaspoon salt
¾ teaspoon gluten-free baking powder*

Put all ingredients in a blender. Blend for 30 seconds. Grease a 10 inch or 9 ½ inch deep dish pie pan. Pour batter into the pan and sprinkle with remaining coconut. Bake at 350°F for 50 to 55 minutes. Cool.

## Cranberry Pake

The name is not a typo. It's a combination of pie and cake. The directions look long to make the pie crust, but it's easy using a food processor. You can use this crust for other pies.

Pie Crust – Use "Our Favorite Pie Crust" or use this recipe below:
1 cup sweet rice flour or fine white rice flour (the sweet rice works better)
½ cup cold butter, cut into 8 pieces
1 medium egg

½ teaspoon salt
½ teaspoon xanthan gum
1 teaspoon gluten-free heavy cream*, milk or gluten-free milk substitute or water

Filling:
2 ½ cups cranberries
¾ cup sugar

½ cup broken walnuts

Batter:
¾ cup butter or gluten-free margarine* (I
    use ½ cup and it works with less)
1 cup sugar (I use ¾ cup sugar)

2 eggs
1 cup Gluten-Free Naturals™ All Purpose
    Flour

Place all pie crust ingredients in a food processor and blend by turning on and off for about 15 seconds or until it forms a ball. If needed, add a little more cream or water. (Or use the traditional method to make pie crust by cutting the butter into the flour using a pastry blender, and then adding the water.) Either roll out crust between 2 sheets of waxed paper or press it into a 10 inch or 9 ½ inch deep dish pie pan with your hands. I find that rolling is easy with this dough and it usually doesn't require any extra rice flour to roll it out. If your dough seems sticky, dust the waxed paper with some Gluten-Free Naturals™ All Purpose flour or rice flour first. Note: do not use smaller than a deep dish pie plate or this pie will boil over and make a mess of your oven.

*For an easy way to put the pie crust in your pie pan, you will need 2 pie pans. You use 1 pie pan as a form and it doesn't get dirty because it only touches the waxed paper. Roll out crust and peel off the top layer of waxed paper. Put it back on. Flip the pie crust over and peel off the waxed paper on this side and put it back on. Now take a pie plate (the one you are using as a form) and put it upside down on the counter. Slide it under the bottom waxed paper of your crust. You have an upside down pie plate, the waxed paper, your layer of crust, and the top piece of waxed paper. Form the crust on the pie plate and remove the waxed paper on top. Now take the other pie plate (the one you will bake the pie in) and lay it upside down over the top. Now flip it over. Remove the first pie plate, remove the waxed paper. You will have your crust perfectly inside the pie plate.*

Put cranberries that have been picked over, washed and dried into the pie shell. Top berries with sugar and nuts. (Do not use less sugar on the cranberries or they will be too sour.) Make batter by adding the ¾ cup butter (or less), 1 cup sugar (or less) and eggs in the food processor. Add the 1 cup Gluten-Free Naturals™ All Purpose Flour and blend in with the processor. Pour batter over cranberries. It will be thick, so spread it over the top using a metal knife. For best results, cover edge of crust with a pie shield or cover with some aluminum foil. This pie has a longer bake time than most, and if you don't cover the edge it will burn. Bake 60 minutes at 350°F. Serves 8 and is delicious when topped with sweetened whipped cream or gluten-free non-dairy topping (Cool Whip®).

## Dutch Apple Tart
This is my mother's recipe. If desired, you can make the crust in a food processor.

Pastry:
2 ½ cups Gluten-Free Naturals™ All
    Purpose flour (do not substitute)
½ cup brown sugar

¼ teaspoon salt
10 Tablespoons butter
1 egg yolk
Grated rind of 1 lemon (optional)

*see gluten-free products list at the end of the book*

Combine flour, salt and sugar. Cut in butter as for pie crust. Add the egg yolk and grated lemon rind, and knead the dough into a ball. Chill and roll out between 2 pieces of waxed paper. Remove the waxed paper. Use the dough to line a 9 inch spring form pan or tart pans.

Filling:                                                     2 eggs
   1 pound of apples                           ½ cup milk
   ¼ cup raisins                               2 Tablespoons sugar
   ¼ cup sugar                                 2 Tablespoons apricot jam*
   1 teaspoon ground cinnamon

Peel, core and slice apples. Arrange apples in the pastry. Sprinkle with raisins, cinnamon, and sugar. Beat the eggs, milk and 2 Tablespoons of sugar together and pour on top of the apples. Bake in a 375°F oven for 50 minutes. When thoroughly cooled, brush with 2 Tablespoons of melted apricot jam.

## Grasshopper Frozen Pie

This is a delicious pie with a brownie crust and light frozen ice creamy mint filling. I've served this to non-celiacs who had no idea it was a gluten-free dessert.

1 Gluten-Free Naturals™ Brownie Mix           1 teaspoon gluten-free mint extract* (I use
   (prepared as directed)                         peppermint)
1 jar of marshmallow crème*                    4 to 6 drops of green food coloring
                                               1 ½ cups whipping cream*

Prepare brownie mix as directed on the package and bake. Allow to cool.

Remove half of the brownies. Crumble these brownies over a 9 inch glass pie plate. Press and form the brownie crumbs into a crust by pressing them on the sides and bottom of the pan, using your fingers. (Save other brownies for another use, or freeze for another time.)

Open the jar of marshmallow cream and add the mint extract and food coloring. Blend it in. The marshmallow crème will deflate somewhat as you mix, so there is room to mix it in the jar.

Whip the cream. I use a heavy duty mixer with a wire whisk attachment. Whip until peaks start to form. Add the marshmallow crème mixture and beat until stiff peaks form. Do not over beat. Pour the cream mixture into the pie crust and spread to fill. Cover with plastic wrap and freeze for 4 hours.

*Variation*: One (8 ounce) tub of Cool Whip® from Kraft® (gluten-free as of this writing) may be substituted for the whipping cream. Beat marshmallow crème, extract, food coloring and whipped topping together with a wire whisk. Fill the brownie shell and freeze 4 hours.

## Lemon Angel Pie

This is a lemon meringue pie that's upside-down, so that the meringue is the crust. I don't make meringues on humid days, because the humidity will make them weep (i.e. droplets form on the surface of the meringue). For this to turn out, make it on a dry weather day.

4 large egg whites (½ cup)
¼ teaspoon cream of tartar
Pinch salt (optional)
1 cup sugar
1 teaspoon gluten-free vanilla* (optional)
4 egg yolks
½ cup sugar
2 to 4 Tablespoons water
Pinch salt (optional)

1 teaspoon grated lemon zest/peel (optional)
4 Tablespoons lemon juice
1 cup gluten-free heavy cream* (or for those that can't have dairy, use Cool Whip® which is gluten-free as of this writing)
2 Tablespoons sugar
Shredded coconut or almonds for garnish (optional)

Beat egg whites and cream of tartar until frothy. Continue beating, gradually adding the 1 cup sugar (adding about 2 Tablespoons at a time). Continue beating thoroughly after each addition. Feel the meringue between your fingers and if there is no grit and it is very stiff it is done. Add vanilla and blend in. Spread in a well greased 9 inch round layer cake pan, making edges slightly higher than center. Bake at 275°F for 1 hour. Turn off the heat and allow the pie shell to remain in the oven for 1 hour with the door slightly ajar. (Alternatively, preheat oven to 450°F. Turn the oven off, put the meringue inside the oven, and leave in the oven for 5 hours.)

Remove the pie shell from the oven and let it cool completely. The center of the crust may rise a little during baking and can be crushed to hold the filling after it has cooled.

Make lemon filling by beating together egg yolks, ½ cup sugar, water, lemon zest and lemon juice. Cook in a non-aluminum pan over low heat until thick and bubbly. (Note: eggs and lemon can react with aluminum, making the filling an ugly greenish color with a metallic taste.) Set aside to cool. Whip the cream until stiff, and add 2 Tablespoons sugar. Spread the lemon filling on the meringue, cover with cream. Refrigerate until ready to serve.

*see gluten-free products list at the end of the book

## Lemon Meringue Pie

My mom used to make lemon meringue pie often in the summer. When she was a newlywed and money was tight, this was the dessert she often made because it is not only very good but inexpensive. I prefer the homemade pudding to the box kind. Most box versions are gluten-free.

Pie Crust, baked (see index) I like "Our
 Favorite Pie Crust" best in this recipe
Pudding:
1 ½ cups sugar
⅓ cup cornstarch
1 ½ cups water
3 egg yolks
1-2 Tablespoons butter

¼ cup lemon juice
1 Tablespoon lemon rind (optional)
Meringue
3 egg whites
¼ teaspoon cream of tartar
6 Tablespoons sugar
½ teaspoon gluten-free vanilla* (optional)

Prepare and bake the pie crust. Put sugar, cornstarch, water, yolks, butter, lemon juice and rind (if using) in a pot that does not have an aluminum interior. (I use a non-stick pot or a stainless steel one.) Cook the filling on medium heat, stirring constantly until thick. I stir it with a whisk. Pour into the prepared pie shell.

Put egg whites and cream of tartar in the bowl of an electric mixer. Begin whipping on high speed. Add the sugar a tablespoon at a time, blending in well after each addition. Meringue is done when you take some between your fingers and don't feel the grit of the sugar. Blend in the vanilla if using.

Top the pudding mixture with the meringue, making sure the meringue goes all the way to the side of the crust. Bake at 400°F for 8 to 10 minutes until meringue is lightly brown on top.

*Variation*: For a butterscotch creamy pie with meringue, substitute this filling: 1 cup sugar, ¼ cup cornstarch, ½ teaspoon salt, 1 cup water, 1 ⅔ cups milk, 3 egg yolks and 1 ½ teaspoons vanilla. Follow as above.

*Variation 2*: For orange meringue pie, substitute orange juice for the lemon juice. Reduce the sugar by ¼ cup.

*Variation 3*: For lime meringue pie, substitute lime juice for lemon and add some green food color to the pudding.

## Peach Pie – Make ahead pie filling

When peaches are in season, buy a half-bushel and prepare this filling to freeze and enjoy come winter.

5 cups peeled, very ripe peaches
¾ cup sugar
1 Tablespoon lemon juice

2 Tablespoons minute tapioca
¼ teaspoon ground cinnamon
Pinch of salt

*see gluten-free products list at the end of the book

Line a pie pan with foil and set aside. Plunge the peaches into boiling water and then into cold water. The peel will now slip right off. Pit and slice peaches into a bowl and combine them with the remaining ingredients. Fit into foil lined pie pan and freeze. When frozen, remove from the pie pan and wrap in freezer wrap.

When it comes time to bake, make a two-crusted pastry. Line pan with pastry, place the frozen peaches over pastry and top with pastry. It makes it easier to do the top crust with the filling frozen. Flute and prick with a fork. Bake in a 400°F oven for 45-50 minutes.

*Variation*: Sometimes I make half this recipe. Instead of freezing it, I put the peaches, sugar, lemon juice, tapioca, cinnamon and salt in a pot. I cook it until it thickens. We enjoy this "pie filling" warm in dishes topped with vanilla ice cream or whipped cream.

If you are cooking it in a pot, cornstarch may be substituted for the minute tapioca. However, cornstarch doesn't freeze well, which is why my mother's original recipe doesn't contain it. If you plan to freeze leftovers, use the minute tapioca.

## Pear Pie
One of our favorite pies we had growing up. It is a delicious change from apple pie.

2 gluten-free pie crusts (see index) to make one 9 inch pie – "Our Favorite Pie Crust" works best in this recipe

1 cup thick applesauce (best with homemade sauce that has ground cinnamon and ground nutmeg added)

½ cup sugar

1 Tablespoon brown sugar

1 teaspoon ground cinnamon (if applesauce doesn't contain cinnamon)

4 cups cored, peeled and sliced fresh pears

Melted sweet butter

Line your pie pan with gluten-free pastry. Mix applesauce, pears, and sugars together. Take filling and add up to 1 teaspoon of cinnamon if needed. Cover with top pastry, flute, and poke a few holes with a fork. Brush top of pie with melted butter. Bake it in a 400°F oven for 30-40 minutes, or until the pie is done.

## Pecan Pie – Crustless Version
This is easy. It forms its own crust on the bottom, has the creamy filling, and the nuts float to the top.

1 ½ cups pecans, chopped (whole pecans can be used but it is more difficult to cut the pie)

¾ cups milk

¾ cups light corn syrup*

1 ½ teaspoons gluten-free vanilla*

4 eggs

¾ cup brown sugar, packed

¼ cup oil

⅓ cup fine white rice flour or Gluten-Free Naturals™ All Purpose Flour

⅛ teaspoon salt

¾ teaspoon baking powder

Whipped cream* for garnish (optional)

Preheat oven to 350°F. Grease a 9" pie plate. Sprinkle nuts in plate. Beat remaining ingredients until smooth in a blender or food processor or mixer. Pour into pie plate. Bake

*see gluten-free products list at the end of the book

for 50-55 minutes until a knife inserted comes out clean. Cool. Best served topped with whipped cream, Cool Whip®, or gluten-free ice cream.

## Pie Crust – Our Favorite

This pie crust is our favorite because it is pie crust with the right taste and texture. It took me years to invent and I think it's better than the real thing! The recipe below is for a single crust, so double it for 2 crust pies. This crust is easy to cut and serve (unlike rice crusts which are very hard) and doesn't get soggy or gritty. There is no need to use a pie shield on this crust since it bakes up just like the wheat crusts you remember. Do not substitute other flour blends or it will not work.

1 cup Gluten-Free Naturals™ All Purpose
    Flour or Gluten-Free Naturals™
    Sandwich Bread Flour
Pinch of salt

⅓ cup butter*, cold from the refrigerator
2 Tablespoons water

Put flour and pinch of salt in a food processor. Cut in the butter with the food processor. Through the feeding tube, slowly add the water. The dough should blend and ball up on one side. (Or the traditional method may be used. Cut the butter into flour using a pastry blender. Blend in the cold water with a fork. Ball up and roll out the dough.)

Remove dough from the processor. Roll out on a piece of waxed paper. Since there is no gluten you do not have to worry about overworking the dough. You can re-roll it if necessary. (If you are having difficulty rolling, refrigerate the dough for 30 minutes.) If you measured carefully, there is no need to put extra flour on the waxed paper before rolling. You don't need a top sheet of waxed paper for rolling.

To easily get it into your pie pan, take a pie plate and turn it upside-down on your counter and slide it under the waxed paper under your pie crust. Use it as a form and center your crust on this pie plate. Now take the pie plate that you will use to make your pie. Turn it upside-down and place it on top of the crust. Flip everything over. Remove the first pie plate and remove the waxed paper. Flute the edges of the crust. Now you are ready to fill your crust. Bake according to your pie filling directions.

For a pre-baked crust, prick the crust with a fork and then bake it at 475°F for 8 to 10 minutes.

For a double crust, double the recipe. Roll out top crust. Fill with pie filling. Put pie crust on top. Seal and flute the edges. Bake according to the pie filling directions.

## Pie Crust – Sweet Version

This is a sweet cookie-like crust using Gluten-Free Naturals™ Cookie Blend. Do not eliminate the sugar or it will not work. Instead you can reduce some sugar in your filling if you wish. This recipe makes enough for a two crust pie. See variation below for directions for a pre-baked single crust. I recommend using a pie shield to prevent the edges from burning.

½ cup butter* or gluten-free margarine*
2 cups Gluten-Free Naturals™ Cookie
 Blend

½ cup sugar (do not eliminate or use a
 sugar substitute)
Pinch of salt
2 eggs

Mix the flour, sugar and salt. Cut in the butter with a pastry blender for best results. If you don't have a pastry blender you can use a fork, or use your food processor. The butter should be the size of small peas. With a metal spoon, mix in the eggs. Use your hands to form the dough into two balls. If too dry, add a little water. Return to your bowl and cover and refrigerate 1 hour.

Take two pieces of waxed paper. Sprinkle some gluten-free flour on it (I prefer using the Cookie Blend). Sprinkle top with a little flour and top with waxed paper. Now take your rolling pin and roll out carefully until thin. Remove top piece of waxed paper. Put crust over your pan and remove bottom piece. Note: If your dough was sticking a lot when you removed the top piece, I suggest you replace the top piece, flip it over, and carefully remove the bottom piece. It may be easier to remove flat on your counter rather than over your pan.

Fill with filling. Use two new pieces of new waxed paper. Roll out top crust and do the same as you did with the bottom crust. In this case I find it easier to loosen both pieces of waxed paper while it's on the counter, since you want a flat one on top.

Flute edges. Bake according to your recipe. About halfway through your baking time, I suggest you check to see if your crust edge is getting too dark. If so, cover edge with foil. I use a pie shield (one of those aluminum rings that cover the pie crust edge so it doesn't get too dark).

For a delicious/easy apple pie, try filling with "delicious apples recipe" [see index]. Since the apples are already cooked, your crust won't overcook. Bake for only 35 minutes at 350°F. For recipes that bake longer than 35 minutes at 350°F, I suggest you cover the crust edges after 35 minutes. If it is a long baking pie, I often put the pie shield on before I put it in the oven.

*Variation*: Make half the recipe for a single crust pie. Bake shell at 350°F for 15 minutes if a pre-baked crust is needed (i.e. for lemon meringue pie).

## Pie Crust – Brownie Crumb, Mock Oreo® Version
I developed this easy to make crust.  No extra butter needed.  No need to grease the pie plate.  This makes enough for 2 pies!  It can be used for any kind of pie that uses a chocolate cookie crumb crust.

1 Gluten-Free Naturals™ Brownie Mix baked and prepared as directed.

Allow brownies to cool.  Take half of the brownies and crumble them over a 9 inch glass pie plate. Press the crumbs to form a crust on the sides and bottom of pan, using your hands.

Repeat with remaining brownies and a second pie plate.  The second crust may be well-wrapped and frozen for another time.  Or instead of preparing a second crust, cut and freeze the leftover brownies and defrost for use at another time.

This crust may be used on baked pies, frozen pies, ready-to-eat pies, and refrigerated pies.  It also works well as a cheesecake crust (see index for recipes).

## Pie Crust – Crepe Version
I developed this easy low calorie crust.  No rolling is needed.  It's not gritty and cuts well.  It's excellent for pumpkin pie, apple pie with streusel topping, and for quiches.  It works well for pies that don't have a top crust and are baked after you add the filling.

| | |
|---|---|
| 1 egg | ¼ cup cornstarch |
| 6 Tablespoons milk | Butter to grease the pan |
| 1 ½ teaspoons oil | |
| ⅛ teaspoon salt | |

Mix all ingredients, except the butter, in a blender.  (I use a hand blender and the mixing cup it comes with.)  Blend well.  Heat a 12 inch Teflon® skillet, add a little butter and swirl it around with your spatula to coat the pan.  (I use my largest fryer pan which has a flat bottom.)  Heat the pan a few minutes then lift it off the heat.  Pour in all the batter into the pan and tip pan from side to side until the bottom is evenly covered with the batter.  Return to medium heat.  Move the pan around on the burner, so that the batter looks dry on top over the entire crepe.  When it looks dry, remove it from heat and take a spatula and make sure it's not stuck anywhere.  With the help of the spatula, slide the crepe from the pan into a 10" of 9 ½" deep dish pie pan.  Carefully move it to center it in the pie pan.  It should be a perfect fit.

Fill with your pie filling (see index) and bake according to your recipe.  The crepe will brown on the top edge but does not burn.  The bottom texture is excellent, light, not gritty and holds up well.  This crust is also low in fat compared to regular pie crust.

*Variation*: Use ¼ cup Gluten-Free Naturals™ All Purpose Flour instead of cornstarch.  The crepe will be smaller and fit an 8 or 9 inch regular pie pan.

## Pie Crust – Cookie Crumb Version
This is a good use for leftover cookies.

¼ cup butter*, melted

1 ¼ cups fine gluten-free gingersnap crumbs or gluten-free vanilla wafer crumbs or other gluten-free cookie crumbs (see index for Gingersnap and Snickerdoodle recipes). You will need about 18 to 20 cookies.

Make cookie crumbs by pulverizing them in a food processor. Some cookies crumble easily, so you can also put them in a heavy plastic bag and a rolling pin to crush them.

Melt the butter in the microwave on the defrost cycle. I put it in a Pyrex® measuring cup because the high sides prevent spatters. Allow to cool a little.

Combine crumbs and butter. Pat into a 9 inch pie pan. Bake at 325°F for 10 minutes and cool. Fill with your favorite filling. It's also good for unbaked pies.

To make an ice cream pie, soften gluten-free ice cream* a little, fill crust, press in ice cream, and refreeze. Take out of the freezer a little before serving so it's easy to slice. Top with gluten-free whipped cream* or whipped topping* if desired.

## Pie Crust – Crumble Version
Easier to make than rolled-out pie crusts and it also makes a nice topping.

1 ½ cups Gluten-Free Naturals™ Cookie Blend (do not substitute)

½ cup sugar (do not eliminate)

Dash of salt

1 stick (½ cup) butter or 6 Tablespoons gluten-free margarine* plus 2 Tablespoons butter

Chopped nuts (optional)

Mix flour with the sugar and salt. Mix in 6 Tablespoons of butter or margarine with a pastry blender or fingers until all is mixed well and crumbs form. Remove half the crumbs and press into the bottom of your pie plate, going up the sides. Do not use a dark colored non-stick type pan or it will burn.

Pour in your filling. Take remaining crumbs. You may mix in some chopped nuts if desired. Take a handful of the crumb mixture and press tightly to form a big compressed lump. Now crumble this lump into good sized crumbs over the filling. Continue until all of the crumb mixture is used. Bake according to the directions on the pie filling recipe. Check half-way through the baking time. If the top gets too dark, cover with foil until it is done.

## Pie Crust – Mock Graham Cracker Crust
The combination of the gluten-free whole grain bread and cinnamon give this crust a flavor that reminds me of graham crackers.  Whenever I have leftover bread, I make dry bread crumbs.  This is a good use for them.

1 to 1 ¼ cups dry bread crumbs made from Gluten-Free Naturals™ Bread
6 Tablespoons sugar
½ to ¾ teaspoon ground cinnamon

¼ cup (½ stick) butter*, melted (I melt it in the microwave using the defrost cycle)

Blend bread crumbs, sugar, cinnamon and melted butter.  Taste the mixture to see if more sugar and cinnamon are needed.  I usually use ¾ teaspoon cinnamon.  Blend well.

Press into a 9 inch pie plate.  I use a rubber spatula.  Press the mixture on the sides and bottom.  For pies that have unbaked fillings (such as ice cream pies or no-bake cheesecake), bake the crust in a preheated 400°F oven for about 10 minutes.  The top edges will start to brown slightly, and the crust will set.  Allow the crust to cool completely before filling.  For pies that are going to be filled and then baked, you can eliminate the baking step, and just fill the crust and bake according to the directions of your pie filling recipe.

*Variation*:  Instead of dry bread crumbs, process 3 to 4 slices Gluten-Free Naturals™ Bread in a food processor.  This makes approximately 1 ½ cups moist crumbs, and because the moist crumbs compress, the extra amount is needed.  Add ¼ cup to 6 Tablespoons finely chopped nuts, such as pecans, walnuts or almonds.  Blend in the sugar, cinnamon and melted butter.  When using this method, I do the whole thing in the food processor.  Because the bread is not dried, the added nuts improve the texture so it is more like graham cracker crumbs.  I prefer the crust made with the dry bread crumbs, but if you don't have any this will work.

*Variation 2*:  Gluten-Free cereal* may be used instead of the gluten-free dry bread crumbs.  Grind it in the food processor to make about 1 ¼ cups of crumbs.

## Pie Crust – Pecan Version
This uses chopped nuts instead of flours.

1 ½ to 2 cups chopped pecans
¼ cup sugar

¼ cup (½ stick) butter or gluten-free margarine*

Chop nuts.  Mix ingredients together and press into a 9 inch pie plate.  For pies that have unbaked fillings (such as ice cream pies), bake crust in a 400°F oven for about 12 minutes.  If the crust slides down the sides, push it back using the back of a metal spoon.  Allow to completely cool.  Fill with filling.  For baked pies (such as baked pumpkin pie), eliminate this baking step.  Just fill and bake according to the directions of your pie filling recipe.

*see gluten-free products list at the end of the book*

## Pie Crust – Roll out Version

This pie crust works but is not as good as "Our Favorite" crust. It is also more difficult to work with.

¼ cup (heaping) cornstarch
¼ cup (heaping) tapioca starch or tapioca flour
¼ cup (heaping) defatted soy flour
2 Tablespoons potato flakes or potato flour (not potato starch)
1 ½ teaspoons xanthan gum

¼ teaspoon salt
2 teaspoons egg white powder
¼ cup sugar
½ cup butter, cold from the refrigerator
1 teaspoon vinegar
1 to 2 Tablespoons cold water (optional)

Blend the gluten-free flours, xanthan gum, salt, egg white powder and sugar. Put in the food processor. Add the cold butter using the cutting blade, pulse to cut the butter into the flours. Add the vinegar and continue pulsing until it forms a ball. If it doesn't form a ball well because it is dry, add the water 1 Tablespoon at a time and continue pulsing. If it is too wet, add a little more of the gluten-free flours. Once it forms a ball, you may now press the dough into the pan using your fingers, or refrigerate the ball for about an hour and roll it out. If pressing it into the pan and it's too wet, sprinkle a little flour on top and work it in. When rolling out I put waxed paper on the counter and sprinkle it with soy flour or cornstarch (or any flours listed above). Sprinkle a little more gluten-free flour on the top, cover with another piece of waxed paper and roll it out.

Once rolled out, remove top piece of waxed paper and then replace it. Flip the crust over. Remove the top waxed paper and replace it. My favorite method is to use a second pie pan as a mold. Slip it upside-down under the bottom waxed paper of the crust while it is on your counter. Form the crust on this pie plate. Remove the top waxed paper and put the pie plate you plan to bake it in upside-down on top. Now flip the whole thing over. Remove the top waxed paper. Your crust is in your pie plate. This is much easier than trying to flip the crust into the pan.

Unlike rice crusts, this will not be as hard to cut. You can make a couple of attempts to roll it or press it back together. You cannot "overwork" a gluten-free crust because there is no gluten which is what makes wheat crusts hard instead of flaky.

Bake at 350°F for about 30 minutes for a pre-baked crust, or fill with filling and bake according to directions. This recipe makes a single crust. If you need a double crust, it is easier to make the bottom crust in the processor and then going back and do the recipe again for the top crust. I often make the pre-baked pie crusts a day or two ahead of time, and fill with the filling the day of the party. Cover edges with a pie shield, or half-way through the baking time, cover your pie with foil so it doesn't burn.

*Variation*: If you don't have a food processor, you can make this crust using the traditional method of cutting the butter into the flours. Add the vinegar and water and blend until it forms a ball. Note: With this traditional method you can use butter at room temperature or Crisco® if you are lactose intolerant.

## Pie Crust – Rice Flour and Potato Flake Version

You can either press this in the pie plate or roll it out (see variation). It is a more crumbly than my other crusts, and doesn't cut as well as the other version.

½ cup sweet rice flour (available at Asian markets) or fine white rice flour
½ cup fine white rice flour
¼ cup potato flakes*

1 Tablespoon cornstarch
6 Tablespoons butter
6 Tablespoons cold water

Put all the dry ingredients into a food processor and pulse to blend. Add the butter, which you have cut into 6 or more pieces. Pulse until butter is cut into fine pieces. Measure the water and turn the processor back on and slowly pour in the water through the feed tube. The pie crust will dough up and form a ball.

Pat the dough into a 10" of 9 ½" deep dish pie pan, covering the bottoms and all the way up the sides. Prick with a fork and bake in a 350°F oven for 15 minutes. Allow it to cool. Note: Bake it the 15 minutes even if you are going to put in a filling that needs additional baking. This will give the crust a nice texture and keep it from getting soggy. You can cover the edges with foil during the second baking if they get too brown, but if you just press it up the sides and don't make fluting, this is not needed.

*Variation*: If you want to roll this crust out, use less water; about 2 or 3 Tablespoons. Roll it out between 2 pieces of waxed paper, to the size of your pan. It usually rolls out easily without adding extra flour to prevent sticking. Follow the directions under other "pie crust rolled out" recipe to get it into your pan. Cut off excess dough around edges. (This crust will crumble if you try to flute the edges). Fill with your filling and bake according to your recipe. I recommend you cover the edges with a pie shield. This crust slices more easily than some other pie crust versions.

## Pie Crust – Rice Flour (Brown and White) Version

My brother-in-law invented this version and it makes enough for a double crust pie. He provided instructions on how he makes such a thin crust, but I admit mine never turns out as good as his. We always enjoy his pies, and it also has less fat than most pie crust recipes. It is difficult to cut. For another rice flour version of pie crust made in a food processor, see Cranberry Pake recipe.

½ cup fine white rice flour
½ cup brown rice flour
1 teaspoon xanthan gum

2 to 3 Tablespoons butter
5 to 6 Tablespoons water

Blend flours and gum. Cut butter into flour using a fork or pastry blender. Slowly add water until the dough holds together.

Put down a piece of waxed paper on your counter. Sprinkle it with rice flour. Top with ½ of the dough. Press dough down a little, sprinkle with rice flour and cover with another piece of waxed paper. Roll until about half the size you need. Lift the waxed paper on top and sprinkle on a little more rice flour to avoid sticking. Do the same on the bottom. Now you can roll it very thin and it won't stick to the waxed paper. Remove top waxed paper,

*see gluten-free products list at the end of the book*

and flip it over your pie plate and remove back waxed paper. (For an easier way to get the crust into your pie plate, see directions in the Cranberry Pake recipe or the Pie Crust Roll out recipe).

Use new waxed paper and repeat for top crust. Follow the directions for your pie filling to get the baking times. Check pie half-way through to make sure the edges are not getting too brown. If so, cover with aluminum foil or a pie shield.

## Pie Crust – Shredded Coconut Version

3 Tablespoons butter*, softened but not melted

1 ½ cups sweetened flaked coconut*

Mix together using your hands and press into an 8" or 9" pie plate. Fill with your favorite filling and bake according to directions. For a baked crust for ice cream or pudding filled pies, bake at 325°F for 10 to 15 minutes until golden. Watch carefully as it can burn easily.

## Pumpkin Pecan Pie – Crustless Version
This pie is very easy to make, and non-celiacs have asked me for the recipe. The nuts give it a nice texture, since there is no crust on the bottom.

15 or 16 ounce can of pumpkin
12 ounce can evaporated milk
2 eggs
2 teaspoons gluten-free vanilla*
½ cup Gluten-Free Naturals™ All
   Purpose Flour
⅛ to ¼ teaspoon salt
1 ½ teaspoons gluten-free baking
   powder*
¼ cup oil

½ cup sugar (This pie is not very sweet. Use up to a ¼ cup more sugar if you prefer things sweeter.)
1 Tablespoon pumpkin pie spice (or I use 2 teaspoons ground cinnamon with ½ teaspoon ground nutmeg and either ½ teaspoon ground ginger or ground allspice)
¾ cup chopped pecans
Cool Whip®or gluten-free whipped cream* (optional)
Ground cinnamon (optional)

Preheat oven to 350°F. Grease a 10" or 9 ½" deep dish pie plate. In a blender or food processor or mixer beat together the pumpkin, evaporated milk, eggs, vanilla, flour, salt, baking powder, oil, sugar and pumpkin pie spice. Stir in pecans. Pour into the pie plate. Bake for 50 to 55 minutes or until a knife inserted in the center comes out clean. Cool completely. Can be made days ahead of time and refrigerated. Before serving, top with cream. Sprinkle with cinnamon if desired.

## Pumpkin Pie – Crustless Version
This pie is very easy to make.  Serve with whipped cream or Cool Whip® for best flavor.

15 or 16 ounce can of pumpkin
12 ounce can evaporated milk
2 Tablespoons oil
2 eggs
¾ cup sugar
⅓ cup fine white rice flour
⅛ teaspoon salt

¾ teaspoon gluten-free baking powder*
2 ½ teaspoons pumpkin pie spice
2 teaspoons gluten-free vanilla*
Gluten-free whipped cream* or Cool
     Whip® for garnish (optional)

Preheat oven to 350°F.  Grease a 10" or 9 ½" deep dish pie plate.  In a large bowl, combine all ingredients except for the whipped cream.  With an electric mixer beat 2 minutes or with a hand blender mix 1 minute or so until well mixed.  Pour the mixture into the pie plate.  Bake for 50 to 60 minutes or until a knife inserted in the center comes out clean.  All to cool and refrigerate before serving.

*Variation*:  When I didn't have pumpkin pie spice, I used 2 teaspoons ground cinnamon, ½ teaspoon ground nutmeg and ¼ teaspoon ground ginger and it was very good.

*Variation 2*:  Gluten-Free Naturals™ All Purpose Flour can be used instead of rice flour.

## Pumpkin Pie
This is a pumpkin pie filling from my mother.  I like this with the Gluten-Free Naturals™ Cookie Blend Crust or the crepe pie crust.  I served it for company recently and they asked me for the recipe.  It has a stronger flavor than other pumpkin pie recipes.

1 recipe pie crust made in a 9" pie pan
     (We like "Our Favorite" crust best, but
     the "Sweet Crust" and the "Crepe
     Crust" also work in this recipe.)
1 ¾ cups canned pumpkin (15 oz. can)
½ cup brown sugar
½ cup white sugar
½ teaspoon salt

1 Tablespoon ground cinnamon (I use 2
     teaspoons)
⅛ teaspoon ground ginger
2 eggs
1 teaspoon molasses (optional)
1 cup evaporated milk
¼ cup orange juice or evaporated milk

Mix all together and pour into a prepared gluten-free pastry shell (see index).  Bake in a preheated 375°F oven.  Place pie on the lower shelf if using my traditional crust or middle shelf for the crepe crust.  Bake for 45-50 minutes or until all but the center 2 inches of filling is set.  It will set when cool.

*Variation*:  For a firmer pie filling, use 3 eggs instead of 2.  Use 1 cup evaporated milk only and eliminate the orange juice.

## Pumpkin Spice and Molasses Pie

This is a good use for leftover gluten-free cookies.  This pumpkin filling uses milk instead of evaporated milk.

¼ cup butter*, melted (I do this in the microwave using the defrost cycle)
20 gluten-free molasses spice cookies, ginger snaps, or other cookies, crushed
1 (15 ounce) can pumpkin (not pumpkin pie filling – ingredients should just be pumpkin)
3 eggs
1 Tablespoon cornstarch
1 teaspoon ground cinnamon

½ teaspoon ground nutmeg
½ teaspoon ground ginger
1 cup sugar
½ teaspoon salt
2 to 4 Tablespoons molasses (depending on your preference)
1 cup milk (I use 2%)
Whipped cream* (optional)

Crush cookies and mix with butter.  (You can crush them using a food processor, or by putting the cookies in a heavy-duty freezer type bag, sealing it, and crushing them with a rolling pin.)  Press into a 9 ½ or 10 inch deep dish glass pie pan.

Mix pumpkin and eggs together in an electric mixer on high for 2 minutes.  Add the rest of ingredients and blend for about 1 minute or until smooth.  Pour into cookie crust.  Bake in a preheated 400°F oven.  Bake for 15 minutes, then reduce oven temperature to 350°F and bake for 25 to 30 minutes more.  All but about the center 2 inches of filling will be set.  It will set when cool.  It's nice served with whipped cream as a garnish.

## Ricotta Pie

This is an Italian cheesecake that is very heavy and dense.  If you're Italian and grew up with this, I'm sure you'll enjoy this recipe.  I do, but I admit that it's an acquired taste.  Not everyone in my family likes it.  My husband prefers the crustless cheese cake recipe (see index) which is much less work and a lot creamier.  As for me, I like leftovers of this for breakfast.

Sweet Pastry:
2 cups Gluten-Free Naturals™ All Purpose Flour or Gluten-Free Naturals™ Cookie Blend
Pinch of salt
3 ½ ounces butter

½ cup sugar
1 egg
1 egg yolk
Grated rind of 1 lemon
Little cold water if needed

Filling:
3 lbs. of gluten-free Ricotta cheese
8 eggs
1 whole orange rind, grated

2 cups sugar
2 Tablespoons gluten-free vanilla*
⅓ cup fine rice flour

Mix together the gluten-free flour, sugar and salt.  Cut in the butter.  Beat egg and egg yolk together, and blend into flour mixture.  Form into a ball.  Mix in a little cold water if dough is too stiff and dry.  I suggest taking your large ball of dough and making 3 balls of dough.

One for the bottom, one for the sides, and one for 5 to 6 strips for the top.  Let dough stand 1 hour covered in the refrigerator before rolling out.

Grease a 10 inch spring-form pan.  Cut a piece of waxed paper, sprinkle with a little Cookie Blend and put less than ½ the dough on it (or one dough balls as noted above).  Top with waxed paper and roll out.  Use this to cover the inside bottom of the pan.  I suggest you flip your dough over, remove bottom waxed paper, replace, flip back over and remove top waxed paper.  Now it will go easily on the bottom.  You can remove the bottom spring-form, put dough on bottom, remove excess dough and replace spring-form.

Now roll out a larger piece of dough (not all of it) using new waxed paper.  Cut into strips as deep as your pan to cover the sides.  (Since our pie crusts are not made with regular flour, you can add any extra dough left from rolling out the bottom.)  Once it's rolled out, repeat as above in removing the waxed paper.  Piece it together using your hands if you have to and press together in the pan.  Press the side and bottom seams together.  Now use a little dough to make 5 or 6 strips (1 inch) to lattice on top of cake.  Remove waxed paper as above.  Then I cut all the strips with a pastry wheel to give a decorative edging.

Blend all the filling ingredients together.  Now place a little at a time in a blender and beat just until smooth.  Pour into shell and continue until all cheese mixture is blended.  Place thin pastry strips on top of Ricotta cheese mixture in a crisscross pattern.  Do not weave, just place them going one way and top with strips going the other way.  Now take a dull knife and push down over filling any side strip dough that is sticking up higher than the filling.  This makes a nice finished edge and keeps that dough from burning.  Brush with beaten egg and bake 350°F for 30 minutes.  Then put the oven at 450°F and bake 10 minutes longer.  (If dough is getting too dark during baking, cover with foil although I have not found this necessary.)

## Strawberry Cloud Pie
This pie has meringue on the bottom for a crust, with strawberries and whipped cream on top.

3 egg whites
½ teaspoon gluten-free baking powder*
1 cup sugar (if berries are very sweet, I use less sugar – about ¾ cup)
¼ cup fine white rice flour
½ teaspoon gluten-free vanilla* or gluten-free vanillin* (optional)

½ cup chopped pecans
1 (1 lb.) box strawberries or 1 quart
½ cup gluten-free heavy cream*, whipped or use gluten-free whipped cream* in a can.

Grease a 9 or 9 ½ inch pie plate.  Whip egg whites and baking powder in an electric mixer until frothy.  Gradually add in the sugar and continue to whip in the electric mixer until you have stiff peaks.  Your meringue will become high and glossy.  I test meringue for doneness by rubbing a small amount between my fingers until I don't feel any grittiness from the sugar.  The secret to a good meringue is having the sugar melt in and become well incorporate with the egg whites.

Now whip in the rice flour a few minutes.  Add the vanilla (optional) and mix it in with the mixer. (I don't use the vanilla).  Fold in chopped pecans by hand using a rubber spatula.  Spread the meringue into your pie plate.  If desired, form it like a crust making an indent in the middle for the berries.  Bake at 300°F for 30 to 35 minutes until set.  Allow to completely cool. (Note – do not cool it quickly in your refrigerator or you will ruin your meringue.  Cool it at room temperature.)

Wash and dry strawberries.  Slice and place on top of meringue crust.  Do not sweeten the strawberries because the crust is already very sweet.  Cover with plastic wrap and refrigerate for several hours.  Immediately before serving, top with gluten-free whipped cream*.  I like to use the type of cream in an aerosol can because you can spray the cream on top in a nice design.

*Variation*:  If you want to use egg white powder* instead of fresh egg whites, I suggest you mix the amount of powder for 3 egg whites with ¼ cup of your sugar and the baking powder.  Add the water needed to reconstitute the powder and mix it in.  Now start whipping it in your mixer.  Gradually add the rest of the sugar and follow the directions as above.  Using this method keeps the egg white powder from clumping; i.e. having lumps that don't mix in.

## Strawberry Tarts, Miniatures

These take some time to make, but they look nice on a dessert table.  I use disposable aluminum mini muffin pans so that it is easier to remove them.  You can press them out from the bottom and they retain their shape.  Mini muffin papers may also be used.

Make pie crust for 2 crusts (see index).
  We prefer "Our Favorite" version in this recipe, since it is easier to work with to make the miniature tarts
3 boxes strawberries
1 cup sugar
3 Tablespoons cornstarch
1 Tablespoon Grand Marnier®*
1 ½ teaspoons lemon juice

Red coloring
6 ounces gluten-free cream cheese*, softened
½ cup sugar
½ cup gluten-free heavy cream*, whipped
½ teaspoon gluten-free vanilla* or gluten-free vanillin*

Prepare pie crust.  Make 50 small balls of dough.  Press into each miniature muffin tin and cover the bottom and the sides.  Freeze the tins, with shells in them, for 10 minutes then bake in a preheated 400°F oven for 15 minutes.  Watch carefully near the end of baking time so that they don't burn. (If using Gluten-Free Naturals™ All Purpose Flour, this is not an issue.)

Go through the strawberries, wash and hull them.  Select 1 box of the least perfect berries to puree.  Measure puree and add enough water to make 1 ½ cups.  Place puree and water into a saucepan and add the 1 cup sugar, cornstarch, Grand Marnier®, lemon juice and few drops red food coloring.  Cook and stir until mixture comes to a boil and thickens.  Set aside.  Dry the perfect berries.  Make filling by mixing the softened cream cheese, ½ cup sugar, whipped cream and vanilla extract together.

*see gluten-free products list at the end of the book

Cool tart shells. (Once cooled, I remove them from the pan. If they are not stuck to the pan, you can remove them later.) Place 1 teaspoon of the cream cheese filling in each. Top each tart with a perfect berry and spoon enough glaze over to cover the filling and glaze berry. Makes 50. This recipe can be cut in half.

## Whipped Lemon Cheese Pie – No Bake Filling

This is lemony no bake cheesecake without eggs. The original recipe called for vanilla yogurt but we found it too sweet so we prefer the plain yogurt. Plain yogurt is gluten-free but some brands of vanilla yogurt are not.

1 gluten-free mock graham cracker crust
  (see index for recipe)
2 envelopes Knox® unflavored gelatin
½ cup cold water
1 (8 ounce) package gluten-free cream
  cheese*, softened
½ cup sugar

2 cups plain yogurt
1 teaspoon gluten-free vanilla* (optional, I
  don't use)
1 (6 ounce) can of gluten-free frozen
  lemonade, thawed
½ cup water

Prepare the gluten-free crust in a 9 or 10 inch pie plate. If you used a crust that you baked, set it aside to cool. The crust can be made ahead of time.

Pour 2 envelopes of gelatin over ½ cup cold water. Let it sit for 2 minutes. Microwave 40 seconds on high and stir to dissolve. If not dissolved, repeat. Set aside.

In a heavy duty mixer, mix the cream cheese and sugar until well incorporated. Turn speed to low and add the gelatin mixture and blend. Scrape sides of bowl and then add the yogurt, ½ cup water, and lemonade on low speed. Once well incorporated, blend on higher speed for several minutes until very smooth and creamy. Fill cooled pie shell. Cover with plastic wrap and chill in the refrigerator. It will take about 4 hours to completely set. I usually make this a day ahead of time.

*Variation*: For key lime cheese pie, substitute gluten-free limeade for lemonade.

# COOKIES

Cookies made with Gluten-Free Naturals™ Cookie Blend are just like the real thing! These are our family-favorite recipes. Use leftover crushed cookies for wonderful cookie crumb crusts for pies. (See index for recipe). Cookies made with Gluten-Free Naturals™ Cookie Blend freeze very well.

When converting your own family recipes, choose recipes that contain granulated sugar. Cookies made using powdered sugar won't hold together as well and will require additional xanthan gum.

You can substitute Gluten-Free Naturals™ All Purpose Flour for the Gluten-Free Naturals™ Cookie Blend in these recipes. The cookies will taste sweeter than with the Cookie Blend.

## Biscotti
These travel well. I enjoy them with a cup of coffee.

1 egg
⅓ cup water
⅓ cup sugar
1 cup Gluten-Free Naturals™ Pancake
  Mix

¼ to ⅓ cup oil (I prefer ¼ cup which
  makes them lower in fat.)
½ teaspoon almond extract (I use a little
  more)
½ teaspoon baking powder
2 heaping Tablespoons sliced almonds

Grease a glass loaf pan. Mix all ingredients together in an electric mixer and pour into prepared pan. Bake at 350°F for 30 to 35 minutes.

Remove from oven, and slice into ½ inch slices. Loosen the edge with your knife and carefully empty the loaf pan onto a cookie sheet. (A dark non-stick cookie sheet may be used to make them extra crunchy.)

Put the slices in a single layer on the pan. Bake for 15 minutes. Turn with a spatula and bake 15 minutes more. Allow to cool completely and store.

*Variation*: To make Anise Toasts, eliminate almonds and almond extract and substitute anise extract.

## Blondies – or Butterscotch Brownies
An easy bar cookie that is especially good for those who don't like chocolate. I have made these for people who do not have celiac disease and they had no idea they were gluten-free. This is also a good cookie for people who can't have chocolate.

¼ cup oil
1 cup brown sugar, packed
1 teaspoon gluten-free vanilla*
1 egg
¾ cup Gluten-Free Naturals™ Cookie
  Blend

½ teaspoon xanthan gum
½ cup chopped nuts
1 teaspoon gluten-free baking powder*
½ teaspoon salt

*see gluten-free products list at the end of the book*

Blend the oil with the sugar, vanilla and egg using a whisk. Add remaining ingredients and blend with a metal or sturdy spoon. Put into a greased 8 x 8 inch pan. Bake at 350°F for 25 to 35 minutes. Cool and cut into squares.

## Brownie Cheesecake Bites

Delicious and decadent. This makes a large pan for a crowd. You can freeze any leftovers, so this is a treat you can make ahead of time and defrost for a party.

1 Gluten-Free Naturals™ Brownie Mix, prepared as directed on the package

4 (8 ounce) packages gluten-free cream cheese*

1 cup sugar

4 eggs

1 teaspoon gluten-free vanilla*

½ cup gluten-free whipping cream*

6 ounces gluten-free semi-sweet chocolate chips*

Prepare brownie mix as directed on package, and spread into a greased 13 x 9 inch baking pan. For best results use a non-stick or glass pan. To blend the brownies easily, use a heavy-duty mixer.

Preheat oven to 350°F. In the same mixing bowl (no need to clean it) blend cream cheese, sugar, vanilla and eggs. Mix until well blended. If you have a heavy duty mixer, you can whip it at high speed to get rid of any lumps, and also make the cheesecake portion lighter in texture. Pour cheese mixture over brownie mixture. Gently spread the cheese layer over the brownie layer. It's ok to get some of the chocolate into the cheese mixture.

Bake for 40 minutes, or until the center is almost set. Allow to cool at least 1 ½ hours before adding the topping. In a microwave safe bowl (I use a 2-cup Pyrex® measuring cup), measure the ½ cup whipping cream and add the 6 ounces of chips. (Note: the two ingredients together measure 1 cup; so you don't have to weigh the chips.) Microwave on the defrost cycle for 6 minutes or until chips are melted. Stir well to blend. Or, put the cream and chips into a saucepan and stir and cook until chips are melted. Be careful not to burn the bottom.

Pour the chocolate mixture over the cheese mixture, and spread to cover. The cheesecake portion will form an edge, so it is easy to keep the chocolate within that edge.

Refrigerate for 3 hours or overnight before serving to set the cheesecake and the chocolate topping. Cut into small pieces and serve. Store the leftovers in the refrigerator or freezer.

## Brownies – Flourless Walnut Truffle Style

Gluten-Free Naturals™ Homemade Brownie Mix is the closest to the real thing. But if you want to make a chocolate dessert without any special gluten-free ingredients, this recipe may be for you. It uses the finely chopped walnuts in place of flour. It is a little crumbly without any added gums, but it has a nice flavor.

4 egg whites
1 Tablespoon sugar
4 egg yolks
¾ cups oil (I use corn or canola oil)
1 cup to 1 ¼ cup sugar

¾ cup cocoa, preferably Dutch processed
½ cup finely chopped (ground) walnuts
2 teaspoons gluten-free vanilla*
Confectioner's sugar for garnish (optional)

With an electric mixer with clean beaters, whip the egg whites and 1 Tablespoon sugar. Beat until stiff with soft peaks.

In another mixer bowl, blend together the egg yolks, oil, cocoa and sugar. Blend in the vanilla and walnuts using the mixer.

Fold the chocolate mixture into the egg white mixture. Pour into a greased 9 inch square pan or an 11 x 17 inch pan and spread until smooth. Bake at 425°F for 20 to 25 minutes, until a cake tester comes out clean. Cool completely. If desired, put them in the refrigerator so that they will be more firm and a little easier to serve. If desired, garnish with Confectioner's sugar.

## Chinese Almond Cookies

This is an old Chinese recipe that I adapted. These are a plain tasting cookie. It reminds me a little of some of the store bought gluten-free cookies that are made with rice flour. You can make these cookies without eggs if you are allergic to eggs.

3 Tablespoons butter, softened
½ cup white rice flour
¼ cup brown sugar, packed

1 cup blanched almonds, ground
About 1 Tablespoon water (or less)
2 teaspoons egg white powder (optional)

Put butter, rice flour, brown sugar and ground almonds in a mixer. Add egg white powder if using. Blend until incorporated. Slowly add the water, adding enough to make the dough hold together. (Depending upon how much almond flour you add, the water needed can vary from a few drops to a Tablespoon.) Blend together. Since this dough has no gluten, you can work it with your hands if needed.

Shape dough into small balls. Use your hands to press the dough together into balls. Place them on a greased cookie sheet and allow space between the cookies. Bake at 350°F for about 15 minutes until golden brown. Makes about 24 cookies.

## Chocolate Chip Cookies

These are the Toll House® cookies that you remember!  I have served these to non-celiacs who thought they were regular homemade chocolate chip cookies, and had no idea they were gluten-free.  These cookies freeze very well and I have successfully stored them for months in freezer bags.  It's nice to have fresh cookies on hand to add to lunches or for a snack.

When using the Gluten-Free Naturals® All Purpose Flour, I pack the measuring cup slightly.  Otherwise the cookies turn out a little flatter and sweeter than the traditional Toll House cookies.

½ cup butter or gluten-free margarine*
6 Tablespoons sugar (¼ cup plus 2 Tablespoons)
6 Tablespoons brown sugar, packed (¼ cup plus 2 Tablespoons)
1 egg
1 teaspoon gluten-free vanilla extract*

1 ¼ cups Gluten-Free Naturals™ Cookie Blend or Gluten-Free Naturals™ All Purpose Flour
¾ teaspoon salt
½ teaspoon baking soda
1 cup gluten-free semi-sweet chocolate chips* (I use a little less)
½ cup nuts (optional, I don't use)

Cream the butter and sugars and blend until fluffy.  Add the egg and vanilla and blend in.  Add the flour, salt, baking soda, and xanthan gum and blend.  Add the chocolate chips (and nuts if using; I prefer without).  Refrigerate dough for 30 to 60 minutes.  (If you don't refrigerate the dough, they turn out flat.)  Drop by teaspoonfuls on to an ungreased baking sheet.  Bake at 375°F for 10 minutes.  Cool 2 minutes on the pan, and then remove to a wire rack.  If they are breaking as you try to get them off the pan, you are removing them too early and let them cool a few more minutes.

These cookies keep as well as the wheat version, but I admit they're usually gone so fast it's hard to tell.  They also freeze very well.  If wrapped well they keep for several months in the freezer.

## Chocolate Chip Cookies, Version 2

These are more difficult to work with than the above recipe, but are good.  They do break apart more easily and do dry out more quickly than the cookies in previous recipe.

1 cup (2 sticks) butter or gluten-free margarine*
¾ cup sugar
¾ cup brown sugar*
2 eggs
2 teaspoons gluten-free vanilla*
¾ cup defatted soy flour
¾ cup white rice flour
¾ cup cornstarch

2 ¼ teaspoons xanthan gum
1 teaspoon methylcellulose (Sure Gel®)
1 teaspoon baking soda
½ teaspoon salt
1 cup chopped walnuts
1 (12 ounce) bag (2 cups) gluten-free semi-sweet chocolate chips

Cream butter and sugars together.  Blend in the eggs and vanilla.  In another bowl, whisk together the flours, xanthan gum, methylcellulose, baking soda, salt, walnuts and chips.

*see gluten-free products list at the end of the book*

Blend the flour mixture into the butter mixture. Cream together until well blended.

Drop by teaspoonfuls onto an ungreased cookie sheet. I use an Airbake® pan. Bake at 375°F for 13 minutes. If using a regular pan, bake them less (about 9 or 10 minutes). They should be golden brown. Remove cookie sheet from oven and let sit for about 3 or 4 minutes. Then remove cookies to a wire rack to cool. If you remove them immediately they will break because they are too fragile when very hot. Delicious!

## Chocolate Chip "Forgotten" Cookies
A melt in your mouth meringue cookie. Since these are very sweet, I don't make the cookies too large.

2 egg whites, or equivalent egg white
   powder plus water
⅛ teaspoon cream of tartar
⅛ teaspoon salt

⅔ cup sugar
1 teaspoon gluten-free vanilla*
1 cup semi-sweet chocolate chips*

Heat oven to 375°F. Grease a cookie sheet. Beat the egg whites with the cream of tartar and salt in a medium bowl until it forms soft peaks. Gradually beat in the sugar, one Tablespoon at a time. Continue beating until stiff peaks form. The egg white mixture will look glossy. Feel it with your fingers and if there is no grit, then the sugar is dissolved and it has been mixed enough. Gently blend in the vanilla and fold in the chocolate chips.

Drop the meringue by teaspoons onto the prepared cookie sheet. Place the cookies in the preheated oven. Turn off the oven and allow the cookies to remain overnight or until the oven has cooled completely. Makes 36 cookies.

## Coconut Brown Sugar Bars
These bar cookies don't use butter or margarine, so it's good for a lactose-free diet. I prefer the coconut dream bar recipe (next recipe) over this one, but this recipe is good for those who can't have butter or margarine.

¼ cup oil
1 cup gluten-free brown sugar
1 egg
¾ cup Gluten-Free Naturals™ Cookie
   Blend or Gluten-Free Naturals™ All
   Purpose Flour
1 teaspoon gluten-free baking powder*

½ teaspoon xanthan gum (eliminate if
   using Gluten-Free Naturals™ All
   Purpose Flour)
⅛ teaspoon salt
½ cup chopped nuts, (I use walnuts or
   pecans)
1 cup grated coconut*

Blend oil, sugar and egg in a heavy duty mixer (such as a KitchenAid®). Add the rest of the ingredients and blend with the mixer. Spread into a greased 9 x 9 inch pan. If difficult to spread, wet the spatula with water. Bake at 350°F for 25 to 35 minutes, until it tests done with a cake tester. Cool completely and cut into squares.

## Coconut Dream Bars (very easy)

These are a family favorite. A mixer makes these cookies quick and easy to put together. Every time I have served them, people love them. No one thinks they are gluten-free. These cookies freeze very well and I have successfully stored them for months in freezer bags.

| | |
|---|---|
| 1 ½ cups Gluten-Free Naturals™ Cookie Blend or Gluten-Free Naturals™ All Purpose Flour | 1 ½ cups packed brown sugar |
| | 3 eggs |
| | 1 teaspoon gluten-free baking powder* |
| ½ cup packed brown sugar | 2 teaspoons gluten-free vanilla* |
| ½ cup butter or gluten-free margarine*, softened | ¼ teaspoon salt |
| | 1 ½ cups gluten-free flaked coconut* |

Preheat oven to 350°. Put the Cookie Blend, 1/2 cup of the brown sugar and the butter in the bowl of a mixer. Mix on low speed until the particles of the butter are fine. Press into the bottom of a greased 9" x 13" non-stick pan. Bake at 350° for 15 minutes.

Using the same mixer bowl (no need to wash it), beat the 1 1/2 cups brown sugar with the eggs just until blended. Mix in the remaining ingredients. Spread over partially baked crust. I spread it to the edges. Bake for 20 to 25 minutes, or until golden brown. Cool completely, and then cut into bars. If they are difficult to cut, cut the entire batch into 4 large pieces, then I remove them from the pan and cut the rest of them using a pizza cutter.

*Variation*: This recipe was featured on the Gluten-Free Naturals™ Cookie Blend because everyone liked it so much. You can substitute Gluten-Free Naturals™ All Purpose Flour in this recipe.

## Coconut Almond Macaroons

| | |
|---|---|
| 2 ⅔ cups flaked coconut | ½ teaspoon salt |
| ⅔ cup sugar | 4 egg whites |
| ¼ cup Gluten-Free Naturals™ Cookie Blend or Gluten-Free Naturals™ All Purpose Flour | 1 teaspoon gluten-free almond extract* |
| | 1 cup almonds, finely chopped |

Combine the coconut, sugar, rice flour and salt in a bowl. Stir in the egg whites and almond extract. Stir in the almonds and mix well. Drop by teaspoonfuls onto lightly greased baking sheets. Bake cookies in a 300°F for 20 to 25 minutes or until the edges are golden brown. Remove immediately to a wire rack and cool.

*Variation*: Fine white rice flour may be substituted for the Cookie Blend in this recipe, for those with allergies.

## Coconut Macaroons (flourless version)

These cookies do not require any special gluten-free ingredients.  They are a good choice if you want a cookie that you can make with items from the grocery store.

3 egg whites
¼ teaspoon cream of tartar
⅛ teaspoon salt
¾ cup sugar

¼ teaspoon gluten-free almond or vanilla extract*
2 cups flaked coconut

Beat the egg whites, cream of tartar and salt until foamy.  Add the sugar, 1 Tablespoon at a time and keep beating until it is stiff and glossy.  When all of the sugar is gone (and when you rub a little of the dough between your fingers and feel no grit) it is done.  Fold in the extract and the coconut.  Drop by teaspoonfuls about 1 inch apart onto a foil-covered cookie sheet.  Bake in a 300°F oven for 20 to 25 minutes.  Cool 10 minutes and remove from the foil.  Store in an airtight container for 2 weeks or freeze.

## Coconut Macaroons made with Sweetened Condensed Milk

This version doesn't require any special gluten-free ingredients, and is also egg-free.  They are very sweet.

1 (15 ounce) can sweetened condensed milk (not evaporated milk)

1 (16 ounce) package shredded coconut
2 teaspoons gluten-free vanilla*

Blend all ingredients in a mixing bowl.  Drop by teaspoonfuls about 1 inch apart onto a foil-covered well-greased cookie sheet.  Bake in a 350°F oven for 8 to 10 minutes or until edges are golden browned.  Cool slightly and remove as soon as you are able to handle them.  Makes about 4 dozen cookies.

*Variation*: Use ⅔ cup sweetened condensed milk, 3 cups coconut, 1 teaspoon gluten-free vanilla* and ¾ teaspoon almond extract* instead of as listed above.  Makes 1 ½ dozen cookies.

## Cornflake Peanut Butter Treats

½ cup sugar
½ cup gluten-free corn syrup*
½ cup gluten-free peanut butter*

½ cup chopped peanuts (optional)
4 cups gluten-free cornflakes*

Line a 9-inch square pan with plastic wrap.  In a saucepan, combine the sugar and syrup.  Cook over medium heat and boil for 1 minute, stirring occasionally.  Remove from heat and add peanut butter (and peanuts, if using).  Pour in cornflakes and coat.  Quickly press it into your pan.  Allow it to cool for 15 minutes or so.  Remove from pan by turning it over onto a large cutting board.  Remove plastic wrap.  Cut into squares.

*see gluten-free products list at the end of the book

## Fortune Cookies

You can have fortune cookies again!  These are crispy, delicious cookies that are fun to make.  They start out like little pancakes and turn into cookies.  No special gluten-free flours are needed for this recipe.

1 large egg
1 to 2 Tablespoons oil (I use the lower
    amount of oil.  If you find that the
    cookies are sticking, increase the oil).
¼ cup sugar
¼ cup cornstarch

¼ teaspoon gluten-free vanilla extract*
    (optional, or orange extract may also be
    used for a different flavor.)
Fortunes written on small papers
    (optional)

Blend the egg, oil and sugar together with a whisk.  Gradually add the cornstarch and whisk it in until smooth.  Blend in vanilla with the whisk.  (A mixer may also be used if a larger batch is being made.)

Heat a Teflon® skillet or fry pan.  Grease it with a little oil, butter or cooking spray.  Pour 1 Tablespoon of batter into the pan.  Use a long handled spoon to spread that amount of batter to make about a 3 inch pancake.

Cook on medium heat until the edges brown.  Flip and cook the other side.  Remove from pan onto a plate.  (At this point I pour my next pancake which allows the one I just removed to cool slightly so I can handle it.)

Place fortune paper in the center of the cookies, if using.  Fold the cookie in half so you have the flat seam on the bottom.  Now hold each outer edge using one index finger on each side.  Push your two thumbs into the middle of the flat seam to form a fortune cookie shape, while pulling down the sides with your index fingers.  Place cookies on a cookie sheet.  Continue until all of your batter is finished.  This amount makes 12 cookies.  (Or, you can use the batter to make 6 large fortune cookies, and insert checks or poems inside as gifts.)  This recipe can be easily doubled.

Preheat your oven to 200°F.  Place the cookies in the oven for about 1 hour to completely dry and crisp them.  Now they will keep for a long time.  Allow to cool completely and enjoy!  (You can skip this step if they are to be eaten immediately, but they will be less crisp.)

Note: Fortune papers are easier to insert before folding, but can be done afterwards.  It's a fun project to have children write up the fortunes.  (Don't reuse fortune papers from gluten containing cookies, or they will contaminate your gluten-free cookies.) Store the leftover cookies in an airtight container, so that they will remain crisp.

*see gluten-free products list at the end of the book

## Gingerbread Cookies

These are the roll out cookies that are perfect for the holidays.  This is my mother-in-law's recipe.  These are the soft gingerbread cookies you remember.

½ cup butter, gluten-free margarine* or
  shortening
½ cup brown sugar
½ cup molasses*
1 egg
1 teaspoon baking powder*
½ teaspoon baking soda
1 teaspoon ground ginger
½ teaspoon ground cinnamon

½ teaspoon ground cloves (or eliminate
  the cloves and double the amount of
  cinnamon)
½ teaspoon ground allspice (optional)
2 ½ cups Gluten-Free Naturals™ Cookie
  Blend (or enough to make stiff dough)
  or Gluten-Free Naturals™ All Purpose
  Flour

Cream the butter and sugar.  Add molasses and egg.  Add baking powder, baking soda, spices and part of the Cookie Blend.  Mix in and then stir in the remaining Cookie Blend.  Add more Cookie Blend, if needed.  Chill dough for easy handling.  (Note: this dough can be made in a heavy-duty mixer.)

Roll dough between waxed paper to a thickness that is between ⅛ to ¼ inch thick.  Don't go any thinner or the cookies will break more easily.  Cut into cookie shapes using cookie cutters.  Since there is no gluten, it is fine to keep re-rolling any leftover dough.  (In wheat cookies re-rolling makes the cookies tough because of the gluten.)  It is easier to cut out cookies using metal open cookie cutters.  If you have the closed type that imprint designs, "flour" those cookie cutters with some Cookie Blend or rice flour so that the cookies don't stick inside them.  For best results choose smaller sized cutters.  Very large size cutters may be used, but if the cookies are stacked in a container they will break more easily.  Store large cookies on a plate and cover with foil or plastic wrap.

Place cookies on a baking sheet.  Bake at 375°F for 10 to 12 minutes.  Cool 2 minutes and remove from pan to a cooling rack.  When cooled, decorate if desired.  Decorator's icing (see sugar cookies – "whiteboys" recipe) may be used.  Makes about 3 dozen.

## Ginger Snaps

Crispy, delicious and they keep well.  They don't fall apart and travel well too.  Leftovers can be pulverized and used to make a nice cookie crumb crust under pumpkin pie.

¾ cup sugar
1 cup brown sugar (light or dark), packed
5 Tablespoons butter*, gluten-free
  margarine* or shortening*
¼ cup molasses*
1 egg
1 teaspoon gluten-free vanilla*
¼ cup water (room temperature not hot)

2 ½ cups Gluten-Free Naturals™ Cookie
  Blend or Gluten-Free Naturals™ All
  Purpose Flour
2 teaspoons ground ginger
1 ½ teaspoons ground cinnamon (or use 1
  teaspoon cinnamon and ½ teaspoon
  ground cloves)
2 teaspoons baking soda
1 teaspoon salt

*see gluten-free products list at the end of the book

-464-

Blend the sugar and brown sugar in a bowl.  If butter is not room temperature, put in the microwave on defrost for about 30 seconds to make it softer.  Cream butter and sugar together.  After well blended, add molasses, egg, vanilla and water and blend well.

Whisk together the Cookie Blend, ginger, cinnamon, baking soda, and salt.  Add to the sugar mixture and blend well.  Refrigerate to make the dough easy to work with.  If you're in a rush, put it in the freezer for about 10 minutes and use the top dough that's chilled.  Return to freezer and repeat until all cookies are made.

Roll dough into 1 inch or smaller balls.  I place on an ungreased light-color Teflon® coated pan.  If you do not have a non-stick type pan, lightly grease the pan.  Place the balls at least 1 inch apart as the dough will spread a lot.  Bake for about 11 minutes at 375°F.  If you made yours smaller than 1", check after 10 minutes; larger than 1" may need 14 minutes.  Cool on pan for 1-2 minutes before removing so that the cookies hold together and don't fall apart.  Don't wait longer than 5 minutes or they will start to stick to the pan.  Cool on racks.  This recipe makes over 100 crunchy cookies that stay crispy.

## Hermits
**A delicious old fashioned molasses type cookie.**

¼ cup milk or gluten-free milk substitute
6 Tablespoons raisins
¼ cup oil
¼ cup molasses*
½ cup brown or white sugar
1 ½ cups Gluten-Free Naturals™ Cookie Blend or Gluten-Free Naturals™ All Purpose Flour

½ teaspoon xanthan gum (eliminate if using Gluten-Free Naturals™ All Purpose Flour)
½ teaspoon ground cinnamon
¼ teaspoon ground nutmeg
½ teaspoon baking soda
¼ teaspoon salt
¼ cup chopped walnuts

Blend the milk, raisins, molasses and oil together.  Set aside so that the raisins plump a little.  Blend together the flour, xanthan gum, spices, baking soda, salt and walnuts.  With a heavy metal spoon, blend together.  Grease an 8 x 8 inch baking pan.  Press the dough evenly into the pan.  Bake in a 350°F oven for 15 to 20 minutes.  Allow to cool, slice and serve.

## Holly Confections

30 large gluten-free marshmallows*
½ cup butter or gluten-free margarine*
1 ½ teaspoons green food coloring

3 cups gluten-free cornflakes* (whole, not crumbs)
Gluten-free cinnamon Red Hots® candy*

Melt marshmallows and butter in a double boiler, or in a Teflon® pot on low heat.  Stir in coloring and remove from heat.  Add cornflakes mixing quickly and gently until all are coated.  Drop from a teaspoon onto waxed paper.  Put two red candies on each for berries immediately.  Let dry one day.  Keep in a closed container.

## Meringue Walnut Kisses
A very sweet cookie.

1 large egg white
½ cup sugar
1 teaspoon gluten-free vanilla extract*

¼ teaspoon salt
1 cup gluten-free cornflakes*
½ cup chopped walnuts

Beat the egg white until frothy. Add the sugar a little at a time, beating well after each addition. Beat in the vanilla and salt. Increase the speed of the mixer and continue beating until stiff peaks form. Fold in the cornflakes and walnuts. Drop by spoonfuls onto greased baking sheets. Bake 20-30 minutes at 375°F until dry to the touch. Allow to cool for 10 minutes on the baking sheets. Transfer to wire racks to cool completely. Makes 24 cookies.

## Molasses Crinkles
A very flavorful spice cookie that requires no butter or margarine, so it is casein-free and has no trans-fats. The original recipe came from Brier Rabbit Molasses®, and has been adjusted to gluten-free. I like the soft version, whereas my husband likes the crispy version. The crispy version keeps for weeks and travel well.

¾ cup oil
1 cup sugar
¼ cup molasses*
2 cups Gluten-Free Naturals™ Cookie
    Blend or Gluten-Free Naturals™ All
    Purpose Flour
2 teaspoons baking soda

¼ teaspoon salt
1 teaspoon ground cinnamon
1 teaspoon ground cloves
½ teaspoon ground ginger
1 egg
Additional granulated sugar to coat
    cookies

Blend oil, sugar and molasses together in a heavy duty mixer. Add the rest of the ingredients and blend until combined. (If you don't have a mixer, you can whisk together the oil and sugars, and then blend in the flour and spices using a sturdy spoon.) Roll the dough in your hands into one-inch balls. If dough is too difficult or sticky to roll, you can refrigerate it first. The original recipe suggested 2 hours, but I found this not necessary.

Put some granulated sugar into a small bowl and roll the cookies in the sugar to coat them. Place them on cookie sheets about two inches apart. I use light gray non-stick cookie sheets by Nordicware®, or, you can line cookie sheets with parchment paper. Bake 10 to 12 minutes at 375°F. This method results in a flat and very crispy cookie.

For a softer cookie that is not flat, freeze the balls in the freezer for 20 to 30 minutes. Then bake as noted above.

Cool on the pan for 2 minutes, then remove to a wire rack to cool. Store in an airtight container when completely cooled.

*Variation*: Melted butter* may be used in place of oil.

*see gluten-free products list at the end of the book

## Neapolitan Cookies

This recipe is my mother's. It makes a lot of cookies and we always enjoy them for the holidays. I admit that they are quite a bit of work, but I think they are definitely worth the effort. They also freeze well. Wrap thoroughly cooled cookies in aluminum foil and then put in a heavy-duty freezer bag.

1 cup (8 ounce) gluten-free almond paste*
    (I use ½ of my egg white almond paste recipe)
1 cup butter
¾ cup sugar
4 eggs, separated
1 ¾ cups Gluten-Free Naturals™ Cookie Blend or Gluten-Free Naturals™ All Purpose Flour

1 teaspoon gluten-free almond extract*
20 drops of gluten-free red food coloring*
13 drops of green gluten-free food coloring*
¼ cup seedless red raspberry jam
¼ cup apricot jam
1 cup gluten-free semi-sweet chocolate chips*

Preheat the oven to 350°F. Grease the bottom of three (9 x 13 inch) pans. Line them with waxed paper or parchment paper and then grease the paper.

In a medium mixer bowl, beat the egg whites with clean beaters. Set aside.

In a large mixer bowl, break up the almond paste into small pieces. Add the butter, sugar and egg yolks. Beat on medium speed. Add the flour and the extract and blend.

Gently fold the egg mixture into the almond mixture. Remove 1 ½ cups and stir in the red color. Turn into one pan. Spread evenly. Remove another 1 ½ cups of batter and add to the green color. Mix well and spread in the second pan. Spread the remaining batter into the third pan.

Bake 8-10 minutes until the edge is slightly brown. Do not over-cook. Invert onto wire racks and remove pans and paper. Turn layers right side up by laying another rack and cool completely.

Now that it's cooled, place the green layer on a large cutting board. Spread raspberry jam evenly on the green layer. Top with the yellow layer. Spread apricot jam on the yellow layer and top with the red layer. Cover with plastic wrap and set a cutting board on top to weigh down and refrigerate overnight.

The next day, melt the chocolate chips (I use a microwave on the defrost cycle) and spread over the top of the red layer. Let it dry and then trim the edges with a sharp knife. Cut into bars 1 ½ inches by ½ inch. Makes 8 dozen. Keep them in the refrigerator or store them frozen to keep fresh longer. They keep better if you don't slice them all until they are needed. I have successfully stored these in the freezer for months by having them well wrapped in foil and then putting them in a freezer bag.

*Variation*: For a different flavor, other flavors of gluten-free jam may be used.

*see gluten-free products list at the end of the book

### "Noatmeal" (no oatmeal) Raisin Cookies

These cookies are mock oatmeal cookies. They are good the day you make them, but we think they taste more like oatmeal cookies the next day. If using the Gluten-Free Naturals™ All Purpose Flour, pack the measuring cup a little when measuring or they will turn out more crispy than chewy.

½ cup (1 stick) butter or gluten-free margarine
¼ cup brown sugar, packed
½ cup sugar
1 egg
1 teaspoon gluten-free vanilla*
1 ¼ cups Gluten-Free Naturals™ Cookie Blend or Gluten-Free Naturals™ All Purpose Flour

½ teaspoon baking soda
¼ teaspoon salt
¼ teaspoon ground cinnamon
⅛ teaspoon ground nutmeg
¼ cup to 6 Tablespoons slivered almonds (Add according to your preference. I like more nuts)
½ cup raisins

Cream butter and sugars. You can use a mixer if you wish. Add the egg and vanilla. Mix in the rest of the flour, baking soda, salt and spices. Gently blend in the almonds and raisins. Do not add them in with a mixer or you lose the texture in the almonds and they won't seem like oatmeal cookies.

Drop the dough by teaspoonfuls on an ungreased cookie sheet. Bake at 350°F for 12 minutes. Cool on the pan for 2 minutes then remove to a cooling rack. Makes over 2 dozen cookies.

### Peanut Butter Cookies

I took these to a Christmas party and they were a hit. Both non-celiac and celiac tasters couldn't get enough of them. I think my nephew ate at least 6, but who's counting?

½ cup butter or gluten-free margarine*
½ cup gluten-free peanut butter*
½ cup sugar
½ cup brown sugar
1 egg

1 ¼ cups Gluten-Free Naturals™ Cookie Blend or Gluten-Free Naturals™ All Purpose Flour
½ teaspoon baking powder
¾ teaspoon baking soda
¼ teaspoon salt

Cream the butter, peanut butter and sugars until well blended. Stir in the egg. Add the rest of the ingredients and blend well. Roll into 3 inch balls. Place on an ungreased cookie sheet and press down in a criss-cross pattern with the tines of a fork. Bake at 375°F for 10 to 12 minutes.

## Peanut Butter Cookies with Chocolate Stars or Kisses
I made these cookies during the holidays, and my guests were surprised to learn that they were gluten-free. They taste like the ones you remember.

½ cup butter or gluten-free margarine*
½ cup gluten-free peanut butter*
½ cup sugar
½ cup brown sugar
1 egg
1 teaspoon gluten-free vanilla*
1 ¼ cups Gluten-Free Naturals™ Cookie Blend or Gluten-Free Naturals™ All

Purpose Flour, plus 2 to 3 or so Tablespoons more if dough is too wet
1 teaspoon baking soda
½ teaspoon salt
1 (4 ¼ oz) box of gluten-free chocolate stars*, approximately 40 per box or Hershey's® Milk Chocolate Kisses, unwrapped (they're gluten-free as of this writing)

In a bowl, cream the butter and sugars together. Add egg, vanilla and peanut butter. Mix together until creamy. In another bowl, whisk together the flour, baking soda and salt. Blend into the butter mixture. If too wet, add additional flour, 1 Tablespoon at a time.

Form into 1 inch balls and roll in sugar. If difficult to roll, refrigerate the dough. Place on an ungreased cookie sheet. Bake at 375°F for 12 minutes. After they come out of the oven, quickly press a candy on top of each one. Cool completely before storing so that the chocolate is firm. Makes over 2 dozen.

## Peanut Butter Cookies, Flourless Version
An easy cookie for children to make. These contain no flour.

2 cups sugar
2 cups gluten-free peanut butter*

1 egg
1 teaspoon gluten-free vanilla*

Blend all ingredients with a sturdy spoon. Roll with your hands into 1 inch balls. Place on a greased cookie sheet and flatten them in a crisscross pattern with the tines of a fork. Bake in a 350°F oven for 10 minutes on an Airbake® pan or in a 325°F oven for 12-14 minutes on a regular pan.

*Variation*: Use 1 ½ cups confectioner's sugar and 1 cup peanut butter instead of what is listed above. Add egg and vanilla. Place on cookie sheet and flatten. Bake at 325°F for 10 minutes. If too sticky, add additional powdered sugar or cornstarch.

*Variation 2*: For chocolate truffle cookies, use 1 cup peanut butter, 1 cup packed light brown sugar, 1 egg, 1 teaspoon baking soda and ½ cup chocolate chips instead of the ingredients above. Blend cookie ingredients, adding chips in last. Put teaspoonfuls on a cookie sheet about 2 inches apart. Do not flatten them. Bake on an ungreased cookie sheet at 350°F for 9 to 10 minutes. Let cookies stay on the cookie sheet 5 minutes before removing them, or they will fall apart. Cool completely on a cooling rack.

## Pecan Pie Bars

This is my favorite version. You need a food processor to make this. I like this better than pecan pie and they are easier to make. I use either chopped pecans or chop them in the processor so that the cookies are easier to cut.

Crust:
1 ½ cups Gluten-Free Naturals™ All
    Purpose Flour or Gluten-Free
    Naturals™ Sandwich Bread Flour
¼ cup sugar

¼ teaspoon salt
6 Tablespoons butter or gluten-free
    margarine*
2 ½ Tablespoons water

Filling:
3 eggs
½ cup sugar (I use a little less)
½ cup light corn syrup (or a little less)

1 Tablespoon butter or gluten-free
    margarine*, melted
1 teaspoon gluten-free vanilla*
¾ cup chopped pecans

In a food processor, put the flour sugar and salt in the processor. Add the cold butter and turn the processor on and cut it in until the butter is in small pieces. Slowly add the water through the feed tube with the processor on. The dough is ready when it balls up on one side of the processor. Press the dough into the bottom and a little up the sides of a 11 x 7 inch pan. Bake 15-20 minutes or until the dough is set.

Mix all of the filling ingredients in the processor until blended. If nuts are already chopped, add them at the end. Otherwise, pulse to chop the nuts. Spread mixture evenly over the crust. Bake 25 minutes at 350°F. The filling will be set. Cool completely and cut into squares.

## Pecan Pie Bars – Version 2

The bottom of this bar cookie is very crumbly but tasty. My nieces and nephews ate a whole batch this past Thanksgiving. This is easier to make than pecan pie. I use chopped pecans because it makes them easier to cut. This is similar to the recipe above except that the crust is not firm.

Crust:
1 ½ cups Gluten-Free Naturals™ Cookie
    Blend or Gluten-Free Naturals™ All
    Purpose Flour

6 Tablespoons butter or gluten-free
    margarine*
¼ cup sugar
¼ teaspoon salt

Filling:
3 eggs
½ cup sugar (I use a little less)
½ cup light corn syrup (or a little less)

1 Tablespoon butter or gluten-free
    margarine*, melted
½ teaspoon gluten-free vanilla* (I use a
    little more)
¾ cup chopped pecans

In a mixer, combine the crust ingredients until crumbly. Press into the bottom an 11 x 7 inch pan. Bake 15-20 minutes or until light golden brown.

Mix all of the filling ingredients in mixer until blended. (I use the same bowl.) Spread mixture evenly over the crust. Bake 25 minutes at 350°F. Filling should be set. Cool completely and cut into squares.

*Variation*: For a firmer crust on the bottom, increase the sugar by ¼ cup. You can decrease the sugar in the filling if you wish to compensate for this.

## Pignoli Cookies
This recipe is from my Aunt.

¼ cup Gluten-Free Naturals™ Cookie Blend or Gluten-Free Naturals™ All Purpose Flour
½ teaspoon baking powder
½ cup granulated sugar
½ cup confectioner's sugar
Dash of salt

2 egg whites, at room temperature (or egg white powder and water)
1 can almond paste* or ½ recipe almond paste (see index)
½ teaspoon almond extract (or use 1 teaspoon for a stronger almond flavor)
Pine nuts

In a mixer, beat the almond paste with the egg whites. Some little lumps may remain, but that is fine. Add extract and dry ingredients. Mix well with a wooden spoon, just until all is mixed in. Or, if you have a heavy-duty mixer you can mix the dry ingredients in with the mixer.

Put nuts in a bowl. Use less than a teaspoon of dough and drop it in the nuts. Coat all and pick up until it forms a ball. Put on a greased cookie sheet or parchment paper. Bake at 325°F for about 20 minutes. As soon as they come out put on a rack to dry. I don't let them get too brown.

## Pinwheel Cookies
These are refrigerator cookies that have a layer of chocolate and vanilla and then are rolled to make the pinwheel design. These were impossible to make gluten-free until I developed the Gluten-Free Naturals™ All Purpose Flour.

¾ cup butter
1 cup sugar
2 eggs
½ teaspoon gluten-free vanilla*
2 ½ cups Gluten-Free Naturals™ All Purpose Flour or Gluten-Free

Naturals™ Sandwich Bread Flour (do not substitute other flour blends)
1 teaspoon salt
1 teaspoon baking powder
2 squares of unsweetened chocolate*

In a mixer, beat together the butter and sugar. Once well blended, add in the eggs and vanilla. Add the flour, salt and baking powder. Blend in. Remove half the dough. Melt the 2 squares of chocolate in the microwave. Allow to cool and blend into the other half of the dough.

Chill the dough. Roll out the dough to 9" x 12", between 2 pieces of waxed paper. Or for a faster method, don't chill the dough. Instead roll out each of the dough between waxed

*see gluten-free products list at the end of the book

paper to the right size, and then chill it laying it on a large baking pan or cutting board so that it is flat.

Remove the top layer of waxed paper on both the vanilla and chocolate layers. Now using the waxed paper to help guide you, turn one layer upside-down and lay it on top of the other. Gently roll the double layer of dough together with a rolling pin so that it sticks together. Then remove the top waxed paper and roll up the dough on the wide side to make a roll that is 12" long and about 2" in diameter. Use the bottom waxed paper to help you roll it. Wrap the dough in waxed paper or plastic wrap and chill it until firm.

Slice the cookies to about ⅛ thick slices. Place on a lightly greased baking sheet. Make sure they are a little bit apart from each other. Bake at 400°F for about 6 to 8 minutes. Cool on a cooling rack.

## Pizzelles

These hold together well and are very tasty. They are very crisp the day you make them but the cookies made with the Cookie Blend will get a little soggy the next day if you don't store them in an airtight container. The cookies made with the Gluten-Free Naturals™ All Purpose Flour stay crisper longer and may be stored in a plastic bag.

I served these cookies at a party, and no one thought they were any different. These are also nice served with ice cream. Break the cookies and dip them in. I enjoy these cookies more than an ice cream cone.

3 eggs
¾ cup sugar
½ cup (1 stick) gluten-free butter or margarine* (I prefer them made with butter)
1 Tablespoon gluten-free vanilla* or gluten-free anise extract*

1 ¾ cups Gluten-Free Naturals™ Cookie Blend or Gluten-Free Naturals™ All Purpose Flour
2 teaspoons baking powder

Beat eggs, adding the sugar gradually. (I use a whisk or an electric mixer may be used.) Beat until smooth.

Melt the butter or margarine in the microwave, using the defrost cycle for about 2 minutes. When cool, add to egg mixture. Add vanilla to egg mixture and stir in. Add flour and baking powder and blend well. (If using the Gluten-Free Naturals™ All Purpose Flour and the dough is a little thin, add 1 to 2 Tablespoons more of the flour to make the dough more workable. I suggest you don't add more than ¼ cup additional flour.)

Cook in a hot, clean (no gluten) pizzelle maker for about 20 to 40 seconds each, depending on your pizzelle maker. Remove with a large pancake turner. The cookies are delicate while hot, and if you try to remove them with a fork or small spatula they will break. Cool on a wire rack. Makes about 30 pizzelles. Store the cookies in an airtight container. This keeps them fresh and crisp.

*see gluten-free products list at the end of the book

*Variation*: For Chocolate Pizzelles, add ¼ cup cocoa, ¼ cup additional sugar and ¼ teaspoon additional baking powder. Cook chocolate pizzelles for 30 to 60 seconds, depending on your pizzelle maker.

## Refrigerator Sugar Cookies
These are nice and buttery. You can make the dough ahead of time, refrigerate, and then slice and bake them later.

1 cup (2 sticks) butter softened
1 cup sugar (or ½ cup brown and ½ cup white sugar)
2 eggs
1 ½ teaspoons gluten-free vanilla*
2 ¾ cups Gluten-Free Naturals™ All Purpose Flour or Gluten-Free

Naturals™ Sandwich Bread Flour (do not substitute other flour blends)
1 teaspoon salt
½ teaspoon baking soda

Cream butter and sugar together using a sturdy spoon or a heavy-duty mixer. Add eggs and vanilla and blend in. Add the dry ingredients and blend in with the mixer or using a sturdy spoon. Drop the entire dough onto a large piece of plastic wrap. Using the outside of the wrap, roll the dough like a log. The roll of dough should be about 2 ½ inches in diameter. Completely cover with the wrap and refrigerate for several hours.

Remove from refrigerator and roll the dough on the counter so that it is a nice round log. Unwrap and slice the dough to make ⅛ inch cookies, and place them apart on an ungreased cookie sheet. Decorate with colored sugar or gluten-free sprinkles if desired. Bake at 400°F for 6 to 8 minutes. Remove from cookie sheet and cool on a cooling rack. If you didn't decorate previously, you can frost with decorators frosting (see index), if you wish.

*Variation*: for cookies that are half chocolate and half vanilla, make 2 rolls in contrasting colors, and chill. (Melt one square of unsweetened baking chocolate and add it to half of the dough before wrapping and chilling.) Once chilled, cut each roll in half lengthwise. Press together the cut surfaces of the 2 halves, to make ½ chocolate and ½ vanilla. If desired, cut in half again, turn dough around, and press cut surfaces together to make cookies that have chocolate and vanilla alternating triangles. Re-wrap and chill the dough. Then slice and bake as directed above.

## Refrigerator Sugar Cookies – Rice Flour Version
These are made with brown rice flour. They are grittier than the previous version but an alternative for those who want to use their own blend of flours.

½ cup (1 stick) butter softened
1 cup sugar
2 eggs
1 teaspoon gluten-free vanilla*
1 cup brown rice flour
½ cup yellow corn flour or sorghum flour

½ cup tapioca starch or tapioca flour
½ teaspoon salt
1 teaspoon baking powder
1 teaspoon xanthan gum

*see gluten-free products list at the end of the book

Cream butter and sugar together using a sturdy spoon or a heavy-duty mixer. Add eggs and vanilla and blend in. Add the dry ingredients and blend in with the mixer or using a sturdy spoon. Drop the entire dough onto a large piece of plastic wrap. Using the outside of the wrap, roll the dough like a log. Completely cover with the wrap and refrigerate for several hours.

Remove from refrigerator and roll the dough on the counter so that it is a nice round log. (Before refrigerating, the dough will be soft and the bottom may be flat.) Unwrap and slice the dough to make round cookies, and place on an ungreased cookie sheet. (I cut them to a size between a ⅛ and ¼ inch thick.) Decorate with colored sugar or gluten-free sprinkles if desired. Bake at 350°F for 10 minutes. I use a light colored, non-stick cookie sheet. Allow to cool on the cookie sheet for 2 minutes before removing so they don't fall apart. Do not leave them on the cookie sheet more than 5 minutes, or they will be difficult to remove. If you didn't decorate previously, you can frost with decorators frosting (see index), if you wish.

*Variation*: You can also use this dough to make roll-out cookies. Refrigerate the dough, roll between waxed paper, cut with cookie cutters and decorate if desired.

## Russian Teacakes
**Since these cookies have no eggs, you need the xanthan gum to hold them together.**

1 cup butter or gluten-free margarine*, softened
½ cup sugar
2 ¼ cups Gluten-Free Naturals™ Cookie Blend or Gluten-Free Naturals™ All Purpose Flour
1 teaspoon xanthan gum (use with Gluten-Free Naturals™ Cookie Blend but eliminate if using the Gluten-Free Naturals™ All Purpose flour)
1 teaspoon gluten-free vanilla*
¼ teaspoon almond extract* (optional)
¾ cup finely chopped nuts (I use almond meal*)
¼ teaspoon salt
Powdered sugar to roll cookies in

Heat oven to 400°F. Mix butter with ½ cup powdered sugar and the vanilla. Add the rest of the ingredients. If dough is too wet, add up to a ¼ cup more gluten-free Cookie Blend. Shape into 1-inch balls using your hands. If difficult to roll, refrigerate dough. Place on an ungreased cookie sheet about 1 inch apart. Bake until set, but not brown, for about 10 to 12 minutes.

Roll in powdered sugar while still warm. Cool. Roll in powdered sugar again.

*see gluten-free products list at the end of the book

## Snickerdoodle Cookies

These are a favorite with both celiacs and non-celiacs.  I put these out at a party and they were gone before the party was over.

1 cup butter
1 ½ cups sugar
2 eggs
½ to 1 teaspoon gluten-free vanilla*
2 ½ cups Gluten-Free Naturals™ Cookie Blend or Gluten-Free Naturals™ All Purpose Flour

2 teaspoons cream of tartar
1 teaspoon baking soda (not baking powder or they will have a sour taste)
½ teaspoon salt
3 teaspoons ground cinnamon
¼ cup sugar

Cream the butter and sugar until fluffy.  Add the eggs and vanilla and blend.  Add the flour, cream of tartar, soda and salt.  Blend well.  In a small dish, blend the cinnamon and sugar together.  Roll into balls that are about 1 inch or a little smaller, and then roll into the cinnamon sugar mixture. (Note: If it is difficult to roll the dough, you may refrigerate it to make it firmer.)  Place on an ungreased cookie sheet and bake at 375°F for 8 to 10 minutes.

## Spritz or Cookie Press Cookies

Traditionally, we like to make Christmas Trees by adding some green food coloring to the batter and sprinkling the cookies with "hundreds and thousands" of sprinkles before baking.

1 cup butter or gluten-free margarine*
⅔ cup sugar
2 ¼ to 2 ½ cups Gluten-Free Naturals™ Cookie Blend or Gluten-Free Naturals™ All Purpose Flour

1 teaspoon gluten-free almond extract* or gluten-free vanilla extract*
½ teaspoon salt
1 egg
Colored sugar or gluten-free sprinkles

Heat oven to 400°F.  Mix the butter and sugar.  Add the remaining ingredients.  If dough is too wet, add up to ¼ cup more Cookie Blend.

Place the dough in your cookie press.  Form cookies on un-greased cookie sheets (I use Airbake® sheets for this, but sometimes you have to bake a little longer.)  Bake 6 to 9 minutes until the cookies are set but not brown.  Remove from the oven and allow to cool on the cookie sheet for a few minutes before removing them.  If you remove them immediately they will break and fall apart.

*Variation*: For chocolate Spritz cookies, add 6 Tablespoons cocoa and 2 additional Tablespoons butter.

*see gluten-free products list at the end of the book

## Spritz Cookies, Version 2

For those who want a cookie made only with brown rice flour. They are slightly gritty, but they seem to melt in your mouth. These are good for people with allergies to other grains.

1 ½ cups butter
1 cup sugar
1 egg
2 teaspoons gluten-free vanilla* or 1
   teaspoon vanilla* and 1 teaspoon
   gluten-free almond extract*

3 ½ to 4 cups brown rice flour
¼ teaspoon salt
1 teaspoon gluten-free baking powder*
Food coloring (optional)

Cream butter and sugar. Add egg, vanilla and extract. Whisk together the flour, salt and baking powder. With a sturdy spoon, blend in the flour mixture. Add the 3 ½ cups flour. If too wet, continue to add rice flour until a good consistency is reached for the cookie press. Add food coloring if desired. (For Christmas I make green cookies in the shape of Christmas trees, and sprinkle on gluten-free colored "hundreds and thousands" of candies to be the ornaments on the trees.)

Fill the cookie press and make the cookies on an ungreased baking sheet. Decorate with sprinkles if desired. Bake at 400°F for 8 to 10 minutes until the cookies are set (not brown). Watch carefully as they can burn easily if left in the oven too long. Allow them to cool a minute or two on the pan, then remove them to a cooling rack.

## Sugar Cookies – Our Favorite Cut-Out Cookies

I have brought these cookies to parties and people didn't realize they were gluten-free. They are the traditional cookies you remember. They are not too sweet so you can decorate or frost them, but we like them as-is too. They took me years to develop and they are easy to make. They get nice and crisp once they cool and are not grainy or dry. See the next recipe for the "paints" to make painted cookies. Or just sprinkle these with colored sugar, or frost after they are cooled.

2 cups Gluten-Free Naturals™ All
   Purpose Flour or Gluten-Free
   Naturals™ Sandwich Bread Flour (do
   not substitute other flour blends)
¼ teaspoon baking powder
¼ teaspoon salt
½ cup butter*, softened
¾ cup sugar

1 egg
1 teaspoon flavoring; either vanilla
   extract* or lemon extract* or half of
   each. Or use half vanilla extract* and
   half almond extract*.
Gluten-free decorations, or see next
   recipe for edible paints (made with egg
   yolks and color)

Blend all ingredients together in a heavy duty mixer. Roll out between 2 pieces of waxed paper and put in the refrigerator until it gets firm. (Or do the traditional method of refrigerating the dough, and then rolling it out. There is no need to add any extra flour for rolling the dough.) I have found that by rolling it first it is easy to roll and doesn't have to be refrigerated as long, since the dough is already thin. Once dough is firm, peel off the top waxed paper and cut out with cookie cutters. Remove the cookies with a metal spatula or pancake turner and put them on non-stick baking sheets. (If you don't have a non-stick pan, then lightly grease the pan.) If dough is difficult to handle, refrigerate it again. Sprinkle

*see gluten-free products list at the end of the book

cookies with colored sugar before baking, if desired.  Bake at 425°F for 5 to 7 minutes.  Remove cookies from pan immediately and place on a cooling rack.  Re-roll any leftover dough and make more cookies.  Since there is no gluten, you can roll it again and again.  They will remain tender.

## Sugar Cookies – Version 2 – to make "Painted" Cookies and Cut Out Cookies

Painted cookies were a tradition in our house every Christmas when we were young. My mother rolled the dough and cut out the cookies while we children decorated them with egg yolk paints before baking.  As children we didn't like the taste of gingerbread so my mother used sugar cookie dough in the shape of gingerbread men and we decorated them too.  She used decorator frosting on those.  (Recipes for edible paints and decorator frosting are at the end of this recipe.)  I developed this cookie recipe using Cookie Blend.  It is good but they are a little bit drier cookies than the previous recipe.  Use any of the sugar cookie recipes in this book to make painted cookies.

2 ¼ cups Gluten-Free Naturals™ Cookie
    Blend
½ teaspoon xanthan gum
2 teaspoons baking powder
½ teaspoon salt
½ cup butter, softened or gluten-free
    margarine*
1 cup sugar

1 egg
¼ teaspoon gluten-free lemon extract*
¼ teaspoon gluten-free vanilla extract*
¼ cup milk or gluten-free milk substitute
Red, yellow and green edible paint (recipe
    follows, made with egg yolks and color)

Whisk the Cookie Blend, xanthan gum and baking powder together and set aside.  Using an electric mixer, cream butter then add sugar and the egg and continue mixing until creamy.  Add flour alternately with milk and extracts, ending with flour, using the least amounts first.  If too wet, add ¼ cup more flour.  If too dry, add 2 Tablespoons more milk.  Chill dough in refrigerator until quite firm to handle.

Remove only about one-third of the dough at a time and roll out in between gluten-free floured waxed paper floured with cornstarch.  (Use a piece of waxed paper on the bottom, dust with cornstarch, sprinkle another piece of waxed paper with cornstarch and cover top of dough with cornstarch side down.)  Roll the dough.  Carefully remove top piece of waxed paper when rolled thin.  Cut into the desired shapes and place on a greased cookie sheet.  (I use sweet butter for this.)  For best results, use smaller size cookie cutters because the cookies will hold together better.  (Sometimes very large shapes may break in half when you stack them in a container.  Very large size cookies should be stored on a flat plate, un-stacked, and covered with foil or plastic wrap.)

Now hand the pan over to your children to decorate the cookies. While they are busy being creative, you can peacefully continue to roll and cut cookies. (See below for decoration recipe.)

When a tray of cookies are completed, bake in a 375°F oven for 8-10 minutes.  Bake 2 to 3 minutes longer if using an Airbake® pan.  Do not brown.  Remove from pans and cool cookies on a rack and you are ready for Santa.  These cookies are colorful and delicious.

*see gluten-free products list at the end of the book

_Edible "Paints"_ – Separate two eggs.  Pour the egg whites into a jar and freeze for another use.  (When the jar gets full, I bake an angel food cake.  The whites can be kept in the freezer for months.)  Lightly beat the egg yolks with a few teaspoons of water and place ⅓ of the mixture into each of 3 custard cups.  Now add food coloring to each cup making one yellow and the others red and green.  Using small paint brushes saved only for this purpose (do not use brushes you have previously used for real paint), the children can paint away.  Just be sure each pot of "paint" has its own brush so colors won't get mixed.  When all are done, I wash these brushes and keep them with my cookie cutters so no one could use them with real paints by mistake.

Note: I recommend using smaller size cookie cutters, since larger cookies tend to crumble when you keep them for awhile.

_Variation_: You can substitute gluten-free almond extract for the lemon.

_Variation 2_:  Instead of making gingerbread men we used this dough.  Cut out with cookie cutters but do not paint.  Instead of painting the cookies you can decorate with decorator's icing when completely cooled.  To make _Decorator's Icing_: blend 1 ¼ cups sifted confectioner's sugar, ⅛ cream of tartar, 1 egg white, ¼ teaspoon vanilla* and food coloring in an electric mixer.  Fill in a decorating tube.  Cover what icing is left with a dampened paper towel to prevent it from drying out.  Decorate cookies when fully cooled.  My mom would make blue icing.  She would decorate the cookies by putting a curl on the forehead, creating the face with eyes, nose, smiling mouth, and making the "clothes" with a bow tie, buttons down the front, cuffs at the sleeves and pants.

_Variation 3_:  One time, by mistake, I made this recipe using 1 ½ cups flour and 2 Tablespoons milk.  I chilled the dough 1 hour.  They were a little more difficult to roll out and I had to keep the dough chilled, but they turned out more delicious and did not fall apart as much as the original recipe.  They were very light and crispy more like a drop cookie.

## Sugar Cookies – Version 3

These cookies hold together better than the previous version, and the dough does not need to be refrigerated.  I think they are good frosted or decorated.  They are a little drier than the second version.  This recipe comes from Wilton® cookie cutters, and I converted it to make it gluten-free.

| | |
|---|---|
| 1 cup butter* or gluten-free margarine*, softened | 2 teaspoons baking powder |
| 1 cup granulated sugar | 3 cups Gluten-Free Naturals™ Cookie Blend or Gluten-Free Naturals™ All Purpose Flour |
| 1 egg | |
| 1 to 2 teaspoons gluten-free vanilla* (I use 2 teaspoons) | |

Cream butter and sugar together, using a sturdy spoon or with an electric mixer.  Mix in the egg and vanilla.  Add the baking powder and 1 cup of Cookie Blend and mix in.  Mix in the next cup of flour.  If you have a heavy duty mixer, you may be able to add the third cup in using the mixer.  For most mixers it will be too much and may strain the motor, so I suggest you add in the final cup by hand using a sturdy spoon.  The dough should be very stiff.

*see gluten-free products list at the end of the book

Divide the dough into 2 balls.  Put down a piece of waxed paper on the counter, put one of the dough balls in the center, cover with another piece of waxed paper and roll until about ⅛th inch thick.  The original recipe said to put flour on the waxed paper, but I found that this is not necessary.  Remove top piece of waxed paper, cut out desired shapes, and put cookies on an ungreased cookie sheet.  Bake in a 400°F oven for 6 to 10 minutes; or until the cookies are lightly browned.

Repeat with second ball of dough.  This recipe works well with either small or large cookie cutters.

<u>Write your own recipes here</u>:

# DESSERTS

## Apples – Baked Apples
I make this for company. Serve them warm topped with gluten-free vanilla ice cream or whipped cream.

Apples
Sugar
Ground cinnamon
Water

Gluten-free apple or orange brandy*
    (optional)
Gluten-free vanilla*

For best results use Rome Beauty or Cortland apples. Core apples and slice away the skin around the stem or top part. Place apples in a pan that holds them nicely leaving only a little space between apples. Pour 1 Tablespoon of water and 1 Tablespoon of brandy (if using) per apple in the bottom of the pan. Also add 1 to 2 teaspoons vanilla to liquid in the pan. Sprinkle each of the apples with 1 teaspoon sugar and enough cinnamon to cover top lightly. Bake at 350°F for about 45 minutes if apples are large or until they test done with a cake tester. Baste 2 or 3 times during baking with pan syrup. These apples are good just the way they come out of the oven but you can top with whipped cream if you like.

## Apple Cobbler with Walnuts or Pecans
This is a delicious dessert. I like as much as apple pie, and it is much easier to make.

½ cup sugar
½ teaspoon ground cinnamon
¾ cup chopped walnuts or pecans (I have used whole pecans and that is good too)
4 cups thinly sliced tart apples (I use green apples)
1 cup Gluten-Free Naturals™ All Purpose Flour
1 teaspoon gluten-free baking powder*

¼ teaspoon salt
¾ cup sugar
1 beaten egg
½ cup evaporated milk or 2% milk
⅓ cup oil or melted butter (I melt the butter in the microwave on the defrost cycle)

In a bowl, mix ½ cup sugar and cinnamon together. Set aside. Wash the apples. Cut and remove the seeds and thinly slice. Place in a greased round casserole. Top with the cinnamon and sugar mixture. Now top with the nuts and arrange them evenly so it looks nice. Use the same mixing bowl used for the sugar. Blend together the All Purpose Flour, baking powder, salt and ¾ cup sugar. Now add the egg, milk and oil or melted butter. Pour over apples and nuts. The batter will begin to sink down and the cobbler will cook in with the apples. Bake at 325°F for 55 minutes. Serve with whipped cream or gluten-free ice cream. Makes 8 servings.

Note: If you're using sweeter apples, you can cut the sugar by a few tablespoons in both the topping and the batter.

*Variation*: You can also substitute ½ cup fine white rice flour for the All Purpose Flour. It will turn out very differently, but still be delicious.

*see gluten-free products list at the end of the book

*Variation 2*: To make it easier, I quarter the apples and remove the seeds. I sometimes leave the peel on, but they are easier to slice if you remove it. Then I used my Salad Shooter® with the slicing blade and shoot the apples right into the prepared casserole dish. Then I put in the grating blade and shoot the pecans right on top of the apples. You can also use a food processor for this.

## Apple Crumble Pie
This is easy to make and has a nice crunchy, crumbly top. Spoon it out and enjoy. It doesn't have any fat in it. This is similar to the Apple Ozark Pudding recipe (see index) but is has a more crumbly cake topping.

½ to ¾ cup sugar (depending on how
   sweet the apples are)
1 egg
½ cup Gluten-Free Naturals™ All
   Purpose Flour
1 teaspoon gluten-free baking powder

¼ teaspoon salt
½ cup chopped nuts
1 teaspoon gluten-free vanilla*
1 cup diced and peeled apples
1 teaspoon ground cinnamon

Grease an 8 inch pie pan. Mix together the sugar, gluten-free All Purpose Flour, baking powder, and salt. Add the egg and blend but do not beat. Add the rest of the ingredients and blend. Pour into pie pan and spread to edges. Bake at 350°F for 30 minutes. Good served with gluten-free ice cream or whipped cream.

*Variation*: Substitute a ½ cup of Gluten-Free Naturals™ Cookie Blend for the All Purpose Flour.

## Apples – "Delicious Apples"
These apples are equally good served with ham or chicken as they are for dessert. I like them served warm for dessert with some gluten-free vanilla ice cream or whipped cream. You can also use these apples as a filling for dessert crepes. This is my mother's recipe and we always enjoy it. They are also a nice low fat alternative to apple pie.

6 Delicious apples
6 Tablespoons sugar
2 tablespoons gluten-free orange brandy*
   (optional)
⅓ cup yellow raisins (sultanas)
¼ cup dark raisins

½ cup water
1 Tablespoon cornstarch
¼ cup water
½ teaspoon ground cinnamon
Some freshly grated nutmeg

Peel, core and quarter the apples. Place in a saucepan with brandy (if using), sugar, raisins, and ½ cup water. Cover and simmer over low heat until apples are tender, but still hold their shape. Mix cornstarch in ¼ cup cold water and add to pan while stirring. Bring to a boil and cook until thick. Add spices and stir in. Good served warm. If you make them ahead of time, reheat in the microwave. I like it served in fancy dessert dishes with whipped cream or ice cream on top.

*see gluten-free products list at the end of the book

*Variation*: You can substitute gluten-free dried cranberries or cherries for the dark raisins.

## Apple Ozark Pudding

The original gluten-containing recipe was made famous by Bess Truman, the wife of former president Harry Truman. This is similar to the "Apple Crumble Pie" recipe but has a little more pudding consistency. I suggest you use less sugar. The original recipe is too sweet for my taste, but I've listed the amount of sugar as Bess had it in her recipe. Rice flour works well in this recipe so this is a good dessert for those allergic to soy and other flours. Or you can use the Gluten-Free Naturals™ All Purpose Flour if you wish.

2 eggs
1 ¼ cups sugar (I use less, especially if I
   use a sweet apple)
2 teaspoons gluten-free vanilla*
¼ cup fine white rice flour or Gluten-Free
   Naturals™ All Purpose Flour

2 ½ teaspoons gluten-free baking
   powder*
½ teaspoon salt
1 apple, chopped into small pieces
1 cup chopped walnuts
Gluten-free whipped cream* or gluten-
   free ice cream*

With a whisk, blend the eggs, sugar and vanilla together in a bowl. Add the flour, baking powder and salt and blend. Stir in the apple pieces and the nuts. Spread into a greased 8 x 8 x 2 inch baking pan. Bake at 350°F for 30-40 minutes. Test with a cake tester after baking 30 minutes. If it does not come out clean, bake 5-10 minutes or so longer. Serve warm with whipped cream or gluten-free ice cream. (I like it best with vanilla ice cream.)

## Applesauce

We use applesauce as a dessert or served with pork, lamb and poultry. It is also good served on gluten-free toast sprinkled with additional sugar and cinnamon for a nutritious snack.

Apples
Sugar
Ground cinnamon

Sprinkling of nutmeg
Cider vinegar

There is no exact recipe for applesauce as all apples are different. You must make it according to your own taste. Peel and core apples and slice them into a pot. Add a little water and cook until apples are mushy. Add sugar and stir, then taste. If not sweet enough add more sugar. If too sweet, add a little cider vinegar. Add a generous amount of cinnamon and a little nutmeg. If apples themselves have a bland taste, cider vinegar will perk the sauce up. Stir sauce well for a home style sauce with some lumps or puree in a blender or with a hand blender.

*see gluten-free products list at the end of the book

## Applesauce Dessert

This recipe comes from my mother. It is a simple dessert. She often made this for us when we were children. I admit that back then I didn't like the jam, but now I do. As a child I also liked this best when my mother layered the cookies and applesauce ahead of time because I liked the way the cookies absorbed the moisture. If you prefer crispier cookie crumbs, do it right before serving.

Crushed gluten-free cookie crumbs
(Homemade or store-bought – plain
cookies are best.)
Applesauce (homemade, canned or jar)

Gluten-free Jam or Jelly of your choice
(optional)
Whipped Cream

Put cookie crumbs in the bottom of some parfait glasses or champagne glasses. Large custard cups may also be used. Cover with applesauce. Put a teaspoon of jam in the middle of each. Cover the entire thing with whipped cream.

*Variation:* Sprinkle with cinnamon and sugar, if desired.

## Apples – Stewed

This recipe comes from my mother's friends.

2 pounds apples
2 Tablespoons butter
½ cup sugar
½ cup water

½ cup white wine
1 small lemon (peel and juice)
1 Tablespoon lemon juice

Wash, peel and core apples. Cut them into thick slices. Sauté in butter 2 to 3 minutes. Sprinkle with sugar and add water, lemon peel and lemon juice. Cover and cook slowly until apples are tender. Serves 6.

## Baked Alaska

When we were children my mother often made baked Alaska for birthday parties and people would rave about it. They seem to have fallen out of favor these days, but maybe after you try this version it will make a come-back.

One layer of cake or one pan of brownies baked in a 9 inch round pan.
I suggest either one Gluten-Free Naturals™ Brownie Mix baked in a round 9" pan (bake for about 25 minutes until it tests done), or Gluten-Free Naturals™ Yellow cake mix prepared as directed or one recipe banana chocolate cake (see index) baked

in a 9" round pan or one recipe sponge cake (see index) baked in a 9" pan).
2 quarts gluten-free ice cream*
6 large egg whites (or use the equivalent egg white powder and water)
½ teaspoon cream of tartar
1 cup sugar

Bake brownies or cake. Use vanilla, strawberry, pistachio or any ice cream combination you like (as long as it's gluten-free). Take a bowl that is 1 inch smaller than the cake and line it

*see gluten-free products list at the end of the book

with plastic wrap. Pack in the 2 quarts of ice cream and freeze. Cool the cake and freeze. (Choose a cake that is not made with a high amount of cornstarch since cornstarch becomes grainy when frozen and your cake will be ruined. Gluten-Free Naturals™ Brownies freeze very well, which is why I prefer them for this recipe. Gluten-Free Naturals™ Yellow Cake also freezes well.) When you are ready to serve, beat the egg whites with cream of tartar until stiff. Add sugar gradually until meringue is stiff and glossy. Rub a little meringue between your fingers to be sure all sugar has melted and you feel no grit. Then you know you will have a good meringue.

Preheat oven to 500°F. Butter the center of a decorative pan or baking dish. Be sure all the cake will be on the buttered spot. Remove ice cream from freezer and invert it on top of cake. Remove plastic wrap. Quickly cover all of the ice cream and cake with meringue leaving no spot uncovered. Place in a very hot oven and bake 5 minutes or until the peaks of the meringue are lightly browned. Serve immediately.

*Variation*: I came up with the idea for a dessert called "Rocky Road to Alaska" by using gluten-free Rocky Road ice cream, brownie on the bottom, and the above recipe. It's delicious!

## Biscuit Tortoni

A very delicious Italian dessert. This was very popular back when my parents were married and this was the dessert they had at their wedding reception. It fell out of favor for years when there became a salmonella problem eating raw eggs. Now with this new method of preparation, you can make this dessert without this risk.

⅔ cup sugar
⅓ cup water
3 egg yolks
Pinch of salt
2 Tablespoons gluten-free Amaretto
   Liqueur (See index for recipe) or use ⅛
   to ¼ teaspoon gluten-free almond

extract (We prefer it with the Amaretto made from the recipe in this book.)
2 cups heavy cream*
3 Tablespoons confectioner's sugar
1 teaspoon gluten-free vanilla*
½ teaspoon gluten-free almond extract*
Crushed gluten-free almond macaroons or ground almonds

Put the sugar and water in a pot. Cook until it becomes a sugar syrup. Set aside and allow to cool a little.

In an electric mixer, beat slowly the 3 egg yolks with the pinch of salt until lemon colored. Then add the syrup slowly while beating in a mixer. Stir in the 2 Tablespoons Amaretto (if using) and refrigerate to cool.

Beat heavy cream with the confectioner's sugar, vanilla and almond extract.

Fold the cream and yolk mixture together and place in 10 to 12 small ramekins (about ¼ cup in each). Top with ground almond macaroons or almonds and freeze.

To serve, remove from freezer and allow to defrost about 10 to 15 minutes before eating.

*see gluten-free products list at the end of the book

## Blintzes with Cheese and Fruit

This recipe comes from Argo® brand Cornstarch, with some changes made by me. Their cornstarch is gluten-free as of this writing.

2 eggs
¾ cup milk
1 Tablespoon oil
¼ teaspoon salt
½ cup cornstarch or Gluten-Free Naturals™ All Purpose Flour
2 Tablespoons powdered confectioner's sugar (optional)

2 (7.5 ounce) packages of gluten-free farmer cheese*
1 egg
3 Tablespoons sugar
2 Tablespoons butter
Gluten-Free Pie filling* or sauce (recipe below)

Mix all ingredients, except the butter, in a blender. (I use a hand blender for this.) Heat a 6 inch Teflon® skillet, add a little butter and swirl it around to coat the pan. Heat the pan a few minutes then lift it off the heat. Pour about 2 Tablespoons or so of batter into the center of the pan and tip pan from side to side until the bottom is covered with the batter. Return to heat. When batter looks dry (about 30 seconds), take a dull table knife and lift one edge of crepe until you can take hold of it with your fingers. Now carefully pull the crepe up and flip it over. Cook a few seconds, lift pan and toss crepe out onto a linen towel or on a plate to cool. Be careful that your pan doesn't overheat. Lower heat and raise heat as needed. Add more butter after every 2 to 3 crepes if needed. (I use a new Teflon pan, so it doesn't need much butter.) This recipe makes about 12 crepes.

Blend together the farmer cheese, egg and sugar. Fill a crepe with 2 Tablespoons of filling. Fold the two sides in, and then roll the other side over to form a closed packet that resembles an egg roll. Continue with the next crepe until all are finished.

Heat a very large skillet with 2 Tablespoons butter. Put the crepes in the skillet, seam down. Cook about 4 or 5 minutes, turn once and cook another 4 or 5 minutes until lightly browned on each side. Meanwhile, warm the pie filling in the microwave. Top blintzes with warmed filling or use the sauce below.

Blueberry sauce:
2 Tablespoons sugar
1 ½ teaspoons cornstarch
¼ cup orange juice

1 ½ cups blueberries, washed and stems removed

Mix sugar, cornstarch and orange juice in a small saucepan. Add berries and bring to a boil. Serve warm over blintzes. Makes about 1 cup sauce.

*see gluten-free products list at the end of the book

## Blueberry Bake
This recipe is from my sister.  It is easier to make than pie.

1 pint blueberries, washed and stems removed (You can use 2 pints if you like more fruit, but be sure to use a deep dish pie pan or it will boil over and make a mess of your oven.)
1 Tablespoon lemon juice
Sprinkling of cinnamon (about ½ teaspoon)

½ cup butter* (you can use a little less)
¾ cup sugar (you can use a little less)
1 cup Gluten-Free Naturals™ All Purpose Flour
Pinch of salt (no need to add if using salted butter)

Rinse berries and remove stems.  Put in a greased deep dish 9 ½ or 10 inch glass pie plate.  Sprinkle berries with lemon juice and cinnamon.  Blend together the butter, sugar, flour and salt to make crumbs.  Top the berries with the crumbs.  Bake at 375°F for 40 minutes.

## Cherry Cobbler
This recipe is from my mother, and I modified it to make it gluten-free.

1 (1 lb.) can red pitted sour cherries
1 Tablespoon cornstarch
½ cup sugar
¼ teaspoon salt
1 cup Gluten-Free Naturals™ All Purpose Flour

1 ½ teaspoons gluten-free baking powder*
½ teaspoon salt
¼ cup sugar
¼ cup butter or gluten-free margarine*
½ cup milk

Drain cherries, reserving ½ cup juice.  Put cornstarch, sugar and salt in the juice and blend.  Place cherries in small buttered baking dish and pour juice mixture over them.  Blend dry ingredients in a food processor.  Add butter and cut in butter as for pastry.  Pour milk in all at once and mix until blended.  Drop dough by spoonfuls over cherries and sprinkle a little sugar over top.  Bake at 375°F for 40 to 45 minutes.  Makes 6 servings.

## Curried Fruit
Nice served on a Holiday buffet.

1 stick (½ cup) butter
1 cup brown sugar

1 teaspoon gluten-free curry powder*
Canned peach halves, or mixed fruit

Melt butter, sugar and curry powder and pour over drained canned fruit.  Put in casserole dish.  Bake in a 350°F oven and let simmer about 1 hour.  Use with meat such as lamb, ham or chicken.

*see gluten-free products list at the end of the book

## Crepes with Fruit Filling

Cornstarch crepes can be made a day or two ahead of time and refrigerated. Then put these together when you're ready to eat them. They may not roll as well as the day they are made, but they are still delicious. I prefer to heat the filling in the microwave until warm, before filling the crepes.

1 recipe for Crepes (see index)
Gluten-free pie filling or "Delicious
   Apples" (see index for recipe)
Cinnamon/sugar (optional)

2 Tablespoons powdered confectioner's
   sugar (optional Gluten-free whipped
   cream* or Cool Whip

Prepare crepes as directed. Warm the pie filling. Fill with 2 to 3 Tablespoons of your favorite gluten-free pie filling (as of this writing Comstock® brand is gluten-free) or some of the apples prepared as directed for "Delicious Apples". Roll up and put on a plate with the seam sides down. Top with some cinnamon/sugar and whipped cream. Or sprinkle with powdered sugar.

*Variation*: If you don't have any fruit filling, the crepes are good spread with jam, some whipped cream, and rolled up.

## Crepes Suzette with Ice Cream and Orange Sauce

Crepes (see index for recipe)
Sauce:
   1 cup orange juice
   2 teaspoons cornstarch
   3 Tablespoons sugar

1 Tablespoon orange peel, freshly grated
   (optional)
2 Tablespoons Grand Marnier® or
   homemade orange liqueur (see index)
1 ½ teaspoons butter
2 cup gluten-free vanilla ice cream*

Make crepes as directed. (I have made the crepes a day ahead of time and refrigerated them.) Blend the orange juice, cornstarch, and sugar in a saucepan. Bring to a boil and simmer, stirring with a whisk until smooth and thick. Add orange rind, the liqueur and the butter and stir to blend in. Pour ½ of the sauce in a deep serving platter or chafing dish.

Take the crepes and put about ¼ cup of ice cream down the middle. Fold over the two sides and put in the serving dish with the seam side down. When all crepes are in the platter, pour remaining sauce over top. Serve immediately.

## Fruit Pudding Upside-down Cake

This recipe comes from one of my mother's friends, and I adapted it to make it gluten-free.  This cake has canned fruit cocktail in it.

½ cup brown sugar
½ cup chopped walnuts
1 cup sugar
1 teaspoon baking powder
1 cup Gluten-Free Naturals™ All Purpose Flour

½ teaspoon salt
1 egg
2 cups canned fruit cocktail (1 large can, well drained)
Gluten-free whipped cream* and gluten-free cherry* garnish (optional)

Grease a 9x9x2 inch pan.  Sprinkle the brown sugar and nuts in the pan and set aside.  Blend together the remaining ingredients in an electric mixer and pour over the sugar and nuts.  (If you want large pieces of fruit in your cake, stir the fruit cocktail in by hand after blending the cake ingredients.  I prefer to have the fruit pulverized by the electric mixer.)

Bake at 300°F for 1 hour.  Cool for 5 minutes and remove from pan.  When ready to serve, cut into 9 squares.  Top with whipped cream and garnish with a cherry if desired.

## Ice Cream – Butter Pecan

There are many brands and flavors of ice cream that are gluten-free.  Here is a way to make your own.  I have the ice cream maker for the KitchenAid® mixer.  I usually put this together at least a day before I want to make it.

½ cup water
1 to 2 Tablespoons butter
¾ to 1 cup brown sugar
⅛ teaspoon salt
1 cup milk

2 to 3 egg yolks or 2 whole eggs
1 Tablespoon gluten-free vanilla*
2 cups of gluten-free heavy cream
3 to 4 Tablespoons chopped pecans

Prepare this mixture at least 6 hours or days before you want to make ice cream, so that you can refrigerate the mixture to get it very cold.  Follow manufacturer's instructions for freezing the ice cream maker.  I prefer if it has been frozen for 24 hours.

Heat the water and butter.  Blend in the sugar and salt until they are dissolved.  Add the milk and warm the mixture a little but do not boil.

In a large Pyrex® measuring cup or bowl, beat the egg yolks or eggs with a whisk.  Pour the hot mixture into the egg mixture, while stirring with a whisk.  This will incorporate the egg and permit it to mix in.  (If you don't follow this method the eggs will cook and become scrambled eggs.)  Now put the mixture back into the pot and cook on medium/low heat until it thickens.  Do not boil and stir with a whisk while heating.  Remove from heat to cool.  Once cooled, add the vanilla, and cream and blend in.  Put in a container, and put in the refrigerator.  (I use the Pyrex® measuring cup and cover it with plastic wrap.)  Put the chopped pecans in the refrigerator so that they will also be cold.  The next day, freeze according to directions on the ice cream maker.  Churn 20 to 30 minutes.  Add the nuts in at the end.

*see gluten-free products list at the end of the book

If you want soft-serve style you can eat it immediately.  Otherwise, for traditional ice cream freeze at least 1 day before serving.

## Ice Cream – Cherry Vanilla
There are many brands and flavors of ice cream that are gluten-free.  Here is a way to make your own. I have the ice cream maker for the KitchenAid® mixer.  I usually put this together at least a day before I want to make it.  I like things less sweet, so you may want to use the full amount of sugar.

1 ½ cups milk
¾ cup sugar (I use 2 Tablespoons less
   because the jam adds sweetness).
⅛ teaspoon salt
¼ cup gluten-free cherry jam
2 to 3 egg yolks or 2 whole eggs

1 Tablespoon gluten-free vanilla*
2 cups of gluten-free heavy cream
¼ cup dried cherries (I cut them into
   smaller pieces using a knife)

Prepare this mixture at least 6 hours or days before you want to make ice cream, so that you can refrigerate the mixture to get it very cold.  Follow manufacturer's instructions for freezing the ice cream maker.  I prefer if it has been frozen for 24 hours.

Scald the milk in a pot, by heating it to 185°F using medium/low heat.  Stir while heating so it doesn't burn.  Do not boil or your milk will curdle and be ruined to make ice cream. Remove from heat.  Add the sugar, salt, and jam, and blend in until sugar is dissolved.

In a large Pyrex® measuring cup or bowl, beat the egg yolks or eggs with a whisk.  Pour the hot mixture into the egg mixture, while stirring with a whisk.  This will incorporate the egg and permit it to mix in.  (If you don't follow this method the eggs will cook and become scrambled eggs.)  Now put the mixture back into the pot and cook on medium/low heat until it thickens.  Do not boil and stir with a whisk while heating.  Remove from heat to cool.  Once cooled, add the vanilla, cream, and dried cherries and blend in.  The cherries will absorb liquid and become softer the next day.  Put in a container, and put in the refrigerator. (I use the Pyrex® measuring cup and cover it with plastic wrap.)  The next day, churn according to directions on the ice cream maker.  Churn 20 to 30 minutes.

If you want soft-serve style you can eat it immediately.  Otherwise, for traditional ice cream freeze at least 1 day before serving.

*Variation*:  For Raspberry ice cream, substitute seedless gluten-free raspberry jam for the cherry.  Eliminate dried cherries.

## Ice Cream – Coffee with Chocolate

There are many brands and flavors of ice cream that are gluten-free. Here is a way to make your own. I have the ice cream maker for the KitchenAid® mixer. I usually put this together at least a day before I want to make it.

2 ½ cups milk

1 ¼ cups sugar (If coffee is very strong, use 1 ½ cups)

½ teaspoon salt

½ cup brewed coffee, cold, regular or decaf

2 whole eggs, beaten

1 Tablespoon gluten-free vanilla*

1 cup of gluten-free heavy cream

¼ cup gluten-free chocolate chips, chopped finely in a food processor. (I prefer semi-sweet but milk chocolate may also be used. Pulse so you chop and don't melt chocolate).

Prepare this mixture at least 6 hours or days before you want to make ice cream, so that you can refrigerate the mixture to get it very cold. Follow manufacturer's instructions for freezing the ice cream maker. I prefer if it has been frozen for 24 hours.

Scald the milk in a pot, by heating it to 185°F using medium/low heat. Stir while heating so it doesn't burn on the bottom. Do not boil or your milk will curdle and be ruined to make ice cream. Remove from heat. Add the sugar and salt and blend in until dissolved. Add the coffee and blend in.

In a large Pyrex® measuring cup or bowl, beat the egg yolks or eggs with a whisk. Pour the hot mixture into the egg mixture, while stirring with a whisk. This will incorporate the egg and permit it to mix in. (If you don't follow this method the eggs will cook and become scrambled eggs.) Now put the mixture back into the pot and cook on medium/low heat until it thickens. Do not boil and stir with a whisk while heating. Remove from heat to cool. Once cooled, add the vanilla, cream, chopped chocolate chips, and blend in. (I use the Pyrex® measuring cup and cover it with plastic wrap.) The next day, freeze according to directions on the ice cream maker. Churn 20 to 30 minutes.

If you want soft-serve style you can eat it immediately. Otherwise, for traditional ice cream freeze at least 1 day before serving.

## Ice Cream – Vanilla

There are many brands and flavors of ice cream that are gluten-free. Here is a way to make your own. I have the ice cream maker for the KitchenAid® mixer. I usually put this together at least a day before I want to make it. I think the egg yolks give a smoother, creamier mouth-feel to plain vanilla ice cream. If adding chips or other additions to ice cream, the whole eggs work well.

1 ½ cups milk

¾ cup sugar

⅛ teaspoon salt

2 to 3 egg yolks or 2 whole eggs

1 Tablespoon gluten-free vanilla*

2 cups of gluten-free heavy cream

Prepare this mixture at least 6 hours or days before you want to make ice cream, so that you can refrigerate the mixture to get it very cold. Follow manufacturer's instructions for freezing the ice cream maker. I prefer if it has been frozen for 24 hours.

*see gluten-free products list at the end of the book

Scald the milk in a pot, by heating it to 185°F using medium/low heat. Stir while heating so it doesn't burn. Do not boil or your milk will curdle and be ruined to make ice cream. Remove from heat. Add the sugar and salt and blend in until sugar is dissolved.

In a large Pyrex® measuring cup or bowl, beat the egg yolks or eggs with a whisk. Pour the hot mixture into the egg mixture, while stirring with a whisk. This will incorporate the egg and permit it to mix in. (If you don't follow this method the eggs will cook and become scrambled eggs.) Now put the mixture back into the pot and cook on medium/low heat until it thickens. Do not boil and stir with a whisk while heating. Remove from heat to cool. Once cooled, add the vanilla and cream and blend in. Put in a container, and put in the refrigerator. (I use the Pyrex® measuring cup and cover it with plastic wrap.) Note: For a smoother texture, you can pour the mixture through a sieve into the container. Cheese cloth can also be used in the sieve if desired.

The next day, freeze according to directions on the ice cream maker. Churn 20 to 30 minutes.

If you want soft-serve style you can eat it immediately. Otherwise, for traditional ice cream freeze at least 1 day before serving.

*Variation:* For chocolate with chocolate chips ice cream, grind up ½ cup gluten-free semi-sweet chocolate chips in a food processor until fine. Stir in half while the mixture is still warm so that the chocolate melts in. Stir in the other half at the end of blending in the ice cream maker.

*Other Variations:* For cookies and cream, add crumbled gluten-free cookies at the end of blending. For chocolate chip ice cream, add ¼ cup chopped gluten-free chocolate chips at the end of blending. For mint chocolate chip, add a few drops of gluten-free peppermint extract and gluten-free chocolate chips. Whatever my add-ins are, I pulse them in the food processor first, so that they are smaller in size and won't be too hard to chew once frozen.

## Mexican Non-Fried Ice Cream

At Mexican Restaurants they often serve Fried Ice Cream for dessert. Here is the flavor without the frying, the work, and the gluten! The cereal topping adds a nice crunch.

Gluten-free Vanilla or Butter Pecan Ice
   Cream*
Honey (Optional)

Gluten-Free Honey Nut Corn Chex®
   Cereal

Scoop Ice Cream into dessert dishes. Drizzle with a little honey. Top with some cereal and serve. I prefer the cereal whole out of the box, but you can crush it if you wish.

*see gluten-free products list at the end of the book*

## Orange Shells

A fancy looking company dessert you can make ahead of time.  Some cans of whipped cream* are gluten-free, so I spray a little of that on the top before serving.  You can toast the almonds ahead of time too.

4 oranges, large and nice orange color
1 quart gluten-free vanilla ice cream*, softened
1 (6 ounce) can frozen orange juice, slightly thawed

¼ cup Grand Marnier® liqueur
¼ cup sliced lightly toasted almonds
Sweetened gluten-free whipped cream*

Halve the oranges and remove the pulp and juice.  (I use a grapefruit knife to help do this.)  Scoop out as much of the pith (white part) as possible without tearing the shell.  Freeze.  The day before serving, mix ice cream, orange concentrate and Grand Marnier together.  It is easy to do if you let the ice cream and juice soften a little.  Fill the frozen orange shells and freeze.  Remove from the freezer 10 minutes before serving.  Top with whipped cream and the toasted sliced almonds.

## Parfait

We didn't make this recipe for a long time because of the salmonella risk with raw eggs.  Now that some brands like Eggland's® have a very low risk I feel comfortable making this again.

2 egg whites
1 cup gluten-free heavy cream*
2 egg yolks (choose eggs that say they don't have salmonella risk, like Eggland's®)
¼ cup sugar
2 teaspoons gluten-free vanilla*
2 egg whites
1 cup gluten-free heavy cream*

2 egg yolks
¼ cup sugar
¼ teaspoon gluten-free almond extract*
¼ cup chopped pistachio nuts
Green food coloring
Gluten-free whipped cream*, gluten-free maraschino cherries* or gluten-free chocolate syrup* for garnish (optional)

Whip egg whites until stiff.  Beat heavy cream until thick.  Beat yolks with sugar and vanilla and fold all together.  Freeze.

Repeat this again with exact ingredients only now omit vanilla and add almond extract, green food coloring and chopped nuts.  Freeze.

Alternate the two mixtures in tall parfait glasses and return to the freezer until a few minutes before serving.  Top with a dollop of sweetened whipped cream*, a gluten-free maraschino cherry* (if desired), or some chocolate sauce.

## Pavlova

This is Australia's national dessert. My mother had this version of the dessert in Australia, and found it to be both colorful and delicious. We enjoyed it long before we knew about the gluten-free diet.

3 egg whites (or equivalent egg white powder and water)
Pinch of salt
¾ cup sugar

2 teaspoons cornstarch
1 teaspoon lemon juice
Extra cornstarch

Beat the egg whites with salt until soft peaks form. Gradually add sugar and continue to beat until sugar melts completely. Test by taking a little meringue between your fingers and see if it feels gritty. If it is gritty continue to beat until it tests smooth and creamy to the touch. Sift cornstarch lightly over top and dribble on the lemon juice. Gently fold into the meringue.

Prepare a Pan by cutting a 9 inch circle of waxed paper or aluminum foil and placing it on a greased cookie sheet. Butter the paper or foil and dust some cornstarch evenly over it. Spread meringue ¼ inch thick on the circle them pipe a decorative border around the outer edge. Place in a preheated 200°F oven and bake one hour. When meringue is completely dry and firm to the touch, it is done. Do not brown. Turn off heat and let it cool in the oven.

Fill the center with fruit. In Australia my mother had it filled with strawberries and kiwi fruit and topped with a generous amount of sweetened whipped cream.

You can also use a spring-form pan. Just grease the bottom and sides. Completely line the pan with paper or foil. Grease the paper or foil and dust with cornstarch as above. Peel off the lining before filling the dessert.

## Peach Cobbler

I make this when peaches are plentiful at the Farmer's Market. This is an egg-free dessert.

¼ cup butter or gluten-free margarine*
½ cup sugar
7 large ripe Freestone peaches
1 ¼ cup or Gluten-Free Naturals™ All Purpose Flour
2 teaspoons gluten-free baking powder*

½ teaspoon salt
¼ cup sugar
¼ cup oil
⅔ cup milk (or gluten-free milk substitute*)

Melt ¼ cup butter in a heavy oven proof 10 inch skillet or baking dish. Remove from heat and sprinkle ¼ cup sugar over top. Set aside.

Boil some water in a large saucepan. Also have some cold water in a large bowl in your sink. When the water boils, put in the peaches and boil just a few minutes. Remove the peaches with a slotted spoon and plunge into the cold water. Now the peach peels will slip off easily. Cut peaches in half and remove the pits. Place the peaches cut side down on top of the butter and sugar. Sprinkle the peaches with ¼ cup sugar.

*see gluten-free products list at the end of the book

Now make the batter by whisking together the gluten-free flour, salt, baking powder and ¼ cup sugar. Add the oil and milk all at once. Blend the ingredients. Drop by spoonfuls on top of the peaches, spreading the dough to cover as much area as possible. Bake in a 400°F oven for 15-20 minutes. Best served warm. Also good topped with gluten-free ice cream*.

## Peach Cobbler – Version 2

This dessert has no eggs. I prefer this made with fresh peaches in the recipe above, but if you are short on time the canned peaches work fine in this recipe.

3 Tablespoons butter or gluten-free margarine*
1 Tablespoon sugar
Sprinkling of cinnamon
1 (29 ounce) can of peaches in light syrup, drained
1 ¼ cups Gluten-Free Naturals™ Cookie Blend or Gluten-Free Naturals™ All Purpose Flour

½ teaspoon xanthan gum (eliminate if using Gluten-Free Naturals™ All Purpose Flour)
2 teaspoons gluten-free baking powder*
½ teaspoon salt
½ cup sugar
¼ cup oil
⅔ cup milk (or gluten-free milk substitute*)

Melt butter in a heavy oven proof 10 inch skillet or baking dish. (A Corningware® dish or Corningware® Simply Lite® pan can be used and the butter can be melted in the microwave.) Sprinkle 1 Tablespoon sugar and some cinnamon over the top of the melted butter. Drain peaches and place on top of the butter and sugar. Now make the batter by whisking together the flour, salt, baking powder and ½ cup sugar together. Add the oil and milk all at once. Blend the ingredients. Pour batter on top of the peaches (it will be loose), spreading the dough to cover as much area as possible. Bake in a 400°F oven for 25 minutes until the top is slightly browned. We enjoy it served warm with gluten-free vanilla or peach ice cream*.

Note: Instead of discarding the syrup from the canned peaches, add it to iced tea for a nice flavor. I brew 4 cups of tea, add the syrup, and add additional sugar to taste. Serve over ice.

## Sherry Almond Mousse

This dessert is my mother's and never had gluten in it. To reduce the risk of salmonella from raw eggs, I use the equivalent of egg white powder and water for the egg whites. (I use egg yolks since they are cooked. I freeze the leftover egg whites from separating the eggs for another use, such as an angel food cake, where they will be cooked.)

1 envelope unflavored gelatin
6 Tablespoons sugar (separated)
2 eggs, separated
2 ½ Tablespoons cream sherry

¼ teaspoon gluten-free almond extract* (I use a little less)
1 cup milk
1 cup gluten-free heavy cream*

Mix 1 cup milk and egg yolks in a saucepan and blend. Add gelatin and ¼ cup sugar and let stand 1 minute. Stir over low heat until gelatin dissolves and mixture thickens slightly. Add sherry and almond extract. Pour into a large bowl and chill, stirring occasionally until mixture slightly mounds when a spoonful is dropped onto a plate.

In another bowl, beat egg whites until stiff and add remaining sugar, gradually to make a stiff meringue. Add to sherry mixture. In the same bowl, beat heavy cream until thick and also add to the sherry mixture. Now fold all together. Lightly oil a pretty 4 cup mold and pour mousse in. Refrigerate overnight. Very nice when served with strawberries and kiwi fruit or topped with a chocolate sauce.

## Strawberry Snow

I use the egg white powder and water for this recipe so that you don't have to worry about the salmonella risk in raw eggs.

2 cups strawberries
Sugar

4 egg whites (or equivalent powdered egg white and water)
¾ cups gluten-free whipped cream*

Crush the strawberries in sugar, reserving some perfect berries for garnish. In the winter gluten-free strawberry jam may be used instead of strawberries and sugar. Beat egg whites until stiff and add the crushed strawberries and whipped cream, folding in and mixing carefully. Pour into dessert bowls and decorate with whole strawberries. This may also be served in champagne or parfait glasses.

## Trifle

This is my mother's favorite dessert. She has had it with canned pineapple in New Zealand, raspberry gelatin in England and without fruit in Australia. They were all delicious but this recipe is her favorite.

3 Tablespoons cornstarch
3 cups milk
6 yolks or 3 whole eggs
6 Tablespoons sugar
1 teaspoon gluten-free vanilla*
1 cup gluten-free heavy cream*
2 teaspoons sugar
Seedless raspberry jam

2 gluten-free sponge cake layers split or Gluten-Free Naturals™ yellow cake mix prepared as directed
½ cup cream (sweet) sherry
1 can (large) sliced peaches, cut into smaller pieces
½ cup sliced almonds, lightly toasted

Make custard by combining cornstarch and ½ cup cold milk. Place remaining milk and sugar in pot and heat to very hot stirring to melt sugar. Pour cornstarch mixture in pot and continue to stir until it thickens. Pour some hot mixture over beaten eggs or yolks and stir rapidly with a whisk. Then pour all back into the pot and heat and stir until you see a few bubbles. Take off the heat immediately and stir in the vanilla. Pour into a bowl and cool, stirring once in a while to prevent a skin from forming on the top.

Split the layers of gluten-free cake and spread with raspberry jam and sandwich together. Place half of cake on the bottom of a pretty glass bowl. Sprinkle ¼ cup sherry over cake. Cover with half the peaches and then half of the custard. Repeat. Cover and refrigerate at

*see gluten-free products list at the end of the book

least 24 hours for flavors to blend. When ready to serve, whip cream with 2 teaspoons sugar and spread over trifle. Garnish with lightly toasted almonds.

## Trifle – Chocolate Kahlua® Version
If you like chocolate, this is a nice change from regular trifle. This is my mother's recipe.

1 package gluten-free chocolate pudding mix* (not instant) prepared according to package directions or see index and make 1 recipe chocolate pudding
1 recipe gluten-free chocolate cake (see index) or a gluten-free cake mix made in a 9" x 12" pan
1 teaspoon gluten-free vanilla*
1 cup gluten-free heavy cream*

1 cup Kahlua® Liqueur (gluten-free as of this writing or see index for recipe)
2 teaspoons sugar
Mini chocolate chips* for decoration (optional)
½ cup sliced almonds, lightly toasted (optional)

Prepare pudding as directed. Cover and set aside to cool, stirring once in a while to prevent a skin from forming on the top

Cut the gluten-free cake into slices. Place half of cake on the bottom of a pretty glass bowl. Sprinkle ½ cup Kahlua over cake. Cover with half the pudding. Repeat. Cover and refrigerate at least 24 hours for flavors to blend. When ready to serve, whip cream with 2 teaspoons sugar and spread over trifle. Garnish with lightly toasted almonds and chocolate chips.

## Twelve Fruit Compote
My mother makes this at Christmas. Not only is it delicious but it also makes the house smell so good while cooking it.

3 cups water
1 pound mixed dried fruits (apricots, peaches, pears). Make sure they are gluten-free. Some dry fruits are coated with flour or oat flour for baking.
1 cup pitted prunes
½ cup raisins or currants
1 cup pitted sweet cherries
2 apples, peeled, cored and sliced
½ cup fresh cranberries

1 cup sugar
1 lemon, sliced
2 (3 inch) cinnamon sticks
6 whole cloves
Sections of one orange
Grated peel of one orange
½ cup seedless grapes
½ cup Grand Marnier®

Combine water, dried fruit, prunes and raisins in a large pot and bring to a boil. Lower heat, cover pan and simmer 20 minutes. Add the cherries, apples, cranberries, sugar, lemon, cinnamon sticks and cloves. Cover and simmer 5 minutes more. Add sections of orange, grapes and Grand Marnier and bring to a boil then remove from heat. Add grated orange peel and remove cloves and cinnamon sticks. Serve warm.

*see gluten-free products list at the end of the book

## Yogurt Parfait
I enjoy this for breakfast or dessert.

Plain Gluten-free Yogurt*
Canned or fresh fruit, cut up
Gluten-free Jam*, in a flavor the same as
    the fruit or compliments the fruit
    (Polaner® All Fruit is labeled gluten-
    free.  Most jams are gluten-free)

Honey-Nut Corn Chex® cereal (now
    gluten-free), slightly crushed if desired
    (optional)
Gluten-free Canned Whipped Cream*
    (optional)

Blend the yogurt with the jam.  Depending on your preferences, use anywhere from 1 to 3 teaspoons per serving.  Sometimes if the fruit is very sweet, I eliminate the jam.

Layer the fruit and yogurt in a parfait glass.  Top with some of the crushed cereal if you want some crunch.  Top with whipped cream if desired.

For a breakfast parfait, I put the fruit in a bowl, top with the yogurt/jam mixture, and top with the cereal.  Or, you can put the fruit and yogurt/jam mixture in a plastic cup, cover and refrigerate it.  Top it with the cereal in the morning so it remains crunchy.

## Zuppa Inglais
Make this a day ahead of time for best results.  Top with cream and garnish it on the day you serve it. This is my mother's recipe.  I also make this when I have leftover gluten-free cake.

6 egg yolks
3 packages of gluten-free vanilla pudding*,
    3 ounce size
4 ½ cups milk
1 gluten-free sponge cake (see index, I
    make the easy sponge cake in a 9" x 11"
    pan or half the sponge cake recipes for

one of the larger cakes.  The cake will be
    about ½" high).
½ cup rum
2 cups gluten-free heavy cream*
4 teaspoons sugar
Chopped pecans
Gluten-free maraschino cherries*
    (optional)

Beat egg yolks in a large saucepan with a rotary beater.  Add the pudding mix and the milk and blend.  Cook until thickened.  Allow to cool.  Cut the sponge cake so they are in slices resembling the size of lady fingers.  Sprinkle the sponge cake with rum and place in a pretty yet large shallow glass dish.  Cover the cake with the cooled pudding.  Whip cream with sugar and cover the top of the dessert.  Sprinkle with chopped nuts, and the well drained cherries if desired.

*Variation*:  Gluten-Free Naturals™ Yellow Cake mix may be used instead of sponge cake.

## Zuppa Inglais – Version 2

For best flavor, put together the cake, rum and pudding a day ahead of time, and cover and refrigerate. Top with mocha whipped cream right before serving. This is my mother's recipe.

1 sponge cake made in a 9 x 11" pan, about a ½" thick in height (see index).
½ cup rum

3 cups custard made as in the Trifle recipe (see index)
1 ½ cups prepared mocha whipped cream (see index)

Sprinkle the rum on the cooled cake. Prepare the custard as for the Trifle recipe and top the cake with it. Allow to cool, cover and refrigerate. The next day prepare the mocha whipped cream and top with it. Slice into squares and serve.

*Variation*: Gluten-Free Naturals™ yellow cake mix prepared as directed may be used instead of the sponge cake.

# PUDDINGS AND CUSTARDS

Puddings are wonderful for dessert, but have you considered them for breakfast? You don't always have to have bread at breakfast. I particularly like Rice Pudding or Custard in the morning. Many brands of pudding are gluten-free (see index) but I prefer my homemade versions.

## Bread Pudding

This is delicious for dessert or breakfast. If using leftover raisin bread, you can use a little less raisins and cinnamon.

5 slices bread, made with Gluten-Free
   Naturals™ Bread Flour (see index)
Gluten-free butter or margarine
⅓ cup raisins (I prefer sultanas)
2 eggs

⅔ cup sugar
2 cups milk
½ teaspoon gluten-free vanilla*
Ground cinnamon

Boil water in a tea kettle. Set aside a large pan, and choose a smaller pan for the bread pudding that will fit into the larger pan to create a water bath for the pudding. Grease the smaller pan.

Line the bottom of the greased pan with raisins. Butter the bread and cut into cubes, and put them over the raisins. Beat together the eggs, sugar, milk and vanilla and pour it over the bread mixture. Sprinkle with cinnamon.

Put the smaller pan into the larger one. Add boiling water to the large pan, about halfway up. Be careful not to spill hot water on yourself and put it into the oven. Bake at 375°F for 1 hour. Remove carefully from the oven because the boiling water can burn you. Serve warm or cool.

*Variation*: A ¼ cup walnuts may be added with the raisins.

## Bread Pudding – Queen's Style

This is a British/Canadian Bread Pudding with a hit of jam and a meringue topping. It is more custard-like than a traditional pudding.

3 cups of cubed day-old bread or stale
   bread, made with Gluten-Free
   Naturals™ Bread Flour (see index for
   bread recipe. Sandwich Bread, Multi-
   grain or even Raisin bread may also be
   used.)
4 cups milk
3 Tablespoons melted butter
¾ cup sugar
½ teaspoon salt
3 egg yolks

1 egg
½ teaspoon gluten-free vanilla*
Boiling water in a kettle for the "bain
   marie"
½ cup jelly or jam (I like black cherry but
   use any flavor you like. Polaner® is
   labeled gluten-free. I use a little less
   than 1/2 cup and make a thin layer.)
3 egg whites
½ cup sugar

*see gluten-free products list at the end of the book*

Grease either an 8 inch square pan or a 9 inch pie pan. (I prefer it made in the pie pan.) Make sure you have a larger pan that your pan will fit into. When you bake it in the oven you have to create a "water bath" or "bain marie" for the pudding.

Put milk in a saucepan and scald it. Add butter and melt it in. Cut bread into cubes and pour the milk over the bread. Add the ¾ cup sugar, salt, egg yolk, egg, and vanilla.

Pour the bread mixture into the prepared baking dish. Set in a larger pan. Fill with 1 inch of hot water in the bottom of the larger pan. (I find it easier to put the pans on the rack in the oven, and pour the water when it is on the rack rather than on the counter.) Bake at 325°F for 45 minutes, or until the pudding is set. You can test it by inserting and knife and seeing if it comes out clean.

Remove from oven. Remove from water bath. Immediately spread a thin layer of jam over the hot pudding.

Take the egg whites and beat them to form soft peaks. Gradually beat in the ½ cup sugar. Beat the meringue until stiff and shiny. To be sure it is done, take a little between your fingers and feel if there is any sugar grit. If there is not it is beaten enough. Spread the meringue over the jam. Bake at 325°F for 20 minutes or until the meringue is lightly browned.

## Butterscotch Pudding
My mother always made puddings from scratch, and this is her recipe.

| | |
|---|---|
| ½ cup boiling water | ⅛ teaspoon salt |
| ½ cup sugar | ½ cup milk |
| 2 Tablespoons butter | 3 Tablespoons cornstarch (use 4 |
| 2 cups milk |    Tablespoons for a firmer pudding) |
| ¼ cup sugar | 1 teaspoon gluten-free vanilla* |

Have the boiling water ready. Take ⅓ cup sugar and place in an iron skillet. Heat and stir with a wooden spoon until the sugar melts and takes a nice amber color. Quickly remove from heat and carefully stir in the boiling hot water. Continue to stir until all the sugar melts into a syrup returning the skillet to the burner if necessary. Add the 2 Tablespoons butter. Pour this into your saucepan.

Measure 2 cups of milk in a large liquid measuring cup. Pour milk in saucepan with the butter mixture. Add the sugar and salt to the milk and stir a few seconds. Heat the milk. While milk is heating, measure ½ cup milk in the same measuring cup and add the cornstarch. Blend well until smooth.

As soon as bubbles appear around the edge of the pan of the heating milk, add the cornstarch mixture and stir (using a whisk) until the pudding is smooth, thick and bubbly. This takes a minute. Remove from heat and stir in vanilla. Pour into 5 or 6 serving dishes and cool. Refrigerate.

*see gluten-free products list at the end of the book

## Chocolate Pudding

The boxed puddings are expensive, considering you're only getting some cornstarch, sugar, and flavorings. I find the homemade more delicious and natural tasting. This is my mother's recipe.

2 cups milk

½ cup sugar

⅛ teaspoon salt

½ cup milk

3 Tablespoons cornstarch (use 4 Tablespoons for a firmer pudding)

2 Tablespoons plus 2 teaspoons cocoa

1 teaspoon gluten-free vanilla*

Measure 2 cups of milk in a large liquid measuring cup. Pour milk in saucepan. Add the sugar and salt to the milk and stir a few seconds. Heat the milk.

While milk is heating, measure ½ cup milk in the same measuring cup and add the cornstarch and the cocoa. Blend well until smooth.

As soon as bubbles appear around the edge of the pan of the heating milk, add the cornstarch mixture and stir (using a whisk) until the pudding is smooth, thick and bubbly. This takes a minute. Remove from heat and stir in vanilla. Pour into 5 or 6 serving dishes and cool. Refrigerate.

## Chocolate Mousse

Light texture and very rich. This is easy to make using the microwave oven.

1 ½ cups gluten-free miniature marshmallows*

⅓ cup milk

1 cup gluten-free semi-sweet chocolate chips*

¼ teaspoon gluten-free almond extract or vanilla extract* (I prefer vanilla)

1 cup (½ pint) cold whipping cream

Chocolate chips for garnish (optional)

Put the marshmallows and milk in a microwave safe container. (I use a 4 cup Pyrex® measuring cup). Microwave it on high for 1 minute in an 800 watt microwave, or on medium or low if you have a higher wattage microwave oven. Stir the mixture with a whisk. Add the extract and chocolate chips and blend them in. (The chocolate chips will melt and blend in.) Set the mixture aside to cool to room temperature.

Whip the cream until stiff. Gently fold it into the chocolate mixture. Fill parfait glasses. This is delicious but very rich. Although the original recipe suggested 4 servings, I use smaller glasses and make 8 smaller servings. Cover with plastic wrap. Refrigerate 3 to 4 hours until stiff. Garnish with additional chocolate chips if desired.

Another way to serve it is slice some fresh strawberries and put a large dab of mousse on it. You don't have to refrigerate the mousse the 3 to 4 hours if using it as a garnish on strawberries.

*Variation*: You can make this on the stove, and make a chocolate and vanilla layer. In a small saucepan, combine the marshmallows and milk. Cook over low heat, stirring constantly, until marshmallows are melted and mixture is smooth. Be careful not to let it

*see gluten-free products list at the end of the book

burn. Remove from the heat. In a medium bowl, pour ⅓ of the marshmallow mixture and add the extract. Set aside. To the remaining mixture, add the chocolate chips. Return to low heat, stirring constantly until the chocolate is melted. Be careful not to burn it. Remove from heat. Cool to room temperature. In a small bowl, beat the whipping cream until stiff. Fold 1 cup whipped cream into the chocolate mixture. Gradually fold remaining whipped cream into reserved mixture. Fill 4 parfait glasses about three-fourths full of the chocolate mixture. Spoon the remaining mixture on top. You will have the chocolate mixture on the bottom, with a white creamy mixture on the top. Refrigerate 3 to 4 hours or until set. Garnish with additional chips if desired.

## Chocolate Mousse, Version 2

This recipe comes from Hershey's® European Style Cocoa, which is my favorite cocoa. It's sometimes hard to find, but you can call them (see list) and they will tell you the stores in your area that carry it.

| | |
|---|---|
| 1 envelope unflavored gelatin | ⅔ cup cocoa |
| ¼ cup cold water | 2 cups (1 pint) cold heavy whipping cream |
| ⅓ cup boiling water | 2 teaspoons gluten-free vanilla* |
| 1 cup sugar | |

Sprinkle the gelatin over the cold water in a bowl. Let stand 2 minutes to soften the gelatin. Add the boiling water and stir until the gelatin is completely dissolved. Cool slightly.

Mix the sugar and the cocoa in a large mixer bowl and add the cream and vanilla. Beat on medium speed and scrape the bottom and sides of the bowl occasionally. Continue to beat, until stiff. Then pour the gelatin in, and beat until well blended.

Spoon into dessert dishes and refrigerate a minimum of 30 minutes. Store covered in the refrigerator until ready to serve. Makes 8 servings.

## Custard – Baked

Delicious as a dessert, or for breakfast! My mother often makes this to bring to people recuperating from an illness because it tastes so good and is so light. This is her recipe.

| | |
|---|---|
| 1 quart milk | Grated nutmeg |
| ½ cup sugar | 1 kettle boiling water for water bath |
| ¼ teaspoon salt | (called bain marie in French or bagno |
| 4 large eggs | maria in Italian) |
| 1 teaspoon gluten-free vanilla* | |

Heat some water in a tea kettle for the water bath for this custard.

Put milk, sugar, and salt into a large saucepan. Stir until sugar melts and heat until milk is very hot. Watch the pot carefully so the milk does not boil over. As soon as milk starts to boil, immediately remove pot from heat.

*see gluten-free products list at the end of the book

Beat 4 eggs slightly in a large bowl and pour the hot milk over them while beating with a whisk. Add vanilla and blend. Pour mixture through a strainer into 10 custard cups. Sprinkle tops of custard with freshly grated nutmeg.

Get out 2 baking dishes each large enough to hold 5 custard cups and place the filled custard cups in them. Pour very hot water halfway. Place in a preheated 325°F oven and bake 25 to 30 minutes. Test for doneness by inserting a knife in the center of one custard. If the knife comes out clean, the custard has cooked enough. Remove from oven and quickly remove the cups from the water bath as the custard will continue to cook and be ruined. Cool and refrigerate.

Note: Use two baking dishes because one is too heavy to handle. Sometimes a little water would spill out and burn my hands.

*Variation*: You can half of this recipe, if desired. I only have 4 large custard cups that hold about ½ cup of milk in each, so I make half the recipe. (My mother's recipe uses 10 smaller size custard cups.) If you use the larger size like I have, you will need to test the custard and bake it a little longer.

*Variation 2*: I have successfully made this by heating the milk in the microwave instead of on the stove. However, watch carefully as it can boil over easily and make a mess.

## Lemon Mousse
If you like lemon desserts, here is an easy one to make.

1 ½ cups of gluten-free heavy cream*
⅓ cup sugar
¼ cup lemon juice (I use bottled, but fresh is even better)

1 teaspoon gluten-free lemon extract* (I use a little less)

Put all ingredients into an electric mixer and whip until light and fluffy. Do not over-beat. (Over-beating cream can make it start to turn into butter and whey, and that will ruin your dessert.)

Spoon the mousse into champagne glasses, to create a fancy looking dessert.

*see gluten-free products list at the end of the book

## Pumpkin Pudding

This is a delicious, creamy pumpkin pie flavored filling with about half the calories of pumpkin pie. It is very fast and easy to make. I enjoy the leftovers for breakfast. The nuts add nice texture since there is no crust.

2 cups milk (I use 1 or 2% milk)
1 cup canned pumpkin (I use half of a 15 ounce can)
½ cup sugar
3 Tablespoons cornstarch
¼ teaspoon salt

1 teaspoon ground cinnamon
¼ teaspoon ground ginger
¼ teaspoon ground nutmeg
1 egg
1 teaspoon gluten-free vanilla*
Walnut halves

*Microwave directions (these were developed using an 800 watt microwave oven)*: In a casserole dish or a 4 cup Pyrex® measuring cup, add the milk, pumpkin, sugar, cornstarch, salt, and spices. Stir together with a whisk. Microwave on high for 8 minutes, and stir with a whisk. (For best results, blend with a whisk after 3 and 6 minutes.) In another bowl, beat egg. Gradually stir and mix in some of the hot mixture into the egg. Then return the egg to the casserole and stir in with a whisk. Microwave 3 minutes more. Stir in vanilla. Pour into individual dessert dishes, custard cups or mini pie plates. Allow to cool. Let it set and top with several walnut halves. Cover with plastic wrap and refrigerate. Fully chill before serving. If desired, top with whipped cream before serving.

*Stove directions*: In a large pot, add milk, pumpkin, sugar, cornstarch, salt and spices. Blend well with a whisk. Cook and stir until thick and bubbly. Lower temperature and cook 2 minutes more. In another bowl, beat egg. Gradually stir and mix in half of the hot mixture into the egg. Return to the pot and stir in. Cook 2 minutes more on low heat and do not boil. Stir in vanilla. Pour into individual dessert dishes or custard cups or mini pie plates. Allow to cool. Let set and top with several walnut halves. Cover with plastic wrap and refrigerate. Fully chill before serving. If desired, top with whipped cream before serving.

*Variation*: Splenda® may be substituted for sugar, to make this an even lower calorie dessert.

## Rice Pudding – Baked

Delicious as a dessert or for breakfast. This is my mother's recipe.

½ cup rice (do not use instant or converted rice)
4 extra large eggs
1 Tablespoon gluten-free vanilla*
6 heaping Tablespoons sugar

Pinch of salt
4 cups hot milk
Freshly grated nutmeg

Cook ½ cup rice according to package directions.

Beat eggs, sugar and salt in a large bowl. Gradually add hot milk to egg mixture, stirring rapidly all the while. Add rice and vanilla and pour into a baking dish. Grate nutmeg over top.

*see gluten-free products list at the end of the book

Place dish in a larger baking dish and pour very hot water into a larger one. Bake at 300°F for 1 hour.

## Rice Pudding – Stovetop Version

Delicious not only for dessert – try some for breakfast! It has rice, eggs, milk and certainly tastes better than cold cereal with milk in the morning. If you want to cut calories, you can substitute a low calorie sweetener for the sugar in this recipe. This is my mother's recipe.

⅔ cup rice (not converted rice or instant rice or it won't work. My Mother uses Carolina® or River® brand.)
2 quarts milk
Dash of salt
4 jumbo eggs

¾ cup sugar
½ teaspoon ground nutmeg
2 teaspoons gluten-free vanilla*
Additional sprinkling nutmeg

Put rice into a large pot and add milk and salt. Bring to a boil, lower the heat and simmer 20 minutes until rice is soft. Stir once in a while to be sure rice is not sticking to the bottom of the pot. While rice is cooking, beat eggs with sugar and nutmeg. When rice is cooked, remove from heat. Add a little milk mixture to egg mixture while beating with a whisk. Now stir egg mixture into the cooked rice. (This method is necessary, or your eggs would cook instead of blending in.) Put pot back over heat and bring to a boil while stirring. As soon as you see a few bubbles, remove from heat and stir in vanilla. Pour mixture immediately into one large or two medium bowls. Sprinkle tops with freshly grated nutmeg.

The secret to good rice pudding is to use rice with a higher starch content. The brands of rice suggested make it a creamier pudding. Don't use converted rice or it won't be good.

## Tapioca Pudding

Good for dessert or for breakfast. To lower calories, you can use a sugar substitute such as Splenda®. Or use Lactaid® milk and use less sugar since Lactaid® milk has a sweeter taste.

2 ¾ cups milk
3 Tablespoons granulated tapioca
⅓ cup sugar (I use about ¼ cup if using Lactaid® milk)

1 egg
Dash of salt
1 teaspoon gluten-free vanilla*

Method 1: Put milk in a pot and heat. Do not boil. Turn off heat and add tapioca and let it soak until it cools down. Mix in egg, sugar, and dash of salt. Boil 1 minute or so. When it looks translucent, it's done. Blend in vanilla.

Method 2: Put the cold milk, tapioca, sugar and egg in a pot. Blend well with a whisk. Let sit 5 minutes. Turn on the heat. Stirring constantly, and bring to a boil. Cook until the tapioca is translucent (about 1 minute). Remove from heat. Add the vanilla and stir in. Stir again after 20 minutes. I often make it this way because I don't have the time to wait for the first method.

*see gluten-free products list at the end of the book

Note: Do <u>not</u> try substituting tapioca starch for the quick cooking tapioca. It will not work. I would only recommend doing it if you wanted to create a totally gross liquid slime for a Halloween party, and you certainly wouldn't want to eat it!

## Vanilla Pudding

Most pudding mixes are gluten-free, but I prefer to make my own. This has a more delicate flavor. It is also less expensive to make your own.

2 cups milk
¼ cup sugar
⅛ teaspoon salt
½ cup milk

3 Tablespoons cornstarch (use 4 Tablespoons for a firmer pudding)
1 teaspoon gluten-free vanilla*

Measure 2 cups of milk in a large liquid measuring cup. Pour milk in saucepan. Add the sugar and salt to the milk and stir a few seconds. Heat the milk. While milk is heating, measure ½ cup milk in the same measuring cup and add the cornstarch. Blend well until smooth. As soon as bubbles appear around the edge of the pan, add cornstarch mixture and stir (using a whisk) until the pudding is smooth, thick and bubbly. This takes a minute. Remove from heat and stir in vanilla. Pour into 5 or 6 serving dishes and cool. Refrigerate.

## Write your own recipes here:

*see gluten-free products list at the end of the book

## Candies, Jams, and Preserves

# CANDIES

Many brands of candy in the U.S. are gluten-free, so I have not included too many recipes to make them. I have listed some store-bought candies that I like in the back of the book. Be careful in Europe and Canada to check with manufacturers because some countries permit them to use flour to prevent sticking and they don't have to list it on the label.

Note that my candy recipes do not involving tempering chocolate. Tempering gives chocolate a glossy finish. It involves raising and lowering chocolate temperatures to exact readings on a candy thermometer. We eat chocolates so quickly that I don't bother doing it. I store chocolates in the freezer in a container to keep them fresh and defrost them before serving them. Sometimes I make nuts dipped in chocolate and those are good frozen or defrosted!

Also note that you should never add water to melted chocolate. It will ruin it. If you need to thin it down, add some shortening to it.

## Candied Almonds or Peanuts

This is an Italian candy that my Mother made at Christmastime. It is less sweet and easier to chew than other "brittles". We enjoyed this before we ever knew about the gluten-free diet.

½ pound whole un-skinned almonds
½ cup sugar
½ teaspoon gluten-free vanilla*
4 teaspoons water

Tiny multi-colored "hundreds and thousands" candies or candy sprinkles (check ingredients)

Butter a cookie sheet (works well on a buttered Teflon® sheet). Place the almonds, sugar, vanilla and water into a saucepan and mix. Put over low heat and stir the whole time while cooking. The sugar will first melt in the water, then the water will evaporate, and then the sugar will crystallize again. Continue to stir and heat and the sugar will melt into a thick brown syrup. As soon as all the sugar melts, immediately remove from heat or your candy will begin to burn. Work very quickly and make little mounds of nuts on the buttered cookie sheet and sprinkle with "hundreds and thousands". Cool and store it in air-tight tins.

*Variation*: Raw peanuts, with or without skins can also be used. You can purchase them at oriental food markets. The nuts get nicely toasted in the hot syrup. Use ¾ pound raw peanuts instead of almonds and you will end up with honey nuts that rival the commercial ones. Don't sprinkle with the candies.

For easy clean up, fill the saucepan with water and bring to a boil.

## Coconut Eggs

There are brands of gluten-free Coconut Easter eggs, but we enjoy making our own. This is my friend's recipe.

1 package (about 21 ounces) shredded coconut* (or for added crunch, toast ½ cup of the coconut and blend it in)
½ cup butter (do not substitute margarine)
1 teaspoon gluten-free coconut flavoring*
1 teaspoon almond flavoring*

½ teaspoon salt (optional)
About 1 cup (¾ of a 14 ounce) can of sweetened condensed milk
Semi-sweet chocolate, melted or gluten-free chocolate candy melts (as of this writing Wilton® chocolate candy melts® are gluten-free)

Combine the sweetened condensed milk and butter in a mixer bowl and mix on medium speed. Blend for about 1 minute. Add the flavorings and salt and blend them in. Mix in the coconut by hand and refrigerate the mixture for 1 hour.

Form or mold the coconut mixture into egg shapes. Place on a cookie sheet lined with waxed paper. Refrigerate for 30 minutes until firm.

Melt the chocolate over hot water, or in the microwave on low. (I microwave using the defrost cycle and check every 20 seconds. Stir to completely melt all chocolate.) Dip the coconut eggs into the chocolate. Refrigerate the coconut eggs to set.

## Copy Pop

This is similar to a snack food called Poppy Cock®. Years ago one of my bosses gave me a decorative container filled with this at Christmastime. We enjoyed is so much that we asked for the recipe. Traditionally popped popcorn made in a pot works best in this recipe, although I have used air popped popcorn successfully. This recipe was created using an 800 watt microwave oven.

1 cup butter
½ cup corn syrup
1 ¼ cups sugar
2 quarts popped corn

1 ½ cups to 2 cups gluten-free nuts (beware some dry roasted nuts contain gluten)
1 teaspoon gluten-free vanilla*

In a 2 or 2 ½ quart mixing bowl combine butter, syrup and sugar. Microwave at high setting (or setting to get 800 watts) for 9 to 15 minutes or until brittle threads form when a small amount is dropped in cold water, stirring every 3 minutes. In a buttered 5 quart container, combine popped corn and nuts. Stir vanilla into cooked syrup and immediately pour over corn mixture. Stir with a meat fork until well coated.

Spread mixture in a single layer on 2 large sheets of waxed paper. Let stand until firm. Break into small pieces and store in an air tight container.

*Variation*: You can also make this on the stove. Heat the mixture as you would for making other candy. Watch carefully so it doesn't get too dark. Poppy Cock® is not dark, and Cracker Jack® is darker. We let it cook too long and it was still good but more like Cracker Jack®.

*see gluten-free products list at the end of the book

## Fudge – Easy Version

This version is delicious, and you don't have to cook it on the stove. It turns out best using a heavy duty mixer, because it can be difficult to stir. This recipe was created using an 800 watt microwave oven.

1 (18 ounce) package of gluten-free semi-sweet chocolate chips*

1 ½ teaspoons gluten-free vanilla*

½ teaspoon gluten-free almond extract* (optional – I prefer it without it)

Pinch of salt

1 (14 ounce) can of sweetened condensed milk

Chopped nuts

Grease a 9 x 9" pan. Line the pan with waxed paper, with it hanging over 2 edges. (Or a good non-stick pan may be used.)

In a large Pyrex® measuring cup, or microwave safe bowl, melt the chocolate chips on defrost/low in the microwave. Heat 5 minutes, then stir. If not melted, repeat and heat 1 or 2 minutes more, then stir. Do not use high temperatures or the chocolate may burn. Add extracts and pinch of salt.

Put melted chips in a heavy duty mixer bowl. Pour the condensed milk in the measuring cup and microwave 1 minute on high. Add it to the mixer bowl. Once you add it you must work quickly or it will get too thick to mix. Turn on the mixer and blend. Pour into prepared pan.

Top with nuts and press them in. Refrigerate for at least 2 hours. When using the non-stick pan, cut it in 4 pieces, remove those pieces and then cut into smaller pieces. If you used the waxed paper, you can lift it out using the waxed paper and then cut into smaller pieces.

## Fudge – Marshmallow Crème version

My husband likes this fudge. He makes a full batch and keeps it in the freezer for snacks.

1 teaspoon gluten-free vanilla*

1 (7 ounce) container marshmallow crème

1 package (12 ounces) gluten-free semi-sweet chocolate chips*

1 ½ cups sugar

1 (10 ounce) can evaporated milk

½ cup (1 stick) butter

Place vanilla, marshmallow crème and chocolate chips in a large mixing bowl and set aside. Mix sugar, evaporated milk and 1 Tablespoon butter in a 3 quart saucepan. Bring to a full rolling boil, stirring constantly over medium heat. Continue boiling until a candy thermometer reaches 233°F (in approximately 8 minutes of boiling).

Add the remaining butter and bring back to a boil, stirring constantly. Immediately pour the hot mixture into the bowl of vanilla, marshmallow crème and chocolate chips. Mix until well blended.

*see gluten-free products list at the end of the book

Pour the fudge into a 9 x 9 inch pan. Cool at room temperature until firm. When cool, cut into squares. (I prefer small pieces, since it is rich.)

## Fudge – Uncooked cream cheese version
We prefer the other versions. I've included this recipe because this version is easier for children to make.

| | |
|---|---|
| 1 (3 ounce) package of gluten-free cream cheese | 2 cups 10X sugar (confectioner's sugar) |
| | 1 teaspoon gluten-free vanilla* |
| 2 squares of bitter cooking chocolate*, melted | Pinch of salt |
| | Nuts |

Remove cream cheese from the refrigerator to soften. In the microwave on the defrost cycle, melt the baking chocolate. Using a sturdy spoon or heavy duty mixer, soften the cream cheese in a bowl and work in the melted chocolate, sugar, salt and vanilla. Spread in a greased 9x9 inch pan. Put in the refrigerator until hardened.

## Irish Potatoes Candy
This recipe is from an Irish friend. They don't contain any potatoes; they just look like tiny potatoes. This is fun for children to make. We serve them on St. Patrick's Day. This recipe can be doubled.

| | |
|---|---|
| 4 ounces (½ of an 8 ounce package) of gluten-free cream cheese | 2 ¾ to 3 cups 10X sugar (confectioner's sugar) |
| ¼ cup (½ stick) butter, softened | Pinch of salt |
| ½ teaspoon gluten-free vanilla* | 1 ¼ cups flaked coconut |
| | Ground cinnamon |

Remove cream cheese and butter from the refrigerator to soften. In a bowl, beat the butter and cream cheese together until smooth. (I use a heavy duty mixer.) Add the vanilla and then add the confectioner's sugar 1 cup at a time. Mix in slowly at first and then beat until smooth. Add the coconut. You may have to mix the coconut into the sugar mixture by using a sturdy spoon. Cover with plastic wrap and refrigerate the mixture for 30 to 60 minutes to make it easier to handle.

Cover the bottom of a small bowl with cinnamon. Roll into the filling into balls or small oblong potato shapes. Roll them in cinnamon. If it is difficult to roll, drop it by teaspoonfuls into the cinnamon and then roll it. We make them look a little bumpy and not perfectly smooth so that they look more like little potatoes. Place on a plate or cookie sheet and chill to set in the refrigerator. Put in a plastic bag and store in the refrigerator until ready to eat.

*Variation*: Use cocoa instead of cinnamon. I prefer the flavor of the cinnamon version, but the cocoa version does look even more like potatoes. The cocoa has a slight bitter taste that dark chocolate lovers like. Since this recipe makes a lot, I often make some with cocoa and some with cinnamon.

*see gluten-free products list at the end of the book

## Marzipan in Chocolate

Most candy is gluten-free, but you have to check to be sure they are not dipped in flour to prevent sticking. In Europe they can make chocolates and use flour to prevent sticking and they don't have to list it on the label. Don't eat imported chocolates without checking if they are gluten-free, even if the ingredients look like they are.

When I was in Belgium years ago, I had wonderful marzipan candy dipped in chocolate and grouped together like a bunch of grapes with a golden paper leaf added. You can do this, or make them separate candies.

½ recipe almond paste, (see recipe under miscellaneous) or 8 ounces (1 cup) of almond paste
2 teaspoons flavoring such as gluten-free almond*, vanilla* or rum flavoring* or 1 Tablespoon liqueur such as Kirschwasser®* or Grand Marnier®* or Kahlua®* (see index). *These liqueurs are gluten-free as of this writing*
Confectioner's sugar (about 1 cup to 1 ¼ cups, or a little more if using liqueur)
Gluten-free chocolate chips*, about 1 cup or chocolate candy melts (as of this writing Wilton® chocolate candy melts® are gluten-free)

Spread confectioner's sugar on a clean counter or board. Take the almond paste, add some of the flavoring, and begin kneading it into the sugar. Continue kneading adding the rest of the flavoring and more sugar. Knead until you have a good consistency. Taste to see if you want to add a flavoring. If adding any of the flavorings, you will use a little more confectioner's sugar. When completely kneaded and a good consistency, make small balls of marzipan.

Take chocolate chips and put them in a microwave safe container (I use a Pyrex® measuring cup.) Heat on defrost 3 minutes. Stir. If not all melted, heat on defrost for 30 seconds more. Stir. Continue if needed. Dip the balls in the chocolate until coated and place on waxed paper placed on a cookie sheet. If your chocolate starts to run low, melt more by repeating the process.

(Note: This method is not "tempering" chocolate which makes the chocolate have a glossy finish. We usually make candies before a party and they are eaten right away, so I don't temper the chocolate. Tempering can be time consuming and requires maintaining exact temperatures.)

Set the candies in a cool place out of the direct sun. When all the candies are dry and cool, you can put them in mini-cupcake liner papers for a nice presentation. (Note: If you put them in while wet, they will stick to the paper and you can get paper stuck to the candy.) Store in a cool place.

If you wish to make the grape bunch pattern, set out a piece of waxed paper on a plate or cookie sheet. While the chocolate is wet, mound them on top of each other until they resemble a bunch of grapes. You can add a leaf while the chocolate is still wet. You can purchase ready-made leaves for baking decoration from specialty shops. Then allow to cool. Store in a cool place.

*see gluten-free products list at the end of the book

*Variation*: Take an almond, wrap some almond paste around it and dip it in the chocolate as above.

## Peanut Brittle
We enjoy this treat. It makes a lot. You can use other nuts if you are allergic to peanuts. This is delicious peanut brittle and be forewarned that it is addictive! This makes a nice gift too. For gifts, put peanut brittle in wide mouth canning jars or decorative food tins.

1 cup corn syrup*
1 cup sugar
¼ cup water
2 Tablespoons butter
2 to 3 cups peanuts (or we use more)

1 teaspoon baking soda (I use a little less)
½ teaspoon gluten-free vanilla* (optional – I only use if the corn syrup doesn't contain vanilla)

Grease a large baking sheet and set aside. In a heavy saucepan, stir together the corn syrup, sugar, water and butter. Cook over medium heat, stirring constantly until the sugar is dissolved and the mixture boils. Once it boils, stop stirring. Insert a candy thermometer and cook until it reaches 280°F. At that point, continue cooking and stir again until the mixture reaches 300°F. Remove from heat.

Stir in peanuts, vanilla and baking soda. Immediately pour into a baking sheet and spread. If you are having difficulty spreading, it may be easier to spread with a greased metal spoon or spatula. It will be hot; be careful not to burn yourself. Cool and break into pieces.

Note: The original recipe told you to add the peanuts at 280°F and continue cooking and stirring until 300°F. We found that when you added the peanuts at that time, the peanuts get too dark. They had a slightly burnt taste because they became too roasted. If you are using roasted peanuts, we found that adding them in at the end resulted in a better tasting peanut brittle.

The baking soda is added so that you have a peanut brittle that you can break apart. If you want a harder brittle, use a little less baking soda. Don't eliminate or it will be too hard, and you will have difficulty breaking it apart. Also, without the baking soda it can be too hard to chew.

*Variation*: Salted or unsalted peanuts can be used. Other nuts can be used, but we like peanuts the best in this recipe.

## Peanut Butter Chocolate Crunch Candies
This recipe comes from my sister-in-law. These candies are decadent! They remind me of a combination of Reese's® Peanut Butter Cups and Nestlé's® Crunch.

3 ½ to 4 cups of gluten-free Rice Chex® or 3 cups of gluten-free crispy rice cereal
½ cup butter, softened
2 cups creamy peanut butter*
3 cups confectioner's sugar

1 cup gluten-free mini semi-sweet chocolate chips*
2 (12 ounce) packages gluten-free semi-sweet chocolate morsels*

*see gluten-free products list at the end of the book

If using Rice Chex®, pulverize them either by putting them in a heavy-duty plastic bag and rolling it with a rolling pin, or by pulsing them in a food processor. If using crispy rice cereal, there is no need to pulverize them.

Cream together the butter and the peanut butter. Blend in the powdered sugar. Stir in the cereal and mini chocolate chips. Roll the mixture into balls. Place on a cookie sheet lined with waxed paper. Put them in the freezer until set.

Melt the semi-sweet chocolate morsels in the microwave oven. Stir until smooth. With a fork, dip the peanut butter balls into the melted chocolate. Place on the cookie sheet lined with waxed paper. Place in the freezer until the chocolate has set. Store the candies in an airtight container at room temperature.

## Peanut Butter Eggs
There are gluten-free brands you can buy, but we enjoy making our own. We usually double the recipe. Gluten-free "candy melt" chocolate can also be used, but we prefer the chocolate chips.)

1 (16 ounce) jar natural peanut butter (Note: do not substitute regular peanut butter or it will not work.)
¼ cup butter (not margarine) at room temperature
1 teaspoon gluten-free vanilla*
¼ teaspoon salt

1 Tablespoon gluten-free corn syrup*
½ pound confectioner's sugar
Semi-sweet chocolate chips*, melted or gluten-free candy melts (as of this writing the Wilton® chocolate candy melts® are gluten-free)

Combine the peanut butter and butter in a mixer bowl. Mix at medium speed for about 1 minute. Add the vanilla, corn syrup and salt, and mix until incorporated. Slowly mix in the Confectioner's sugar until it is dough consistency. I mix some of it in by hand first, and then use the mixer to finish blending it. Refrigerate the peanut mixture for about 1 hour.

When the peanut mixture is easy to handle, shape it into egg shapes. Place on a pan lined with waxed paper. Refrigerate for 30 minutes before dipping them in chocolate.

Melt the chocolate over hot water in a double boiler, or in the microwave on low. (I microwave using the defrost cycle and check every 20 seconds. Stir to completely melt all chocolate.) Dip peanut butter eggs into the chocolate and set on your tray covered with waxed paper. Refrigerate to set.

## Smores® (also called "Some Mores") Candy

Store-bought gluten-free cookies and crackers break easily. This is a good use for the broken ones.

1 (12 ounce) package of semi-sweet
    chocolate chips*
½ cup miniature marshmallows*

1 cup of broken gluten-free crackers,
    cookies or cereal (I use gluten-free Rice
    Chex®)

Melt the chocolate over hot water, or in the microwave on low. (I microwave using the defrost cycle and check every 20 seconds. Stir to completely melt all chocolate.)

Remove from heat and add the marshmallows and broken crackers or cereal.

Drop by teaspoons onto waxed paper. Allow them to cool completely. Refrigerate to set.

## Sweet Pecans or Walnuts

A friend made these for me for my birthday. These are a nice treat to serve at a party or during the Christmas holiday.

1 Tablespoon egg white
⅛ to ¼ teaspoon gluten-free vanilla*
2 cups whole pecans or walnuts

2 to 4 Tablespoons sugar (I use 2
    Tablespoons)
2 to 4 Tablespoons brown sugar (I use 2
    Tablespoons)
1 teaspoon ground cinnamon

Mix the egg white with the vanilla. Add the nuts and blend until they are coated and sticky. Mix together the sugars and cinnamon. Sprinkle it over the nuts. Stir until the sugar mixture coats the nuts.

Spread on an un-greased non-stick cookie sheet. Bake at 300°F for 20 minutes. Immediately use a spatula to un-stick the nuts from the pan. Allow to cool before storing. Clean up the pan with hot water.

These make a nice presentation by putting them in a decorative tin, and placing nut clusters in mini-cupcake or candy papers. Or put them in a decorative jar as a gift.

*Variation*: To make sweet and spicy nuts, use ¼ cup each of regular and brown sugar. Decrease the cinnamon to ½ teaspoon. Eliminate the vanilla. Add 1 to 1 ½ teaspoons salt, 1 ½ teaspoons chili powder, and a pinch of cayenne pepper. Bake 10 minutes longer if you want the nuts to be more toasted. Note: As you eat these nuts you will taste the sweet and then get a zing of spicy at the end. The heat does build as you eat more of them, so be warned!

*Variation 2*: Other nuts such as peanuts can be used.

*Variation 3*: Egg white powder and water can be used in place of the egg white.

*see gluten-free products list at the end of the book

*Variation 4*:  Use the lower amounts of sugar (or just ¼ cup of regular sugar), eliminate the vanilla, and use them as a topping on salads.

*Variation 5*:  Silpat® silicon non-stick pan lining can be used.  This made it easier because it was non-stick, but I had to double the baking time.

## Ruth's Baby Bars

Baby Ruth® candy bars from Nestle® are gluten-free as of this writing, but here's a way to make a candy with a similar flavor.  This recipe is from my cousin.

½ cup sugar
½ cup brown sugar
1 cup white corn syrup
¾ cup peanut butter
5 cups gluten-free cornflakes*

⅔ cup peanuts* (I use regular roasted since dry roasted may not be gluten-free)
1 cup chocolate chips*

Put the sugar, corn syrup and peanut butter in a pot.  Heat and stir.  When creamy, add the cornflakes, peanuts and chocolate chips.  Mix and put in a buttered 13 inch pan.  Pack in and cool.  Cut into squares and serve.

## Write your own recipes here:

# JAMS / PRESERVES

Since most preserves are gluten-free, I do not usually make many of my own. Here are a few unusual recipes from my mother for preserves you can't easily find in stores.

If you have the Zojirushi® bread machine, you can make preserves using the jam cycle. It is easy to do. You add the ingredients into the pan and the machine cooks it at the right temperature and stirs it until done. I have successfully made them by following the instructions that come with the machine.

I have also used the recipes that come in the box with Sure-Jell®, and adapted the quantities for the bread machine. My experience is 2 to 3 cups of crushed fruit works in the bread machine. Homemade preserves are good for those allergic to corn, in order to avoid high fructose corn syrup.

Remember, that those who eat wheat cannot dip knives or spoons that touched gluten into your jar of preserves, or it will be contaminated.

## Banana Butter

Make this when you have some very ripe bananas on hand. This is good on hot gluten-free toast with or without peanut butter. It's a nice change from jam. This is my mother's recipe.

| | |
|---|---|
| 4 ripe bananas | ¼ cup lemon juice |
| ⅔ cup sugar | ½ cup orange juice |
| 3 eggs | 1 Tablespoon grated lemon peel (optional) |
| 6 Tablespoons butter | |

Start boiling water in the bottom of a double boiler. Place bananas one at a time in your blender to puree. Break eggs into the top part of the double boiler. Add juices, sugar and grated peel (if using.) Add banana puree and place pot on top of the boiling water. Simmer and stir until mixture is smooth and rather thick. You will know it is done when the mixture coats a metal spoon. It does not take very long. When cooked, quickly remove top from boiling water and pour into sterilized jars and seal. Refrigerate. Makes 3 ½ cups. Since this is a smaller amount, I don't bother with sterilizing. It keeps well in the refrigerator a week to 10 days un-sterilized.

## Blueberry Jam made in the Zojirushi® Bread Machine

I make this jam in the summer when blueberries are plentiful at the farmer's market. It is very easy to make jam in the bread machine because it cooks it at the right temperature and stirs it for you.

| | |
|---|---|
| 2 cups of crushed blueberries (about 1 and ½ pints) | Half of a (1.75 ounce) box of Sure-Jell® pectin (If you like thicker jam, you can use the whole box, which is what I do) |
| 2 cups sugar | |

Wash and remove stems from blueberries. Carefully crush berries with a potato masher. Put in the bread machine with the sugar and pectin. Cook using the jam cycle. Carefully put the hot jam in clean, sterilized jars and cover. After it has cooled, store it in the refrigerator. It keeps a long time refrigerated. Otherwise, follow directions in the Sure-Jell® box and process the jam in a canner so it will be shelf-stable.

*see gluten-free products list at the end of the book*

## Grape Jelly made in the Zojirushi® Bread Machine
This is a good use of leftover grapes.

1 ½ lbs of grapes (you can use less)
Bottled grape juice (about ¾ cup)
3 ½ cups sugar

Half of a (1.75 ounce) box of Sure-Jell®
  pectin (If you like thicker jam, you can
  use the whole box, which is what I do.)

Wash and remove stems from grapes. Process the grapes in a food processor using the cutting blade until fine. Add enough grape juice to make 2 ½ cups total. Put in the bread machine with the sugar and pectin. Cook using the jam cycle. Carefully put the hot jam in clean, sterilized jars and cover. After it has cooled, store it in the refrigerator. It keeps a long time refrigerated. Otherwise, follow directions in the Sure-Jell® box and process the jam in a canner so it will be shelf-stable.

## Lemon Butter
Fruit butters are nice served on toast or quick breads. They are easy to prepare yet very expensive to buy at gourmet shops. This is my mother's recipe.

4 eggs
¾ cup sugar
½ cup fresh lemon juice

¼ cup water
2 teaspoons grated rind
4 ounces (1 stick) butter

Follow the method for making banana butter. Makes 3 cups.

## Pepper Jelly
This is good to use as an appetizer with cream cheese. This is my mother's recipe.

4 large thick green or red peppers, seeded
  and chopped coarsely to get 2 cups
1 ½ cups cider vinegar
6 ½ cups sugar

1 bottle of Certo® pectin or Sure-Jell®
A few drops of gluten-free hot sauce* or a
  small hot pepper, chopped

Put the peppers, sugar, vinegar and hot sauce or hot pepper in a large pot. Stir and simmer and bring to a rolling boil. Add a bottle of pectin and stir to cook another 3 minutes. If color is too light, add a few drops of vegetable coloring when adding the pectin. Skim off foam and ladle into sterilized jars. Seal with paraffin.

Serve this jelly over a block of gluten-free cream cheese. Spread it on gluten-free crackers for an easy appetizer. Or use the jelly alone as an accompaniment for meats.

*see gluten-free products list at the end of the book

## Strawberry Jam made in the Zojirushi® Bread Machine

2 ½ cups of crushed strawberries (2 pints)          Half of a (1.75 ounce) box of Sure-Jell®
3 ½ cups sugar                                                      pectin (If you like thicker jam, you can
                                                                           use the whole box)

Wash and remove stems from strawberries.  Slice and carefully crush berries with a potato
masher.  Put in the bread machine with the sugar and pectin.  Cook using the jam.  Carefully
put the hot jam in clean, sterilized jars and cover. (Caution:  It will be hot!)  After it has
cooled, store it in the refrigerator.  It keeps a long time refrigerated.  Otherwise, follow
directions in the Sure-Jell® box and process the jam in a canner so it will be shelf-stable.

## Write your own recipes here:

## Beverages and Miscellaneous

# BEVERAGES

Many beverages are gluten-free, but you have to check. I have provided some lists in the back of this book. Below are some favorites from my mother, which we always enjoy. She prefers making her own liqueurs for use in desserts, because they have a more delicate flavor.

### Amaretto Liqueur

Since some brands of amaretto may contain gluten in their flavorings, here is a way to make your own. Liqueurs are easy to make. I like to use liqueurs in desserts.

6 Tablespoons boiled water

2 Tablespoons light brown sugar (or dark brown sugar for darker color)

¼ cup sugar

¼ cup gluten-free corn syrup (Plain or with vanilla added may be used. If your syrup is very thick then add 1 additional Tablespoon of water.)

¾ cups vodka (I use potato vodka)

½ teaspoon gluten-free teaspoon vanilla* (use less or eliminate if your corn syrup contains vanilla)

1 ½ teaspoons gluten-free almond extract*

Boil water and measure 6 Tablespoons into a glass jar. (I use a cleaned out mayonnaise jar.) Add the sugars and corn syrup and stir until dissolved. If it is not dissolving well enough, heat in the microwave for 30 seconds and stir again. Repeat if necessary. Once dissolved, add the rest of the ingredients and blend in. Store covered with the lid. It is better if you allow it to age a day or two so the flavors blend.

You can use this Amaretto in the Biscuit Tortoni recipe in this book.

### Cherry Liqueur

Chambord® was not gluten-free at the time I checked because the flavorings, but this may have changed. Here's a way to make your own cherry liqueur. This is my mother's recipe.

1 quart cherries (fresh)

½ pound sugar cubes

1 Tablespoon ground allspice

1 Tablespoon ground cinnamon

1 Tablespoon clove stems, remove heads

1 pint (2 cups) gluten-free vodka or other gluten-free alcohol*

Wash cherries and remove stems. Fill a large jar alternately with a thick layer of cherries then sugar and a little spice. Repeat until all ingredients are used. Add vodka, cover and let stand in a dark place for 2 months or more to age. Strain and enjoy. It tastes better aged longer.

*see gluten-free products list at the end of the book

## Chocolate Syrup for Milk

Hershey's® brand chocolate syrup is gluten-free as of this writing. In case you can't find a gluten-free brand (or prefer not to have corn syrup), here's a way to make your own. This uses sugar instead of corn syrup, so this is perfect for people with corn allergies. It stores well, covered in the refrigerator.

1 cup sugar
2 squares bitter chocolate* or ½ cup
   cocoa
⅛ teaspoon salt

1 cup cold water
1 ½ teaspoons gluten-free vanilla*

Place sugar and water in a saucepan and boil hard for 5 minutes. Watch that it doesn't boil over. Add unsweetened chocolate and salt, and stir until chocolate melts and is blended in. Simmer another 10 minutes.

If using cocoa, blend all ingredients, except the vanilla, together in a saucepan using a whisk. Simmer 15 minutes. Be careful that it doesn't boil over.

Remove from heat and add vanilla. Store in the refrigerator and use 2 Tablespoons per glass of milk.

## Cocoa or Hot Chocolate

This makes enough for 2 cups. Many brands of the instant hot chocolate are gluten-free, but sometimes you just want to have the real thing. This is also good made with Lactaid® milk. I use a little less sugar if using Lactaid® milk.

2 Tablespoons cocoa
3 Tablespoons sugar (or more if you like it
   sweeter)
¼ cup water

1 ¾ cups milk
½ teaspoon gluten-free vanilla*

Mix the cocoa and the sugar together in a small saucepan. Stir in the water with a whisk. Put it on the stove and cook this mixture until it comes to a good boil. Remove from heat. Add the milk and blend in with a whisk. Return to a low heat and heat through but don't boil it. When heated, remove from heat and add vanilla and stir.

## Coffee Liqueur

Kahlua® is gluten-free as of this writing, but here's a way to make your own.

2 cups water
4 cups sugar
1 (2 ounce) jar very strong instant coffee
   (I use a brand-new, freshly opened, jar;
   it gives it a much better flavor.)

1 bottle (750 ml or 25.4 ounce) of gluten-free vodka*
1 vanilla bean

*see gluten-free products list at the end of the book

Boil all except vodka. Cool. Place vodka and vanilla bean into a half gallon glass container. Pour boiled ingredients over and mix together. Cap loosely and keep at room temperature for 30 days.

## Daiquiri (Easy)
This is quick to put together in a blender. Be sure to use a very flavorful jam or it will be too bland. Makes 2 servings.

3 ounces of gluten-free rum*

1 teaspoon sugar

4 teaspoons lime juice (I use bottled)

8 to 10 teaspoons gluten-free jam* (I use 3 Tablespoons peach or strawberry jam)

1 ½ to 2 cups crushed ice (I use 2 cups)

Put all in blender in the order given, and blend until ice is fine. If too thick you can add a little juice or water. Serve immediately.

## Lemon Cordial
Lemoncello® is gluten-free as of this writing, but here's a way to make your own. This is little lighter in flavor and less sweet. I also like using it in cooking. This is my mother's recipe.

6 lemons

3 cups gluten-free vodka* or other gluten-free alcohol*

3 cups water

1 ½ cups granulated sugar

Wash lemons and peel very carefully with a potato peeler to assure that you remove only the lemon part and none of the white pith. Put the peels into a ½ gallon glass jar with the vodka for 10 days. After days, strain and reserve the liquid. Reserve the peel in the strainer. Make a syrup of the sugar and water by heating on the stove until the sugar melts. Stir until dissolved and boil 3 minutes. Take the strainer containing the lemon peels, and now pour the sugar syrup into the vodka mixture through the strainer. This warm liquid running through the peel will get additional flavor and color from the peels. Store covered with a tight lid at room temperature for 3 days. Use and enjoy over sorbets (sherbet) or in fruit salads. After that, store in the freezer to maintain flavor. Use within one year. Makes 6 cups. I usually make half of the recipe.

## Orange Cordial or Liqueur
Grand Marnier® is gluten-free as of this writing, but here's a way to make your own. This is my mother's recipe and it is a little lighter in flavor. I like it used in cooking and baking.

1 dozen oranges

1 quart gluten-free vodka* or other gluten-free alcohol. (My mother's original recipe used Southern

Comfort®, but I have been unable to confirm whether or not it's gluten-free.)

1 pound granulated sugar

Wash oranges and peel very carefully with a potato peeler to assure that you remove only the orange part and none of the white pith. Put the peels into the vodka for 6 weeks. After 6 weeks, strain the beverage. Make a syrup of the sugar and a little water by heating on the

*see gluten-free products list at the end of the book

stove until the sugar melts. Add to the orange flavored vodka and then bottle it. This can be used to make "Orange Cup" (see index).

## Orange Julie

I like this better than the drink you can get at the mall. (I have not been able to confirm if that drink is gluten-free or not.) You know this is safe when you make it yourself. You need a blender that can crush ice to make this. It's refreshing on a hot summer day.

1 ½ cups orange juice
1 cup water
¼ cup sugar (or 6 packets sugar substitute)

1 teaspoon gluten-free vanilla*
1 teaspoon egg white powder
1 to 1 ½ cups ice

Put the juice, water, sugar, vanilla and egg white powder in a blender and blend for 30 seconds. Add the ice and blend 30 seconds more until ice is crushed. It will be frothy and delicious.

## Orangeade

An nice alternative to lemonade.

4 cups water
2 cups orange juice

¼ cup lemon juice (reconstituted can be used, but fresh is better)
½ to ¾ cup sugar (I use less sugar)

Mix together. Serve over ice. Garnish with orange slices if desired.

## Punch – My Mother's Favorite

My mother's original recipe contained whiskey for a delicious whiskey sour type of punch. If whiskey is distilled properly, it is safe. Check with the manufacturer to be sure that no mash goes back into the product. For example, as of this writing Jack Daniels (www.jackdaniels.com) says that gluten is removed in the distilling process. If you prefer to stay with products not made from gluten grains, use potato vodka to make a vodka sour punch.

2 cups gluten-free alcohol spirits* (I use vodka* made from corn or potatoes or gluten-free whiskey* may be used)
2 quarts gluten-free ginger ale*
24 ounces of orange juice
26 ounce can of pineapple juice
6 ounces lemon juice (I use reconstituted)

1 bottle of gluten-free cherries* plus ½ the juice from the jar or no cherries and ¼ to ½ cup of Juicy Juice® cherry juice* (which is gluten-free as of this writing)
Orange slices for garnish (optional)

Chill all ingredients except the alcohol. Mix all but ginger ale in a large punch bowl over a block of ice. (I usually blend juices ahead of time for a party.) If you cannot find gluten-free cherries, use the cherry juice instead. Add ginger ale just before serving.

*see gluten-free products list at the end of the book

## Russian Tea

Years ago, "Russian Tea" made with Tang® orange drink powder was very popular. This version made with orange juice is better in flavor, and you know it is safe. Remember that regular orange juice is gluten-free, but some with additives (such as calcium added) may not be safe.

1 cup sugar
1 quart water
1 cinnamon stick
3 Tablespoons tea leaves (be sure they're gluten-free) or equivalent tea bags may be used.

1 ½ teaspoons whole cloves
1 cup orange juice
½ cup lemon juice
12 ounces pineapple juice

Boil sugar, water and spices together. Remove from heat. Add the tea and steep 5 minutes. Heat the juices in a large pot and add the tea mixture to the juices through a strainer. Serve hot.

## Sangria

This reminds me of the Sangria served in restaurants. This makes enough for 2 people. Double or triple it to make a pitcher for a party. If you have any leftover, store it in the refrigerator. It will be a little less fizzy the next day, but still good.

1 cup red wine (I prefer a sweeter red wine instead of a dry one)
¼ cup orange juice*
¼ cup cherry juice* (I use Juicy Juice® cherry flavor. If you use the juice from

a jar of gluten-free maraschino cherries*, use half the amount)
Juice from ¼ of a fresh lime
1 (12 ounce) can of lemon-lime soda (I use Sprite®)
Crushed ice

Blend wine with juices. Squeeze in the lime juice. Pour in the can of soda and gently blend together. Fill tall glasses about ½ to ⅔rds full of crushed ice. Pour Sangria into glasses and serve.

## Sangria – Version 2

This version makes a large pitcher full and uses club soda instead of lemon-lime soda. This is similar to the Sangria that I had in Spain.

¼ cup sugar (or more to taste)
1 Tablespoon water
4 cups red wine, chilled (I prefer a sweeter red wine instead of a dry one)
½ cup orange juice*
¼ cup lemon juice (I use bottled)
¼ cup lime juice (I used bottled)

¼ to ½ cup Grand Marnier®* (I use ¼ cup). Grand Marnier is orange brandy and is gluten-free as of this writing. Another gluten-free fruit flavored brandy could be used.
1 ½ to 2 cups club soda, chilled
1 orange, sliced for garnish
Crushed ice

Blend sugar, water, wine, juices and Grand Marnier together. Add club soda and float orange slices in the sangria before serving. Fill tall glasses or large wine glasses about ½ to

*see gluten-free products list at the end of the book

⅔rds full of crushed ice. (I use more ice and fill the glasses about ¾ full of ice.) Pour Sangria into glasses and serve. If desired, garnish glasses with some orange slices.

## Vodka or Whiskey Sour Punch

Another of my mother's punch recipes. For a whiskey sour punch, you can substitute gluten-free whiskey for the vodka. (Alcohol that is distilled properly is safe. Check that no mash is put back in after the distillation process or it will be contaminated with gluten. As of this writing, Jack Daniels® www.jackdaniels.com says all gluten is removed in the distillation process.)

1 (12 ounce) can orange juice concentrate
1 (12 ounce) can frozen lemonade concentrate
2 cans gluten-free vodka* (fill the two cans you just emptied to get 24 ounces)

or use gluten-free whiskey* for whiskey sour punch
2 cans water (24 ounces)
2 bottles of chilled club soda

Pour all but soda over a block of ice in a punch bowl. Add soda just before serving.

## Write your own recipes here:

# MISCELLANEOUS

## Almond Paste, egg white version

*Some brands of almond paste may have gluten, so here is a way to make your own. This version is very good to use it in baked goods. I use a ½ recipe to make the Neapolitan Cookies (see index).*

½ pound slivered blanched almonds (or I use ½ pound of almond meal*)
1 ½ cups confectioner's sugar

1 egg white (I use the equivalent egg white powder and water)
1 Tablespoon water
½ teaspoon almond extract
Tiny pinch of salt (optional)

Grind the almonds in a blender or food processor. If using almond meal, add it to the food processor. Add the confectioner's sugar and blend well. Combine the egg whites, water and extract. With the blade going, add in a steady stream. Continue to blend until a smooth paste is formed. Put the paste in a clean heavy duty plastic freezer bag and store in the refrigerator. You can also freeze it for several months.

## Almond Paste, candy version

*Some brands of almond paste may have gluten, so here is a way to make your own. This makes 1 pound of almond paste. I use a candy thermometer and a food processor to make this. This recipe is good to make candies.*

½ pound blanched slivered almonds
1 cup sugar
½ cup water
1 heaping Tablespoon light corn syrup

½ teaspoon gluten-free almond extract (you can use less, depending on your taste) or 1 Tablespoon Rose water (available in specialty shops; it gives it that special marzipan taste).

In a food processor, grind the almonds. They will be finely ground and just a little oily.

(If you cannot find blanched almonds, put whole almonds in boiling water for a few minutes, and then in cold water. The skins should fall right off. Place the almonds on a baking sheet to dry out all day or place them in the oven at 250°F for 8 minutes, stirring after 4 minutes to dry. Grind in a food processor as above. I have found that the whole ones do not grind as finely as the sliced blanched ones. Your final product will be good but not quite as smooth.)

In a saucepan, blend the sugar, water and corn syrup. Cook until it reaches the soft ball stage (235-240°F, according to the mark on your thermometer.) Remove from heat. Add the extract and blend. You can mix in the almonds with a very strong spoon. I prefer to blend them together in the food processor. With the food processor on, add the syrup in a slow stream. It will ball up in the processor. Allow to cool a little so you can handle it. Wrap it the shape of a log in plastic wrap. Store in the refrigerator for about a month, or in the freezer for 6 months or so.

*\*see gluten-free products list at the end of the book*

If you make it a few days in advance, I think the flavors blend better. To make it pliable again, you can work it with your hands or set it on top of your stove with the oven on to warm it. You can also microwave it very briefly on defrost, but only do so 10 seconds at a time. You want to soften it, not melt it. Be careful because if you overheat it the sugar can get very hot and burn you.

## Boiled Eggs – Foolproof method

If you find that often when you boil eggs they are overcooked in the center, or the outer edges of the yolks look green, this is a foolproof method for cooking them.

The secret to making eggs that are easy to peel is to purchase them one week before you plan to boil them. When eggs are too fresh, the shells stick to the eggs so that they are difficult to peel and unattractive looking. You will be using your eggs within the selling date on the carton, but purchasing them a week earlier makes a big difference in your results.

Place eggs in cold water in a pot. Put on the stove and bring to a rolling boil. Lower the heat and simmer for 5 minutes. Remove from heat. Cover the pot and set a timer for 15 minutes.

When timer sounds, remove the lid and drain the water. Cover with cold water and add some ice cubes. They should cool quickly. Crack and peel the eggs. They should be cooked to perfection.

*Variation*: For large parties when I boil over 2 dozen eggs in one pot to make deviled eggs, I reduce the time the eggs sit to only 10 minutes instead of 15. Since it takes so much longer to boil the larger quantity of water, it cooks the eggs more. Reducing the time by 5 minutes solves the problem.

## Cheese Sandwiches – Open Melt

Gluten-free American cheese*
Gluten-free bread* (see recipes in this
   book, or the bread or pizza mix from
   www.gfnfoods.com)

Sliced tomatoes
Gluten-free bacon* cut into 1 ½ inch
   pieces

Heat the oven to 350°F. Place as many slices of bread as you want on the baking pan and toast in the oven until lightly browned. Watch carefully. This takes about a few minutes. Turn bread over and place 1 slice of cheese on top of each slice of bread. Top with tomato slice and a piece of bacon. Bake until cheese melts and bacon is cooked. Serve immediately. If you cut the skin off the tomato on one side before cooking, you can remove the skin before serving.

*see gluten-free products list at the end of the book*

## Cheese Steak Sandwiches

I buy good sandwich steaks at the meat counter. I don't use the frozen variety that are made of compressed meat bits because they shrink too much and often have added fat. If you are afraid that the meat will be tough, you can sprinkle on some gluten-free meat tenderizer and pound with a mallet. I make rolls using recipes from this book, or use the pizza mix from www.gfnfoods.com. Or use gluten-free corn tortillas to make your own hot wraps.

Sandwich steaks
Gluten-Free Rolls (see recipes in this book) or use Gluten-Free Corn Tortillas*

1 large Spanish onion, sliced into rings
Gluten-free American cheese* at room temperature so it melts better
Oil, salt and ground black pepper

You will need two skillets. Sauté onion in a little oil until tender and sprinkle with salt and pepper and keep hot. Heat the second skillet a minute, add a little oil and heat another minute. Brown 2 steaks quickly, turn over and place 1 or 2 slices of cheese on top of each steak. Have 2 rolls cut open and ready to fill. Quickly place the steaks on the gluten-free rolls or on corn tortillas* (see below for instructions). Put the steak side down on either the roll or tortilla (cheese side on top). Put hot onions on top of cheese, fold closed, and serve. The hot onions and the steak help melt the cheese.

Note: To heat tortillas, place on a microwave safe dish. Cover with a damp paper towel and heat in the microwave on High Power for 1 minute. Alternatively, to grill tortillas, place them one at a time in a skillet with some oil and heat on both sides. (An iron skillet works best for heating tortillas.) Immediately fill grilled tortillas as explained above, since they will get hard once they cool. Another method is to grill one side of the tortilla and flip it over. Top with meat, cheese and onions while still in the pan. Fold over using a spatula (careful, it will be hot) and heat on each side until cheese melts.

## Chicken Fat

This recipe is from my mother. She lived through the depression and people wasted nothing.

Whenever you buy a super-fat chicken, remove all the lumps of yellow fat and place them in a heavy saucepan with a cover. Heat the fat over low heat until it melts (this is called rendering). Then pour the golden liquid through a sieve into a jar and let it cool. If I am going to use it soon, I refrigerate the fat. If not, I place it in the freezer.

This fat keeps well and has many uses. Chicken fat is low in cholesterol and tasty. You can use 2 Tablespoons of it when making a piecrust. If it is a chicken potpie, use even more to give a nice chicken flavor. It is also good to fry potatoes and can be used in Gingerhen Bread (see index). You can also use it in Chicken Ala King or in Liver Pate.

## Cinnamon Applesauce Ornaments

A gluten-free dough ornament for children to make. They smell good too. Do not eat. These are for decoration only.

1 cup ground cinnamon plus more if        ¾ cup applesauce
   needed                                    2 Tablespoons white glue (optional)

Put the applesauce in a bowl and mix in cinnamon to make a dough. If too wet, add more cinnamon. If you want to keep these ornaments a while and make them a little less fragile, add the glue and some extra cinnamon. When it is a good consistency to roll out, put some on a sheet of waxed paper. Cover with another sheet and roll out using a rolling pin. Don't make them too thin or the ornaments will break when they dry. They should be the thickness of cut out cookies. Cut out using cookie cutters (gingerbread men work well). Use a drinking straw to make a hole at the top for hanging.

Dry the ornaments for several days. When completely dry, add some eyes or use glitter to decorate. Hang with a ribbon or string.

If you plan to store them for next year, store in an airtight jar. You may want to spray them with clear spray paint to help preserve them.

*Variation*: Set out some raisins to dry at the same time you are drying the ornaments. They can be glued on for decoration after the ornaments dry. Red Hots* can also be glued on for decoration. Or use some of those plastic eyes that you can get at craft stores.

## Cornstarch Modeling Dough

This is a good alternative to those wheat based modeling clay. This dough will dry and can be used for Christmas ornaments.

½ cup cornstarch                          Additional cornstarch for kneading
1 cup baking soda                         Ground cinnamon or food coloring for color
¾ cup cold water                             (optional)
½ Tablespoon oil

For microwave method: Mix the cornstarch and baking soda together in a microwave-safe pan. Add the oil and water. Blend until smooth. Microwave on high for 2 minutes, uncovered. Stir. Microwave 3 to 4 minutes more. Stir. The mixture should have the consistency of dry mashed potatoes.

For stovetop method: Mix the cornstarch and baking soda together in a pan with sides. Add the water and oil all at once and blend until smooth. Cook the mixture over medium heat. Cook until it is the consistency of dry mashed potatoes. (As it cooks. it will boil, thicken in lumps and then become a thick dough that holds its shape.) Do not overcook.

For both methods: Take the dough out of the pan, put it on a plate and cover it with a damp cloth. Let it cool down until it is cool enough to handle.

*see gluten-free products list at the end of the book

Put some cornstarch on your counter or a large plate. Knead the dough on this surface, adding more cornstarch if needed. If you want your dough to be brown instead of white, add some cinnamon. If you want it to be a color, you can add some food coloring. Knead it in. If the dough is not going to be used immediately, store the cooled clay in an airtight freezer type bag or container.

The dough can be rolled into a ¼ inch thickness and cut with cookie cutters. Use a straw to make a hole at the top for Christmas ornaments. Any dough you are not working with should be kept covered with a damp cloth so that it stays pliable. Place ornaments on a wire rack to dry. You can leave them on the racks overnight to dry. To speed drying, put the racks on a pan and place in a preheated 350°F oven and then turn the temperature off. Turn the ornaments sometime during the drying process to help them dry evenly. Leave them in the oven until the oven is cold. If they are still not dry, repeat the process.

The dough can also be used as modeling clay to make ropes, snakes, balls, etc. Some very thick pieces may dry unevenly and crack. If you plan to save your creation and dry it, it may be better to make smaller pieces and glue them together when dry. Items may be painted, decorated with markers, glue and glitter, etc. You may want to coat the items with clear acrylic spray if you want to preserve them.

## Curry Powder

Curry is actually a blend of spices. Some brands may contain wheat flour to make it free flowing. In recent years many brands have changed their formulations and no longer have wheat in them. Wheat flour would have to be listed on the ingredients list. Here is a recipe to make your own curry powder. I think this version is strong, so I use it sparingly.

1 teaspoon ground coriander
½ teaspoon ground turmeric
¼ teaspoon ground cumin
¼ teaspoon ground mustard
¼ teaspoon ground ginger

¼ teaspoon chili powder
¼ teaspoon ground cinnamon
¼ teaspoon ground cardamom
⅛ teaspoon ground black pepper

Blend all ingredients. This makes about 1 Tablespoon of curry powder. You can double the recipe and store leftover curry powder in an airtight container.

## Easter Eggs

Most Easter Egg color is gluten-free, but we found this worked much better and is a lot less expensive. We use this for our annual egg coloring event. Children and adults all decorate eggs.

Place desired number of eggs in a pot with cold water to cover. Heat pot and boil for 12 minutes. Remove from heat and place eggs in cold water. Set aside. (Or see "Boiled Eggs – Foolproof Recipe" to make your boiled eggs).

Get one mug for each color. In each mug, add the following:

¾ cup warm water
5 drops food coloring*

2 teaspoons apple cider vinegar

*see gluten-free products list at the end of the book

Place egg in the color with a spoon. Remove eggs after 2-4 minutes (until desired color). Dry with fresh paper towel. Refrigerate eggs until ready to use.

If desired, color eggs with non-toxic crayons (such as Crayola®) before putting them in the egg color.

## Grilled Cheese Sandwiches

Gluten-Free Naturals™ bread works well for grilled cheese sandwiches. This method insures that your cheese melts properly without your bread becoming too browned. My mother shared this secret with me when I was a little girl helping her in the kitchen.

| | |
|---|---|
| 4 slices gluten-free bread (preferably made from Gluten-Free Naturals™ Bread Flour) | Butter<br>2 to 4 slices gluten-free cheese (we like American or Muenster cheese) |

Place 4 slices of bread on a clean griddle. (Gluten can transfer to your food from an unclean griddle, so be sure it is clean.) Spread butter on the top side of the bread. Turn on heat. Warm the unbuttered side of the bread until the butter on the top starts to melt.

Now, turn 1 slice over on the griddle. Top with cheese. Put the second slice of bread on top of the cheese, with the buttered side on top. (The warmed sides of the bread are near the cheese, so it melts nicely.) Repeat for second sandwich. Grill until golden brown. Flip and grill the other side of the sandwich until golden brown. Serve.

*Variation*: Add some gluten-free ham with the cheese. I like to put it in-between 2 slices of cheese. (The cheese melts even better if you heat or grill the ham first.)

## Peanut Butter

Most brands of peanut butter are gluten-free. Here is a way to make your own to avoid trans-fats, too much sugar, or to use a different type of nut (such as cashews, almonds, etc). Note: Use caution if purchasing dry roasted peanuts or flavored peanuts as those may contain gluten.

| | |
|---|---|
| 2 cups salted peanuts or other salted nuts<br>2 to 3 Tablespoons oil | 1 Tablespoon honey |

Put nuts in a food processor and blend on high until nuts are coarsely chopped. Drizzle in the oil through the feeding tube and continue to blend until smooth. Add the honey and continue blending until smooth and creamy.

Store it in the refrigerator. Your peanut butter may seem a little warm and thin after processing it, but it will thicken after it is refrigerated. This recipe makes 1 cup of peanut butter.

## Muesli/Oat-Free Granola

We like to take this when traveling since it is nice as a breakfast cereal or sprinkled on top of gluten-free yogurt. It's high in protein. It can be addictive to munch on, so I pack it in serving size zipper sandwich bags for trips. If it gets crushed in the suitcase, we still enjoy it and the texture is even more like granola. This is one of those recipes that you can vary according to your preferences.

3 to 4 Tablespoons oil (I use 3 Tablespoons)

½ cup honey (you can use more, this is not very sweet)

About 5 cups of gluten-free Rice Chex® cereal (I use almost ⅔ of a 12.8 ounce box), or other gluten-free cereal such as cornflakes. Use more or less cereal depending on your preferences.

½ cup sesame seeds (I use less, about ¼ cup)

½ cup gluten-free hulled sunflower seeds (regular or salted work fine)

½ cup slivered or chopped almonds (I prefer slivered)

½ cup walnuts or other nuts (I like pecans)

1 cup shredded coconut (optional, I don't use)

1 cup raisins or other gluten-free dried fruit

For best results use a non-stick baking pan. I use a 9 x 13" size. Preheat oven to 300°F. Put oil and ¼ cup of the honey in pan and heat several minutes until honey melts. Stir in the seeds, nuts, and coconut if using. Spread into a layer in the pan. (Do not add fruit or raisins until the end or they will get too hard.)

Bake the nut mixture for 10 to 15 minutes to roast them. Then add the cereal and mix it in. Top with the remaining honey and bake for 20 to 30 minutes more, stirring the mixture about every 10 minutes. We find that baking in this manner helps toast the seeds, nut, and coconut so they are more flavorful. When finished baking, add raisins or dried fruit, and stir to incorporate.

Immediately pour mixture out onto waxed paper to cool. (If you leave it in the pan it will get hard and stick to the pan, and you'll have to reheat it.) *Note: Be very careful removing it from the pan. The honey gets very hot and can burn you. I suggest you wear oven mitts on both hands to avoid getting burned.* Once cooled, store in an airtight container so that the cereal stays crispy.

*Variation:* Substitute ½ cup maple syrup for honey. Other nuts can be used, such as peanuts, hazelnuts or pecans. Instead of raisins, you can substitute gluten-free apricots, Craisins® (gluten-free as of this writing), or gluten-free dates. Or use a gluten-free dried fruit mix.

*Variation 2:* Use a Silpat® non-stick silicon pad to make this easier to prepare. Spread the cereal on the pad in a pan. Drizzle on ¼ cup honey and 3 Tablespoons oil all over the cereal. Add the seeds and nuts and sprinkle them on to distribute. Drizzle on the remaining ¼ cup honey. Bake at 325°F for 30 minutes. Stir and then bake it 15 minutes more. Remove from the oven and carefully stir as it cools so it doesn't stick. (Wear oven mitts, it will be hot!) Allow to completely cool on the pan, and put into a container or Ziploc® bag. This eliminates the steps of stirring the cereal more frequently, and also removing it from the pan onto waxed paper to cool.

*\*see gluten-free products list at the end of the book*

*Variation 3*:  I have not tried this, but I am told that using gluten-free textured soy protein for the cereal works well, and has the consistency of oats.  You could probably substitute 3 to 4 cups of the textured soy protein instead of using the cereal.  Additional oil may be needed to help toast the soy protein.  Store it in an airtight container.

*Variation 4*:  For a sugar-free version, substitute gluten-free/sugar-free syrup for honey.

*Variation 5*:  There are some new companies that sell gluten-free oats (uncontaminated oats).  Some doctors are allowing their patients to add them into their gluten-free diet under their supervision.  The doctors that say you can add oats recommend that you start slowly and consume no more than a ½ cup per day.  They also recommend that you get another endoscopy to check the health of your villi to be sure you are tolerating them.  Some celiacs cannot tolerate oats, while others can.  Since my husband is doing so well without oats and doesn't miss eating them, he decided not to go that route.  There are still some conflicting studies on oats, and it is somewhat controversial.  If you want to use gluten-free oats in this recipe, increase the oil to ⅓ to ½ cup.  Toast the oats with the nuts, and follow the rest of the recipe.

## Taco Seasoning Mix
Many brands of taco seasoning mix contain gluten.  Here is a way to make your own.  This is less expensive and makes enough for several times.

3 Tablespoons chili powder
1 to 2 Tablespoons paprika
2 Tablespoons gluten-free flour (Gluten-Free Naturals™ All Purpose flour, fine white rice flour, gluten-free yellow cornmeal, yellow corn flour or cornstarch may be used.)

3 to 4 teaspoons ground cumin (optional)
2 teaspoons salt
1 teaspoon sugar
½ teaspoon garlic powder
¼ teaspoon ground red pepper (optional)

Blend all and store in an airtight jar.  Or reuse and label an old spice jar.

Directions to make taco filling:  Brown 1 pound of ground meat in a skillet.  Drain any excess fat.  Add 1 to 1 ½ Tablespoons of this seasoning mix and ¼ cup water.  If desired, add 1 Tablespoon dried minced onion or onion flakes when you add the water.  [Or instead of adding ¼ cup water, add a (14 ounce) can of undrained diced tomatoes for more flavor.]  Simmer a few minutes, until it thickens and minced onions are cooked.

## Tarragon Vinegar

Some brands of Tarragon vinegar may contain gluten because of the flavorings used. Here is a way to make your own. Every year my mother plants tarragon in her garden to make this. This is her recipe. You can use this in salad dressings, or to make Tarragon Grilled Chicken (see index). Try it in Italian Salad dressing or in Chicken Marinade. Bottles of this vinegar make nice gifts.

2 cups fresh Tarragon
½ gallon wine vinegar

Extra sprigs for garnish (optional – needed 2 weeks later)

Briefly wash the tarragon and cut it up. In a pot, heat the vinegar and tarragon. This helps to release the tarragon flavor. After heating, pour into glass containers. (I use old glass mayonnaise jars with a plastic top or old pickle jars that have been cleaned.) Cover and let set 2 weeks. (If using a glass jar with a metal lid, I put a larger piece of plastic wrap over the top and then screw on the lid.)

After 2 weeks, pour the vinegar through a sieve into a bowl to remove the tarragon pieces. Then pour into pretty vinegar bottles. (Use bottles that are food safe. Wine bottles with corks are a good choice. Small-mouth canning jars can also be used.) If desired place a fresh clean sprig of tarragon in the bottle. This sprig of tarragon is just for decoration.

## Vanilla Extract

Most vanilla extract is gluten-free because alcohol that is distilled properly is safe. When we initially started the diet there was controversy about distilled alcohol, but it was shown that properly distilled alcohol is safe for people with celiac disease. For those who are purists and want to be sure the alcohol never originated from wheat, here is a way to make your own.

1 vanilla bean, split lengthwise with seeds exposed (keep bean ends intact)
½ cup gluten-free vodka* (I like potato vodka)

Using a cutting board carefully cut the vanilla bean with a knife to expose the seeds but don't cut through the ends. Place the vanilla bean in a bottle with a lid. Add the vodka and shake well. Store it covered in a cool dark place for at least four to six weeks. (I keep it in my pantry.) During that time shake the bottle a few times a week. Keep it stored at room temperature. It will get better the longer it sits. Leave the bean in there and just pour off the liquid to use in recipes. Do not reuse the bean when the liquid is gone.

I also like a small dash of vanilla extract poured on coffee grounds before making coffee. A lot of flavored coffees have gluten, but this is a way to have your own gluten-free version of "French Vanilla" coffee that is delicious.

*Variation*: Rum* may be used instead of potato vodka, but we prefer the flavor with the vodka. (Note: Rum* (without the vanilla bean soaked in it) may also be used in recipes in place of vanilla, if you prefer that flavor.)

Write your own recipes here:

# Gluten-Free Products List; Products Used in Creating this Book

This list is <u>not</u> inclusive of all gluten-free products.  There are a lot more out there!

NOTE:  USE THIS LIST WITH EXTREME CAUTION!  THERE IS NO GUARANTEE THAT THEY ARE GLUTEN-FREE <u>NOW</u>.  Also, these lists are for products available in the <u>United States</u> and formulations may be different in other countries.  We cannot be responsible for manufacturer's changes or possible errors in this list.  It is your responsibility to check for yourself to be sure you are safe.  You can use this as a guideline to call manufacturers before you go shopping.  On some manufacturer's websites under FAQ they list gluten-free status.  Others you will have to choose "contact us".  Many companies will also send you lists.  Items are listed either by my preference or the timing when I discovered the foods were gluten-free.

These websites may keep more up-to-date lists, but you should still verify the information for yourself.
http://forums.delphiforums.com/celiac/start  (I discovered this wonderful list after I prepared my list)
http://www.celiac.com
http://www.glutenfreeinfo.com
http://www.clanthompson.com (you can purchase a gluten-free list, or lists for your phone, palm or pocket pc)
http://www.gfcfdiet.com (contains lists for gluten-free and casein free diet)
http://homepage.mac.com/sholland/celiac/GFfoodlist.pdf (list from a celiac group in Chicago)

| Ingredient | Brand(s) | Contact Information |
|---|---|---|
| All Purpose Flour (gluten-free) | GFN Foods™ makers of Gluten-Free Naturals™ | 1-866-761-6147 www.gfnfoods.com |
| Almond Extract | McCormick's® (all extracts) | 1-800-632-5847 www.mccormick.com |
| Almond Meal | Blue Diamond | www.bluediamond.com |
| Almond Paste | Blue Diamond | www.bluediamond.com |
| Bacon (most regular bacon is gluten-free, but some with flavors or low fat may contain gluten). | Hormel® Value Brand, Black Label, & Microwave<br>Hormel® Canadian Bacon (list on web)<br>Hormel® Bacon bits and pieces<br>Oscar Mayer®<br>Hillshire Farms®<br>Boars Head®<br>Jennie-O® Extra Lean Turkey Bacon<br>Hatfield® Regular, Thick Sliced & Reduced Sodium | 1-800-523-4635 www.hormelfoods.com<br>1-800-523-4635 www.hormelfoods.com<br>1-800-523-4635 www.hormelfoods.com<br>1-800-222-2323 www.oscarmeyer.com<br>1-800-328-2426<br>1-800-352-6277<br>1-800-523-4635 www.hormelfoods.com<br>1-800-523-5291 www.hatfieldqualitymeats.com |
| Baked Beans | B&M® from B&G Foods® (list on web)<br>Hunt's® Pork & Beans<br>Bush's Best Baked Beans (<u>not</u> their Chili Beans, Homestyle Chili or Chili Magic®line) | 1-973-401-6500 www.bgfoods.com<br>1-800-585-6392<br>www.bushbeans.com (listed on website) |
| Baking Powder (check ingredients.) | Calumet® by Kraft®<br>Davis®<br>Rumford® | www.kraftfoods.com<br>www.jelsert.com<br>www.hulman.com |
| Beans, canned black, kidney, etc. | Goya® blue label<br>Joan of Arc® from B&G Foods<br>Most store brands are gluten-free, check ingredients | 1-800-275-4692 www.goya.com<br>1-973-401-6500 www.bgfoods.com |
| Bologna | Louis Rich® Turkey Variety Pack (ham, bologna, cotto salami)  Kraft Foods says any allergens are noted on ingredients list<br>Hatfield® Ring Bologna, Regular, German & Lebanon<br>Jennie-O® Refrigerated Sliced Lunchmeat (Turkey, Smokey Turkey, Bologna, Salami) | 1-800-323-0768, www.kraftfoods.com<br><br>1-800-523-5291 www.hatfieldqualitymeats.com<br><br>1-800-523-4635 www.hormelfoods.com |

Use this list with extreme caution and as a guideline only for finding products.
It is your responsibility to check the gluten-free status of all foods yourself.
There is no guarantee that they are gluten-free now.

| Ingredient | Brand(s) | Contact Information |
|---|---|---|
| Bouillon or soup base | Better Than Bouillon® <br> Tone's®, chicken flavor only (at Sam's club) <br> McCormick Real Chicken & Beef Base (at Costco) <br> Herb Ox® by Hormel® (check varieties) Beef, Chicken, Vegetable, Spicy Chicken, Garlic Chicken and low sodium Beef and Chicken. (They are now labeled gluten-free and listed on their webpage). | www.superiortouch.com <br> 1-800-247-5251 www.spiceadvice.com <br> 1-800-632-5847 www.mccormick.com <br> 1-800-333-6339 www.hormelfoods.com |
| Brandy | Grand Marnier® | www.grand-marnier.com (under FAQ on web) |
| Bread | GFN Foods™ makers of Gluten-Free Naturals™ <br> Kinnikinnick® bread <br> Food for Life® Rice Almond Bread (g-f on label) | 1-866-761-6147, www.gfnfoods.com <br> www.kinnikinnick.com <br> www.foodforlife.com |
| Bread Flour (gluten-free) | GFN Foods™ makers of Gluten-Free Naturals™ | 1-866-761-6147www.gfnfoods.com |
| Broth (check ingredients) | Swanson's® Ready to Serve Beef & Chicken only | 1-800-257-8443 |
| Buckwheat Flour | Pocono® brand from The Birkett Mills® (listed on web page, designated mill.) <br> Hodgeson Mill® (mills wheat but cleans between lines) | www.thebirkettmills.com <br><br> 217-347-0105 ext 31 |
| Butter (most real butter including store brands are gluten-free. Some unsalted butter may contain natural flavorings, so check those.) | Land O Lakes® <br> Keller's® and Hotel Bar® | 1-800-328-4155 www.landolakes.com <br> 1-800-535-5371 www.butter1.com |
| Buttermilk | Friendship® <br> Hood® | www.friendshipdaries.com <br> 1-800-662-4468 www.hphood.com |
| Buttermilk Powder | Saco® | 1-800-373-7226 www.sacofoods.com |
| Candy – hard type | LifeSavers® (check ingredients) | 1-800-622-4726 www.candystand.com |
| Capers | B &G® (list on web page) | 973-401-6500 www.bgfoods.com |
| Cereal | Cream of Rice® <br> Cornflakes – Nature's Path® (gluten-free on label) <br> Rice Chex®, Corn Chex® and Honey Nut Chex® (new – gluten-free on label) from General Mills® | www.kraftfoods.com <br><br> 1-800-328-1144 www.generalmills.com |
| Cheese, American | Borden® <br> Kraft® (ingredients clearly marked) | 1-888-337-2407 www.elsie.com <br> 1-800-543-5335 www.kraftfoods.com |
| Cheese, Blue (check ingredients) | Treasure Cave® <br> Stella® | www.treasurecavecheese.com <br> www.stellacheese.com |
| Cheese, Cheddar (and other types) | Kraft® (brick) (ingredients clearly marked) <br> Land O Lakes® (natural cheeses only) <br> Many store brands are gluten-free. Check ingredients. | 1-800-538-1998 www.kraftfoods.com <br> 1-800-328-4155 www.landolakes.com |
| Cheese, Cottage Cheese | Breakstone's® from Kraft <br> Hood® <br> Friendship® (regular 4%, 2%, low fat) | 1-800-538-1998 www.kraftfoods.com <br> 1-800-662-4468 www.hphood.com <br> www.friendshipdairies.com |
| Cheese, Cream | Philadelphia® from Kraft <br> Many store brands are gluten-free. Check ingredients. | 1-800-538-1998 www.kraftfoods.com |
| Cheese, Farmer | Friendship® | www.friendshipdairies.com |
| Cheese, Mozzarella | Sargento® (real only, imitation has wheat) <br> Polly-O® from Kraft <br> Borden® <br> Bel Gioioso® regular and fresh mozzarella (all of their cheeses are gluten-free) | 1-800-243-3737 www.sargentocheese.com <br> 1-800-323-0768 www.kraftfoods.com <br> 1-888-337-2407 www.elsie.com <br> 1-920-863-2123 www.belgioioso.com |
| Cheese, Mozzarella, shredded | Borden® <br> Sargento® (real only, not taco flavored) | 1-888-337-2407 www.elsie.com <br> 1-800-243-3737 www.sargentocheese.com |
| Cheese, Parmesan | Kraft® (allergens clearly labeled) | 1-800-323-0768 www.kraftfoods.com |
| Cheese, Ricotta | Polly-O® from Kraft <br> Sargento® (contains triple distilled vinegar) | 1-800-323-0768 www.kraftfoods.com <br> 1-800-243-3737 www.sargentocheese.com |
| Cheese, Shelf-Stable | The Laughing Cow® and Mini-Baby Bel® <br> Swiss Knight® Wedges | 1-800-272-1224 www.laughingcow.com <br> www.emmiusa.com |
| Chicken broth, canned | Swanson® | 1-800-257-8443 www.campbellsoup.com |

Use this list with extreme caution and as a guideline only for finding products.
It is your responsibility to check the gluten-free status of all foods yourself.
There is no guarantee that they are gluten-free now.

| Ingredient | Brand(s) | Contact Information |
| --- | --- | --- |
| Chicken, canned and shelf-stable | Valley Fresh® from Hormel® shelf-stable packets and cans | www.valleyfresh.com or www.hormelfoods.com |
| Chicken, fresh (Most fresh chicken is gluten-free. Most store brands are gluten-free. Beware of "added" solutions or "enhanced with" in some brands. ) | Perdue® Tyson® (Note: check ingredients when purchasing meats at Wal-Mart®, since they add solutions to some of their meats). | 1-800-473-8383 www.purdue.com 1-800-233-6332 |
| Chicken, roasted (Beware of wheat in some ready to serve products) | Tyson® Whole Roasted Heat and Eat (natural flavorings are essence of rosemary) | 1-800-233-6332 |
| Chili Powder (many brands are gluten-free. Check ingredients) | McCormick® (since ingredients may change, check the ingredients list on the package). | 1-800-632-5847 www.mccormick.com |
| Chili Sauce | Heinz® (In 2008 I found out this became gluten-free) | 1-800-255-5750 www.heinz.com |
| Chocolate candy (stay away from those containing rice crispy pieces or cookies. Outside the US they don't have to list wheat to prevent sticking) | Hershey's® (certain varieties only) Nestlé's® (certain varieties only) Russell Stover® fudge, but contains vanilla which could possibly be made from grains Baci® After Eight Mints Ghirardelli (certain varieties only; some items may share equipment with items containing malt.) | 1-800-468-1714 www.herseys.com 1-800-637-8536 www.nestle.com 1-800-777-4028 www.russellstover.com  www.nestleeuropeanchocolate.com www.nestleeuropeanchocolate.com 1-800-877-9338www.ghirardelli.com |
| Chocolate chips/bits, semi-sweet or milk chocolate | Hershey's® Nestlé's® | 1-800-468-1714 www.hersheys.com 1-800-637-8536 www.nestle.com |
| Chocolate syrup | Hershey's® regular and special dark Nestlé's® Fox's U-Bet (all varieties) [For those with corn allergies, their specially labeled Kosher for Passover products contain sugar, not corn syrup.] | 1-800-468-1714 www.hersheys.com 1-800-441-2525 www.nestle.com 1-718-385-4600 www.foxs-syrups.com |
| Chocolate, bitter | Baker's® | 1-800-323-0768 www.kraftfoods.com |
| Chutney | Patak's® Mango Chutney Major Grey's®/Crosse and Blackwell® | 1-800-523-4635 www.hormelfoods.com 1-888-643-7219 www.crosseandblackwell.com |
| Clams, canned | Bumblebee® (all canned seafood except ready to eat salad containing crackers) | www.bumblebee.com |
| Cocktail Frankfurters | Hormel® Smokies® Hillshire Farms® Li'l Smokies® | 1-800-523-4635 www.hormelfoods.com 1-800-328-2426 |
| Cocktail Sauce | Crosse & Blackwell® Cocktail and Shrimp sauce by J.M. Smucker Co.® Golden Dip Cocktail Sauce by McCormick Heinz® (in 2008 I found out this became gluten-free) | 1-888-643-7219 www.crosseandblackwell.com  1-800-632-5847 1-800-255-5750 www.heinz.com |
| Coffee, flavored (check ingredients) | Nescafe® from Nestle® Melitta® all flavors | 1-800-637-8536 www.nestle.com www.melitta.com |
| Coffee-Mate® | Coffee-Mate® Powder and Liquid | www.coffee-mate.com |
| Cognac (made from grapes) | Remy Martin® | www.remy-cointreau.com |
| Communion Wafers | Ener-G® Benedictine Sisters of Perpetual Adoration (approved for Catholics; contains below 100 ppm gluten) CM Almy Church Supply Catalog | www.ener-g.com 1-800-223-2772 e-mail: altarbreads@benedictinesisters.org www.almy.com |
| Cool Whip® | Cool Whip from Kraft (specific varieties) | 1-800-268-7808, www.kraft.com |
| Cookie Blend (gluten-free) | GFN Foods®, makers of Gluten-Free Naturals™ | 1-866-761-6147, www.gfnfoods.com |
| Cooking spray (Check labels, many store brands are gluten-free). | Pam® (not the version containing flour!) | 1-800-544-5680 |
| Corn Cakes (like Rice Cakes, but thinner) | Corn Thins® by Real Foods® (gluten-free on label) | www.realfoods.com.au/products.html |

Use this list with extreme caution and as a guideline only for finding products.
It is your responsibility to check the gluten-free status of all foods yourself.
There is no guarantee that they are gluten-free now.

| Ingredient | Brand(s) | Contact Information |
|---|---|---|
| Corn, creamed | DelMonte® | www.delmonte.com |
| Cornflakes | Nature's Path® (gluten-free on label)<br>Corn Chex® (gluten-free on label) I use these as a substitute for crushed cornflakes in recipes | |
| Corn Flour | Bob's Red Mill® (read carefully to purchase the gluten-free version) | www.bobsredmill.com |
| Cornmeal and Polenta | Albers® from Nestle USA<br>Hodgeson Mill® (mill wheat but clean between lines)<br>Bob's Red Mill® Polenta/Yellow Corn Grits | 1-800-441-2525<br>217-347-0105 ext 31<br>www.bobsredmill.com |
| Corned Beef | Appleton® from Aldi® stores (gluten-free on label)<br>Freirich®<br>Hormel® canned corned beef | www.freirich.com<br>1-800-523-4635 www.hormelfoods.com |
| Corn Syrup | Karo® – Light and Dark Syrup | 1-866-430-5276 www.karosyrup.com |
| Cornstarch | Argo® or Kingsford® (they say no contamination) | www.cornstarch.com |
| Crabmeat, canned | Bumblebee® (all canned seafood except ready to eat salad containing crackers) | www.bumblebee.com |
| Cream | Hood ® (all Hood® creams) including heavy, whipping and cans<br>Cool Whip® from Kraft (specific varieties)<br>Reddi Wip® Original & Extra-Creamy in cans from ConAgra®<br>(Note: when I called Land O'Lakes® brand in 2004 they said they do not know if the ingredients added to their gourmet whipping cream were safe or not, so they said do not use it. This may have changed.) | 1-800-662-4468 www.hphood.com<br><br>1-800-268-7808, www.kraft.com<br>1-800-745-4514, www.reddi-wip.com |
| Cream Cheese | Philadelphia Brand® from Kraft<br>Many store brands are also gluten-free – check labels | www.kraft.com |
| Curry Powder | Durkee®<br>McCormick® (no longer contains wheat) | 1-800-247-5251<br>1-800-632-5847 www.mccormick.com |
| Deli Meats (prepackaged) | Hillshire Farms® from Sara Lee<br>Oscar Mayer® (certain varieties) from Kraft<br>Jenny-O® (certain varieties) from Hormel (see web)<br>Hatfield® (ones labeled gluten-free) | 1-800-328-2426<br>1-800-222-2323 www.oscarmayer.com<br>1-800-523-4635 www.hormelfoods.com<br>1-800-523-5291 www.hatfieldqualitymeats.com |
| Dried Fruit | Craisins® | 1-800-662-3263 www.oceanspray.com |
| Egg White Powder | Just Whites® (contains only egg whites) | |
| Elbow Macaroni | Tinkyada®<br>Mrs. Leeper's® corn elbows<br>DeBoyles® | www.tinkyada.com<br>www.mrsleeperspasta.com<br>1-800-749-0730 |
| Extracts | McCormick's® (all extracts) | 1-800-632-5847 www.mccormick.com |
| Food Coloring | Durkee® | 1-800-247-5251 |
| Frankfurters or Hot Dogs | Oscar Mayer® (Kraft® doesn't hide gluten on labels)<br>Ball Park® from Sara Lee<br>Hatfield® Franks, Original Hotdog, Beef Franks<br>Jennie-O® Turkey Franks | 1-800-222-2323 www.oscarmayer.com<br>513-936-2000 or 1-800-328-2426<br>1-800-523-5291 www.hatfieldqualitymeats.com<br>1-800-523-4635 www.hormelfoods.com |
| Gelatin | Jello Brand® from Kraft | 1-800-431-1001 www.jell-o.com |
| Gin | Popov® Gin<br>Tanqueray® Gin<br>Gordons®, Gordons® Citrus & Gordons® Wildberry | www.diegeo.com<br>www.diegeo.com<br>www.diegeo.com |
| Grits (beware of contamination in some brands) | Albers® from Nestle USA | 1-800-441-2525 |
| Ham | Hatfield® Country Made boneless Ham, traditional honey or maple hamsteaks (list on web)<br>Hormel® Black label (throw out the flavor packet)<br>Hormel® Cure 81 (Boneless, Bone-in, Spiral)<br>Smithfield®<br>Louis Rich® Turkey Variety Pack (Ham, Bologna, cotto | 1-800-523-5291 www.hatfieldqualitymeats.com<br><br>1-800-523-4635 www.hormelfoods.com<br>1-800-523-4635 www.hormelfoods.com<br>1-757-357-1376<br>1-800-323-0768, www.kraftfoods.com |

Use this list with extreme caution and as a guideline only for finding products.
It is your responsibility to check the gluten-free status of all foods yourself.
There is no guarantee that they are gluten-free now.

| Ingredient | Brand(s) | Contact Information |
|---|---|---|
| | salami) Kraft Foods says any allergens are noted on ingredients list | |
| | Underwood® Deviled Ham Spread | 1-973-401-6500 www.bgfoods.com |
| | Hormel® Natural Choice® (gluten-free on label) | www.hormelfoods.com |
| Horseradish | Boar's Head® | 1-800-352-6277 www.boarshead.com |
| | Woeber's® Horseradish Sauce | 1-800-548-2929 www.woebermustard.com |
| Hot Dogs or Frankfurters | Oscar Mayer® (Kraft® doesn't hide gluten on labels) | 1-800-222-2323 www.oscarmayer.com |
| | Ball Park® from Sara Lee | 513-936-2000 or 1-800-328-2426 |
| | Hatfield® Franks, Original Hotdogs, Beef Franks | 1-800-523-5291 www.hatfieldqualitymeats.com |
| | Jennie-O® Turkey Franks | 1-800-523-4635 www.hormelfoods.com |
| Hot Sauce | Tabasco® (contains distilled vinegar) | www.tabasco.com |
| | Trappey's® Hot Sauce | 1-973-401-6500 www.bgfoods.com |
| | Frank's® Original Red Hot Sauce, Xtra Hot, Red Hot | 1-800-841-1256 www.franksredhot.com |
| | Buffalo Wing Sauce & Chili n Lime | |
| Ice Cream | Friendly's (certain flavors only) – list on web | 1-800-966-9970 www.friendlys.com |
| | Hood® Grand (certain flavors only) – list on web | 1-800-662-4468 www.hphood.com |
| | Edy's® Grand (certain flavors only) – list on web | 1-888-590-3397 www.edys.com |
| | Turkey Hill® (certain flavors only) – will send list | 1-800-mydairy www.turkeyhill.com |
| | Breyer's® (certain flavors only) | www.breyers.com |
| | Philly Swirl® (gluten-free on label) | |
| Italian Ice | Luigi's Italian Ice | 1-800-294-4196 ext 18 |
| | Wyler's® Authentic Italian Ice | www.jelsert.com |
| Jams/Jellies | Polaner® All fruit, jellies, jams, preserves (gluten-free on label) | 1-973-401-6500 www.bgfoods.com |
| Juice Blends | Juicy Juice® all flavors, from Nestle® | 1-800-637-8536 www.nestle.com |
| | Ocean Spray® Juices and Drinks, all varieties | 1-800-662-3263 www.oceanspray.com |
| | V8® Splash and V8® V-Fusion, all varieties | www.v8juice.com or www.campbellsoup.com |
| | V8® Splash Smoothies; Orange Creme, Peach Mango, and Strawberry Mango only. | |
| Ketchup | Heinz® | 800-255-5750 www.heinz.com |
| | DelMonte® | www.delmonte.com |
| Kielbasa/Smoked Sausage | Hillshire Farms® from Sara Lee (all varieties except corn dogs and those with beer) | 1-800-328-2426 www.hillshirefarm.com |
| | Hatfield® (see list on web for varieties) | www.hatfieldqualitymeats.com |
| Lasagna | DeBoles® from Hain (no boil lasagna) | 1-800-749-0730 |
| | Tinkyada® (gluten-free on label) | www.tinkyada.com |
| Lemoncello | Sogno di Sorrento® Lemoncello | 617-227-3193 |
| Liqueur | Kahlua® (coffee) | www.kahlua.com |
| | Kirschwasser® (cherry) | www.clearcreekdistillery.com |
| | Black Haus® Blackberry Schnapps | www.diageo.com |
| | Rumple Minze® Peppermint Schnapps | www.diageo.com |
| Liquid Smoke | Haddon House® | www.haddonhouse.com |
| | Wrights® (use ½ the amount with this brand) Hickory and Mesquite flavors | 1-888-887-3268 www.bgfoods.com |
| Liverwurst | Hatfield® Regular and Reduced Sodium | 1-800-523-5291 www.hatfieldqualitymeats.com |
| Macaroons | Jenny's® (says gluten-free on the label) | |
| Maraschino cherries | Cherry Man® (check as suppliers can change) | 503-359-7121 www.cherryman.com |
| | Bell View® (gluten-free on label) | 800-223-2848/800-872-9029 www.bellview.com |
| Margarine | Fleischmann's from ConAgra (some are casein-free) | 1-800-988-7808 www.fleischmanns.com |
| | Fleischmann's Light & unsalted Soft Spread & stick (dairy free & gluten-free) | 1-800-988-7808 www.fleischmanns.com |
| | Fleishman's made with olive oil | 1-800-988-7808 www.fleischmanns.com |
| | Fleishman's original stick & soft spread | 1-800-988-7808 www.fleischmanns.com |
| | Blue Bonnet from ConAgra | 1-800-988-7808 |
| | Parkay from ConAgra | 1-800-988-7808 |
| | Earth Balance® Buttery Spreads (lactose & gluten-free) | www.earthbalance.net |

Use this list with extreme caution and as a guideline only for finding products.
It is your responsibility to check the gluten-free status of all foods yourself.
There is no guarantee that they are gluten-free now.

| Ingredient | Brand(s) | Contact Information |
|---|---|---|
| Marinade | EZ Marinader – Mr. Yoshida's Teriyaki | www.heinz.com |
| Marshmallows | Jet Puffed® from Nabisco® | 1-800-225-7321 www.kraftfoods.com |
| | Camp Fire® from Doumak® | www.campfiremarshmallows.com |
| Mayonnaise | Hellman's® or Best Food's® | 1-800-338-8831 or www.unilever.com |
| Milk/dairy substitutes/ and Lactose Free Milk | Vance's® Darifree | 1-800-497-4834 www.vancesfoods.com |
| | Silk® Soymilk by White Wave® | 1-800-488-9283 www.silksoy.com |
| | Cremora® nondairy creamer | www.cremora.com |
| | Carnation® nonfat dry milk | 1-800-637-8536 www.nestle.com |
| | Coffee Mate® | 1-800-637-8536 www.nestle.com |
| | Carnation® instant breakfast | 1-800-637-8536 www.nestle.com |
| | Hood® Premium Chocolate Milk (full fat and low fat) | 1-800-662-4468 www.hphood.com |
| | Hood® Simply Smart® Milk | 1-800-662-4468 www.hphood.com |
| | Hood® Golden EggNog | 1-800-662-4468 www.hphood.com |
| | Lactaid® milk (made by Hood® dairies) | 1-800-522-8243 (Lactaid®) or 1-800-662-4468 |
| | Almond Breeze® all flavors | 1-800-662-4468, www.hphood.com |
| | SoyDream® from Hain® – all varieties | www.bluediamond.com |
| | Rice Dream® from Hain® – certain varieties only | www.tastethedream.com |
| | EdenSoy® Unsweetened and EdenBlend® (Organic Rice/Soy Blend) only | www.tastethedream.com www.edenfoods.com |
| Molasses | Brier Rabbit® mild, full and blackstrap molasses | 1-800-887-3268 www.bgfoods.com |
| | Grandma's® molasses | 1-800-426-4891 |
| Monosodium Glutamate (MSG) | Accent® from B&G Foods | 1-973-401-6500 www.bgfoods.com |
| Mustard (note: you can substitute 1 tsp. prepared mustard = ¼ tsp. dry in most recipes) | Hellman's® Dijonnaise® | 1-800-338-8831 or www.unilever.com |
| | French's® mustard (all flavors) | 1-800-841-1256 www.frenchsfoods.com |
| | Boar's Head® Deli & Honey Mustard | 1-800-352-6277 |
| | Plochman's® | www.plochman.com |
| | Woeber's® mustard | 1-800-548-2929 www.woebermustard.com |
| Mustard, Dry | McCormick's® | 1-800-632-5847 www.mccormick.com |
| | Durkee® | 1-800-247-5251 |
| Non-Dairy Creamer | Coffee-Mate® Liquid and Powder | www.coffee-mate.com |
| Noodles | Glutano® (gluten-free on label) | www.glutano.com |
| Olives | Pearl Brand® (black or green w/pimientos) | 1-800-523-9828 www.olives.com |
| | Peloponnese Kalamata Olives from Hormel® | 1-800-523-4635 www.hormelfoods.com |
| | Diomede® Spanish Olives (available at Aldi®) | 1-888-401-9880 www.sevilleimports.com |
| | B&G® black and green olives | 1-973-401-6500 www.bgfoods.com |
| Orange Juice | Store brands and name brands that have orange juice as their only ingredient. Check any that have additives. (For example, some with added calcium may be unsafe.) | |
| Paprika | McCormick's® | 1-800-632-5847 |
| | Durkee® | 1-800-247-5251 |
| Pasta | Tinkyada® (gluten-free on label) | www.tinkyada.com |
| | Mrs. Leeper's® corn and rice pastas | www.mrsleeperspasta.com |
| | DeBole's rice pasta | 1-800-749-0730 |
| | Rizopia® (gluten-free on label) | www.rizopia.com |
| | Notta Pasta® and A Taste of Thai® (g-f on label) | www.atasteofthai.com |
| | Sam Mills® Pasta d'Oro (gluten-free on label) | |
| Peanut Butter and nut spreads | Skippy® (regular & honey roasted) – Unilever | 1-800-338-8831 |
| | Peter Pan® from ConAgra | 1-877-528-0745 |
| | Nutella® hazelnut spread | 1-800-nutella |
| | Smucker's® All Natural peanut Butter | 1-888-550-9555.www.smuckers.com |
| Peanuts (check labels) | Planter's® (roasted – not dry roasted) | 1-800-NABISCO (622-4726) |
| Pectin | Sure-Jell® and Certo® from Kraft | www.kraftfoods.com |
| Pepperoni | Hormel® (gluten-free on label) | 1-800-523-4635 www.hormelfoods.com |
| Peppers (jar variety) | B & G® Foods | 1-973-401-6500 www.bgfoods.com |

Use this list with extreme caution and as a guideline only for finding products.
It is your responsibility to check the gluten-free status of all foods yourself.
There is no guarantee that they are gluten-free now.

| Ingredient | Brand(s) | Contact Information |
|---|---|---|
| Pickles and Relish | Vlasic® <br> B & G® Pickles, Peppers, Relishes (list on web) [Note: Some of their products are no longer made in the U.S.] | 1-800-421-3265 <br> 1-973-401-6500 www.bgfoods.com |
| Pie filling | Comstock® and Wilderness® (all varieties – modified food starch is corn) | 1-800-270-2743 www.birdseyefoods.com |
| Popcorn <br> (Plain popcorn that you pop yourself is gluten-free) | Jiffy Pop® <br> Act II <br> Orville Redenbacher® (specific varieties) <br> Utz® popped snack (flavors: Butter, Cheese, and White Cheddar Popcorn; gluten-free on label) <br> Bachmann® popped snack; plain and flavored (see web) | 1-712-239-1232 www.jollytime.com <br> www.actii.com <br> 1-800-328-6286 <br> www.utzsnacks.com 1-800-367-7629 <br><br> www.bachmanpretzels.com |
| Pork, fresh and w/marinade | Hatfield® (see gluten-free list on web) | 1-800-523-5291 www.hatfieldqualitymeats.com |
| Potato Buds/Flakes | Betty Crocker® <br> Idaho Supreme® | 1-800-828-3291 www.bettycrocker.com <br> www.idahosupreme.com |
| Potato Chips – check for contamination | Utz® (plain made on dedicated lines) – Home Style, Kettle Classic, Grandma Utz, (list on web and labeled "a gluten-free food" on the bag.) <br> Wise® – plain and unseasoned, Wise, Riggies, lightly salted, Regular Delis and Crunchers <br> French's Potato Sticks, Original, BBQ, Pizza Party & Cheeze Cheddar <br> Martins Chips® (all potato chips and popcorn are gluten-free and all equipment is gluten-free) <br> Bachmann® Golden Crisp All Natural and Golden Wavy | www.utzsnacks.com 1-800-367-7629 <br><br><br> www.wisesnacks.com 1-800-438-9473 or 1-888-759-4401 <br> 1-800-841-1256 www.frenchsfoods.com <br><br> www.martinschips.com <br><br> www.bachmanpretzels.com |
| Potatoes, frozen | OreIda® (specific varieties only.) <br> (Beware of natural flavor in toaster hash browns. This may have changed in 2006.) | 1-800-892-2401 |
| Pretzels | Ener-G® <br> Snyder's of Hanover® Gluten-Free Pretzel Sticks | www.ener-g.com <br> www.snydersofhanover.com |
| Pudding | Royal® and My-T-Fine® Pudding (cooked & instant) <br> Jell-O Brand® (cooked & instant) check ingredients <br> Kozy Shack® ready-made (those labeled gluten-free) | www.jelsert.com <br> 1-800-431-1001 www.jell-o.com <br> www.kozyshack.com |
| Red Hot candy | Red Hots® by Ferrara Pan <br> Hot Tamales® by Just Born® | www.ferrarapan.com <br> 1-800-445-5787 |
| Refried Beans | Ortega® (check labels) <br> Taco Bell® Fat Free Refried Beans | www.oretga.com |
| Rice, white, brown, instant, jasmine <br> Note: Plain rice is gluten-free, so you can use store brands. Use caution purchasing any rice blends, rice pilafs, or with flavoring packets. Rice with pasta is unsafe. | Carolina®: long grain white rice/brown rice/instant white rice/Carolina Gold (Parboiled) Authentic Spanish Rice Mix/Long Grain and Wild Rice Mix, Saffron Yellow Rice Mix (listed on web page) <br> Mahatma® Rice, River® Rice, and Success® Rice (check web page for specific varieties.) <br> Uncle Ben's® Original Converted Rice, Instant rice, Boil-in-Bag, Whole Grain Brown Rice, Instant Brown Rice, Long Grain & Wild Rice (must discard packet), Ready Rice: Original/Long Grain/Whole Grain Brown/Spanish Rice. | www.riviana.com, www.carolinarice.com <br><br><br> www.mahatmarice.com, www.riverrice.com, www.successrice.com <br> 1-800-548-6253 www.unclebens.com |
| Rice Cakes | ShopRite® plain and salted | 1-800-shoprite, www.shoprite.com |
| Rice Crackers | Asian® Gourmet Brand (says gluten-free on the label) <br> Blue Diamond® Nut Thins (say gluten-free on label) | 1-800-257-6174 ext. 225 |
| Rice Flour | Ener-G® <br> Mochiko® Blue Star Brand Sweet Rice Flour <br> Erawan® Brand (at Asian Markets --3 elephants in the logo on label). Sometimes Asian Rice Flour may be too fine a grind for yeast breads, and cause some bread | www.ener-g.com <br> www.kodafarms.com <br> www.choheng.com |

Use this list with extreme caution and as a guideline only for finding products.
It is your responsibility to check the gluten-free status of all foods yourself.
There is no guarantee that they are gluten-free now.

| Ingredient | Brand(s) | Contact Information |
|---|---|---|
| | items to fall when they cool.  If using, you may have to adjust the rice flour amounts in baking recipes. | |
| Roasted Red Pepper | Peloponnese® Roasted Sweet Peppers/Hormel® B & G® Foods | 1-800-523-4635 www.hormelfoods.com 1-973-401-6500 www.bgfoods.com |
| Rum | Bacardi® (made from sugar) Captain Morgan® Rums (except Parrot Bay FMBs) | www.bacardi.com www.diageo.com |
| Salad Dressings (I use the recipes in this book, so I rarely purchase salad dressings. If you buy them, check ingredients). | Wish Bone® (certain varieties only) Seven Seas® Viva Italian Kraft® (certain varieties only) Kraft policy is they don't hide gluten containing ingredients on labels.  In 2008 I checked Ranch and Balsamic vinaigrette and they were safe. Emeril's® House Herb Vinaigrette | 1-800-697-7887 www.wish-bone.com 1-800-543-5335 1-800-323-0768 www.kraft.com 1-973-401-6500 www.bgfoods.com |
| Salsa, Picante, and Taco Sauce (Note: as of October 2008 Pace® Picante and Salsas are no longer gluten-free) | Chi-Chi's® Taco Sauce  (list on web) Chi-Chi's® Picante, Fiesta, Natural, Garden, and Original Salsa (contains distilled vinegar) Herdez® Canned Salsa Ortega (specific varieties) from Nestle Herr's® Mild and Medium | 1-800-523-4635 www.hormelfoods.com 1-800-523-4635 www.hormelfoods.com 1-800-333-7846 1-800-225-2270 www.herrs.com |
| Saltine Crackers | Ener-G® | www.ener-g.com |
| Sauerkraut (read labels, most canned or fresh is safe) | B&G® DelMonte® Hatfield® in pouch | 1-973-401-6500 www.bgfoods.com 1-800-543-3090 www.hatfieldqualitymeats.com |
| Sausage | Hatfield® fresh sweet Italian and hot sausage (see web page for a list of all gluten-free products) Johnsonville® (not Beer 'n Bratwurst or Brown Sugar & Honey Breakfast – those have wheat). Jones Dairy Farm® original pork sausage roll (call for the entire list of their gluten-free products) Hormel® Little Sizzlers® sausage links and patties Jennie-O Turkey Store® Fresh Dinner Sausage, Sweet Italian, Hot Italian, Cheddar Turkey Bratwurst, Lean Turkey Bratwurst (see list on web page under FAQ for many more items) Jamestown® Bulk Sausage (e-mail Smithfield for a list of their other gluten-free products) Boar's Head® Bratwurst (listed on web page) | www.hatfieldqualitymeats.com 1-888-556-2728 www.johnsonville.com 1-800-563-1004 www.jonesdairyfarm.com 1-800-523-4635 www.hormelfoods.com 1-800-523-4635 www.hormelfoods.com www.smithfield.com 1-800-352-6277 www.boarshead.com |
| Semi-sweet chocolate | Hershey's® Nestlé's® | 1-800-468-1714 1-800-637-8536 www.nestle.com |
| Sherbet | Hood® all varieties | 1-800-662-4468 www.hphood.com |
| Shortening | Crisco® | 1-800-766-7309 www.crisco.com |
| Shrimp, canned | Bumblebee® (all canned seafood except ready to eat w/crackers) | www.bumblebee.com |
| Smoked Sausage | Hillshire Farms® from Sara Lee (all varieties of Kielbasa.  Some smoked sausage is labeled that it contains wheat.  Also, no corn dogs and items with beer) Hatfield® Smoked Sausage and Kielbasa 1 lb. loop (see list on web page) | 1-800-328-2426 1-800-523-5291 www.hatfieldqualitymeats.com |
| Soft Drinks | Coca Cola® classic, regular and diet, caffeine free, vanilla, and cherry, Sprite® regular and diet, Fresca® A&W® Root Beer , Country Time® , Dr Pepper®, Canada Dry Ginger Ale®, 7 Up® Pepsi® products such as Sierra Mist®, Pepsi®, Pepsi Blue®, Mug® Root Beer, and Mug® Cream Turkey Hill® (all beverages) Wyler's® Drink Mixes and Wyler's® Light | www.cocacola.com 1-800-696-5891, www.dpsu.com 1-800-433-2652, www.pepsi.com www.turkeyhill.com www.Jelsert.comt |

Use this list with extreme caution and as a guideline only for finding products.
It is your responsibility to check the gluten-free status of all foods yourself.
There is no guarantee that they are gluten-free now.

| Ingredient | Brand(s) | Contact Information |
|---|---|---|
| Soup | Progresso® Creamy Mushroom (check ingredients) | 1-800-200-9377 www.progressosoup.com |
| Soup Base | Better Than Bouillon®<br><br>Tone's® (chicken only)<br>Major® | www.superiortouch.com<br>1-800-247-5251 www.spiceadvice.com<br>www.majorproducts.com |
| Sour Cream | Breakstone's® from Kraft<br>Land O Lakes®<br>Friendship® (regular, not flavored)<br>Hood (all varieties) | 1-800-538-1998 www.kraftfoods.com<br>www.landolakes.com<br>www.friendshipdairies.com<br>1-800-662-4468 www.hphood.com |
| Soy Flour | Ener-G®<br>Hodgeson Mill® (mill wheat but clean between lines) | www.ener-g.com<br>217-347-0105 ext 31 |
| Soy Sauce | LaChoy® from ConAgra (Regular and Lite)<br>Chung King® | 1-800 252-0672 www.conagrafoods.com |
| Spaghetti | Tinkyada® (gluten-free on label, g-f facility)<br>DeBoles® (certain varieties, gluten-free on label)<br>Bi-Aglut® (gluten-free on label)<br>Rizopia® (gluten-free on label, wheat free facility)<br>Sam Mills® (gluten-free on label) | www.tinkyada.com<br>www.deboles.com<br>www.biaglut.com (web page is in Italian)<br>www.rizopia.com |
| Spices<br>Many spices are gluten-free. Check labels. If it is pure spice it is safe. | McCormick®<br>Tone's®/ Durkee® | 1-800-632-5847 www.mccormick.com<br>1-800-247-5251 www.tones.com |
| Sugar, confectioner's, granulated and brown | Domino® (none of their sugars contain gluten)<br>Check ingredients, most store brands are gluten-free. Confectioner's sugar usually contains cornstarch which is safe. Brown sugar usually contains caramel color from sugar which is safe. | www.dominosugar.com |
| Sugar substitute | Splenda® (all varieties)<br>Sweet N Low® granulated sugar substitute | 1-800-777-5363 www.splenda.com<br>www.sweetnlow.com |
| Syrups | Aunt Jemima® by Quaker Oats®, all syrups<br>Hungry Jack®<br>Vermont Maid®<br>Karo® – Light and Dark, and Pancake Syrup<br>Maple Grove Farms of Vermont®: Raspberry, Strawberry, Blueberry, Apricot, and pure Maple<br>Log Cabin® Country Kitchen | 1-800-407-2247 www.auntjemima.com<br>1-800-767-4466<br>1-973-401-6500 www.bgfoods.com<br>1-866-430-5276 www.karosyrup.com<br>1-973-401-6500 www.maplegrove.com<br><br>1-877-852-7424 www.pinnaclefoodscorp.com |
| Taco Shells made from Corn | Old El Paso® from General Mills®<br>Mission Foods® (all corn products are safe) | 1-800-300-8664 www.generalmills.com<br>1-800-600-8226 www.missionfoods.com |
| Tapioca starch or tapioca flour | Ener-G®<br>Erawan® Brand (in Asian markets – has 3 elephants in logo on the label).<br>Bob's Red Mill | www.ener-g.com<br>www.choheng.com<br><br>www.bobsredmill.com |
| Tartar Sauce | Hellman's® | 1-800-338-8831 www.unilever.com/brands/ |
| Tea | Lipton® regular and decaf Tea bags and Lipton Iced Tea mixes and ready-to-drink teas<br>Nestea® iced tea mixes from Nestle, including their new liquid concentrate<br>Snapple® Iced Tea (they reformulated lemon tea to remove gluten ingredient)<br>Turkey Hill® bottled drinks | 1-888-547-8668 www.liptont.com<br><br>1-800-441-2525<br><br>1-800-Snapple  www.snapple.com<br><br>www.turkeyhill.com |
| Thai food ingredients | A Taste of Thai® (as of 10/01/08 their website says all products are gluten-free, but read labels carefully. I found that some products still on stores shelves were unsafe. For example, their Pad Thai for Two kit in a store on 4/30/09 contained wheat.) | www.atasteofthai.com |
| Tomato Crushed or Strained or Peeled or Diced | Redpack® and Tuttorusso® (citric acid is from corn)<br>DelMonte®<br>Hunts® (except diced w/green chilies) | 1-877-748-9796 www.redgold.com<br>1-800-543-3090<br>1-800-858-6392 |

Use this list with extreme caution and as a guideline only for finding products.
It is your responsibility to check the gluten-free status of all foods yourself.
There is no guarantee that they are gluten-free now.

| Ingredient | Brand(s) | Contact Information |
|---|---|---|
| Tomato Juice (Many store brands are just tomatoes and ascorbic acid which is safe) | V8® from Campbell's®, all varieties<br>Sacramento® original from Redgold® | www.campbellsoup.com or www.v8juice.com<br>1-877-748-9796 www.redgold.com |
| Tomato Puree | Redpack®<br>Tuttorusso®<br>DelMonte®<br>Hunts® | 1-877-748-9796 www.redgold.com<br>1-877-748-9796 www.redgold.com<br>1-800-543-3090<br>1-800-858-6372 |
| Tomato Sauce<br>(8 oz. cans) | Contadina®<br>Hunt's® (except varieties containing meat)<br>Tuttorusso®, and Redpack®<br>DelMonte® (all except sauce flavored w/ meat)<br>Wal-Mart® store brand (gluten-free on label)<br>Shop-Rite® store brand<br>Aldi® store brand (gluten-free on label) | www.contadina.com<br>1-800-858-6392 www.hunts.com<br>1-877-748-9796 www.redgold.com<br>1-800-543-3090<br><br>1-800-ShopRite |
| Tomato Sauce (jar)<br>(note: as of Oct. 2008, Prego® is not longer gluten-free) | Aunt Millie's® all varieties (from Heinz® foods)<br>Classico® (all red and white varieties)<br>Ragu® (certain varieties only, but Unilver® products have allergens & rye, oats, barley clearly listed on labels). Natural variety has easier labels to check.<br>Five Brothers® Fresh Tomato & Basil<br>Emeril's® Home Style Marinara (see others on web)<br>Francesco Rinaldi® Traditional, Hearty, Garden, & Organic Tomato Sauces (not Premium Sauces which are Vodka and Alfredo sauces)<br>Barilla® (certain varieties only) | 1-888-337-2420<br>1-888-337-2420 www.classico.com<br>1-800-328-7248<br><br><br>1-800-328-7248<br>1-973-401-6500 www.bgfoods.com<br>www.francescorinaldi.com (e-mail on the contact us page for a response)<br><br>1-800-9-barilla |
| Tomatoes, Stewed | Tuttorusso® and Redpack®<br>Contadina®<br>Hunts®<br>DelMonte® | www.redgold.com<br>www.contadina.com<br>www.hunts.com<br>www.delmonte.com |
| Tortilla chips – check for contamination | Mission® Rounds (all corn products gluten-free and no cross-contamination. These include corn tortillas, corn tortilla chips, taco shells, tostadas, corn gorditas and sopes.)<br>Chi-Chi's® by ConAgra Foods (dedicated lines)<br>Utz® Foods (certain varieties – will say gluten-free on labels or see web page) White Corn Tortilla Chips, Restaurant Style, Corn Chips (They wash between lines, with flavorings added last. Some flavors have gluten, so check.)<br>Bachmann® (see list on web) 21g Wholegrain<br>Chipitos® Black bean Salsa, Thai BBQ, Sweet Chili Lime, and plain<br>Grande® All Natural Tortilla Chips (labeled GF) | 1-800-600-8226 www.missionfoods.com<br><br><br>1-502-772-2500<br>1-800-367-7629 www.utzsnacks.com<br><br><br><br>www.bachmanpretzels.com<br><br><br>www.snydersofhanover.com |
| Tortillas (corn only) | Mission® – gluten-free on label (dedicated lines)<br>Pepito® corn tortillas (made by Mission®)<br>Mex-America® | 1-800-600-8226 www.missionfoods.com<br>1-800-600-8226 www.missionfoods.com<br>1-814-781-1447 www.mexamericanfoods.com |
| Tuna, canned and foil packs These 3 major brands say that their vegetable broth does not contain wheat. | Star-Kist® (all varieties <u>except</u> lunch kits with crackers)<br>Bumblebee® (all of canned seafood <u>except</u> crackers in the ready to eat with crackers)<br>Chicken of the Sea® (all varieties <u>except</u> imitation crabmeat [Crab-tastic®] and tuna salad kits containing bread crumbs or crackers). | 1-800-252-1587 www.starkist.com<br><br>www.bumblebee.com<br><br>www.chickenofthesea.com |
| Turkey | Shady Brook Farms® (listed on web site); whole turkey, fresh ground turkey, and certain varieties of turkey tenderloin roasts<br>Butterball® if you discard the gravy packet<br>Butterball® Smoked, precooked (tastes like Ham)<br>Pilgrim's Pride® Hotel Style Turkey Breast (Wampler®) | www.shadybrookfarms.com<br><br><br>1-800-288-8372 www.butterball.com<br>1-800-288-8372 www.butterball.com<br>1-800-824-1159 www.pilgrimspride.com |

Use this list with extreme caution and as a guideline only for finding products.
It is your responsibility to check the gluten-free status of all foods yourself.
There is no guarantee that they are gluten-free now.

| Ingredient | Brand(s) | Contact Information |
|---|---|---|
| | Jennie-O® Prime Young Turkey (throw out packet), Fresh Ground Turkey, lean, extra lean, Italian, and Mexican and Fresh Lean Turkey Patties, Frozen Ground Turkey (see list on Hormel® website) | 1-800-523-4623 www.hormelfoods.com |
| | Norbest® (gluten-free on label) | www.norbest.com |
| Turkey Cold cuts | Louis Rich® Smoked Turkey Variety Pack (Ham, Bologna, cotto salami) Kraft Foods says any allergens are noted on ingredients list. | 1-800-323-0768, www.kraftfoods.com |
| | Hormel® Natural Choice® (gluten-free on Label) | www.hormelfoods.com |
| Whiskey | Jack Daniels® (says all gluten is removed in the distillation process.) | www.jackdaniels.com |
| | Johnnie Walker® (all) | www.diageo.com |
| | Crown Royal® | www.diageo.com |
| | Seagram's® 7 and Seagram's® VO | www.diageo.com |
| Vanilla or Vanillin | McCormick® | 1-800-632-5847 www.mccormick.com |
| Vinegar (All Malt Vinegar is unsafe. Most store brand vinegars are safe. Check for possible additives.) | Heinz® distilled white (from corn), red wine, apple cider – (the cider flavored vinegar, which is different than apple cider vinegar, had gluten in 2006 but this has changed) | 800-255-5750 www.heinz.com |
| | Regina® from B&G Foods, all varieties | 1-973-401-6500 www.bgfoods.com |
| Vodka | Smirnoff® Vodka, Black & Twist | www.diageo.com |
| | Popov® Vodka | www.diageo.com |
| | Tanqueray® Vodka | www.diageo.com |
| | Gordons® | www.diageo.com |
| | Luksusowa® Vodka (potatoes) | Labeled that it is made only from potatoes |
| Worcestershire Sauce | Lea & Perrins® | 1-800-987-4674 www.lea-perrins.com |
| | French's® | 1-800-841-1256 www.frenchsfoods.com |
| Yeast | Red Star® (also provides recipes & baking advice) | 1-800-4-celiac www.redstaryeast.com |
| | Fleishmann's® | www.breadworld.com |
| Yogurt, plain | LaYogurt® plain only (whole, lowfat, fat free) | www.johannafoods.com |
| | Friendship® plain lowfat yogurt (all of their products are gluten-free) | www.friendshipdairies.com |
| | Dannon® (plain only) | 1-877-326-6668 www.dannon.com |
| | Stonyfield® plain (New lowfat plain with inulin is gluten-free – inulin is made from chicory) | 1-800-776-2697 www.stonyfield.com |
| | Fage® | www.fageusa.com |
| Yogurt, flavored | CascadeFresh® (available at Wild Oats® markets) Stabilizers are from tapioca and apple pectin. | 1-800-511-0057 www.cascadefresh.com |
| | Yoplait®, Columbo®, and Go-Gurt® from General Mills® | 1-800-967-5248 www.yoplait.com |
| | Breyers® yogurt from Coolbrands Inc. | 1-800-661-5338 www.breyersyogurt.com |
| | Stonyfield® yogurts, smoothies and soy yogurts (now all labeled gluten-free) except Yobaby® plus fruit and cereal | www.stonyfield.com |
| | Fage® (all yogurts) | www.fageusa.com |

Use this list with extreme caution and as a guideline only for finding products.
It is your responsibility to check the gluten-free status of all foods yourself.
There is no guarantee that they are gluten-free now.

## Medical References

Endnotes:

1. www.biblegateway.com New International Version c, 1978, and 1984, International Bible Society.
2. Fasano A, Berti I, Gerarduzzi T, et al. Prevalence of celiac disease in at-risk and not-at-risk groups in the United States: a large multicenter study. Arch Intern Med 2003;163(3):286-92.
3. Castano L BE, Ortiz L, Nunez J, Bilbao JR, Rica I, Martul P, Vitoria JC. Prospective population screening for celiac disease: high prevalence in the first 3 years of life. J Pediatr Gastroenterol Nutr 2004 2005;39((1)):80-4.
4. Accomando S, Cataldo F. The global village of celiac disease. Dig Liver Dis 2004;36(7):492-8.
5. Gomez JC, Selvaggio GS, Viola M, et al. Prevalence of celiac disease in Argentina: screening of an adult population in the La Plata area. Am J Gastroenterol 2001;96(9):2700-4.
6. http://www.celiachealth.org/. Educational Site on Celiac Disease. 2004.
7. Granot E, Korman SM, Sallon S, Deckelbaum RJ. "Early" vs. "late" diagnosis of celiac disease in two ethnic groups living in the same geographic area. Isr J Med Sci 1994;30(4):271-5.
8. Tatar G, Elsurer R, Simsek H, et al. Screening of tissue transglutaminase antibody in healthy blood donors for celiac disease screening in the Turkish population. Dig Dis Sci 2004;49(9):1479-84.
9. Fasano A, Catassi C. Current approaches to diagnosis and treatment of celiac disease: an evolving spectrum. Gastroenterology 2001;120(3):636-51.
10. Catassi C, Rossini M, Ratsch IM, et al. Dose dependent effects of protracted ingestion of small amounts of gliadin in coeliac disease children: a clinical and jejunal morphometric study. Gut 1993;34(11):1515-9.
11. Biagi F, Campanella J, Martucci S, et al. A milligram of gluten a day keeps the mucosal recovery away: a case report. Nutr Rev 2004;62(9):360-3.
12. Thorn MM, RN, CCRC. Celiac Disease. The most common underdiagnosed autoimmune disease. Advance Online Editions for Nurses 2005:1.
13. Collin P, Thorell L, Kaukinen K, Maki M. The safe threshold for gluten contamination in gluten-free products. Can trace amounts be accepted in the treatment of coeliac disease? Aliment Pharmacol Ther 2004;19(12):1277-83.
14. Hadjivassiliou M, Williamson CA, Woodroofe N. The immunology of gluten sensitivity: beyond the gut. Trends Immunol 2004;25(11):578-82.
15. Chin RL, Sander HW, Brannagan TH, et al. Celiac neuropathy. Neurology 2003;60(10):1581-5.
16. Furse R. M. MAS. Atypical Presentation of Coeliac Disease. British Medical Journal 2005;330:773-4.
17. Lippincott WW. Stedman's Medical Dictionary. 2004.
18. Pruessner HT. Detecting celiac disease in your patients. Am Fam Physician 1998;57(5):1023-34, 39-41.
19. Nelsen DA, Jr. Gluten-sensitive enteropathy (celiac disease): more common than you think. Am Fam Physician 2002;66(12):2259-66.
20. Merck. Merck Manual Second Home Edition. Chapter 125 2004;Malabsorption(on-line version).
21. Farrell RJ, Kelly CP. Diagnosis of celiac sprue. Am J Gastroenterol 2001;96(12):3237-46.
22. Pietzak M. Follow-up of Patients with Celiac Disease: Achieving Compliance with Treatment. Gastroenterology 2005;128(Supplement):S135-S41.
23. Rickels MR, Mandel SJ. Celiac disease manifesting as isolated hypocalcemia. Endocr Pract 2004;10(3):203-7.
24. Kavak US, Yuce A, Kocak N, et al. Bone mineral density in children with untreated and treated celiac disease. J Pediatr Gastroenterol Nutr 2003;37(4):434-6.
25. Stenson WF, Newberry R, Lorenz R, Baldus C, Civitelli R. Increased prevalence of celiac disease and need for routine screening among patients with osteoporosis. Arch Intern Med 2005;165(4):393-9.
26. Vasquez H, Mazure R, Gonzalez D, et al. Risk of fractures in celiac disease patients: a cross-sectional, case-control study. Am J Gastroenterol 2000;95(1):183-9.
27. Boyles S. Drug for Bone Disease Linked to "Jaw Death". WebMD Medical news 2005.
28. Ficarra G, Beninati F, Rubino I, et al. Osteonecrosis of the jaws in periodontal patients with a history of bisphosphonates treatment. J Clin Periodontol 2005;32(11):1123-8.
29. Lenart BA, Lorich DG, Lane JM. Atypical fractures of the femoral diaphysis in postmenopausal women taking alendronate. The New England journal of medicine 2008;358(12):1304-6.
30. Neviaser AS, Lane JM, Lenart BA, Edobor-Osula F, Lorich DG. Low-energy femoral shaft fractures associated with alendronate use. Journal of orthopaedic trauma 2008;22(5):346-50.

31. Rude RK, Olerich M. Magnesium deficiency: possible role in osteoporosis associated with gluten-sensitive enteropathy. Osteoporos Int 1996;6(6):453-61.

32. Bergman EA, Massey LK, Wise KJ, Sherrard DJ. Effects of dietary caffeine on renal handling of minerals in adult women. Life Sci 1990;47(6):557-64.

33. Mazariegos-Ramos E, Guerrero-Romero F, Rodriguez-Moran M, Lazcano-Burciaga G, Paniagua R, Amato D. Consumption of soft drinks with phosphoric acid as a risk factor for the development of hypocalcemia in children: a case-control study. J Pediatr 1995;126(6):940-2.

34. Fitzpatrick LaH, RP. Got Soda? Journal of Bone and Mineral Research 2003;18(9):1570.

35. Massey LK, Bergman EA, Wise KJ, Sherrard DJ. Interactions between dietary caffeine and calcium on calcium and bone metabolism in older women. J Am Coll Nutr 1994;13(6):592-6.

36. Fernando GR, Martha RM, Evangelina R. Consumption of soft drinks with phosphoric acid as a risk factor for the development of hypocalcemia in postmenopausal women. J Clin Epidemiol 1999;52(10):1007-10.

37. Kozanoglu E, Basaran S, Goncu MK. Proximal myopathy as an unusual presenting feature of celiac disease. Clin Rheumatol 2004.

38. Tursi A. Gastrointestinal motility disturbances in celiac disease. J Clin Gastroenterol 2004;38(8):642-5.

39. Bilezikian JP. The role of estrogens in male skeletal development. Reprod Fertil Dev 2001;13(4):253-9.

40. De Carolis S, Botta A, Fatigante G, et al. Celiac disease and inflammatory bowel disease in pregnancy. Lupus 2004;13(9):653-8.

41. Ludvigsson JF, Ludvigsson J. Coeliac disease in the father affects the newborn. Gut 2001;49(2):169-75.

42. Ludvigsson JF, Montgomery SM, Ekbom A. Celiac disease and risk of adverse fetal outcome: a population-based cohort study. Gastroenterology 2005;129(2):454-63.

43. Hernandez MA, Colina G, Ortigosa L. Epilepsy, cerebral calcifications and clinical or subclinical coeliac disease. Course and follow up with gluten-free diet. Seizure 1998;7(1):49-54.

44. Pratesi R, Modelli IC, Martins RC, Almeida PL, Gandolfi L. Celiac disease and epilepsy: favorable outcome in a child with difficult to control seizures. Acta Neurol Scand 2003;108(4):290-3.

45. Zelnik N, Pacht A, Obeid R, Lerner A. Range of neurologic disorders in patients with celiac disease. Pediatrics 2004;113(6):1672-6.

46. Kleopa KA, Kyriacou K, Zamba-Papanicolaou E, Kyriakides T. Reversible inflammatory and vacuolar myopathy with vitamin E deficiency in celiac disease. Muscle Nerve 2004.

47. Volta U, De Giorgio R, Petrolini N, et al. Clinical findings and anti-neuronal antibodies in coeliac disease with neurological disorders. Scand J Gastroenterol 2002;37(11):1276-81.

48. Serratrice J, Disdier P, de Roux C, Christides C, Weiller PJ. Migraine and coeliac disease. Headache 1998;38(8):627-8.

49. NIH. Consensus Development Conference Statement on Celiac Disease, National Institutes of Health, June 28-30, 2004, Final Statement August 9, 2004 4:00 pm. 2004.

50. Bushara KO. Neurologic presentation of celiac disease. Gastroenterology 2005;128(4 Suppl 1):S92-7.

51. Carta MG, Hardoy MC, Boi MF, Mariotti S, Carpiniello B, Usai P. Association between panic disorder, major depressive disorder and celiac disease: a possible role of thyroid autoimmunity. J Psychosom Res 2002;53(3):789-93.

52. Sategna-Guidetti C, Volta U, Ciacci C, et al. Prevalence of thyroid disorders in untreated adult celiac disease patients and effect of gluten withdrawal: an Italian multicenter study. Am J Gastroenterol 2001;96(3):751-7.

53. Rabsztyn A, Green PH, Berti I, Fasano A, Perman JA, Horvath K. Macroamylasemia in patients with celiac disease. Am J Gastroenterol 2001;96(4):1096-100.

54. Potocki P, Hozyasz K. [Psychiatric symptoms and coeliac disease]. Psychiatr Pol 2002;36(4):567-78.

55. Thomson. PDR (Physicians Desk Reference). wwwthomsonhccom 2004.

56. Patinen P, Hietane J, Malmstrom M, Reunala T, Savilahti E. Iodine and gliadin challenge on oral mucosa in dermatitis herpetiformis. Acta Derm Venereol 2002;82(2):86-9.

57. Ojetti V, Aguilar Sanchez J, Guerriero C, et al. High prevalence of celiac disease in psoriasis. Am J Gastroenterol 2003;98(11):2574-5.

58. Michaelsson G, Gerden B, Hagforsen E, et al. Psoriasis patients with antibodies to gliadin can be improved by a gluten-free diet. Br J Dermatol 2000;142(1):44-51.

59. Michaelsson G, Ahs S, Hammarstrom I, Lundin IP, Hagforsen E. Gluten-free diet in psoriasis patients with antibodies to gliadin results in decreased expression of tissue transglutaminase and fewer Ki67+ cells in the dermis. Acta Derm Venereol 2003;83(6):425-9.

60.    Abdo A, Meddings J, Swain M. Liver abnormalities in celiac disease. Clin Gastroenterol Hepatol 2004;2(2):107-12.

61.    Kaukinen K, Halme L, Collin P, et al. Celiac disease in patients with severe liver disease: gluten-free diet may reverse hepatic failure. Gastroenterology 2002;122(4):881-8.

62.    Schmidt B, Novacek G, Brichta A, Vogelsang H, Wrba F, Ferenci P. Sonographic diagnosis of coeliac disease in a case with suspected acute liver failure. Eur J Gastroenterol Hepatol 2005;17(9):995-8.

63.    Leffler D, Saha S, Farrell RJ. Celiac disease. Am J Manag Care 2003;9(12):825-31; quiz 32-3.

64.    Hervonen K, Vornanen M, Kautiainen H, Collin P, Reunala T. Lymphoma in patients with dermatitis herpetiformis and their first-degree relatives. Br J Dermatol 2005;152(1):82-6.

65.    Buess M, Steuerwald M, Wegmann W, Rothen M. Obstructive jaundice caused by enteropathy-associated T-cell lymphoma in a patient with celiac sprue. J Gastroenterol 2004;39(11):1110-3.

66.    Green PH, Jabri B. Celiac disease and other precursors to small-bowel malignancy. Gastroenterol Clin North Am 2002;31(2):625-39.

67.    Saadah OI, Zacharin M, O'Callaghan A, Oliver MR, Catto-Smith AG. Effect of gluten-free diet and adherence on growth and diabetic control in diabetics with coeliac disease. Arch Dis Child 2004;89(9):871-6.

68.    Ventura A, Magazzu G, Greco L. Duration of exposure to gluten and risk for autoimmune disorders in patients with celiac disease. SIGEP Study Group for Autoimmune Disorders in Celiac Disease. Gastroenterology 1999;117(2):297-303.

69.    Buckley O, Brien JO, Ward E, Doody O, Govender P, Torreggiani WC. The imaging of coeliac disease and its complications. Eur J Radiol 2007.

70.    GIG. Associated Autoimmune Disease with Celiac Disease and Dermatitis Herpetiformis. Gluten Intolerance Group 2003:2.

71.    Aydemir S, Tekin NS, Aktunc E, Numanoglu G, Ustundag Y. Celiac disease in patients having recurrent aphthous stomatitis. Turk J Gastroenterol 2004;15(3):192-5.

72.    wikipedia. Maladies caused by gluten. wwwwikipediaorg/wiki/gluten 2005.

73.    Kero J, Gissler M, Hemminki E, Isolauri E. Could TH1 and TH2 diseases coexist? Evaluation of asthma incidence in children with coeliac disease, type 1 diabetes, or rheumatoid arthritis: a register study. J Allergy Clin Immunol 2001;108(5):781-3.

74.    Barcia G, Posar A, Santucci M, Parmeggiani A. Autism and Coeliac Disease. J Autism Dev Disord 2007.

75.    Rubio-Tapia A, Murray JA. The liver in celiac disease. Hepatology (Baltimore, Md 2007;46(5):1650-8.

76.    Usai P, Serra A, Marini B, et al. Frontal cortical perfusion abnormalities related to gluten intake and associated autoimmune disease in adult coeliac disease: 99mTc-ECD brain SPECT study. Dig Liver Dis 2004;36(8):513-8.

77.    Tunc T, Okuyucu E, Ucleri S, et al. Subclinical celiac disease with cerebellar ataxia. Acta Neurol Belg 2004;104(2):84-6.

78.    Pfaender M, D'Souza WJ, Trost N, Litewka L, Paine M, Cook M. Visual disturbances representing occipital lobe epilepsy in patients with cerebral calcifications and coeliac disease: a case series. J Neurol Neurosurg Psychiatry 2004;75(11):1623-5.

79.    Goodwin FC, Beattie RM, Millar J, Kirkham FJ. Celiac disease and childhood stroke. Pediatr Neurol 2004;31(2):139-42.

80.    Freeman HJ. Collagenous colitis as the presenting feature of biopsy-defined celiac disease. J Clin Gastroenterol 2004;38(8):664-8.

81.    Pynnonen PA, Isometsa ET, Verkasalo MA, et al. Gluten-free diet may alleviate depressive and behavioural symptoms in adolescents with coeliac disease: a prospective follow-up case-series study. BMC Psychiatry 2005;5(1):14.

82.    Sumnik Z, Kolouskova S, Malcova H, et al. High prevalence of coeliac disease in siblings of children with type 1 diabetes. Eur J Pediatr 2004.

83.    Silano M, Volta U, Vincenzi AD, Dessi M, Vincenzi MD. Effect of a Gluten-free Diet on the Risk of Enteropathy-associated T-cell Lymphoma in Celiac Disease. Dig Dis Sci 2007.

84.    Emami MH, Taheri H, Kohestani S, et al. How frequent is celiac disease among epileptic patients? J Gastrointestin Liver Dis 2008;17(4):379-82.

85.    Ojetti V, Nucera G, Migneco A, et al. High prevalence of celiac disease in patients with lactose intolerance. Digestion 2005;71(2):106-10.

86.    Pengiran Tengah CD, Lock RJ, Unsworth DJ, Wills AJ. Multiple sclerosis and occult gluten sensitivity. Neurology 2004;62(12):2326-7.

87.   Patel RS, Johlin FC, Jr., Murray JA. Celiac disease and recurrent pancreatitis. Gastrointest Endosc 1999;50(6):823-7.

88.   Thomson A. Celiac disease as a cause of pancreatitis. Gastroenterology 2005;129(3):1137.

89.   Woo WK, McMillan SA, Watson RG, McCluggage WG, Sloan JM, McMillan JC. Coeliac disease-associated antibodies correlate with psoriasis activity. Br J Dermatol 2004;151(4):891-4.

90.   Cuomo A, Romano M, Rocco A, Budillon G, Del Vecchio Blanco C, Nardone G. Reflux oesophagitis in adult coeliac disease: beneficial effect of a gluten-free diet. Gut 2003;52(4):514-7.

91.   Manchanda S, Davies CR, Picchietti D. Celiac disease as a possible cause for low serum ferritin in patients with restless legs syndrome. Sleep medicine 2009.

92.   Hwang E, McBride R, Neugut AI, Green PH. Sarcoidosis in Patients with Celiac Disease. Dig Dis Sci 2007.

93.   El Moutawakil B, Chourkani N, Sibai M, et al. [Celiac disease and ischemic stroke.]. Revue neurologique 2009.

94.   Trucco Aguirre E, Olano Gossweiler C, Mendez Pereira C, Isasi Capelo ME, Isasi Capelo ES, Rondan Olivera M. [Celiac disease associated with systemic sclerosis.]. Gastroenterologia y hepatologia 2007;30(9):538-41.

95.   Bahloul M, Chaari A, Khlaf-Bouaziz N, et al. [Celiac disease, cerebral venous thrombosis and protein S deficiency, a fortuitous association?]. Journal des maladies vasculaires 2005;30(4 Pt 1):228-30.

96.   Kallel L, Matri S, Karoui S, Fekih M, Boubaker J, Filali A. Deep venous thrombosis related to protein S deficiency revealing celiac disease. Am J Gastroenterol 2009;104(1):256-7.

97.   Treem WR. Emerging concepts in celiac disease. Curr Opin Pediatr 2004;16(5):552-9.

98.   Arentz-Hansen H. Public Library of Science, Mentioned at WebMD http://my.webmd.com/content/article/95/103344.htm. 2004;1:001-9.

99.   Sollid LM, Gray GM. A role for bacteria in celiac disease? Am J Gastroenterol 2004;99(5):905-6.

100.  Forsberg G, Fahlgren A, Horstedt P, Hammarstrom S, Hernell O, Hammarstrom ML. Presence of bacteria and innate immunity of intestinal epithelium in childhood celiac disease. Am J Gastroenterol 2004;99(5):894-904.

101.  Molberg O, Uhlen AK, Jensen T, et al. Mapping of gluten T-cell epitopes in the bread wheat ancestors: implications for celiac disease. Gastroenterology 2005;128(2):393-401.

102.  Pizzuti D, Buda A, D'Odorico A, et al. Lack of intestinal mucosal toxicity of Triticum monococcum in celiac disease patients. Scand J Gastroenterol 2006;41(11):1305-11.

103.  Spaenij-Dekking L, Kooy-Winkelaar Y, van Veelen P, et al. Natural variation in toxicity of wheat: potential for selection of nontoxic varieties for celiac disease patients. Gastroenterology 2005;129(3):797-806.

104.  Campaign CA. Spring/Summer Newsletter. http://celiacnihgov/NewsletterSpring08aspx 2008.

105.  Tursi A, Brandimarte G, Giorgetti G. High prevalence of small intestinal bacterial overgrowth in celiac patients with persistence of gastrointestinal symptoms after gluten withdrawal. Am J Gastroenterol 2003;98(4):839-43.

106.  Initial Assessment and Follow-up Care of Celiac Patients (presentation on 9/29 to Westchester celiac sprue support group), summaried by Sue Goldstein. www.celiac.com, 1995. (Accessed at

107.  Baker AL, Rosenberg IH. Refractory sprue: recovery after removal of nongluten dietary proteins. Ann Intern Med 1978;89(4):505-8.

108.  Green PH, Jabri B. Coeliac disease. Lancet 2003;362(9381):383-91.

109.  Lee SK, Brar P, Bhagat G, Lewis SK, Green PH. Budesonide for the Treatment of Porly Responsive Celiac Disease. Celiac Disease Center at Columbia University Summer 2005 Newsletter 2005;1(2):7.

110.  Culliford AN, Green PH. Refractory sprue. Curr Gastroenterol Rep 2003;5(5):373-8.

111.  Abdulkarim AS, Burgart LJ, See J, Murray JA. Etiology of nonresponsive celiac disease: results of a systematic approach. Am J Gastroenterol 2002;97(8):2016-21.

112.  Tursi A, Brandimarte G, Giorgetti GM. Sorbitol H2-breath test versus anti-endomysium antibodies for the diagnosis of subclinical/silent coeliac disease. Scand J Gastroenterol 2001;36(11):1170-2.

113.  Tursi A, Brandimarte G, Giorgetti GM. Sorbitol H2-breath test versus anti-endomysium antibodies to assess histological recovery after gluten-free diet in coeliac disease. Dig Liver Dis 2002;34(12):846-50.

114.  http://www.celiacdiseasecenter.columbia.edu. Celiac Disease Center at Columbia University. 2006.

115.  http://labtestsonline.org. Celiac Disease Lab Tests. 2006.

116.  Hospital BIDMC-B. Beth Israel Deaconess Medical Center – Boston – Answers to Commonly Asked Question about Celiac Disease. wwwbidmcharvardedu/displayasp?leaf_id=11884 2005.

117. Tamaro G, Perticarari S, Princi T, et al. A problem solving in driving tests which method for carbohydratedeficient transferrin (cdt) in adolescents affected by celiac disease? Biomedical sciences instrumentation 2008;44:525-30.

118. Dickey W, Kearney N. Overweight in celiac disease: prevalence, clinical characteristics, and effect of a gluten-free diet. Am J Gastroenterol 2006;101(10):2356-9.

119. Baker T, Medical College of Georgia. Compound that helps rice grow reduces nerve, vascular damage from diabetes. https://mymcgedu/portal/page/portal/News/archive/2008/53162EF70C212CC7E0440003BAD149FF 2008.

120. Usuki S, Ariga T, Dasgupta S, et al. Structural analysis of novel bioactive acylated steryl glucosides (ASGs) in Pre-germinated brown rice bran. Journal of lipid research 2008.

121. Usuki S, Ito Y, Morikawa K, et al. Effect of pre-germinated brown rice intake on diabetic neuropathy in streptozotocin-induced diabetic rats. Nutrition & metabolism 2007;4:25.

122. Hagiwara H, Seki T, Ariga T. The effect of pre-germinated brown rice intake on blood glucose and PAI-1 levels in streptozotocin-induced diabetic rats. Bioscience, biotechnology, and biochemistry 2004;68(2):444-7.

123. Arakeri G, Arali V, Brennan PA. Cleft lip and palate: An adverse pregnancy outcome due to undiagnosed maternal and paternal coeliac disease. Med Hypotheses. 2010 Feb 24.

124. Fasano A, Counts D. Editorial: commentary on "anti-pituitary antibodies in children with newly diagnosed celiac disease: a novel finding contributing to linear growth". Am J Gastroenterol. 2010 Mar;105(3):697-8.

125. Delvecchio M, De Bellis A, Francavilla R, Rutigliano V, Predieri B, Indrio F, De Venuto D, Sinisi AA, Bizzarro A, Bellastella A, Iughetti L, Cavallo L. Anti-pituitary antibodies in children with newly diagnosed celiac disease: a novel finding contributing to linear-growth impairment. Am J Gastroenterol. 2010 Mar;105(3):691-6. Epub 2009 Nov 10.

126. Peroni DG, Paiola G, Tenero L, Fornaro M, Bodini A, Pollini F, Piacentini GL. Chronic urticaria and celiac disease: a case report. Pediatr Dermatol. 2010 Jan 1;27(1):108-9.

127. Kearby R, Bowyer S, Scharrer J, Sharathkumar A. Case Report: Six-Year-old Girl With Recurrent Episodes of Blue Toes. Clin Pediatr (Phila). 2010 Jan 28.

128. St Clair NE, Kim CC, Semrin G, Woodward AL, Liang MG, Glickman JN, Leichtner AM, Binstadt BA. Celiac disease presenting with chilblains in an adolescent girl. Pediatr Dermatol. 2006 Sep-Oct;23(5):451-4.

129. Bartyik K, Várkonyi A, Kirschner A, Endreffy E, Túri S, Karg E. Erythema nodosum in association with celiac disease. Pediatr Dermatol. 2004 May-Jun;21(3):227-30.

130. Song MS, Farber D, Bitton A, Jass J, Singer M, Karpati G. Dermatomyositis associated with celiac disease: response to a gluten-free diet. Can J Gastroenterol. 2006 Jun;20(6):433-5.

131. Pinals RS. Arthritis associated with gluten-sensitive enteropathy. J Rheumatol. 1986 Feb;13(1):201-4.

132. Falcini F, Ferrari R, Simonini G, Calabri GB, Pazzaglia A, Lionetti P. Recurrent monoarthritis in an 11-year-old boy with occult coeliac disease. Successful and stable remission after gluten-free diet. Clin Exp Rheumatol. 1999 Jul-Aug;17(4):509-11.

133. Rabsztyn A, Green PH, Berti I, Fasano A, Perman JA, Horvath K. Macroamylasemia in patients with celiac disease. Am J Gastroenterol. 2001 Apr;96(4):1096-100.

134. Barera G, Bazzigaluppi E, Viscardi M, Renzetti F, Bianchi C, Chiumello G, Bosi E. Macroamylasemia attributable to gluten-related amylase autoantibodies: a case report. Pediatrics. 2001 Jun;107(6):E93.

135. Haussmann J, Sekar A. Chronic urticaria: a cutaneous manifestation of celiac disease. Can J Gastroenterol. 2006 Apr;20(4):291-3.

136. Jordá FC, Vivancos JL. Fatigue as a Determinant of Health in Patients With Celiac Disease. J Clin Gastroenterol. 2009 Nov 20.

137. Siniscalchi M, Iovino P, Tortora R, Forestiero S, Somma A, Capuano L, Franzese MD, Sabbatini F, Ciacci C. Fatigue in adult coeliac disease. Aliment Pharmacol Ther. 2005 Sep 1;22(5):489-94.

138. Goodman BP, Mistry DH, Pasha SF, Bosch PE. Copper deficiency myeloneuropathy due to occult celiac disease. Neurologist. 2009 Nov;15(6):355-6

139. Goel NK, McBane RD, Kamath PS. Cardiomyopathy associated with celiac disease. Mayo Clin Proc. 2005 May;80(5):674-6.

140. Narula N, Rawal P, Manoj Kumar R, Ram Thapa B. Association of Celiac Disease with Cardiomyopathy and Pulmonary Hemosiderosis. J Trop Pediatr. 2009 Nov 6.

141. Curione M, Barbato M, Viola F, Francia P, De Biase L, Cucchiara S. Idiopathic dilated cardiomyopathy associated with coeliac disease: the effect of a gluten-free diet on cardiac performance. Dig Liver Dis. 2002 Dec;34(12):866-9.

142. Lodha A, Haran M, Hollander G, Frankel R, Shani J. Celiac disease associated with dilated cardiomyopathy. South Med J. 2009 Oct;102(10):1052-4.

143. Leslie C, Mews C, Charles A, Ravikumara M. Celiac Disease and Eosinophilic Esophagitis: A True Association. J Pediatr Gastroenterol Nutr. 2009 Oct 13.

144. Olén O, Montgomery SM, Elinder G, Ekbom A, Ludvigsson JF. Increased risk of immune thrombocytopenic purpura among inpatients with coeliac disease. Scand J Gastroenterol. 2008;43(4):416-22.

## Ingredient Substitution Chart

Use this chart to substitute an ingredient in baking and cooking. These substitutions work, but keep in mind that they may not work as well as the original ingredient.

This chart can come in handy if you run out of an ingredient. It can also be helpful if you have food allergies. For example, if you are allergic to corn, you can make a ketchup substitute without corn sweeteners for a barbeque sauce recipe.

| INGREDIENT | SUBSTITUTE |
|---|---|
| 1 teaspoon baking powder | ½ teaspoon cream of tartar plus ¼ teaspoon baking soda |
| 1 cup honey or 1 cup corn syrup | 1 cup sugar plus ¼ cup water |
| 1 cup milk | 1 cup gluten-free soy milk* or 1 cup gluten-free potato milk* or 1 cup gluten-free almond milk* or ⅓ cup non-fat dry milk plus 1 cup water or ¼ cup gluten-free non-dairy creamer* plus 1 cup water (blend creamer into dry ingredients first, and add water in recipe). |
| 1 cup buttermilk for baking | 1 cup gluten-free plain yogurt* or 1 cup milk plus 1 teaspoon vinegar or lemon juice. Plus I recommend 1/16 to ⅛ teaspoon of xanthan gum blended in, since gluten-free baking often utilizes the thickness of buttermilk. |
| 1 cup sour milk for baking | 1 cup milk plus 1 teaspoon vinegar or lemon juice |
| 1 cup heavy cream (not for whipping, but for use in baking) | ¾ cup milk plus ⅓ cup butter |
| 1 cup sour cream (not for dips, but for baking) | ⅞ cup sour milk plus 3 Tablespoons butter plus I recommend 1/16 to ⅛ teaspoon of xanthan gum. |
| 1 cup sweetened condensed milk | 1 (12 ounce) can evaporated milked with ½ pound (1 cup) of sugar slowly added, cooked and stirred constantly until desired thickness. |
| 1 ounce square unsweetened baking chocolate | 3 Tablespoons cocoa plus 1 Tablespoon butter or shortening |
| 4 ounce bar of sweet baking chocolate | 3 Tablespoons cocoa plus 3 Tablespoons butter or shortening plus 4 ½ Tablespoons sugar |
| 6 ounces semi-sweet chocolate baking bar or 1 cup semi-sweet chips (melted and added to baking) | 6 Tablespoons cocoa plus ¼ cup butter or shortening plus 7 Tablespoons sugar |
| 1 cup ketchup (for use in recipes such as barbeque sauce) | 1 cup gluten-free tomato sauce plus ⅓ cup sugar plus 2 Tablespoons vinegar |
| 1 teaspoon mustard | ¼ teaspoon dry mustard |

| INGREDIENT | SUBSTITUTE |
|---|---|
| 1 teaspoon Italian seasoning | ¼ teaspoon each oregano, basil, rosemary, thyme |
| 1 medium onion | 1 Tablespoon dried minced onion or 1 teaspoon onion powder |
| 1 clove garlic | ⅛ to ¼ teaspoon garlic powder or granulated garlic |
| 1 Tablespoon fresh herbs (such as basil oregano, sage, etc.) | 1 teaspoon dried herbs |
| 1 cup chicken broth | 1 cup water plus 1 teaspoon gluten-free bouillon or gluten-free soup base. Use less salt in recipe if using bouillon, since it can be salty. |
| 1 teaspoon vinegar | 1 teaspoon lemon juice |
| Juice of one lemon | 2 to 3 Tablespoons bottled lemon juice |
| Juice of one orange | 6 to 8 Tablespoons orange juice |

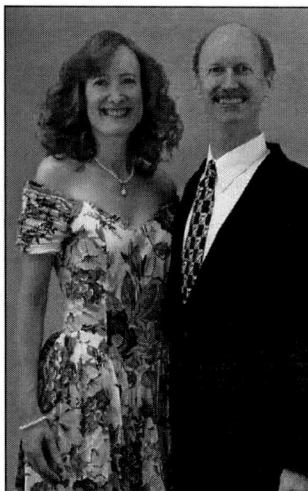

About the Author: Anita Jansen invents products for GFN Foods™, the makers of Gluten-Free Naturals™, and comes from a family with a long history of culinary talent. After her husband was diagnosed with celiac disease in 2000, she spent years experimenting and creating delicious gluten-free foods. Her passion for good food was the inspiration for GFN Foods™. The company was founded in 2004 by a member of her family and is based on her recipes.

Anita works for a major pharmaceutical company in the clinical research department, which inspired her to thoroughly research celiac disease. She credits the caring doctors that she works with for helping her husband to be accurately diagnosed. She also is thankful to her co-workers for taste testing many of the baked goods she developed for this book.

Anita uses both her knowledge of food and science to educate patients and physicians.

What other people are saying about this book:

"The medical information in this book is more comprehensive than anything I have read on celiac disease. It gave me an understanding why this diet is important for my health and signs to look for. It gave me knowledge so that I could talk to my doctor and make the right decisions for my health. A book like this has been long overdue."

John, Research Scientist

"I never realized that all of the strange symptoms I was getting were because of my restaurant food choices, until I read this book. I unknowingly ate some gluten regularly, but since reading this book now I don't and I feel great! The recipes are so good and unlike other books, these recipes turn out perfectly. The diet can be a lot easier than I thought. This book has also saved me money. Before I found this book I used to try a lot of recipes and throw things away. This book not only helped me to improve my health, but it ended my failed recipe frustration!"

Eileen, Retired

"I was one of Anita's taste testers when she developed products for GFN Foods™. Her gluten-free products were better than anything else that I tried and I have tried a lot of products! I have been anxiously awaiting this book because I knew if her recipes were as good as those that she had developed for GFN Foods™, that this book would be a winner. These recipes are just as wonderful as the Gluten-Free Naturals™ products made by GFN Foods™."

Christina, Physician

"You can make the recipes for your entire family. Not only will they enjoy them, they won't notice the difference. In many cases we liked these recipes better than the originals! You can tell that this book was written with a lot of love, and that the recipes were all tested, because everything I have tried turned out perfectly."       Lisa, Realtor

"My daughter has Asperger's Syndrome, and even though this book is directed to celiac patients, it has been a God-send to me. The recipes are wonderful. My 6-year old daughter always asks if it is something from Anita before trying something new. If it is one of Anita's recipes she wants to try it because she knows it will be good. Our whole family has been enjoying her recipes. My daughter sometimes can be particular about textures and she likes the fact that Anita's food has good texture and is not gritty. My son doesn't have Asperger's, but he always wants to try her food and he enjoys it too. So does the rest of our family."       Lauren, working Mother of 2

"These are delicious! What are they supposed to be missing?"

Bud, non-celiac taste-tester
and Business Owner